# Pharmaceutical Inorganic Chemistry

***Second Edition***

COVERS LATEST PCI SYLLABUS

# Pharmaceutical Inorganic Chemistry
## *Second Edition*

**V. Alagarsamy**
M. Pharm., Ph.D., FIC, DOMH,
Professor and Principal,
MNR College of Pharmacy,
Sangareddy, Hyderabad.

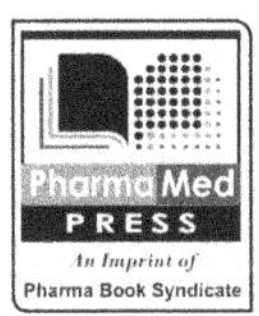


**PharmaMed Press**
*An imprint of Pharma Book Syndicate*
**A unit of BSP Books Pvt. Ltd.**
4-4-309/316, Giriraj Lane,
Sultan Bazar, Hyderabad - 500 095.

**Pharmaceutical Inorganic Chemistry,** ***Second Edition*** **by** ***V. Alagarsamy***


*Second Edition,* 2018
*First Edition,* 2014



***Published by***

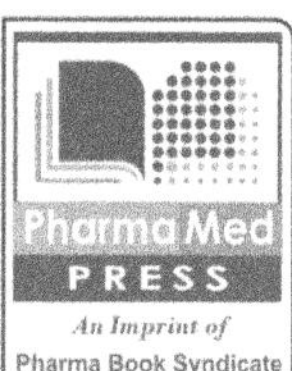


**PharmaMed Press**
*An imprint of Pharma Book Syndicate*
**A unit of BSP Books Pvt. Ltd.**
4-4-309/316, Giriraj Lane, Sultan Bazar, Hyderabad - 500 095.
Phone: 040-23445600, 23445688; Fax: 91+40-23445611
E-mail: info@pharmamedpress.com
www.pharmamedpress.com/pharmamedpress.net

**ISBN: 978-93-86819-68-0 (Hardback)**

# Contents

## CHAPTER 2

## BASICS OF PHARMACEUTICAL INORGANIC CHEMISTRY

## Chapter 4

## Quantitative Analysis (Volumetric and Gravimetric Analysis)



## Chapter 5

## Quality Control and Test for Purity

## CHAPTER 6

## INORGANIC PHARMACEUTICALS (INORGANIC COMPOUNDS USED IN PHARMACY)

## CHAPTER 8

## COORDINATION COMPOUNDS

# Preface to Second Edition

The author and publisher are presenting this second edition of the "Pharmaceutical Inorganic Chemistry" with great pleasure.

Since its first edition, in 2015, the Pharmaceutical Inorganic Chemistry book serves as a reliable source for the Pharmaceutical Inorganic Chemistry. The overwhelming response to the first edition throughout India is due to its comprehensive content (especially the Chemical reactions and assay).

The positive feedback received from faculty members and student's community all over India as shown below have inspired us to present this Pharmaceutical Inorganic Chemistry, Second Edition.

- The simple language used and the hints given for remembering methods of different assays are first of its kind.
- The book is presented in a down-to-earth fashion and hence easy to read and reproduce perfectly in examination.
- This book is comprehensive to learn all aspects of Pharmaceutical Inorganic Chemistry.
- The book is presented in attractive and easy-to-read manner and hence the fresher of graduate students are able to read without hesitation.
- The book is presented in student friendly style and approach.
- This is a perfect textbook. It helps faculty to teach students methodically.

**New to this edition**

The major goal of the author is to provide all aspects of inorganic drugs i.e. preparation, test for purity, assay and medicinal importance. As the methods of assay are many, I have presented a simple way to remember with easy language and chemical reactions which distinguish this book from other books in market. The following are the new features with updated information.

- Thoroughly revised Volumetric Analysis with the additional information on the basics, errors in analysis and applications are first of its kind.
- Gravimetric Analysis topic has been enriched with additional information.
- Covered all chapters as per PCI syllabus.

I hope this new edition of the Pharmaceutical Inorganic Chemistry will be welcomed by the teachers and all students of pharmacy, pharmaceutical chemistry, chemistry & allied field.

**Dr. V. Alagarsamy**

# Preface to First Edition

Pharmaceutical Inorganic Chemistry was evolved due to the applications of inorganic compounds in the pharmacy for treating many of the ailments of human and veterinary. Most of the pharmaceutical inorganic compounds are ionic compounds, consisting of cations and anions formed by ionic bond. It is a versatile area encompassing the chemical, biochemical, biological (Pharmacological) and pharmaceutical features of medicinally useful inorganic compounds. Due to the recent advancements and developments in chemical and analytical techniques and pharmacological screening programs, the inorganic compounds are standardized and find their way into medicine.

As the students entering graduate course, understanding of Pharmaceutical Inorganic Chemistry is always been a difficult task especially the assay of different kind of inorganic compounds. Hence my efforts have been devoted to authoring a book by equipping with the challenging requirements of the subject for the new generations of the teachers all over India, which is easy to read for students who are not necessarily of Pharmacy program, but mainly for the first time reading chemistry of inorganic compounds, their analysis and the pharmacological applications.

Methodical description of each chapter, enriching chemical and pharmaceutical background of the medicinally important inorganic compounds, proceeding each inorganic compound in a systematic way in easy-to-understand style in the larger interest of the students without any difficulty and making the reader acquainted thoroughly with Chemistry of Inorganic Compounds is the unique feature of this book. Covering all the pharmaceutical, analytical and chemical aspects of the medicinally useful inorganic compounds is the first of its kind.

In preparing this textbook, I have tried to enrich the inorganic compounds with the pharmaceutical application, so that the anticipated audience of this book will feel the importance of inorganic compounds and to make the book a comprehensive. The students of pharmacy and students of science graduates of our country faced with the scarcity of books to serve their needs. Few of the authors dealt well about the preparation, but principles of the assay of inorganic compounds are untouched which are needed to know and some of the books of Pharmaceutical Inorganic Chemistry fail to give the chemical equations for all reactions, hence the students are unable to understand the reactions clearly. Hence the content of this book is made as a humble attempt to cater the needs of academicians belonging to all Indian Universities by incorporating the chemical structure of all reactions and enriching the principles of assay of each inorganic pharmaceutical.

The book is divided into 8 chapters; chapter 1 to 5 deals about the basic aspects of Pharmaceutical Inorganic Chemistry and the chapter 6 provides the detailed information about the inorganic pharmaceuticals. Based on the therapeutic use inorganic compounds are further classified, in each chapter, an overview of the individual chapter, classification and individual compound preparation, official standard, test for purity [the test for common impurities present in most of the inorganic pharmaceuticals are described in one place (Chapter 5) which can be applied for all compounds is the first of its kind], test for identification, properties, assay and therapeutic uses are described. Chapter 7 deals about Radio Pharmaceuticals and the last chapter describe Coordination compounds.

In order to help the students to reproduce well in exams, the style and presentation are followed in a stereotype, especially in the assay part, if the student study the principles of ten compounds, all the inorganic compounds assay can be written using this format. In some places abbreviations are used to make still easier e.g., Known Excess Standard is abbreviated as KES to remember well, similarly Excess Unreacted Reagent is abbreviated as EUR. These small inputs help a lot for the freshers who enter into pharmacy.

We hope that this special volume will be a good source of information and reference for not only to graduates, Pharm-D., and post-graduate students but also for basic and applied researchers in this field. I welcome suggestions and constructive criticism from all corners of scientific community.

***-Author***

## Acknowledgements

A warm response to my earlier Books on “The Text Book of Medicinal Chemistry”, “Pharmaceutical Chemistry of Natural Products” (Published by Elsevier) and “Practical Pharmaceutical Inorganic Chemistry” (Published by PharmaMed Press) prompted me to write this Book on ‘Pharmaceutical Inorganic Chemistry”, covering all the topics suggested by the PCI, AICTE and various universities in India for graduate students. I dedicate this book to the many hundreds of pharmacy students, whom I have taught over the years and my Teachers who have encouraged me to convert my class notes into the textbook in order to reach into wide range of academic community.

It is my pleasure to place on record my heartfelt thanks to everyone who have made this book possible, especially my beloved teachers who taught me Pharmaceutical Inorganic Chemistry in my D.Pharm. and B.Pharm., who made me to read the subject in a simplified manner.

I am immensely grateful to Prof. K. Chinnaswamy, Dr. B. Suresh, Dr. R.K. Goyal, Dr. Rajani Giridhar and Dr. M.R. Yadav for their constant support, inspiration and initiation extended to me to author the book.

I gratefully acknowledge the constant and continuous encouragement and moral support extended by Shri M.N. Raju, Chairman, and Mr. M. Ravi Varma, Vice Chairman, MNR Educational Trust, Hyderabad, for my entire academic and research pursuit, is a great motivation for me in taking up this new challenge.

I Thank Prof. R. Shyam Sunder, Prof. A. Ravinder Nath and Prof. D. Jaya Prakash, Dr. P. Shashikala, Faculty of Technology, Osmania University, Hyderabad for their constant support in all my academic activities.

I express my sincere appreciation to my students, research scholars and friends especially, Dr. V. Raja Solomon, Mrs. M.T. Sulthana, Mr. B. Narendhar, Mrs. K. Manasa, Mr. B. Chandrasekar, Mr. G. Saravanan, Dr. P. Parthiban, and Dr. S. Murugesan for their untiring support in making this book.

I thank Mr. Anil Shah, Managing Director, PharmaMed Press for recognizing and inviting me to writing this book. The friendly interaction I had experienced with the PharmaMed Press team, Mr. Naresh, Mr. Chandra Sekhar and Mrs. Sandhya who had offered a cordial support, which always made me to give my inputs in order to make this Book one of the Best. Getting such a cooperative and energetic team encourage the author to continue their writing always. I thank them whole heartedly for accepting all my views while designing the book and helping me reach this target.

In all my academic efforts the stimulation I gain from my father, mother, sister, brothers and wife to reach this goal is like the nature provides plenty of inorganic salts for healthy maintenance of humanity, and the patience and cooperation extended by my children, Aish and Abhi made me think of the goal without any diversion. To express my thankfulness, I pray the Almighty to bless my children with teachers like those I got in my life so that they too are inspired by their teachers and dedicate to the field of Pharmacy and, in turn, serve for the mankind.

***-Author***

# Abbreviations

| | | |
|---|---|---|
| A | - | Antiport carrier for $HCO_3^-$ and $Cl^-$ |
| $A^0$ | - | Armstrong |
| Ac | - | Adenylate cyclase |
| ACE | - | Angiotensin Converting Enzyme |
| α | - | Alpha |
| AMU | - | Atomic Mass Unit |
| ANS | - | Autonomic Nervous System |
| Atm Pressure | - | Atmospheric Pressure |
| AP | - | Anaphase |
| API | - | Active Pharmaceutical Ingredient |
| ATP | - | Adenosine TriPhosphate |
| AsT | - | Arsenic free |
| Aq | - | Aqueous |
| B.P. | - | British Pharmacopoeia |
| BPC | - | British Pharmacopoeia Commission |
| BPC | - | British Pharmaceutical Codex |
| BHA | - | Butylated Hydroxy Anisole |
| BHT | - | Butylated Hydroxy Toluene |
| BP | - | Blood Pressure |
| BMR | - | Basal Metabolic Rate |
| β | - | Beta |
| BAL | - | British Anti Lewisite |
| cAMP | - | Cyclic Adenosine Monophosphate |
| CA | - | Carbonic Anhydrase |
| CNS | - | Central Nervous System |
| CTZ | - | Chemoreceptor Trigger Zone |
| C/s | - | Counts per second |
| C/m | - | Counts per minute |
| C | - | Curie |

| | | |
|---|---|---|
| $cm^2$ | - | Centimeter square |
| CCR | - | Corrected Counting Rate |
| CFT | - | Crystal Field Theory |
| $^{o}C$ | - | Degree centigrade |
| $DAB_{12}$ | - | Deoxy Adenosyl cobalamine |
| DNA | - | Deoxyribo Nucleic Acid |
| DMF | - | Di Methyl Formamide |
| d/s | - | Disintegrations per second |
| d/m | - | Disintegrations per minute |
| $d_N$ | - | Change in number of atoms N |
| $d_T$ | - | Change in time |
| **EUR** | - | **Excess Unreacted Reagent** |
| EDTA | - | Ethylene Diamine Tetra Acetate |
| ECL | - | Entero Chromatin Like cells |
| ECF | - | Extra Cellular Fluid |
| EP | - | European Pharmacoepia |
| ESR | - | Erythrocyte Sedimentation Rate |
| EMRS | - | Electro Magnetic Radiation Source |
| eV | - | ElectronVolts |
| FAS | - | Ferric Ammonium Sulphate |
| FDA | - | Food and Drug Administration |
| $FADH_2$ | - | Flavin Adenine Dinucleotide |
| GEPD | - | Gastro Easophageal reflux Disease |
| gm | - | Gram |
| GIT | - | Gastro Intestinal Tract |
| GR | - | Gastrin Receptor |
| GABA | - | Gamma Amino Butyric Acid |
| GMP | - | Good Manufacturing Practices |
| G-M | - | Geiger Muller Counter |
| g | - | Gas |
| $\gamma$ | - | Gamma |
| GFR | - | Glomerular Filtration Rate |
| HPLC | - | High Performance Liquid Chromatography |
| HPV | - | Human Papilloma Virus |
| HSAB | - | Hard and Soft Acid Base concept |
| H | - | Histamine (its receptor $H_2$) |

| | | |
|---|---|---|
| H.Pylori | - | Helicobacter Pylori |
| IP | - | Indian Pharmacopoeia |
| IND.P. | - | Indian Pharmacopoeia |
| IPC | - | Indian Pharmacopoeia Commission |
| I.M. | - | Intramuscular |
| I.V. | - | Intravenous |
| IR | - | Infrared |
| IL-1 | - | Interleukin-1 |
| INN | - | International Non-proprietary Name |
| IUPAC | - | International Union of Pure and Applied Chemistry |
| J/Kg | - | Joules/ kilogram |
| **KES** | - | **Known Excess Standard** |
| Keq | - | Equilibrium constant |
| Ka | - | Ionizatioon constant for acid |
| LFT | - | Ligand Field Theory |
| l | - | Liquid |
| L | - | Litre |
| M | - | Molarity/Molality |
| ml | - | Milli litre |
| mg | - | Milli gram |
| mmol/L | - | Milli mole/litre |
| mV | - | milli Volts |
| meq/kg | - | milliequvalents/kilogram |
| M.P. | - | Melting Point |
| mmHg | - | millimetre of mercury |
| mEq/L | - | milliEqivalents/ Litre |
| methyl $B_{12}$ | - | Methylcobalamin |
| MP | - | Metaphase |
| mCi | - | milli curie |
| μCi | - | microcurie |
| μgm | - | microgram |
| mm | - | millimetre |
| MeV | - | Milli electron Volts |
| MOT | - | Molecular Orbital Theory |
| Mol. Formula | - | Molecular Formula |
| Mol.Wt | - | Molecular Weight |

| | | |
|---|---|---|
| NSAIDS | - | Non Steroidal Anti Inflammatory Drugs |
| N | - | Normality |
| NF | - | National Formulary |
| nm | - | Nanometre |
| NADH | - | Nicotinamide Adenine Dinucleotide |
| NMR | - | Nuclear Magnetic Resonance |
| $N_t$ | - | Number of atoms present at 't' time |
| $N_0$ | - | Number of atoms present at zero time |
| ORS | - | Oral Rehydration Salt |
| ORD | - | Optical Rotatory Dispersion |
| OEC | - | Oxygen Evolving Complex |
| $\lambda$ | - | Proportionality Constant (decay constant) |
| P | - | Proton pump ($H^+/K^+$ ATPase) |
| PK | - | Protein Kinase activated |
| ppm | - | Parts Per Million |
| PCT | - | Potassium Cupric Tartarate |
| PCT | - | Proximal Convoluted Tubules |
| $pCO_2$ | - | Partial pressure of carbon dioxide |
| PAPS | - | Phosphor Adenosine Phosphor Sulphate |
| PP | - | Prophase |
| p | - | Para |
| $P^H$ | - | Ionisation constant |
| $P^{Ka}$ | - | Dissociation constant |
| PMT | - | Photo Multiplier Tube |
| q.s. | - | Quantity sufficient |
| RNA | - | Ribonucleic Acid |
| RA | - | Rheumatoid Arthritis |
| RS | - | Reference Solution |
| RAD | - | Radioactive Absorbed Dose |
| $R_f$ | - | Retention factor |
| S | - | Solid |
| $ST_2$ | - | Somatostatin receptor |
| SMFP | - | Sodium Mono Fluro Phosphate |
| STP | - | Standard Temperature and Pressure |
| PC II | - | Transcobalamin II |
| THFA | - | Tetra Hydro Folic Acid |

| | | |
|---|---|---|
| TLC | - | Thin Layer Chromatography |
| TP | - | Telophase |
| TNF | - | Tumor Necrosis Factor |
| $t_{1/2}$ | - | Half life |
| torr | - | Pressure |
| USP | - | United States Pharmacopoeia |
| USSRT | - | Union of Soviet Socialist Republic Pharmacopoeia |
| UV | - | UltraViolet |
| UK | - | United Kingdom |
| UKAEA | - | United Kingdom Atomic Energy Authority |
| Vol | - | Volume |
| v/v | - | Volume/Volume |
| V | - | Volts |
| VBT | - | Valence Bond Theory |
| w/v | - | Weight/Volume |
| w/w | - | Weight/Weight |
| WHO | - | World Health Organisation |

CHAPTER 1

# INTRODUCTION TO PHARMACEUTICAL INORGANIC CHEMISTRY

## 1.1 PHARMACEUTICAL CHEMISTRY

Pharmaceutical Chemistry is a branch of chemistry that deals with the chemical, biochemical and pharmacological aspects of drugs. It includes synthesis/isolation, identification, structural elucidation, structural modification, Structural Activity Relationship (SAR) studies, study of the chemical characteristics, biochemical changes after drug administration and their pharmacological effects.

### 1.1.1 Inorganic Chemistry

Inorganic chemistry is the study of all the elements and their compounds except carbon and its compounds (which is studied under organic chemistry). Inorganic chemistry describes the characteristics of substances such as nonliving matter and minerals which are found in the earth except the class of organic compounds. Branches of inorganic chemistry include coordination chemistry, bioinorganic chemistry, organometallic compounds and synthetic inorganic chemistry. The distinction between the organic and inorganic are not absolute, and there is much overlap, especially in the organometallic chemistry, which has applications in every aspect of the pharmacy, chemical industry–including catalysis in drug synthesis, pigments, surfactants and agriculture. In short, Inorganic chemistry is the branch of chemistry that deals with inorganic compounds. In other words, it is the chemistry of compounds that do not contain hydrocarbon radicals.

### 1.1.2 Inorganic Compounds

These are traditionally viewed as compounds being synthesized by the geological systems and lack hydrocarbon (carbon-hydrogen). In contrast, organic compounds are those found in biological systems. In general organic chemists say any molecule containing carbon as an organic compound and hence this means that inorganic chemistry deals with the compounds or molecules which lack carbon atom. Berzelius, the 19$^{th}$ century chemist, described inorganic compounds as inanimate. The first important synthetic inorganic compound was ammonium nitrate for soil fertilization. Inorganic compounds are found in nature as minerals. Soil contain iron sulfide as pyrite or calcium sulfate as gypsum. They are also found multitasking as biomolecules: As electrolytes (sodium chloride), in energy storage (ATP) or in construction (the polyphosphate backbone in DNA). Inorganic compounds are synthesized for use as drugs such as cisplatin, magnesium hydroxide, catalysts such as vanadium (V) oxide and titanium (III) chloride, or as reagents in organic chemistry such as lithium aluminium hydride.

Medicinally useful substances are derived from either organic or inorganic sources. Naturally obtained compounds attracted the attention of humans always, in which inorganic chemicals contributing significantly in some of the ailments, even after the development of many drugs from synthetic and plant sources. Many of the inorganic salts (antimony, arsenic and mercury) are known to be poison, still they are used in medicine cautiously. Some of them are replaced by the organic medicines.

**Study of pharmaceutical applications of the inorganic compounds led to the establishment of a new avenue called Pharmaceutical inorganic chemistry**, which deals with the study of both non-essential and essential elements about their preparation, standards of purity, test for identification, limit tests to be performed for determining the quality and extent of purity, storage, different formulations and their storage conditions and therapeutic uses.

The term 'Pharmaceutical' is used for any chemical substance useful in preventive or therapeutic or which finds use in the preparation of medicament. Some find use only in the laboratory during the preparation but may not be present in the final product, these are also incorporated under pharmaceuticals. Quality of all these pharmaceuticals must be carefully controlled. For this reason specifications of quality are mentioned for each pharmaceutical. These descriptions are reported in the pharmacopoeia.

### 1.1.3 Importance of Inorganic Pharmaceuticals

Inorganic pharmaceuticals are useful in any of the following ways.

1. Useful medicinally for their therapeutic purpose. Example: Astringents and antimicrobials etc.
2. Useful as pharmaceutical aids. Example: Bentonite, talc etc.
3. To change the reaction of body fluid. To acidify or alkalise. Example: Antacids, alkalis, mineral acids.
4. Replacing or replenishing the normal content of body fluids. Example: Sodium, potassium, calcium, chloride, phosphate etc.
5. Useful as reagents to carry out the reactions. Example: Catalysts (platinum, nickel) oxidizing and reducing agents (lithium aluminium hydride).
6. Useful in Pharmaceutical analysis. Example: Titrants such as potassium permanganate etc.

Various uses of inorganic pharmaceuticals in pharmacy are presented herein

***Abrasives:*** Drugs which are used for the cleaning and whitening of teeth. Example: Dibasic calcium phosphate.

***Absorbents:*** Drugs which are used to absorb the toxins and bacteria in the GIT. Example: Calcium carbonate.

***Acidifiers:*** Drugs which are used to enhance the acidity temporarily in GIT. Example: Dilute hydrochloric acid.

***Adsorbents:*** Drugs which are used in the treatment of mild dysentery or diarrhoea or other disturbances of GIT due to their ability to adsorb gases, toxins, and bacteria. Example: Bismuth subcarbonate, Bismuth subnitrate.

***Alkalizers:*** Drugs which are used to induce the alkaline condition or used in acidic condition of body. Example: Sodium citrate.

***Anaesthetics:*** Drugs which are used to produce reversible loss of sensation. Example: Nitrous oxide.

***Analgesic:*** Drugs which are used to relieve pain. Example: Nitrous oxide.

***Antacids:*** These are drugs which are usually alkaline substances, used for neutralizing excess acid in the stomach. Example: Aluminium hydroxide gel, Calcium carbonate, Magnesium carbonate.

***Anthelmintics:*** Compounds used for the treatment of worm infestations or schistosomiasis. Example: Ammoniated mercury, Sodium antimony tartarate.

***Antibacterial:*** Drugs which are used in the treatment of bacterial infections. Example: Yellow mercuric oxide (ophthalmic).

***Anticonvulsants:*** Drugs which are used for the treatment of epilepsy. Example: Potassium bromide.

***Anti coagulants:*** Drugs which are used to prevent blood clotting. Example: Sodium citrate.

***Anti depressants:*** Drugs which are used in the treatment of depression. Example: Lithium carbonate.

***Antidotes:*** Drugs which are used in the treatment of poison. Example: Sodium nitrite, Sodium thiosulphate.

***Antifebriles:*** Drugs which are used to relieve pain or reduce fever. Example: Ammonium acetate.

***Antifungal agents:*** Drugs which are used in the treatment of fungal infections. Example: Zinc undecylenate (topical use), Potassium iodide.

***Antihypercalcemic agents:*** Drugs which are used in the treatment of abnormal calcium concentration in the body. Example: Sodium acid phosphate.

***Anti infectives:*** Drugs which are used in the treatment of local infections. Example: Potassium permanganate, Silver nitrate, Hydrogen peroxide, Boric acid.

***Anti inflammatory agents:*** Drugs which are used in the treatment of inflammatory pain (Rheumatoid arthritis). Example: Sodium aurothiomalate.

***Anti irritant agents:*** Drugs which are used to prevent irritation or allergic reactions. Example: Aluminium metal powder.

***Antiseptics:*** Drugs which are used to inhibit the growth and development of micro organism without killing. Example: Strong iodine solution.

***Antiperspirants:*** Drugs which are used to remove the bad odour in body. Example: Aluminium sulphate.

***Anti-protozoals:*** Drugs which are used in the treatment of protozoal infections or Leishmaniasis. Example: Sodium antimony gluconate.

***Anti pruritics (topical):*** Drugs which are used in the production of soothing effect in the skin. Example: Calamine.

***Anti rheumatics:*** Drugs which are used in the treatment of rheumatism. Example: Sodium aurothiomalate.

***Anti thyroids:*** Drugs which are used in the treatment of thyrotoxicosis. Example: Potassium perchlorate.

***Anti tumor agents:*** Drugs which are used in the treatment of cancer. Example: Cisplatin (Testicular and ovarian cancer).

***Anti schistosomal agents:*** Drugs which are used in the treatment of schistosomiasis. Example: Sodium antimony tartrate.

***Antioxidants:*** Substances that prevents or delays oxidation. Some formulations, vegetable oils and prepared foods contain antioxidants. Example: Sodium bisulphate, sodium metabisulphite, sodium sulphite.

***Astringents:*** These are the substances which bring about protein precipitation. Astringent action is evidenced by contraction and wrinkling of tissue and by blanching. Example: Calamine, Aluminium citrate.

***Bactericides:*** Drugs which are used to kill bacteria. Example: Potassium permanganate.

***Bacteriostatics:*** Drugs which are used to prevent the growth of bacteria. Example: Alum, borax (local bacteriostatic).

***Bleaching agents:*** Drugs which are used in the cleansing of wounds or bleaching. Example: Hydrogen peroxide.

***Buffers:*** Substance which prevents the change in pH upon addition of acid or base. Example: Acetate buffer (pH – 3.9), Sodium citrate buffer.

***Calcium supplements:*** Drugs which are used as a calcium source. Example: Calcium lactate, Calcium gluconate.

***Cathartics:*** Drugs which are used to enhance defecation, removes constipation and expulsion of intestinal parasites. Example: Calomel, Magnesium sulphate.

***Chlorine source:*** Substance which liberates chlorine. Example: Chlorinated lime, Chlorinated soda.

***Dentifrices:*** Drugs which are used in cleaning the surface of the teeth. Example: Calcium carbonate, Magnesium peroxide.

***Depilatory agents:*** Drugs which are used to remove hair. Example: Barium sulphide.

***Diagnostic agents:*** Drugs which are used in diagnose the diseased conditions of the organs. Example: Barium sulphate.

***Diaphoretics:*** Drugs which are used to promote sweating. Example: Potassium citrate.

***Disinfectants:*** Drugs which are used to kill the microbes in nonliving things. Example: Ammonium acetate.

***Diuretics:*** Drugs which are used to increase the urine output. Example: Ammonium chloride, Ammonium iodide.

***Dressing material:*** Substances which are used for the dressing of burns. Example: Aluminum metal foil.

***Dusting powders:*** Substance which are used to have soothing effect on the skin. Example: Talc, Zinc stearate, Light kaolin.

***Electrolyte replenishers:*** Compounds used to treat acid base imbalance conditions in the body. Example: Sodium chloride, Ringer lactate solution, Potassium chloride.

***Emetics:*** Drugs which are used to induce vomiting. Example: Zinc sulphate, Copper sulphate.

***Expectorants:*** Drugs which are used in the treatment of cough. They promotes the ejection of mucus (sputum) from the lungs, bronchi and trachea by increasing its fluidity (reducing viscosity). Example: Potassium iodide (sedative expectorant), Eucalyptus, Lemon (stimulant expectorant), Ammonium chloride, Potassium iodide.

***Fillers:*** Drugs which are used to fill the dental cavities. Example: Gold and Silver metals.

***General anaesthetics:*** Drugs which are used to produce reversible loss of sensation. Example: Nitrous oxide.

***Germicides:*** Drugs which are used to kill the germs. Example: Chlorinated lime.

***Haematinics:*** Drugs which are used in the treatment of anaemia. Example: Ferrous sulphate, Ferric ammonium citrate and other iron compounds.

***Haemostatic:*** Drugs which are used to arrest the flow of blood. Example: Alum.

***Inhalants:*** Inhalants are the drugs or chemicals which in the vapour form are inhaled or administered through the respiratory system in the body. Example: Oxygen, $CO_2$, Ammonium carbonate, Nitrous oxide, Helium.

***Iodine supplements:*** Drugs which are used in the treatment of iodine deficiency. Example: Potassium iodide.

***Laxatives:*** Drugs which are used to promote the evacuation of bowel. Example: Magnesium Sulphate, Sodium phosphate.

***Protectives:*** Substance which tend to form a coating and protect the exposed skin or mucus membrane from harmful stimuli. Example: Zinc stearate, Zinc oxide.

***Purgatives:*** Drugs which are used to defecate. These agents relieve constipation and helps in the expulsion of intestinal parasites. Example: Magnesium sulphate.

***Radiation shields:*** Compounds which are used to prevent the entry of radiations. Example: Lead sheets, Wall lining.

***Radio isotope tracers:*** Radioactive element or compound added to material to monitor the material's distribution as it progresses through a system. Example: Carbon-14, Tritium.

***Radiotherapeutic agents:*** Radioisotopes used for the treatment of diseases. Example: Iodine-121, Cr- 52 and Gold- 198.

**Rubifacients:** Substances which causes reddening of skin by dilating blood vessels and increasing blood circulation in the applied area. Example: Ammonia.

**Scabicides:** Drugs which are used in the treatment of scabies. Example: Sulphur.

**Sedatives:** Substance which causes CNS depression and produces sedation. At higher dose they produce sleep. Example: Potassium bromide, Lithium carbonate.

## 1.2 PHARMACOPOEIA

The word Pharmacopoeia is derived from Greek words 'pharmakon' means a drug (both remedy and poison) and 'poiein' means to make or create. Pharmacopoeia is a book containing directions for the identification of samples and the preparation of compound medicines, and published by the authority of a government or a medical or pharmaceutical society. For this reason Pharmacopoeia is a legislation of a nation which sets standards and mandatory quality indices for drugs, raw materials used to prepare them and various pharmaceutical preparations.

### 1.2.1 Monograph

In simple way monographs are descriptions of pharmaceutical preparations. In broader way it is a reference work for pharmaceutical drug specifications. It is a complete description of a specific pharmaceutical, which includes chemical formulae, atomic and molecular weight, definition, statement of content, category, dose, usual strength, description, solubility, identification tests, assay, other test, limits of impurities, quantities, and conditions for storage. The appendices include standards for apparatus, reagents and solutions, indicators, reference substances, test animals, calculation of results, other chemicals techniques, processes etc. of the concerned pharmaceuticals.

By the direction of the council of the pharmaceutical society of the certain nations, the world's most comprehensive source of drug information in a single volume is published periodically in the society's department of pharmaceutical sciences.

It is the traditional activity, to help the practicing pharmacists and physicians aiming to provide unbiased concise reports on the actions and uses of most of the world's drugs and medicines. By reflecting clinical practice, every publication of Pharmacopoeia monographs are accurately organized based on the updated needs of today's pharmacist. In the form of new monographs the details are provided for new compounds and some of the previous monographs which are not in continued use are deleted. The overall effect is to provide an increase in the average of drugs with typographically improvements to assist the reader in locating sections of a monograph.

With the search for an effective treatment of diseases a few of the developing therapeutics are revised continuously in Pharmacopoeia. Example: Anti HIV agents. In Pharmacopoeia the drug's distinguished features are updated, renewed and discussed for the treatment of infections and development of antiviral, antiprotozoal and antibacterial therapy. Along with novel approaches in the treatment advances in the cardiovascular group of drugs are included. The other areas like anti-malarial drugs, anti-neoplastic agents, anti-parkinsonism drugs etc. are also included in Pharmacopoeia.

Based on the published information, Pharmacopoeia is divided in to three different major parts. Each part is comprised of several chapters.

**Part I:** Generally the drugs that have similar use or actions are bringing together by part I of Pharmacopoeia. In related chapters to guide reader the cross references is used to find out the drug that may be of interest. The common actions of the groups of drugs are provided as background information in many of the chapters.

**Part II:** Monographs of new drugs, drugs under investigation, drugs which are not easily classified and obsolescent drugs still of interest are presented in part II of Pharmacopoeia. It also provides details regarding effects of required drug therapy.

**Part III:** Composition of the proprietary medicines that are advertised to the public in different countries are documented with omission of herbal medicine in part III of Pharmacopoeia.

Only the pharmaceuticals which are commonly and currently in use are included in the Pharmacopoeia; whereas the substances which are found to be undesirable and are not currently in use are excluded. Moreover part of Pharmacopoeia may also comprise the pharmaceuticals which are used for application or internal consumption by human beings.

In the Pharmacopoeia only minimum standards are prescribed for pharmaceuticals, but with more stringent standards the manufacturer may supply these substances. Hence a drug has to obey strictly the standards prescribed by any one of the Pharmacopoeias. The medication may be considered as substandard if it does not obey these standards and usually it is not prescribed by medical practitioners.

### 1.2.2 History of Pharmacopoeia

Each country has legislation on pharmaceutical preparations which sets a standards and required quality indices for medicament, raw materials and preparations employed in the manufacture of drugs. These regulations are presented in separate articles. General and specific matters relating to individual drugs are published in the form of a book called a Pharmacopoeia.

On $15^{th}$ December 1820, the first United State Pharmacopoeia (U.S.P) was released. In 1864, the first British Pharmacopoeia (B.P) was published with inclusion of monographs on benzoic acid, gallic acid, tartaric acid, tannic acid, camphor, lactose, sucrose and seven alkaloids along with their salts.

## 1.3 INDIAN PHARMACOPOEIA

British Pharmacopoeia was utilized as the official book of standards in India before independence. The actual process of publishing the first Indian Pharmacopoeia started in the year 1944 under the chairmanship of Col. R. N. Chopra. The Indian Pharmacopoeia list was first published in the year 1946 and was put forth for approval. The government of India constituted a permanent Indian Pharmacopoeia Committee in 1948 for the preparation of the Indian Pharmacopoeia and established a central Indian Pharmacopoeia Laboratory at Ghaziabad, Uttar Pradesh to keep it up to date. The Indian Pharmacopoeia is published in fulfillment of the requirements of the Drugs and Cosmetics act, 1940 and rules there under.

The drugs and cosmetics act 1940 stated that the Indian Pharmacopoeia is the book of standards for drugs included therein and the standards as included in the Indian Pharmacopoeia would be official. If considered necessary, these standards can be amended and the secretary of the Indian Pharmacopoeia committee is authorized to issue such amendments.

Government of India, Ministry of Health and Family welfare publishes Indian Pharmacopoeia based on the recommendation of Indian Pharmacopoeia committee (in accordance with Drugs and Cosmetics Acts 1940, Dangerous Drugs Act 1930, and Poisons Act 1919 and the rules framed there under). In general, the general notices and appendices included in the Indian Pharmacopoeia and as amended in addendum apply both to the matter contained in the Indian Pharmacopoeia and to the matter contained in this Addendum.

After independence, the first edition of the Indian Pharmacopoeia (I.P) was published in the year 1955 under the chairmanship of Dr. B. N. Ghosh. Supplement for first edition of Indian Pharmacopoeia was published in the year 1960. This Pharmacopoeia contained both western and traditional system drugs commonly used in India. The same policy was continued while preparing the Indian Pharmacopoeia 1966. After eleven years, under the chairmanship of Dr. B. Mukherji the second edition of Indian Pharmacopoeia was released in 1966 with some modification. The supplement to the second edition of Indian Pharmacopoeia was published in 1975.

There had been a phenomenal growth and development of Indian pharma industry especially from early 1970 both in the range of active pharmaceutical ingredients (APIs) and the dosage forms produced. In view of these rapid advances, it was decided to publish a new edition of the Pharmacopoeia and its addenda at regular and shorter intervals for which the Indian Pharmacopoeia Committee was reconstituted in 1978. The third edition of the Indian Pharmacopoeia got published in 1985 under the chairmanship of Dr. Nityanand. Addendum/supplement I and II to third edition has been published in 1989 and 1991 respectively. In this Pharmacopoeia inclusion of traditional system of drugs was limited. However, most of the new drugs manufactured and/or marketed were included while only those herbal drugs which had definite quality control standards had got place in it.

In view of the continuing rapid increase in the range of drugs produced in India eleven year later the fourth edition of the Indian Pharmacopoeia was published under the chairmanship Dr. Nityanand in 1996. Addendum to fourth edition has been published initially in 2000 followed by in 2002 and 2005. In addition, supplement 2000 for veterinary products are also released. The addendum 2005 was published by the Indian Pharmacopoeia

Committee which included a large number of antiretroviral drugs, and raw plants commonly used in making medicinal products not covered by any other Pharmacopoeias and attracted much global attention. The Indian Pharmacopoeia Committee decide to delete the obsolete or less used product monographs and added monographs based on the therapeutic merit, medicinal need and extent of use of such articles in the country.

The Indian Pharmacopoeia Commission (IPC) has been established in the year 2005. The IPC provided systematic approach and practices for publication of Indian Pharmacopoeia 2007 with focus on those drugs and formulations that cover the National health care programs and the national essential medicines. It contained monographs on antiretroviral, anticancer, anti- tubercular and herbal drugs. It further emphasized on biological monographs such as vaccines, immunosera for human use, blood products, biotechnological and veterinary (biological and non biological) preparations. Addendum 2008 to the Indian Pharmacopoeia 2007 was published which had taken care of the amendments to Indian Pharmacopoeia 2007 and also incorporated 72 new monographs.

The sixth edition of Indian Pharmacopoeia published in accordance with the principles and designed plan decided by the scientific body of the IPC. To establish transparency in setting standards for this edition, the contents of new monographs, revised appendices and other information have been published on the website of IPC, besides following conventional approach of obtaining comments. The feedback and inputs were reviewed by the relevant expert committee to ensure the feasibility and practicability of the standards and methods revised. The principle of openness, justice and fairness is kept in mind during compiling and editing the contents of this edition.

The IPC secretariat and Indian Pharmacopoeia laboratory staff, with the support of different advisory expert committee, and expert members of the scientific body have examined the suitability of the standards. In order to make Indian Pharmacopoeia 2010 user friendly, the existing formatting pattern has been suitably revised. The standards prescribed in this edition are encouraged to adhere with the concept of harmonization, keeping in view the technological status for manufacture and analysis of drugs and pharmaceuticals in the country without compromising with the quality of the products. It strives to update the existing monographs as well as incorporating the new monographs of drug substances based on clinical use of medicines in India and improving their test protocols.

The Indian Pharmacopoeia 2010 has been considerably revised and improved in respect of the requirements of monographs, appendices and testing protocols by introducing advanced technology. The contents of appendices are by and large revised in consonance with those adopted internationally. The monographs of special relevance disease of this region have been given special attention.

In addition emphasis has been put to bring out harmonization in appendices to establish a sound connection between individual monographs and the relevant appendices, so as to make this edition precise and well structured. Number of monographs and appendices are expanded further to incorporate the latest technological advancement and regulatory compliance. Constant efforts have been made to unify the national drug standards and to bring them in line with the international standards progressively, by addition of monographs of new drugs and adopting current methodology.

### 1.3.1 Features of various Editions of Indian Pharmacopoeia

| S. No. of Edition | Year of publication | Year of addendum released | Features of edition |
|---|---|---|---|
| First | 1955 | 1960 | Contains both western and traditional system drugs commonly used in India. |
| Second | 1966 | 1975 | Contains both western and traditional system drugs commonly used in India. |
| Third | 1985 | 1989 ($1^{st}$)<br>1991 ($2^{nd}$) | In this Pharmacopoeia inclusion of traditional system of drugs was limited. However, most of the new drugs manufactured and/or marketed were included while only those herbal drugs which had definite quality control standards had got place in it. |
| Fourth | 1996 | 2000 ($1^{st}$)<br>2002 ($2^{nd}$)<br>2005 ($3^{rd}$) | Which included a large number of antiretroviral drugs, and raw plants commonly used in making medicinal products not covered by any other Pharmacopoeias and attracted much global attention. The Indian Pharmacopoeia Committee decide to delete the obsolete or less used product monographs and added monographs based on the therapeutic merit, medicinal need and extent of use of such articles in the country. |
| Fifth | 2007 | 2008 | It focuses on those drugs and formulations that cover the National health care programmes and the national essential medicines. It contained monographs on antiretroviral, anticancer, anti-tubercular and herbal drugs. It further emphasized on biological monographs such as vaccines, immunosera for human use, blood products, biotechnological and veterinary (biological and non biological) preparations. |
| Sixth | 2010 | 2012 | It comprises of three volumes. Each volume has got different features. Volume I comprises notices, preface, about Indian Pharmacopoeia Commission, acknowledgements, introduction, general chapters and reference data. Volume II contains general notices, dosage forms (general monographs), drug substances, dosage forms and pharmaceutical aids (A to M). Volume III includes general notices, drug substances, dosage forms and pharmaceutical aids (N to Z), vaccines and immunosera for human use, herbs and herbal products, blood and blood related products, biotechnology products, veterinary products and index. |
| Seventh | 2014 | - | It is presented in four volumes. Included products of biotechnology, indigenous herbs and herbal products, veterinary vaccines and additional antiretroviral drugs and formulations, inclusive of commonly used fixed-dose combinations. Standards for new drugs and drugs used under National Health Programmes are added and the drugs as well as their formulations which are not in use now a days are deleted from this edition. The IP 2014 incorporates 2548 monographs of drugs among this 577 are new monographs consisting of APIs, excipients, dosage forms, antibiotic monographs, insulin products and herbal products etc. 19 New Radiopharmaceutical Monographs and 1 General chapter is first time being included in this edition. |

### 1.3.2 Indian Pharmacopoeia 2010

This new edition of Indian Pharmacopoeia entitled sixth edition (Indian Pharmacopoeia 2010) was published by the IPC. It supersedes the fifth edition but any monograph of the earlier edition that does not figure in this edition continues to be official as stipulated in the second schedule of Drugs and cosmetics act, 1940.

**Presentation**

The Indian Pharmacopoeia 2010 comprises of three volumes. Each one volume has got different features. Volume I comprises notices, preface, about Indian Pharmacopoeia Commission, acknowledgements, introduction, general chapters and reference data. Volume II contains general notices, dosage forms (general monographs), drug substances, dosage forms and pharmaceutical aids (A to M). Volume III includes general notices, drug substances, dosage forms and pharmaceutical aids (N to Z), vaccines and immunosera for human use, herbs and herbal products, blood and blood related products, biotechnology products, veterinary products and index.

The scope of Pharmacopoeia has been extended to include products of biotechnology, indigenous herbs and herbal products, veterinary vaccines and additional antiretroviral drugs and formulations, inclusive of commonly used fixed dose combinations. Standards for new drugs and drugs used under national health programs are added and the drugs as well as their formulations not in use nowadays are omitted from this edition. The number of monographs of excipients, anticancer drugs, herbal products and antiretroviral drugs has been increased in this edition. Monographs of vaccines and immunosera are also upgraded in view of the development of latest technology in the field. A new chapter on liposomal products and a monograph of liposomal Amphotericin B injection is added advantage in view of latest technology adopted for drug delivery. A chapter on NMR is incorporated in appendices. The chapter on microbial contamination is also updated to a great extend to harmonize with prevailing international requirements.

### 1.3.3 Format

In an effort to make the Indian Pharmacopoeia more user's friendly, design of the texts of the monographs and of the test methods are kept same like Indian Pharmacopoeia 2007. Cross referencing has been avoided to make each monograph complete in itself thus making it convenient to the analyst.

**Basis of pharmaceutical requirements**

As in the past, this compendium provides a publicly available statement concerning the quality of a product that can be expected and demonstrated at any time throughout the accepted shelf life of the article. The standards laid down represent the minimum with which the article must comply and it is inculcate on the manufactured in accordance with the GMPs. It is essential that sufficiently stringent limits are applied at the time of release of a batch of a drug substance or drug product so that the pharmacopoeial standards are met until its expiry date when stored under the storage conditions specified.

It must be noted that a valid interpretation of any requirement of Indian Pharmacopoeia should be done in the context of the monographs as a whole, the relevant general monograph, where appropriate, the specified tests and methods of analysis including any reference to relevant general notices. Familiarity with the general notices will facilitate the correct application of the requirements.

### 1.3.4 Changes

Keeping in view the essential requirement under the Drugs and Cosmetics Act, 1940 and rules there under in the information on category of a drug, dosage and usual available strengths of dosage forms have been kept in this edition.

General chemical tests for identification of an article have been almost eliminated and the more specific infrared and ultraviolet spectrophotometric tests have been given emphasis. The concept of relying on published infrared spectra as a basis for identification has been continued.

The use of chromatographic methods has been greatly extended to cope with the need for more specificity in assays and in particular, in assessing the nature and extend of impurities in drug substances and drug products. Most of the existing assays and related substances tests are upgraded by liquid chromatography method in view to have more specificity and to harmonize with other international Pharmacopoeias.

The test for pyrogens involving the use of animals has been virtually eliminated. The test for bacterial endotoxins introduced in the previous edition is now applicable to more items. The test for abnormal toxicity is now confined to certain vaccines.

### 1.3.5 General Chapters

Volume I is devoted mainly to test methods that are applicable to all the articles of the Indian Pharmacopoeia and general information pertaining to the quality requirements of medical substances. It also includes reference data such as reference spectra, typical chromatograms etc. The test methods reflect the sophistication of analytical methodology and instrumentation.

Analytical methods are, in general, in harmony with those adopted internationally for monitoring the quality of drugs. The steps taken for harmonization have been initiated by the need to cope with the increasing demand for drugs manufactured in the country to meet globally accepted standards.

The trend towards controlling the microbial quality of all medicinal products have been recognized and the requirement regarding limits of bacterial contamination even of products for oral administration and topical application so that adequate controls are exercised by manufactures by the adoption of Good Manufacturing Practices (GMPs) has been continued.

The chapter on vaccines: General requirements has been updated. Minor corrections have been made in the appendices entitled tests on chicken flocks free from specified pathogens for the production and quality control of vaccines and general provisions. Avian viral vaccines – tests for extraneous agents in seed lot. The peptide mapping test for inactivated

Hepatitis B vaccine has been deleted. Wherever appropriate, other corrections has also been incorporated and over all presentation improved.

In view of considering the microbiological quality, the whole microbiological general chapter comprising of effectiveness of antimicrobial preservatives, microbial contamination in non sterile products and microbiological quality of raw material, dosage forms, herbs, processed herbs and herbal products have been extensively revised. For the first time in this chapter the analysis of certain *Shigella boydii* (strain of tropical region of our country) is made essential as it causes acute dysentery.

The chapter on biotechnology derived therapeutic products has been fully revised. Special emphasis given on monoclonal antibodies and antisera.

The standards prescribed in the Indian Pharmacopoeia are to establish the compliance with regulatory requirements on article. The criteria to be adhered are; a) The interpretation of a monograph must be in accordance with all the general requirements, testing methods, texts and notices pertaining to it, in the Indian Pharmacopoeia. b) A product is not of standard quality unless it complies with all the requirements of the monograph.

This edition of Indian Pharmacopoeia 2010 supersedes the Indian Pharmacopoeia 2007 edition. The Indian Pharmacopoeia 2010 incorporated 287 new monographs consisting of APIs, excipients, dosage forms and herbal products, etc. This Indian Pharmacopoeia edition plays a significant role in improving the quality of medicines which in turn promote public health and accelerate the growth and development of pharma sector.

In Pharmacopoeia under a monograph each pharmaceutical agent has been described. In appendices of the Pharmacopoeia the various standards for chemical apparatus, technique processes etc. are described. Appendices are considered as important as the main body monographs for a pharmaceutical chemist and an analyst. In the Pharmacopoeia those pharmaceuticals which are commonly used in the recent past have been included. Substances which have proved to be undesirable from past experience are removed from Pharmacopoeia. In general due to idleness, substances which are commercially available in excellent purity and are commonly used for other purposes are also not included. In case, if such substances find use internally then they are included in the monographs. The standards prescribed for a chemical are the minimum. It does not prevent a manufacturer from supplying these with more stringent standards. In the Pharmacopoeia if a substance has not been included it does not imply that it cannot be used or marketed. Such non official substances must correspond to standards prescribed either in the earlier editions of the Indian Pharmacopoeia or in other recognized pharmacopoeia (of other countries).

Generally in India products corresponding to the British Pharmacopoeia (BP) and United States Pharmacopoeia (USP) are marketed. Other better known Pharmacopoeias are International Pharmacopoeia (IP), European Pharmacopoeia (EP) and Union of Soviet Socialist Republics Pharmacopoeia (USSRP). To avoid confusion with International Pharmacopoeia, Indian Pharmacopoeia sometimes abbreviated as IND.P. or PI Generally IP will be understood as Indian Pharmacopoeia unless otherwise specified in our country. The various other compendia prescribing standards for pharmaceuticals are British

Pharmaceutical Codex (BPC) and National Formulary (NF). In the interest of proper health any substance which fails to correspond to any official standard should not be used.

**Official substances:** In the latest edition of the Pharmacopoeia those drugs and pharmaceuticals are termed as official substances in that country of Pharmacopoeia. It is very important to understand the difference between an official substance and chemical individual with same name. The individual chemical can be pure to any specified purity. The official substance is a commercial product which is required to comply with standards specified in the Pharmacopoeia and may often have some other substances added for specific reasons. For example, to prevent the formation and to inactivate any poisonous phosgene (carbonyl chloride) gas that may be formed in contact with the air during storage of chloroform of the Pharmacopoeia contains 1-2 % of added ethyl alcohol.

### 1.3.6 Pharmacopoeial Description/Presentation

Most of the Pharmacopoeias including Indian Pharmacopoeia consist of the three major sections namely

(a) Introduction including general notices

(b) Monographs of the official drugs

(c) Appendices.

**(a)** ***Introduction:*** It is a useful pointer to pharmaceutical progress since last edition. It summarizes the different changes including additions/deletions in the current edition compared to last edition. To avoid misinterpretation and misunderstanding of later parts of the text, attention should be paid to general notices at the outset.

**(b)** ***Monographs:*** The general monographs for dosage forms of active pharmaceutical ingredients (APIs) are grouped together at the beginning of volume II of Indian Pharmacopeia 2010. They are followed by the monographs for the APIs, pharmaceutical aids and individual dosage forms all in alphabetical order. Monographs for other articles of a special nature such as vaccines and immunosera for human use, herbs and herbal products, blood and blood related products, biotechnology products, veterinary products are given in separate sections in volume III of Indian Pharmacopeia 2010.

The written study of a subject was implied by the word “monograph”. These are considered as very important because medicinal substances are used for the cure and/or prevention of diseases. Therefore their written studies appear as monographs in the Pharmacopoeia. These monographs are arranged in the alphabetical order of their names and are somewhat stereotyped in style. The following information about the drugs and pharmaceutical aids are described in Pharmacopoeial monographs.

### 1.3.7 General Monographs

General monographs on dosage forms include requirements of general application and apply to all preparations within the scope of the introduction section of the general monograph, except where a preamble limits the application. The requirements are not necessarily comprehensive for a given specific preparation, additional requirements may sometimes be given in the individual monograph for it.

### 1.3.8 Production

Statements given under the heading production relate to particular aspects of the manufacturing process and are not necessarily comprehensive. However, they are mandatory instructions to manufacturers. For example, they may relate to source materials, to the manufacturing process and its validation and control, to any process testing that is to be carried out by the manufacturer on the final product either on selected batches or on each batch prior to release. All this cannot be verified on a sample of the final product by an independent analyst. It is for the licensing authority to verify that the instructions have been followed.

The absence of a section on production does not imply that attention to features such as those given above is not required. An article described in a monograph of the Pharmacopeia is to be manufactured in accordance with the principles of good manufacturing practice and in accordance with the requirements of the Drugs and Cosmetic Rules, 1945. The general principles applicable to the manufacture and quality assurance of drugs and preparations meant for human use equally to veterinary products as well.

### 1.3.9 Manufacture of Drug Products

The opening definitive statement in certain monographs for drug product is given in terms of the active ingredient(s) only. Any ingredient(s) other than those included in the statement, must comply with the general notice on excipients and the product must conform to the Pharmacopoeial requirements.

Official preparations are prepared only from ingredients that comply with the requirements of the Pharmacopoeial monographs for those individual ingredients for which monographs are provided.

### 1.3.10 Excipients

Any substance added in preparing an official preparation shall be innocuous, shall have no adverse influence in the therapeutic efficacy of the active ingredients and shall not interfere with the tests and assays of Pharmacopoeia. Care should be taken to ensure that such substances are free from harmful organisms.

### 1.3.11 Individual Monographs

Drug products that are the subject of an individual monograph are also required to comply with the tests given in the general monographs.

1. ***Title:*** The main title for a drug substance is the International Non-proprietary Name (INN) approved by World Health Organization (WHO). The official name of the compound in English is stated in the title. In place of the main title, sometimes sub titles are given which are synonyms/subsidiary names; where included, they have the same significance as the main title. For example, calcium carbonate can also be called precipitated chalk; iron and ammonium citrate can also be called ferric ammonium citrate and milk of magnesia can also be called magnesium hydroxide mixture.

When a product contains one or the other different salts of an active molecule, the main title is based on the full name of the active ingredient. For example, chloroquine phosphate tablet and chloroquine sulphate tablets.

2. ***Chemical formulae:*** When the chemical structure of an official substance is known or generally accepted, the graphic and molecular formulae are normally given at the beginning of the monograph for information. To specify the absolute stereo chemical configuration International Union of Pure and Applied Chemists (IUPAC) systems have been used. If the substance is enantiomer, the sign of optical rotation has been attached to the systematic name.

3. ***Atomic and molecular weight:*** The atomic and molecular weight is shown, as and when appropriate at the top right hand corner of the monograph. For example, magnesium chloride (Molecular weight: 202.30) and potassium permanganate (Molecular weight: 158.03). In general if the correct chemistry is not known or the compound is of indefinite composition these two items are not provided. For example chemical formula and molecular weight for iron ammonium citrate are not provided.

4. ***Definition:*** The opening statement of a monograph is one that constitutes an official definition of the substance, preparation or other article that is the subject of the monograph. In some monographs of pharmaceutical preparations the statement is given in terms of principle ingredient(s). In monographs on vegetable drugs, the definition indicates whether the subject of the monograph is, for example, the whole drug or the drug in powdered form. Certain pharmaceutical substance and other articles are defined by reference to a particular method of manufacture.

5. ***Statement of content:*** The limits of content stated are those determined by the method described under assay.

6. ***Category:*** This part of monograph expresses the pharmacological or therapeutic or pharmaceutical application of the compound. Although the compound may have other applications usually this part describes the main application. Analgesics, antibiotic, antacid, laxative etc. are some of the main categories for inorganic pharmaceuticals in the Pharmacopoeia.

7. ***Dose:*** Dose mentioned in the Pharmacopeia is intended merely for general guidance and represent, unless otherwise stated, the average range of quantities which are generally regarded as suitable for adults when administered by mouth. It provides the quantity guidance to the prescriber or the physician to achieve the desired therapeutic effects in adults. The dose can be altered as and when required. For example the dose of calcium carbonate is 1 – 5 gm.

   This is omitted for substances not used for internal administration. Usual strength may be given for pharmaceutical dosage forms like injection etc. which is the most commonly marketed dosage strength.

8. ***Usual strength:*** It indicates the strength(s) usually marketed for information of the pharmacist and the medical practitioner.

9. ***Description:*** This part of monograph is not to be interpreted in a strict sense and is not to be regarded as official requirements. It illustrates a physical description of the substance such as amorphous nature or crystalline, odor, color and taste etc. In the preliminary evaluation of the integrity of an article these properties help and not themselves the standards or tests or purity. For example, Calcium carbonate is a fine white microcrystalline powder, odorless and tasteless.

10. ***Solubility:*** The solubility mentioned in Indian Pharmacopeia is the approximate solubility at a temperature between 15 °C and 30 °C, unless otherwise stated, and are not to be considered as official requirements. In the Pharmacopoeia under general notices solubility is described. The solubility of a substance in water, hot or boiling water, alcohol, glycerol, other organic solvent, acid and alkali were given.

11. ***Test methods:*** References to general methods of testing are indicated by test method numbers in brackets immediately after the heading of the test or at the end of the text.

12. ***Identification:*** These identification tests are not a proof of identity. This usually involves specific chemical test or tests for identifying the substance. It provides a means of verifying that the identity of the material under examination is in accordance with the label on the container. In certain monographs alternative series of tests are given; compliance with either one or the other set of tests is adequate to verify the identity of the article. In general for inorganic pharmaceuticals color reactions, precipitation reactions and gas evolving reactions are used. For example, Phenol gives violet color with ferric chloride.

13. ***Tests and assay:*** These are the official methods upon which the standards of Pharmacopoeia depend. The requirements are not framed to take into account all possible impurities. Tests and assay are prescribed for the minimum sample available on which the attributes of the article should be measured. Assurance of quality must be ensured by the manufacture by the use of statistically valid sampling and testing programs.

14. ***Tests:*** In general the assays and test are carried out at a temperature between 20 °C and 30 °C unless otherwise stated. Precaution should be taken to avoid exposure to direct sunlight or other strong light where it is directed that an analytical operation is to be carried out "in subdued light". Similarly precaution should be taken to exclude actinic light by the use of low actinic glassware, working in a dark room or similar procedures where a procedure is directed to be performed "protected from light". For preparations other than those of fixed strength, the quantity to be taken for a test or an assay is usually expressed in terms of the active ingredient. It means that the quantity of the

active ingredient expected to be present and the quantity of the preparation to be taken are calculated from the strength stated on the label.

15. ***Other tests:*** In the monographs on dosage forms and certain preparations, under the sub heading "other tests" it is stated that an article complies with the tests stated under the general monograph of the relevant dosage form or preparation. Details of such tests are illustrated in the general monographs.

16. ***Limits:*** The limits given are based on data obtained in normal analytical practice. They take into account normal analytical errors, of acceptable variations in manufacture and of deterioration to an extent that is acceptable. No further tolerances are to be applied to the limits for determining whether or not the article under examination complies with the requirements of the monograph.

17. ***Quantities:*** Unless otherwise stated, in tests with numerical limits and assays, the quantity stated to be taken for testing is approximate. Volumes stated in microliters (µl) are measured using a micropipette or micro syringe. The term "transfer" is used generally to indicate a quantitative operation.

18. ***Apparatus:*** Measuring and weighing devices and other apparatus are described in the chapter entitled "apparatus for tests and assays". Unless otherwise stated, comparative tests are carried out using identical Nessler cylinders.

19. ***Reagents and solutions:*** The reagents required for the tests and assays of the drugs in the Pharmacopoeia are defined in the various chapters showing their nature, degree of purity and the strengths of the solutions to be made from them.

20. ***Indicators:*** Where the use of an indicator solution is mentioned in an assay or test, approximately 0.1 ml of the solution shall be added, unless otherwise directed.

21. ***Reference substances:*** These are the authentic specimens chosen and verified on the basis of their suitability for intended use as prescribed in the Pharmacopoeia and not necessarily suitable in other circumstances.

22. ***Test animals:*** Unless otherwise directed, animals used in test or assay shall be healthy and are drawn from a uniform stock, and have not been previously treated with any material that will interfere with the test or the assay.

23. ***Calculation of results:*** The results should be calculated to one decimal place more than the significant figures stated and then rounded up or down as follows; if the last figure calculated is 5 – 9, the preceding figure is increased by 1; if it is 4 or less, the preceding figure is left unchanged.

24. ***Storage:*** These directions are useful in preserving the activity of the chemical. Specific directions are given in some monographs with respect to the temperatures at which Pharmacopoeial article should be stored, where it is considered that usage at a lower or higher temperature may produce undesirable results. The storage conditions are defined

by the following terms; a) Store in a dry, well ventilated place at a temperature not exceeding 30 °C, b) Store in a refrigerator (2 °C to 8 °C) and do not freeze, c) store in a freezer and d) Store in a deep freezer (below -18 °C). The storage conditions not related to temperature are indicated in the following terms; a) Store protected from light and b) Store protected from light and moisture. Where no specific storage directions or limitations mentioned, it is to be understood that the storage conditions include protection from moisture, freezing and excessive heat (any temperature above 40 °C). For example insulin injection store in multiple dose containers at a temperature between 2 °C to 8 °C. It should not be allowed to freeze.

25. ***Storage containers:*** The storage containers in the Pharmacopoeia are indicated in the following terms; a) Well closed containers: This implies the substance is stable and gets protected from dust, dirt, insects etc, getting into the container, b) Tightly closed container: The substances in such cases get affected by atmospheric oxygen or moisture or carbon dioxide. For example, reducing agents, hygroscopic substances, strong bases etc. must be stored in tightly closed containers. It may also include such compounds are volatile or contain dissolved gases etc. c) Light resistant container: Substances which are affected by light are stored in amber or dark colored containers, d) Single dose containers: This is generally prescribed for some injectables which once opened should not be used again. For example, Ferrous fumarate (Store in a light resistant container).

26. ***Labeling:*** The labeling of drugs and pharmaceuticals is governed by the Drugs and Cosmetics Rule, 1945. The statements that are given in the monographs under the side heading "labeling" are not comprehensive. Only those that are necessary to demonstrate compliance or otherwise with the monograph have been given and they are mandatory. For example, in the monograph on betamethasone sodium tablets the labeling statement is "The label states the strength in terms of the equivalent amount of betamethasone". Any other statements may also include as recommendations.

(c) ***Appendices:*** A comprehensive section of appendices are presented followed by the general notices and monographs. The apparatus that are needed for various Pharmacopoeial tests and assays are described in the appendix 1. Biological tests and assays are described in appendix 2. The details of various chemical tests and assays are included in appendix 3. The details of microbiological tests and assays are included in appendix 4. In the appendix 5, some physical tests and determinations like loss on drying, determination of pH, melting range etc are described. Appendix 6 includes the useful directions on cleaning glassware. Appendix 7 describes the reagents and solutions needed for the various tests and assays, their method of preparation, standards etc. Appendix 8 describes reference substances. Appendix 9 have been described fully the names, symbols used in the Pharmacopoeia for weights and measures and of elements and their atomic weights have been described.

### 1.3.12 Representative example of a Monograph of Indian Pharmacopoeia 2010

**Ferrous Gluconate**

$$Fe^{++}\left[\begin{array}{c} COO^{-} \\ H-C-OH \\ HO-C-H \\ H-C-OH \\ H-C-OH \\ CH_2-OH \end{array}\right]_2$$

Mol. Formula $C_{12}H_{22}FeO_{14}.xH_2O$ Mol. Wt: 446.1 (anhydrous)

Ferrous Gluconate is ferrous di (D-gluconate).

Ferrous Gluconate contains not less than 95.0 percent and not more than 102.0 percent of $C_{12}H_{22}FeO_{14}$, calculated on the dried basis.

***Category:*** Haematinic.

***Dose:*** Prophylactic, 600 mg daily; therapeutic, 1.2 to 1.8 g daily, in divided doses.

(300 mg of ferrous gluconate is approximately equivalent to 35 mg of ferrous iron).

***Description:*** A yellowish grey or pale greenish–yellow, fine powder or granules, odour, slight, resembling that of burnt sugar.

**Identification**

(a) Dissolve 5 gm in *carbon dioxide –free water* at 60 °C, cool and dilute to 50 ml with water. 1 ml of the resulting solution gives reaction A of ferrous salts.

(b) Determine by thin layer chromatography, coating the plate with *silica gel G.*

*Mobile phase.*A mixture of 10 volumes of *concentrated ammonia*, 10 volumes of *ethyl acetate*, 30 volumes of *water* and 50 volumes of *ethanol (95 percent).*

*Test solution.* Dissolve 20 mg of the substance under examination in 2 ml of *water* heating if necessary in a water-bath at 60 °C.

*Reference solution.* Dissolve 20 mg of *ferrous gluconate RS* in 2 ml of *water*, heating if necessary in water-bath at 60 °C.

Apply to the plate 5 µl of each solution. After development dry the plate at 105 °C for 20 minutes and spray with 5 percent w/v solution of *potassium dichromate* in a 40 percent w/v solution of *sulphuric acid.* The principle spot in the chromatogram obtained with the test solution corresponds to that in the chromatogram obtained with the reference solution.

**Tests**

***Appearance of solution:*** Dissolve 5.0 gm in *carbon dioxide- free water* at 60 °C, cool and dilute to 50 ml with the same solvent (solution A). Dilute 2 ml of solution A to 10 ml with *water*. When examined against the light, the resulting solution is clear.

***pH:*** 4.0 to 5.5, determined in solution A, 3 to 4 hours after preparation.

**Arsenic:** To 5.0 gm add 15 ml of *water* and 15 ml of *stannated hydrochloric acid*, distil 22 ml and add to the distillate 40 ml of *water* and 0.2 ml of *stannous chloride solution AsT*. The resulting solution complies with the limit test for arsenic (2 ppm).

***Heavy metals:*** Warm 2.0 gm gently with 10 ml of *nitric acid* until reaction begins and allow to stand until the evolution of nitrous fumes subsides. Boil gently to complete oxidation, adding a further 5 ml of *nitric acid*, if necessary, and continue boiling until the volume is reduced to about 5 ml. Add 20 ml of *hydrochloric acid*, boil gently for 1 minute, cool and extract with three quantities, each of 20 ml, of *ether*. If the acid solution is still more than faintly yellow, extract with a fourth quantity of 20 ml of *ether* and discard the ether extracts. Transfer the acid solution to a narrow - necked flask, rinse the separator with 5 ml of *water*, and add the rinsing to the flask. Heat to remove the dissolved *ether* and part of the *hydrochloric acid*. Cool and dilute to 50 ml with *water*. 25 ml of the resulting solution complies with the limit test for heavy metals, method A (20 ppm).

***Chlorides:*** 0.4 gm complies with the limit test for chlorides (625 ppm).

***Sulphates:*** 0.3 gm complies with the limit test for sulphates (500 ppm).

***Barium:*** Dissolve 0.1 gm in 50 ml of *distilled water*, and 5 ml of *dilute sulphuric acid*, and allow to stand for 5 minutes. The solution is not more opalescent than a mixture of 10 ml of solution A and 45 ml of *distilled water*, when examined against the light.

***Ferric iron:*** Not more than 1.0 percent, determined by the following method. Weigh accurately about 5.0 gm, transfer to a glass-stoppered flask and dissolve in a mixture of 100 ml of freshly boiled and cooled *water,* 10 ml of *hydrochloric acid*. Add 3 gm of *potassium iodide*, shake well and allow to stand in the dark for 5 minutes. Titrate the liberated iodine with *0.1M sodium thiosulphate* using *starch solution*, added towards the end of the titration as indicator. Repeat the operation without the substance under examination. The difference between the titrations represents the amount of iodine liberated by the ferric iron.

1 ml of *0.1M sodium thiosulphate* is equivalent to 0.005585 gm of ferric iron.

***Oxalic acid:*** Dissolve 1 gm in 5 ml of *water*, add 2 ml of *hydrochloric acid* and transfer to a separator. Extract with two quantities, each of 20 ml, of *ether*. Evaporate the combined ether extracts to dryness on a water-bath and dissolve the residue in 5 ml of *water*. Add 0.05 ml of *acetic acid* and 3 ml of *calcium chloride solution*; no turbidity is produced.

***Reducing sugar:*** Dissolve 0.5 gm in 10 ml of *water* and make alkaline with *dilute ammonia solution*. Pass *hydrogen sulphide* into the solution and allow to stand for 30 minutes. Filter and wash the precipitate with two quantities, each of 5 ml of *water*. Combine the filtrate and the washings and acidify with *dilute hydrochloric acid*. Add 2 ml of *dilute hydrochloric acid* in excess. Boil the solution until the vapors no longer darken *lead acetate paper* and, if necessary, boil further to concentrate the solution to about 10 ml. Cool and add 10 ml of *sodium carbonate solution*, set aside for 5 minutes, filter and dilute the filtrate to 100 ml with *water*. To 5 ml of the filtrate add 2 ml of *potassium cupric-tartrate solution* and boil for 1 minute; no red precipitate is formed.

***Loss on drying***: 5.0 per cent to 10.0 per cent determined on 1.0 gm by drying in an oven at 105 °C.

***Microbial Contamination:*** Total viable aerobic count, not more than 1000 micro- organisms per gm, determined by plate count.

***Assay:*** Dissolve 0.5 gm of *sodium bicarbonate* in a mixture of 70 ml of water 30 ml of *1M sulphuric acid*. When effervescence ceases, add about 1.0 gm, of accurately weighed substances under examination, shake gently to dissolve and titrate with *0.1M ceric ammonium nitrate*, using 0.1 ml of *ferroin solution* as indicator, until the red colour disappears.

1 ml of *0.1M ceric ammonium nitrate* is equivalent to 0.04461gm of $C_{12}H_{22}FeO_{14}$.

***Storage:*** Store protected from light.

### 1.3.13 Indian Pharmacopoeia 2014

**Highlights**

- It is effective from 1st January, 2014
- Presented in 4 hard bound volumes with DVD
- Total monographs 2548, 577 new Monographs included.
- For the first time in this edition 19 new Radiopharmaceutical monographs and 1 general chapter is included.
- Presented in user friendly format and cross referencing has been avoided
- Veterinary products monographs are the integral part of this edition
- Use of chromatographic methods has been greatly extended
- More specific IP and UV Spectrophotometer tests have been introduced and classical chemicals tests for identification of an article have been almost eliminated.
- Test for pyrogen almost eliminated
- Obsolete monographs have been omitted
- More herbal drugs monographs has been added
- Included several new monographs not included in any other major pharmacopoeias of the world.

## 1.4 EXTRA PHARMACOPOEIA (MARTINDALE)

Pharmacopoeia possesses wealth of information with no explanation. The person must familiarize himself with the general notices and the various appendices of Pharmacopoeia to consult the Pharmacopoeia. From the extra Pharmacopoeia (Martindale), one can obtain most complete information on every type of pharmaceutical or drug. This book was rich especially with therapeutic and clinical information of the drugs. For inorganic pharmaceuticals there are several other useful literature references are included.

A practicing pharmacist William Martindale in the year 1883 published the extra Pharmacopoeia. To provide practical and up to date information concerning drugs and galenicals included in the British Pharmacopoeia was its main aim. In the span of three years four editions of Martindale were published.

Due to the accumulation of information up to the year 1910 the subject matter to be divided into two volumes in the initial editions of Martindale. The first double volume edition was published in 1912. In December 1933, the pharmaceutical society of Great Britain acquired the copy right of the Extra Pharmacopoeia upon the death of Dr W.H Martindale son of William Martindale. Thereafter the society is continuing to issue it under the editorship of the director of pharmaceutical sciences department. 23$^{rd}$ edition of volume II was published in 1955 and the 24$^{th}$ edition of volume I was published in 1958. Supplement for 24$^{th}$ edition was published in 1961. In February 1967 the 25$^{th}$ edition was published by the pharmaceutical society of Great Britain. While the 26$^{th}$ edition was released in July 1972.

The 30$^{th}$ edition of Martindale contains up to date authoritative information on drugs and medicine which are used throughout the world was published in 1993. It is written for all those involve in use of drugs and medicines including practicing pharmacists and physicians.

In order to meet the requirements of today's reader the latest edition of Martindale has been markedly changed. It includes a significant shift to a more clinical emphasis an increase in the number of referenced reviews and a massive increase information on proprietary medicines. In addition usual period between editions was shorten to meet the need for up to date information.

## 1.5 BRITISH PHARMACOPOEIA

The section 54 of Medical Act of 1858 stressed the need of publication of a book having a list of medicines and compounds, and the manner of preparing them together with true weights and measures by which they are to be prepared and mixed. Hence the British Pharmacopoeia was decided to publish. In the year 1864 the first British Pharmacopoeia was published by combining the three old and reputed Pharmacopoeias namely Pharmacopoeia Londinensis (1618) Edinburgh Pharmacopoeia (1699) and Dublin Pharmacopoeia (1807). New editions and addendum was released quickly. The 2$^{nd}$ edition was released in 1867. The 3$^{rd}$ and 4$^{th}$ edition was published in the year 1885 and 1898 respectively. Addendum to 2$^{nd}$ and 3$^{rd}$ edition was released in the year 1874 and 1890 respectively.

Separate parts such as preparation of compounds are included in the 1864 British Pharmacopoeia. As per practice of several other Pharmacopoeias in this edition of British Pharmacopoeia the contents had been arranged alphabetically. A gap in revision belated the next edition of British Pharmacopoeia until 1914.

In Britain it was realized that technical complexity of the drug specifications was increasing and a different kind of set up was needed to prepare the Pharmacopoeias after publication of the British Pharmacopoeia 1914. Hence the further edition was published in 1928 and 1932. There after the commission was recommended to revise the British Pharmacopoeia every ten years once.

A range of diagnostic materials was included in 1932 revision. An important addition was inclusion of standards and tests for antitoxins and insulin. Seven addenda covered the interim between 1932 and next edition of 1948. In this 1948 edition ($7^{th}$), for substances newly introduced into medicine, generic names were provided. Methods of analysis such as disintegration tests for tablets and sterilization methods were expanded. Many new monographs related to sex hormones and penicillin's were included. Due to the rapid development of pharmaceutical and pharmacological progress at this time it was decided that the normal interval between new editions should be five instead of ten years.

The next edition was released in the year 1953. In this edition of British Pharmacopoeia, the titles of drugs and preparations were given in English instead of Latin. Abbreviated Latin title was retained as a synonym. Capsules, constituted as new group of formulation and the implant methods for sex hormones and their standards were also described in this edition. The $9^{th}$ edition (1958) contains 160 new monographs. Spectrophotometric analysis and inclusion of tranquillizing drugs are the other features of this edition. The next i.e., tenth edition was published in 1963.

The duties of the British Pharmacopoeia commission were defined clearly in medicines order 1970. The first edition of British Pharmacopoeia that was prepared strictly under the provisions of Medicines Act was the thirteenth edition which was published in the year 1980. Due to an expansion of drug information latter the British Pharmacopoeia was decided to publish in two volumes.

Authoritative standard for the quality of many substances preparation and articles used in medicine and pharmacy for some 130 years was provided in 1993 edition of British Pharmacopoeia. For the convenience of user this edition consolidates and extends the 1988 edition with its 1989, 1991, and 1992 addenda. Moreover monographs of the European Pharmacopoeia were also included in this particular edition.

The last year edition of the British Pharmacopoeia i.e., British Pharmacopoeia 2013 comprises six volumes which contain nearly 3,000 monographs for drug substances, excipients and formulated preparation, together with supporting general notices, appendices (test methods, reagents etc.) and reference spectra used in the practice of medicine. All are comprehensively indexed and cross-referenced for easy reference. Items used exclusively in veterinary medicine in the UK are included in the BP (Veterinary).

The volume I and II deals with medicinal substances, whereas volume III describes about formulated preparations, blood related preparations, immunological products, radiopharmaceutical preparations, surgical materials and homeopathic preparations. The volume IV contains appendices, infrared reference spectra and index. The volume V is for veterinary purpose i.e., British Pharmacopoeia (Veterinary). The volume VI is the CD-ROM version of British Pharmacopoeia, British Pharmacopoeia (Veterinary) and British approved names.

The 2013 edition of British Pharmacopoeia is available as a printed volume and electronically in both on line and CD-ROM versions, the electronic products use sophisticated search techniques to locate information quickly. For example, pharmacists referring to a monograph can immediately link to other related substances and appendices referenced in the content by using 1,30,000 plus hypertext links within the text.

The British Pharmacopoeia 2013 package comprises five volumes of the British Pharmacopoeia 2013 and a single volume of the British Pharmacopoeia (Veterinary) 2013, along with a fully searchable CD-ROM and online access which provided flexible resources.

The British Pharmacopoeia 2013 was legally effective from 1 January 2013 and contains 41 new British Pharmacopoeia monographs, 40 new European Pharmacopoeia monographs, 619 amended monographs, 6 new and 1 amended infrared reference spectra and European Pharmacopoeia 7$^{th}$ edition material up to and including Supplement 7.5. In addition updates in January, April and July to harmonise with the European Pharmacopoeia was also provided.

The current edition of the British Pharmacopoeia i.e., British Pharmacopoeia 2014 comprises five volumes and a single volume of the British Pharmacopoeia (Veterinary) 2014, along with a fully searchable CD-ROM and online access to provide with flexible resources.

### 1.5.1 Highlights of British Pharmacopoeia 2014

- Legally effective from 1 January 2014
- 40 new BP monographs are included
- 272 amended monographs
- Three new Supplementary Chapters are included
- Four new BP (Vet) monographs are included
- One new BP (Vet) Supplementary Chapter is included
- Free in-year updates in April and July to harmonise with the European Pharmacopoeia

## 1.6 EUROPEAN PHARMACOPOEIA

An official book of standards adopted by Germany, France, Italy, Netherlands, Switzerland and Belgium is European Pharmacopoeia. In July 1964, the council of Europe issued an order, to frame out European Pharmacopoeia. 1969 onwards in the respective member countries it was appeared as official standard book for medicinal substances and other drugs. Later on it was revised continuously to keep the information up to date.

## 1.7 PHARMACOPOEIA INTERNATIONALS (INTERNATIONAL PHARMACOPOEIA)

In various countries there are no uniformity in terminology and strengths of pharmaceutical preparations used. In the year 1874, a view had been expressed that some world uniformity in the standards for potent drugs must necessary to overcome various problems. These views got further support in second international conference held in 1925 where an international agreement on the Unification of formulae for seventy seven potent drugs and preparations got reached. In 1936 the Health Organization of the League of Nations established a technical commission of Pharmacopoeial experts. The work was undertaken by the WHO after the World War II which was ended in 1946. Finally volume I of the long awaited International Pharmacopoeia was published in 1951 by Latin with translation into English and French. This International Pharmacopoeia contains monographs for over two hundred drugs and chemicals, with appendices on reagents tests and biological assays. Latter in the year 1955 the second volume was published which contains formulae for preparations having various drugs and substances already present in volume I. In 1959 the supplement for first edition was released with incorporation of some newer drugs and substances with its method of preparations and the appropriate tests. In 1967 the second edition of International Pharmacopoeia got published, followed by a supplement in 1971. Third edition of International Pharmacopoeia was published in the form of several volumes, in which volume I appeared in 1979.

The Pharmacopoeial authorities of all countries are expected to give due considerations to its standards so as for achieving uniformity of standards as far as practicable even though the International Pharmacopoeia cannot be imposed legally on any country.

## 1.8 UNITED STATES PHARMACOPOEIA (USP)

In 1817, Dr. Lyman spalding proposed a plan to publish a National Pharmacopoeia to the medical society of the country at New York. 15$^{th}$ December 1820 the first edition of United States Pharmacopoeia was published with 217 drugs in about 272 pages. After the gap of ten years further editions of USP appeared. The 19$^{th}$ edition of USP was published in the year 1905. However, it was given the title of USP VIII as to show that it was 8th revision. Pharmacopoeia must be revised every 5 years was suggested in the 1940 convention.

On July 5 of 1974, unification of the USP and NF (National Formulary) was announced. Afterwards in the subsequent editions consolidated USP and NF into a single volume was published. USP covers all drug substances and drug products; whereas NF covers only pharmaceutical ingredients.

In January 1990, the 22$^{nd}$ edition of USP combined with 17$^{th}$ edition of NF was published.

The current version of USP–NF standards deemed official by USP are enforceable by the United States Food and Drug Administration (US-FDA) for medicines manufactured and marketed in the United States. The latest edition, USP 36–NF 31, published on November 1, 2012 in English, and became official from May 1, 2013. The highlights and features are it contains more than 4,600 monographs with specifications for identity, strength, quality, purity, packaging, and labeling for substances and dosage forms. It also comprise more than 260 general chapters providing clear, step-by-step guidance for assays, tests, and procedures. More over it also focus, specific charts and a combined index which help us to find the information.

## 1.9 PHARMACEUTICAL INDEX

Its 12th edition has been completely revised and incorporated updated material as well as entirely fresh subject areas. The new codex provides a reference source on all aspects of pharmaceutical science and technology.

Part I covers the multidisciplinary nature of pharmaceutics and demonstrates how quality is built into medicines from conception ideas and to develop and for production and use. The chapters broadly encompass the pharmaceutics content of the syllabus for pharmacy undergraduates and also provide direction and support for the continuing education of graduates with special emphasis on the product development and the innovation. Part II includes an extensive collection of pharmaceutical data arranged in monograph form. It is edited by staff of the Royal pharmaceutical society by inviting known experts to write individual chapters.

## 1.10 THE DRUGS AND COSMETICS ACT 1940

### 1.10.1 Scope

The Drugs and Cosmetics Act 1940 has been enacted for the purpose of proper enforcement and the purpose is that no substandard drugs be sold in the market and no one will sell even genuine drug without license.

This Act mainly concerned with the standard and quality of drugs manufactured in this country and therefore controls the manufacture, sale and distribution of drugs. This act is not related to excise duty or impositions on narcotic drugs.

### 1.10.2 Objectives

In view of the commitment undertaken by the Government of India the objects of Drugs and Cosmetics Act 1940 are as follows.

I. Regulation of international traffic in all the drugs covered by the convention.
II. Regulations of manufacture and internal traffic of certain specified drugs such as cocaine and morphine.

### 1.10.3 Features of Drugs and Cosmetics Act 1940

***Definitions:*** As per Drugs and Cosmetics Act 1940 the drugs and cosmetics are defined as follows,

***Drugs (Ayurvedic Unani or siddha):*** It include all medicines intended for internal or external use for or in the diagnosis treatment, mitigation or prevention of disease of disorder in human beings or animals and manufactured exclusively in accordance with the formulae described in the authoritative book, Ayurvedic siddha and unani, tibb system of medicine specified in the first schedule.

***Cosmetics:*** It means any article intended to be rubbed, poured, sprinkled or sprayed in on or introduced into or otherwise applied to the human body or any part for cleansing, beautifying, promoting attractiveness or alternating the appearance. It also includes any articles intended for use as a component of cosmetics.

## 1.10.4 Standard of Quality

In relation to a drug that the drug complies with the standard set out. Cosmetics also complies with standard as recommended.

**Misbranded drugs**

A drug shall be termed to be misbranded:

(a) If it so colored, powdered or polished that damage is concealed or if it is made to appear of better or greater therapeutic value than it really is; or

(b) If it is not labeled in the prescribed manner; or

(c) If its label or container or anything accompanying the drug bears any statement design or

(d) If its label or container or anything accompanying the drug bears any statement design or device which makes any false claim for the drug or which is false or misleading in any particular manner.

***Adulterated drugs:*** The drug shall be termed to be adulterated.

(a) If it consists in whole or in part of any filthy putrid or decomposed substance; or

(b) If it has been prepared packed or stored under insanitary conditions whereby it may have been contaminated with filth or whereby it may have been rendered injurious to health, or

(c) If it contains any harmful or toxic substance which may render injurious to health; or

(d) If it bears or it contains for the purposes of coloring only, a color other than one which is prescribed or

(e) If any substance has been mixed therewith so as to reduce its quality or strength.

***Spurious drugs:*** A drug shall be termed to be spurious:

(a) If it is imported under a name which belongs to another drug; or

(b) If it is an imitation of or is a substitute for another drug or resembles another drug in a manner likely to deceive or bears upon it or upon its label or container the name of another drug unless it is plainly and conspicuously marked so as to reveal its true character and its lack of identity with such other drug or

(c) If the label or container bears the name of an individual or company purporting to be the manufacturer of the drug, which individual or company is fictitious or does not exist; or

(d) If it has been substituted wholly or in part by another drug or substance or

(e) If it purports to be the product of a manufacturer of whom it is not truly a product.

### 1.10.5 License to Sell, Stock, Exhibit or Offer for Sale or Distribute Drugs by Retail other than those Specified in (Schedules c, c (1) and (x))

License form 20 is to be filled by the official drug distributor in the following proforma:

1. Is hereby licensed to sell, stock or exhibit for sale or distribute by retail drugs other than those specified in of the Drugs and Cosmetics Rules 1945 and to operate a pharmacy on the premises situated at subject to the conditions specified below and to the provisions of the Drugs and Cosmetics Act 1940 and the rules there under.
2. The license shall be in force from to
3. Names of qualified person in charge
4. Categories of drugs

### 1.10.6 Conditions for License

1. This license shall be displayed in a prominent place in a part of the premises open to the public.
2. The license shall comply with the provisions of the Drugs and Cosmetics Act 1940 and the rules there under for the time being in force.
3. No drug shall be sold unless such drugs are purchased under cash or credit memo from a duly licensed dealer or a duly licensed manufacturer.
4. No sale of any drug shall be made to a person not holding the requisite license to sell stock or exhibit for sale or distribute the drug provided that this condition shall not apply to the sale of any drug.
5. An officer or authority purchasing on behalf of government or
6. A hospital medical, educational or research institution or a registered medical practitioner for the purpose of supply to his patient or
7. A manufacturer of beverages confectional biscuits and other non medical products where such drugs are required for processing those products.

The licensee shall inform the licensing authority in writing in the event of any change in the constitution of the firm operating under license. Where any change in the constitution of firm takes place, the current license shall be deemed to be valid for a maximum period of three months from the date on which the change takes place unless a fresh license has been taken from the licensing authority in the name of firm with the changed constitution.

## 1.11 CLASSIFICATION OF INORGANIC PHARMACEUTICALS

Inorganic Pharmaceuticals can be classified in two ways

1. Based on their uses,
2. Based on their application in therapy.

Classification based on their uses is described already.

Classification based on their applications (therapeutic classification) is described below.

***Acidosis:*** Acidosis is a pathologic condition resulting from accumulation of acid and hydrogen ions. Inorganic drugs used in this condition are all electrolyte replenishers like sodium chloride, potassium chloride and others.

***Acne:*** Acne is a very common chronic inflammatory dermatosis in adolescent in both sexes. The lesions are seen on face, upper chest and upper back. Inorganic drugs used in this condition are sulphur and its compounds

***Alkalosis:*** Alkalosis is a pathologic condition resulting from accumulation of base and characterized by decrease in hydrogen ion concentration. Inorganic drugs used in this condition are all acidic electrolyte replenishers like sodium chloride, potassium chloride.

***Allergic diseases:*** Allergic disease is a state of hypersensitivity induced by exposure to a particular antigen (allergen) resulting from immunologic reaction. An inorganic drug used in this condition is magnesium thiosulphate.

***Anaemia:*** Anaemia is defined as decreased hemoglobin concentration in blood below the lower limit of the normal range of individual. Inorganic drugs used in this condition are, all iron compounds (Haematinics: Ferrous Sulphate, Ferrous gluconate, Ferric ammonium citrate etc.).

***Anoxia:*** It is a condition characterized by an absence of oxygen supply to an organ or a tissue. Oxygen is used in this condition.

***Arthritis:*** It is a chronic systemic disease manifested as inflammation of peripheral joints and hematological, pulmonary, cardiovascular and neurological abnormalities. Inorganic drug used in this condition is sodium aurothiomalate.

***Asphyxia:*** A condition in which extreme decrease in the concentration of oxygen in the body accompanied with increase in the concentration of carbon dioxide level leads to unconscious or death. Oxygen is used in this condition.

***Asthma:*** Asthma is characterized by hyper responsiveness of bronchial smooth muscle to a variety of stimuli, resulting in narrowing of air tubes accompanied by increased secretions; symptoms include wheezing, cough, and dyspnoea. Organic drugs like salbutamol is used in this condition.

***Athlete's foot (Tinea pedis):*** It is a superficial fungal infection of stratum corneum of skin, located in the web spaces between toes. Inorganic drugs used in this condition are sodium pyrophosphate.

***Boils:*** Bacterial infection of hair follicles and surroundings. An inorganic drug used in this condition is magnesium sulphate.

***Burns:*** Injuries to the tissues caused by frictions, heat, radiation, electricity or chemicals. Inorganic drugs used in this condition are silver nitrate, oxygen, zinc peroxide.

***Carbuncles:*** Carbuncle is a bacterial infection spread under the skin and subcutaneous tissue with oozing of pus. Inorganic drug used in this condition is magnesium sulphate.

***Cholecystitis:*** It is an inflammation of gall bladder, which begins with obstruction, followed by infection of gall bladder. It is of acute and chronic.

***Cleaning aids (surgical scrub):*** An Inorganic drug used in the cleaning of wounds and ulcers or affected area. Example chlorinated soda.

***Conjunctivitis:*** It is characterized by inflammation of conjunctiva (Conjunctiva is a delicate membrane that lines the eyelids and covers the exposed surfacc of sclera). Inorganic drug used in this condition is silver protein.

***Corns (Korn):*** Corn is a horny thickening of stratum corneum of skin of toes, caused by friction and pressure from poorly fitting shoes. Inorganic drugs used in this condition are silver nitrate, copper oleate.

***Dandruff:*** Dandruff is a dry scaly material desquamated from scalp. Inorganic drugs used in this condition are selenium sulphide, antimony sulphide, cadmium sulphide.

***Dental Caries:*** Dental caries is a disease of teeth caused by acids produced by action of microorganisms on carbohydrates. It is characterized by decalcification of tooth accompanied by foul mouth odour. Inorganic drugs used in this condition are sodium fluoride, strontium and other fluorides.

***Dermatitis:*** Dermatitis is an inflammatory response to a variety of agents acting on skin from outside or within the body such as chemicals, drugs, hypersensitivity to various agents and haptens etc. Inorganic drug used in this condition is cadmium sulphide.

***Diarrhoea:*** Increased frequency or decreased consistency of bowel movement. Inorganic drugs used in this condition are oral rehydration salts, bismuth subcarbonate, calcium carbonate, electrolyte replenishers.

***Dysentery:*** It means diarrhoea with abdominal cramps, tenesmus and passage of mucous in the stools. It is of bacillary and amoebic types. Inorganic drugs used in this condition are all bismuth compounds (Bismuth subcarbonate and Bismuth subgallate)

***Eclampsia:*** It is a serious condition related to high blood pressure caused by pregnancy leads to convulsions, coma, before or during or shortly after child birth. An inorganic drug used in this condition is magnesium sulphate.

***Eczema:*** It is an inflammatory response to a variety of agents acting on skin from outside or within the body such as chemicals and drugs, hypersensitivity to various antigens and haptens. Inorganic drugs used in this condition are iodine (All solutions), fuller's earth and calamine.

***Eye infections:*** Infection of sebaceous gland of the eye lid hordeolum. Inorganic drugs used in this condition are boric acid, silver nitrate, borax, silver protein, yellow mercuric oxide, zinc sulphate.

***Flatulence:*** It is the process of release excess amount of gases like hydrogen, methane, carbon dioxide from the intestine to the anus during final stage of digestion. An inorganic drug used in this condition is activated charcoal, magnesium silicate etc.

***Gangrene (Tissue necrosis):*** It is a form of necrosis of tissue super added putrefaction, caused due to ischemia. An inorganic drug used in this condition is zinc peroxide.

***Gingivitis:*** Inflammation of gums (Gums are red and puffy). An inorganic drug used in this condition is zinc iodide

***Hemodialysis:*** Removal of certain elements from the blood by diffusion phenomena and to retain the normal constituents in it. Inorganic drugs used in this condition are all electrolyte replenishers.

***Hyperacidity:*** Excessive acid secretion in stomach. Inorganic drugs used in this condition are antacids (aluminium hydroxide and magnesium hydroxide).

***Hypercalcemia:*** It is the excess of calcium in blood with the symptoms like muscle weakness, fatigue, depression, nausea, anorexia and constipation. Inorganic drugs used in this condition are sodium phosphate, sodium sulphate.

***Hyperhidrosis:*** It is a disorder caused by excessive sweating. An inorganic drug used in this condition is sodium pyrophosphate.

***Hyperthyroidism:*** Also called as Thyrotoxicosis. It is a hypermetabolic, clinical and biochemical state caused by excess production of thyroid gland in cases of graves' disease, a toxic adenoma and toxic multinodular goiter. An inorganic drug used in this condition is potassium perchlorate.

***Hypomagnesemia:*** It is abnormally low magnesium content of blood plasma as a result of malabsorption, dehydration, alcoholism or renal disease with the symptoms like neuromuscular activity. An inorganic drug used in this condition is magnesium chloride.

***Intracranial pressure:*** Pressure inside the skull and thus in the brain and CSF. An inorganic drug used in this condition is hypertonic saline.

***Iron deficiency:*** It occurs due to increased metabolism of iron, malabsorption from diet or high excretion of iron from the body resulting in hypochromic anemia. Inorganic drugs used in this condition are all iron compounds (ferric ammonium citrate, ferrous Sulphate and ferrous fumarate)

***Leishmaniasis:*** Several different illness caused by an organism protozoan. An inorganic drug used in this condition is sodium antimony gluconate.

***Malignant wounds:*** These are the result of cancerous cells infiltrating the skin and its supporting blood. Oxygen is used in this condition.

***Manic Depression:*** Cyclic alteration of manic and depressive phases bipolar disorder. An inorganic drug used in this condition is lithium carbonate.

***Muscular excitability:*** The ability of a muscle fiber to respond rapidly to stimulating agent. An inorganic drug used in this condition is calcium gluconate.

***Osteoporosis:*** Reduction in the amount bone mass due to loss of bone proteins and calcium, lead into fractures after trauma. Inorganic drugs used in this condition are all calcium compounds and fluorides.

***Peritoneal dialysis:*** It is a technique performed across the membrane of peritoneal cavity and is used to remove toxic chemicals from the body. Inorganic drugs used in this condition are sodium and potassium acetate, electrolyte replenishers.

***Pharyngitis:*** Inflammation of the mucous of the pharynx. Inorganic drugs used in this condition are iodine and its solutions (Aqueous iodine solution, strong iodine solution, weak iodine solution).

***Poisoning:*** A drug substance, when ingested or inhaled or absorbed or applied or injected into or developed within the body, has chemical action that causes damage to the structure or disturbance of function, producing symptoms, illness or death. Inorganic drugs used in this condition are (antidotes are used in this case)

| | | |
|---|---|---|
| Cyanide poisoning | - | Sodium thiosulphate. |
| | | Sodium nitrite |
| Digitalis poisoning | - | Potassium chloride injection |
| Gaseous poisoning | - | Oxygen |
| Insecticide poisoning | - | Fuller's earth |

***Pruritis:*** An unpleasant cutaneous sensation that desire to stretch the skin to obtain relief. Inorganic drugs used in this condition are calomel, ammoniated mercury.

***Psoriasis:*** It is a chronic inflammatory dermatitis with lesions characterized by brownish red papules and plaques which are covered with fine, silvery, white scales. Inorganic drugs used in this condition are calomel, ammoniated mercury.

***Ring worm infection:*** Common fungal infection of the skin. Inorganic drugs used in this condition are sulphur, iodine solution.

***Scabies:*** A contagious dermatitis of humans and various wild and domestic animals caused by a mild "*sarcoptes scabiei*". An inorganic drug used in this condition is sulphur.

***Shock:*** A life threatening clinical syndrome of cardiovascular collapse characterized by an acute reduction of effective circulating blood volume (hypotension) and an inadequate perfusion of cells and tissues (hypoperfusion). Organic drug like adrenaline is used in this condition.

***Skin infection:*** Any infection or allergy due to pathogens. Inorganic drug used in this condition is zinc undecylenate.

***Sore throat:*** Bacterial or viral infection in the throat, such as common cold. Inorganic drugs used in this condition are iodine.

***Sun burns:*** Allergic reactions affecting living tissue skin (rashes). Inorganic drugs used in this condition are calamine, titanium dioxide.

***Thyroid deficiency/Hypothyroidism:*** It is a hypometbolic clinical state resulting from inadequate production of thyroid hormones for prolonged periods or rarely from resistance from peripheral tissues to the effect of thyroid hormones. Inorganic drugs used in this condition are hydroiodic acid, potassium iodide.

***Thyrotoxicosis:*** It is a hyper metabolic and biochemical state caused by excess production of thyroid hormones. Inorganic drugs used in this condition are iodine solutions.

***Tonsillitis:*** It is caused by bacteria called *staphylococci* or *streptococci*, may be acute or chronic, characterized by redness, enlargement and inflammation of the tonsil glands.

Inflammation of throat is due to bacterial or viral infection. Inorganic drug used in this condition is iodine.

***Tumors:*** A new growth of tissue in which multiplication of the cells is uncontrolled and progressive and also called as "neoplasm". An inorganic drugs used in this condition is cisplatin.

***Ulcers:*** It is an exudation of surface of an organ or tissue, which is produced by sloughing of inflammatory necrotic tissue.

***Duodenal ulcer:*** Ulcers formed due to excessive secretion of hydrochloric acid with symptoms like steady or burning pain in upper abdomen that can be relieved by ingestion of food, antacid or cold milk. This may be an infection caused by bacteria (*H. Pylori*). An inorganic drugs used in this condition is aluminium hydroxide gel.

***Gastric or peptic ulcer:*** These are the areas of degeneration and necrosis of gastrointestinal mucosa exposed to acid-peptic secretions; symptoms are vomiting, sepsis and burning pain in upper abdomen. Inorganic drugs used in this condition are bismuth compounds, magnesium trisilicate.

***Skin or topical ulcer:*** An inorganic drug used in this condition is zinc oxide.

***Uremia:*** Excess of urea, creatinine and other nitrogenous end products of proteins and amino acid metabolism in the blood. Drugs used in this condition are haemodialysis fluid (or) peritonical dialysis fluid.

***Urethritis:*** Inflammation of urethra (painful or difficult for urination). An inorganic drug used in this condition is zinc permanganate.

***Urticaria:*** Urticaria or hives is the presence of transient, recurrent, pruritic wheals (raised erythematous areas of edema) on skin and oral, laryngeal and gastrointestinal mucosa. An inorganic drug used in this condition is calamine.

***Varicose veins (Varicocele):*** It is the dilation, elongation, tortuosity of veins of pampiniferous plexus in the spermatic cord. Inorganic drug used in this condition is lead-oleate.

***Warts:*** Common viral lesions of the skin caused by *Human papillomavirus* (HPV) a small, rough growth typically on a human's hand or feet. An inorganic drug used in this condition is silver nitrate.

***Wounds:*** Injury or damage to the skin. Inorganic drugs used in this condition are hydrogen peroxide, zinc peroxide.

## 1.12 PHARMACEUTICAL AIDS

The following agents which are not used in therapy but they play important role in the manufacture or storage of pharmaceuticals are called as pharmaceutical aids.

***Absorbents:*** Substances used to absorb gases. Inorganic substances used for this purpose are activated charcoal, soda lime.

***Adsorbents:*** Substances used to adsorb gases, coloring matters etc. Inorganic substances used for this purpose are aluminium phosphate, fuller's earth.

***Acidifiers:*** Substances used to make acidic condition. Inorganic substance used for this purpose is dilute hydrochloric acid.

***Alkalisers:*** Substances used to make alkaline condition. Inorganic substances used for this purpose are sodium carbonate, ammonia solutions.

***Antioxidants:*** Substances used to prevent the oxidation of pharmaceuticals. Inorganic substances used for this purpose are sodium bisulphite, hypophosphorous acid.

***Buffers:*** Substances used to maintain pH. Inorganic substances used for this purpose are phosphate buffer, borate buffer.

***Chelating agent:*** Substances used to make complexation. Inorganic substance used for this purpose is EDTA.

***Decolorizing agent:*** Substances used to remove colors. Inorganic substances used for this purpose are fuller's earth, activated charcoal.

***Desiccants:*** Substances used to absorbs moisture and provide dry micro atmosphere in containers of pharmaceuticals. Inorganic substances used for this purpose are calcium chloride, silica gel.

***Excipients:*** Substances used to increase the bulk of a solid mass, which carries a drug. Inorganic substances used for this purpose are di and tri basic calcium phosphate.

***Filter aids:*** Substances used for clarification purpose. Inorganic substances used for this purpose are kieselguhr, fuller's earth.

***Opacity agent:*** Substances used for making high reflectance of capsules. Inorganic substance used for this purpose is titanium dioxide.

***Solvents or vehicles:*** Substances used as a vehicle for liquid dosage forms and injectables. Inorganic substances used for this purpose are purified water and water for injection.

***Tonicity adjusting agents:*** Substances used to adjust the tonicity of injectables. Inorganic substance used for this purpose is sodium chloride.

***Thickening agents or suspending agents:*** Substances used to stabilizes suspensions. Inorganic substances used for this purpose are silica gel, colloidal silica.

***Water softeners:*** Substances used to soften water. Inorganic substance used for this purpose is sodium carbonate.

## PROBABLE QUESTIONS

1. Define pharmaceutical chemistry?
2. Explain the various aspects of pharmaceutical chemistry.
3. Explain the importance of inorganic chemistry in pharmacy.
4. Define pharmaceuticals and explain about their uses.

5. Explain about various pharmacopoeias.
6. Write the salient features of recent edition of Indian Pharmacopoeia.
7. Define the following terms:

| | | | |
|---|---|---|---|
| (i) | Misbranded drug | (ii) | Adulterated drug |
| (iii) | Standard of quality | (iv) | Spurious drug. |

8. Define the term monograph and explain with any one official drug.
9. Briefly explain about the storage conditions of drugs.
10. Describe the development of Pharmacopoeias.
11. Briefly explain about Drugs and Cosmetics Act 1940.
12. Classify pharmaceutical inorganic compounds based on their applications with examples.
13. Classify pharmaceutical inorganic compounds based on their therapeutic uses with examples.
14. Explain about pharmaceutical index.
15. Briefly explain the history of Indian Pharmacopoeia.

CHAPTER 2

# BASICS OF PHARMACEUTICAL INORGANIC CHEMISTRY

## 2.1 ATOMIC SYMBOLS

Atoms of the different elements are represented by using symbols. Atomic symbol is one or two letter notation used to represent an atom corresponding to a particular element. The atomic symbol consists of the first letter capitalized, from the name of the element, some times with an additional letter from the name in lower case. For example, fluorine has the symbol "F" and chlorine has the symbol of "Cl". Many symbols are also derived from a name in another language (Latin). Example sodium is represented by the symbol "Na" derived from its Latin name Natrium. Symbols of some selected elements are listed in Table 2.1.

**Table 2.1** Symbols of elements and their physical appearance

| Name of the element | Atomic symbol | Physical appearance of element* |
|---|---|---|
| Aluminium | Al | Silvery white metal |
| Barium | Ba | Silvery white metal |
| Bromine | Br | Reddish brown liquid |
| Carbon<br>Graphite<br>Diamond | C | Soft, black solid.<br>Hard, colorless crystal. |
| Chlorine | Cl | Greenish-yellow gas |
| Chromium | Cr | Silvery-white metal |
| Cobalt | Co | Silvery-white metal |
| Copper (Cuprum) | Cu | Reddish metal |
| Fluorine | F | Pale yellow gas |
| Gold (Aurum) | Au | Soft yellow metal |
| Helium | He | Colorless gas |
| Hydrogen | H | Colorless gas |
| Iodine | I | Bluish black solid |
| Iron (Ferrum) | Fe | Silvery-white metal |

**Table 2.1** *Contd...*

| Name of the element | Atomic symbol | Physical appearance of element* |
|---|---|---|
| Lead (Plumbum) | Pb | Bluish-white metal |
| Magnesium | Mg | Silvery white metal |
| Manganese | Mn | Grey white metal |
| Mercury (Hydragyrum) | Hg | Silvery white liquid metal |
| Neon | Ne | Colorless gas |
| Nickel | Ni | Silvery white metal |
| Nitrogen | N | Colorless gas |
| Oxygen | O | Colorless gas |
| Phosphorous (white) | P | Yellowish white, waxy solid |
| Potassium (Kalium) | K | Soft, silvery white material. |
| Silicon | Si | Grey, lustrous solid. |
| Silver (Argentum) | Ag | Silvery white metal |
| Sodium (Natrium) | Na | Silvery white metal |
| Sulphur | S | Yellow solid |
| Tin (Stannum) | Sn | Silvery white metal |
| Zinc | Zn | Bluish white metal |

*Common form of the element under normal conditions (Standard Temperature and Pressure).

## 2.2 EMPIRICAL FORMULA

An empirical formula for a compound is the formula of a substance which expresses its percentage composition. It indicates about the ratio of number of atoms in the compound but does not indicate the actual number of atoms of each element present in it.

**Steps for calculating the empirical formula**

1. Divide the percentage of elements (obtained or determined by suitable methods) by its atomic mass (weight), which will give the relative number of moles of various elements present in the compound.
2. Divide the quotients obtained in the above step by smallest of them so as to get a simple atomic ratio (Minor values being neglected).
3. Multiply the figures, so obtained by a suitable integer of necessary in order to obtain whole number ratio.
4. Finally write down the symbols of various elements side by side and put the above numbers as the subscripts to the lower right hand of each symbol, which represent the empirical formula.

**Example 1:** A compound has the following composition. It contains 9.76% of Mg, 13.01% of sulphur, 26.01% of oxygen and 51.22% of water.

Calculate its empirical formula

**Step1:** Divide the percentage composition of each element by its relative atomic weight (calculation of relative number of Moles)

Magnesium (Mg) = 9.76/24 = 0.406

Sulphur (S) = 13.01/32 = 0.406

Oxygen (O) = 26.01/16 = 1.625

Water ($H_2O$) = 51.22/18 = 2.846

**Step 2:** Calculation of simple ratio moles

Mg = 0.406/0.406 = 1

$O_2$ = 1.625/0.406 = 4

S = 0.406/0.406 = 1

$H_2O$ = 2.846/0.406 = 7

**Step 3:** Calculation of simplest whole number ratio.

Mg = 1

S = 1

$O_2$ = 4

$H_2O$ = 7

Hence the empirical formula is $MgSO_4$. $7H_2O$

## 2.3 MOLECULAR FORMULA

The molecular formula of a substance refers the actual number of atoms of each element present in its molecule. It may be same as that of the empirical formula of the substance and exact multiple of it.

Molecular formula = n x empirical formula.

Where n =1, 2, 3, when n =1, the molecular formula coincide with empirical formula.

Molecular weight = Empirical formula weight x n

n = Molecular weight/Empirical formula weight

**Steps for writing molecular formula**

(a) Calculate the empirical formula.

(b) Calculate the empirical formula mass by adding the atomic mass of all the atoms present in the empirical formula of the compound.

(c) Divide the molecular mass (determined experimentally) by the empirical formula mass and find out the value of "n" which is whole number.

(d) Multiply the empirical formula of the compound with "n" so as to find out the molecular formula of the compound.

**Example 1:** A compound on analysis gave the following percentage composition. Na = 14.31%, S = 9.97%, H = 6.22%. Calculate the molecular formula of the compound on the assumption that all the hydrogen in the compound is present in combination with oxygen as water of crystallization. Molecular mass of the compound is 322 (Table 2.2).

**Table 2.2** Molecular formula calculation

| Element | Percentage | Relative number of moles | Simple ratio number | Simplest whole number ratio |
|---|---|---|---|---|
| Na | 14.31 | 14.31/23 = 0.62 | 0.62/0.31 = 2 | 2 |
| S | 9.97 | 9.97/32 = 0.31 | 0.31/0.31 = 1 | 1 |
| H | 6.22 | 6.22/1 = 6.22 | 6.22/0.31 = 20 | 20 |
| O | 69.5 | 69.5/16 = 4.34 | 4.34/0.31 = 14 | 14 |

**Solution 1: Calculation of Empirical Formula**

Now the empirical formula is $Na_2SH_{20}O_{14}$

**Calculation of Molecular formula:** According to the definition of molecular mass

n = Molecular mass/Empirical formula Mass

= 322/322 =1

Hence molecular formula = (Empirical formula) x n

n = 1

So, molecular formula = $(Na_2SH_{20}O_{14})_1$

Here all hydrogen atoms are present as $H_2O$ in the compound it means 20 hydrogen atoms must have combined. It means 20 hydrogen atoms must have combined with 10 oxygen atoms to forms 10 water molecules for water of crystallization. The remaining 4 oxygen atoms should be present within the rest of the compound.

So the molecular formula = $Na_2SO_4.10H_2O$

## 2.4 MOLECULAR WEIGHT

The molecular weight of a compound is the weight of one molecule of it as compared to the weight of an atom of hydrogen as 1.

or

It is the sum of the atomic weight of all of the atoms in a molecule of the substance.

**Example:** Molecular weight of $H_2O$ is 18.0 amu

$2 \times H = 2 \times 1.008 = 2$

$1 \times O = 1 \times 16 = 16$

Molecular weight = 18

Methods for determining molecular weight of substances are classified in to two types.

1. Physical methods.
2. Chemical methods.

**Physical methods**

1. Victor Meyer method.
2. Dumas method.
3. Hoffman method.
4. Freezing point and Boiling point method.

**Chemical methods**

1. Platinichloride method for bases.
2. Silver salt method for acids.
3. Volumetric method for acids and bases.

## 2.5 STOICHIOMETRIC EQUATIONS

Stoichiometric equation is a short scientific representation of a chemical reaction.

**Stoichiometry:** It is the calculation of quantities of reactants and products involved in the chemical reaction.

## 2.6 CHEMICAL EQUATIONS

An important feature of atomic theory is its explanation of a chemical reaction as a rearrangement of the atoms of the substances.

**For example:** Hydrogen reacts with oxygen and gives water molecule which involves the combination of hydrogen and oxygen. Similarly the reaction between sodium metal with chlorine gas involves the rearrangement of the atoms of sodium and chlorine to give the new combination of atoms in the product of sodium chloride. These types of combination or rearrangement of atoms are conveniently represented by a chemical equation by using chemical formulas.

**Chemical equation** is the symbolic notation of a chemical reaction in terms of chemical formulas.

**For example:** Burning reaction between sodium and chlorine to give sodium chloride is written as

$$2\,Na + Cl_2 \longrightarrow 2\,NaCl$$

The formulas on left side of the equation represents reactants (starting material in a chemical reaction).

The formulas on the right side of the equation represent products (substance obtained from a reaction).

The coefficient of 2 in front of the formula Na, and NaCl indicates the relative number of molecules or units involved in the reaction.

In many cases the state or phases of the elements involved in the particular chemical reaction is mentioned in the reaction by placing appropriate labels following the formulas of substances.

The following symbols are used as phase labels.

(g) = gas, (l) = liquid, solid = (s)

Aq = aqueous (water solution)

When we use the above phase labels the previous equation becomes

$$2\ Na_{(s)} + Cl_{2(g)} \longrightarrow 2\ NaCl_{(s)}$$

In an equation conditions under which a reaction carried out also should be indicated. If the reactants are heated, then the condition of this reaction is indicated by putting the symbol Δ (delta) above the arrow. For example:

$$2\ NaNO_3 \xrightarrow{\Delta} 2\ NaNO_{2(s)} + O_{2(g)}$$

Important other conditions such as temperature, pressure, catalyst etc may be noted above or below the arrow of the equation.

## 2.7 BALANCING OF CHEMICAL EQUATIONS

### 2.7.1 Balanced Equation

When the co-efficient in a chemical equation are correctly given, the number of atoms of each element is equal on the both sides of the arrow, then the equation is said to be balanced equation. The chemical equation should be balanced by following atomic theory.

For example, consider the following equation, hydrogen atom combines with bromine and gives hydrogen bromide. The skeletal equation of the reaction is represented as follows.

$$H_2 + Br_2 \longrightarrow HBr$$

The number of hydrogen and bromine atom in the left hand side is two, but the right hand side is one so the number of molecules of HBr is multiplied by two in the right hand side of the equation.

$$H_2 + Br_2 \longrightarrow 2\ HBr$$

Now the above equation is said balanced or stoichiometric equation.

In the following example, the reaction between potassium permanganate and hydrochloric acid, the skeleton of the equation is written as follows

$$KMnO_4 + HCl \longrightarrow KCl + MnCl_2 + Cl_2 + H_2O$$

If an element is present only one substance in the left hand side of the equation and if the same element is present only one of the substance in the right side, it may be taken up first while the balancing equation.

or

Balance first the atoms for element that occur in only one substance on each side of the equation. This method is called as inspection method of balancing equation.

According to the above rule, the equation is balanced by the following way or balancing the equation is started with K, Mn, O or H but not with Cl.

| Left hand side | Right hand side |
|---|---|
| K = 1 | 1 |
| Mn = 1 | 1 |
| O = 4 | 1 |

So the equation becomes

$$KMnO_4 + 8\,HCl \longrightarrow KCl + MnCl_2 + Cl_2 + 4\,H_2O$$

Now there are 8 hydrogen atoms on the right side of the equation, so we must write 8 HCl. Among the eight chlorine atoms on the left side, one is present in KCl, 2 is present $MnCl_2$ leaving five free chlorine atoms. Therefore, the above equation becomes

$$KMnO_4 + 8\,HCl \longrightarrow KCl + MnCl_2 + 5/2\,Cl_2 + 4\,H_2O$$

All the stoichiometric equations are written with whole numbers coefficient and so the equation is multiplied throughout by 2, then the equation becomes

$$2\,KMnO_4 + 16\,HCl \longrightarrow 2\,KCl + 2\,MnCl_2 + 5\,Cl_2 + 8\,H_2O$$

### 2.7.2 Balancing Redox Reaction Equations

The concepts of oxidation and reduction reaction are important for understanding to this topic.

**Redox reaction:** In day today life, we come across process like fading of the color of the clothes, burning of the combustible substances like cooking gas, wood, coal etc. like that the number of industrial processes like electro plating, extraction of metals etc., all of these reactions or processes fall in the category of specific type of reactions called oxidation-reduction or redox reaction. Redox reactions are also forms the basis of electrochemical and electrolytic cells.

According to the basic concept

Oxidation is defined as "process of addition of oxygen or removal of hydrogen".

Reduction is a process of "removal of oxygen or addition of hydrogen".

**Example:** Reaction of $Cl_2$ with $H_2S$

Oxidation ($H_2$ atom is removed from $H_2S$)

$$H_2S + Cl_2 \longrightarrow 2\,HCl + S$$

Reduction (Hydrogen atom added to the chlorine atom)

So $H_2S$ gets oxidized and $Cl_2$ gets reduced.

### 2.7.3 Electronic Concept of Oxidation and Reduction

According to the electronic concept

**Oxidation** is a process in which an atom loses one or more electrons. This loss of electrons leads to increase of positive charge or decrease the negative charge of the species.

$$Cu \longrightarrow Cu^{2+} + 2e^- \text{ [Increases the positive charge]}$$

$$Fe \longrightarrow Fe^{3+} + e^- \text{ [Increases the positive charge]}$$

**Oxidizing agents or oxidants:** The species which undergo gaining of electrons during the reactions are called oxidizing agents or oxidants.

**Reduction:** It is a process in which an atom gains one or more electrons, leads to increase the negative charge or decrease the positive charge of the species which involves in the chemical reaction.

$$Fe^{3+} + e^- \longrightarrow Fe^{2+} \text{ [Decreases the positive charge]}$$

$$Zn^{2+} + 2e^- \longrightarrow Zn \text{ [Decreases the positive charge]}$$

**Reducing agents:** The species which undergo loss of electrons during the reaction are called as reducing agents.

**Oxidation Number:** It is defined as the residual charge that an atom appears to have, when all other atoms from the molecule are removed as ions.

Atoms can have positive, zero or negative values of oxidation numbers depending upon their state of combination. General rules for assigning oxidation number to an atom are represented in Table 2.3.

Balancing of oxidation reduction equation by inspection method is too difficult, so the reaction is balanced by using another method called half reaction method.

**Table 2.3** Oxidation numbers of the elements

| Rules | Applies to | Statement |
|---|---|---|
| 1 | Elements | The oxidation number of an atom in an element is zero. |
| 2 | Mono atomic ions | The oxidation number of an atom in a mono atomic ion equals the charge on the ion. |
| 3 | Hydrogen | The oxidation number of hydrogen is +1, in most of the compounds. (But it is -1 in binary compound with metal e.g., $CaH_2$) |
| 4 | Oxygen | The oxidation number is -2 in most of the compounds (but -1 in other peroxides) |
| 5 | Halogen | The oxidation number of fluorine is -1 in all of its compounds. But each of the other halogens ($Cl^-$, $Br^-$, $I^-$) are -1 in binary compounds, except when the other element is another halogen above it in the periodic table or the other element is oxygen. |
| 6 | Compounds and ions | The sum of the oxidation number of the atoms in a compound is zero. The sum of the oxidation numbers of the atoms in a polyatomic ion is equal to the charge on the ion. |

This method consist of two steps

1. Separating the equation into two half reactions one for oxidation and the other for reduction.
2. Then balance each half reaction and then combine them to obtain a balanced oxidation reduction reaction.

Essential information needed for describing the skeleton equation for oxidation reduction reaction is as follows.

What species is being oxidized and reduced?

What product is result from the oxidation and reduction?

Does the reaction occur in either acidic or basic medium?

**Steps in balancing oxidation reduction reaction in acidic condition**

1. Assign oxidation numbers to each atom which one is oxidized and which one is reduced.
2. Split the skeleton equation in to two equations as like as the species containing the element that increases in oxidation number and write those species to give the oxidation half reaction. Similarly, note the species containing the element that decreases in oxidation number and write the reduction half reaction.
3. Complete the separation and balance each half reaction.
   (a) Balance all atoms except O and H.
   (b) Balance hydrogen atoms by adding $H^+$ ions to one side of the equation.
   (c) Balance O atoms by adding $H_2O$ (water) molecules to one side of the equation.
   (d) Balance electric charge by adding electrons ($e^-$) to the more positive side.

4. Combine the two half reactions to get a final balanced equation.
   (a) Multiply each half reaction by a factor such that when the half reactions are added, the electrons are canceled (because electrons cannot present in the final equation).
   (b) Simplify the balanced equation by cancelling species that occur on both sides and reduces the co efficient, to smallest whole numbers. Then checking the equation is indeed balanced.

**Example 1:** Oxidation of ferrous ion by potassium permanganate (permanganate ion) in acidic solution, the skeleton equation of the reaction is written as follows.

$$\underset{(aq)}{\overset{(+2)}{Fe^{2+}}} + \underset{(aq)}{\overset{(+7)}{MnO_4^-}} \longrightarrow \underset{(aq)}{\overset{(+3)}{Fe^{3+}}} + \underset{(aq)}{\overset{(+2)}{Mn^{2+}}} \text{ (acidic solution)}$$

According to step (1), we write the incomplete oxidation half reaction. First of all iron (II) is oxidized to iron (III) it is indicated by

$$\underset{(aq)}{\overset{(+2)}{Fe^{2+}}} \longrightarrow \underset{(aq)}{\overset{(+3)}{Fe^{3+}}}$$

Note that the above equation is balanced in ferrous as it stands (step 3a). According to the step 3b and 3c require that the half reaction be balanced in O and H, but these atoms are not present in the above equation, so ignore that equation. Then according to the step 3d, we need to balance the half reaction in electric charge, this step is done by adding one electron to the more positive side. So the final oxidation half reaction is

$$\underset{(aq)}{Fe^{2+}} \longrightarrow \underset{(aq)}{Fe^{3+}} + e^-$$

Now the above equation is balanced in respect of Fe and electrical charge.

Next step is writing a reduction half reaction. According to the step (2), we write the species containing the atom for which the oxidation number decreases.

$$\underset{(aq)}{\overset{(+7)}{MnO_4^-}} \longrightarrow \underset{(aq)}{\overset{(+2)}{Mn^{2+}}}$$

Now the equation is balanced in Mn as it stands. For step 3c, you add four water molecules to the right side of the equation then it becomes

$$\underset{(aq)}{\overset{(+7)}{MnO_4^-}} \longrightarrow \underset{(aq)}{\overset{(+2)}{Mn^{2+}}} + \underset{(l)}{4\,H_2O}$$

According to step (3), to balance the hydrogen atom by adding $H^+$ ions, add eight $H^+$ ions to the left side of the equation (because the reaction takes place in the presence of acidic solution, if the reaction takes place in the presence of basic solution means, $OH^-$ ions are added).

$$\underset{(aq)}{\overset{(+7)}{MnO_4^-}} + 8\,H^+ \longrightarrow \underset{(aq)}{\overset{(+2)}{Mn^{2+}}} + \underset{(l)}{4\,H_2O}$$

Finally, the above half equation is balanced in respect to that of electric charge. Note that the left side has the charge of +7 (-1, +8), whereas the right side has the charge of +2. So you add five electrons to the left side. So the final reduction half reaction is

$$\underset{(aq)}{MnO_4^-} + 8\,H^+ + 5\,e^- \longrightarrow \underset{(aq)}{Mn^{2+}} + \underset{(l)}{4\,H_2O}$$

The above final half reaction is balanced in the different kind of atoms and in electric charge.

According to step 4a, you need to multiply each half reaction by a factor, in such a way when the two half reactions are added, the electrons are cancel. Then multiply the oxidation half reaction by 5 (the number of electrons in the reduction half reaction) and multiply the reduction half reaction by 1 (the number of electrons in the oxidation half reaction).

Then add the two half reactions.

$$5 \text{ x } (Fe^{2+} \longrightarrow Fe^{3+} + e^-)$$

$$1 \text{ x } [MnO_4^- + 8\,H^+ + 5e^- \longrightarrow Mn_2^+ + 4\,H_2O]$$

$$5\,Fe^{2+} + MnO_4^- + 8\,H^+ + \cancel{5e^-} \longrightarrow 5\,Fe^{3+} + Mn^{2+} + 4\,H_2O + \cancel{5e^-}$$

$$5\,Fe^{2+} + MnO_4^- + 8\,H^+ \longrightarrow 5\,Fe^{3+} + Mn^{2+} + 4\,H_2O$$

**Example 2:** Zinc ion reduces nitrate ion to ammonium ion in the presence of concentrated acidic solution.

The skeleton equation for the above reaction is

$$\underset{(s)}{\overset{0}{Zn}} + \underset{(aq)}{\overset{(+5)}{NO_3^-}} \longrightarrow \underset{(aq)}{\overset{(+2)}{Zn^{2+}}} + \underset{(aq)}{\overset{(-3)}{NH_4^+}}$$

**Step1:** Separate the equation in to two half reactions. Here zinc is oxidized (oxidation number increases) and nitrogen is reduced (oxidation number decreases). The two incomplete half reactions are

$$\underset{(s)}{\overset{0}{Zn}} \longrightarrow \underset{(aq)}{Zn^{2+}} \quad \text{(Oxidation reaction)}$$

$$\underset{(aq)}{NO_3} \longrightarrow \underset{(aq)}{NH_4^+} \quad \text{(Reduction reaction)}$$

**Step2:** Balance the oxidation half reaction, it is balanced in zinc as it stand (step 3a). There is no oxygen and hydrogen atoms, so ignore step 3b and 3c. Follow step 3d, add electrons to the more positive side of the equation to balance the charge.

$$Zn_{(s)} \longrightarrow Zn^{2+}_{(aq)} + 2e^- \quad \text{(Oxidation half reaction)}$$

**Step3:** Balance the reduction half reaction. The reduction half reaction is balanced in N, but not complete in either 'O' or 'H'. So add three water molecules to the right side of equation to balance 'O' atoms and add ten $H^+$ ions to the left side to balance the four H atoms in the $NH_4^+$ ion and the six H atoms in the $H_2O$ we just added (step 3c).

$$10H^+_{(aq)} + NO_3^-{}_{(aq)} \longrightarrow NH_4^+{}_{(aq)} + 3\,H_2O_{(l)}$$

Now, add electrons to the more positive side to balance the charge.

$$10H^+_{(aq)} + NO_3^-{}_{(aq)} + 8e^- \longrightarrow NH_4^+{}_{(aq)} + 3\,H_2O_{(l)}$$

The above reaction is balanced (reduction –half reaction) in charge and different kinds of atoms.

**Step 4:** Then multiply the two half reactions by factors so that when added, cancel the electrons. We multiply the oxidation half reaction by 4 and the reduction half reaction by 1.

$$4 \times (Zn \longrightarrow Zn^{2+} + 2e^-)$$

$$10H^+ + NO_3^- + 8e^- \longrightarrow NH_4^+ + 3\,H_2O$$

$$4\,Zn + 10H^+ + NO_3^- + \cancel{8e^-} \longrightarrow 4\,Zn^{2+} + \cancel{8e^-} + NH_4^+ + 3\,H_2O$$

Finally, the balanced equation is written as follows.

$$4\,Zn_{(s)} + 10H^+_{(aq)} + NO_3^-{}_{(aq)} \longrightarrow 4\,Zn^{2+}_{(aq)} + NH_4^+{}_{(aq)} + 3\,H_2O_{(l)}$$

To balance the oxidation reduction equation in basic solution we begin by balancing the equation as if it were a reaction in acidic solution then add the following steps.

(a) Instead of adding $H^+$ ions in the equation add the number of $OH^-$ ions to both sides of the equation.

(b) Simplify the equation by noting that $H^+$ reacts with $OH^-$ gives $H_2O$. Cancel only water molecules that occur on both sides of the equation and write the equation into simplest form.

**Example:** Oxidation of sulfite ion by permanganate ion in basic solution:

The skeleton equation of the reaction is

$$MnO_4^- + SO_3^{2-} \longrightarrow MnO_2 + SO_4^{2-}$$

First complete and balance the equation as if were in acidic solution similar to that of the previous examples. Then follow the rule step 1 mentioned in the above paragraph, add many $OH^-$ ions to the both sides of the equilibrium as there are $H^+$ ions. After noting that $H^+$ ions react with $OH^-$ ions to give water, to get the simplified form of the equation. After balance the equation similar to that of acidic solution, we get the following equation.

Then add $OH^-$, to both sides of the equation

$$2\,MnO_4^- + 3\,SO_3^{2-} + 2\,H^+ \longrightarrow 2\,MnO_2 + 3\,SO_4^{2-} + H_2O$$

Add 2 $OH^-$ groups to both sides of the equation.

$$2\,MnO_4^- + 3\,SO_3^{2-} + \underbrace{2\,H^+ + 2\,OH^-}_{2H_2O} \longrightarrow 2\,MnO_2 + 3\,SO_4^{2-} + 2\,OH^- + H_2O$$

Then replace $2H^+ + 2OH^-$ by $2H_2O$ molecules on the left side of the equation, then cancel one of these water molecules with right side.

The final balanced equation is

$$2\,MnO_4^- + 3\,SO_3^{2-} + H_2O \longrightarrow 2\,MnO_2 + 3\,SO_4^{2-} + 2\,OH^-$$

## 2.8 PERIODIC TABLE

A tabular arrangement of elements in rows and columns highlighting the regular repetition of the elements is called as periodic table.

All compounds are present in nature; no two elements possess identical chemical and physical properties. But some small groups of elements are having very close similarity in chemical properties, but not in physical properties. According to these properties the elements are arranged in the periodic table as groups and periods. The periodic table was first independently suggested by the Russian chemist Dmitri Mendeleev (1834) and the German chemist Lothar Meyer (1830-1895). They independently gave similar discoveries. They found that, when they arranged the elements according to their atomic weight by placing them in horizontal rows, one row under the other, so that the elements in each vertical column possesses similar properties. This periodic table is called as short table. Next the development of long table was introduced by Thomson Bohr.

But the Modern periodic Law states that "The elements are arranged in the periodic table according to their atomic numbers", because the properties of the elements are based primarily upon the valence shell electrons.

The table according to the above modern periodic law referred as a long form periodic table. The horizontal row of the table is mentioned as periods and the vertical columns are mentioned as groups. Table 2.4 commonly referred as a long form of the periodic table since A and B sub groups are spreads across the chart.

## Table 2.4 The periodic table of the elements

Atomic Symbol — Symbols — Atomic Number (number of protons)

Name: ___ium

Widgets: How it is (or was) used or where it occurs in nature

- Solid / Liquid / Gas (at room temperature)
- The color of the symbol is the color of the element in its most common pure form. Examples: metallic solid; red liquid; colorless gas
- Human Body: top ten elements by weight
- Earth's Crust: top eight elements by weight
- Magnetic: ferromagnetic at room temperature
- Noble Metals: corrosion-resistant
- Radioactive: all isotopes are radioactive
- Only Traces Found in Nature: less than a millionth percent of earth's crust
- Never Found in Nature: only made by people

Transition Metals

| Periods | Alkali Metals Group IA | Alkali Earth Metals IIA | IIIB | IVB | VB | VIB | VIIB | VIII | VIII | VIII | IB | IIB | Boron Group IIIA | Carbon Group IVA | Nitrogen Group VA | Oxygen Group VIA | Halogens Group VIIA | Noble Gases 0-Group |
|---|---|---|---|---|---|---|---|---|---|---|---|---|---|---|---|---|---|---|
| 1 | H 1 Hydrogen<br>Sun and Stars | | | | | | | | | | | | | | | | | He 2 Helium<br>Balloons |
| 2 | Li 3 Lithium<br>Batteries | Be 4 Beryllium<br>Emeralds | | | | | | | | | | | B 5 Boron<br>Sports Equipment | C 6 Carbon<br>Basis of Life's Molecules | N 7 Nitrogen<br>Protein | O 8 Oxygen<br>Air | F 9 Fluorine<br>Toothpaste | Ne 10 Neon<br>Advertising Signs |
| 3 | Na 11 Sodium<br>Salt | Mg 12 Magnesium<br>Chlorophyll | | | | | | | | | | | Al 13 Aluminum<br>Airplanes | Si 14 Silicon<br>Stone, Sand, and Soil | P 15 Phosphorus<br>Bones | S 16 Sulfur<br>Egg Yolks | Cl 17 Chlorine<br>Swimming Pools | Ar 18 Argon<br>Light Bulbs |
| 4 | K 19 Potassium<br>Fruits and Vegetables | Ca 20 Calcium<br>Shells and Bones | Sc 21 Scandium<br>Bicycles | Ti 22 Titanium<br>Aerospace | V 23 Vanadium<br>Springs | Cr 24 Chromium<br>Stainless Steel | Mn 25 Manganese<br>Earthmovers | Fe 26 Iron<br>Steel Structures | Co 27 Cobalt<br>Magnets | Ni 28 Nickel<br>Coins | Cu 29 Copper<br>Electric Wires | Zn 30 Zinc<br>Brass Instruments | Ga 31 Gallium<br>Light-Emitting Diodes (LEDs) | Ge 32 Germanium<br>Semiconductor Electronics | As 33 Arsenic<br>Poison | Se 34 Selenium<br>Copiers | Br 35 Bromine<br>Photography Film | Kr 36 Krypton<br>Flashlights |
| 5 | Rb 37 Rubidium<br>Global Navigation | Sr 38 Strontium<br>Fireworks | Y 39 Yttrium<br>Lasers | Zr 40 Zirconium<br>Chemical Pipelines | Nb 41 Niobium<br>Mag Lev Trains | Mo 42 Molybdenum<br>Cutting Tools | Tc 43 Technetium<br>Radioactive Diagnosis | Ru 44 Ruthenium<br>Electric Switches | Rh 45 Rhodium<br>Searchlight Reflectors | Pd 46 Palladium<br>Pollution Control | Ag 47 Silver<br>Jewelry | Cd 48 Cadmium<br>Paint | In 49 Indium<br>Liquid Crystal Displays (LCDs) | Sn 50 Tin<br>Plated Food Cans | Sb 51 Antimony<br>Car Batteries | Te 52 Tellurium<br>Thermoelectric Coolers | I 53 Iodine<br>Disinfectant | Xe 54 Xenon<br>High-Intensity Lamps |
| 6 | Cs 55 Cesium<br>Atomic Clocks | Ba 56 Barium<br>X-Ray Diagnosis | 57 - 71<br>Rare Earth Metals | Hf 72 Hafnium<br>Nuclear Submarines | Ta 73 Tantalum<br>Mobile Phones | W 74 Tungsten<br>Lamp Filaments | Re 75 Rhenium<br>Rocket Engines | Os 76 Osmium<br>Pen Points | Ir 77 Iridium<br>Spark Plugs | Pt 78 Platinum<br>Labware | Au 79 Gold<br>Jewelry | Hg 80 Mercury<br>Thermometers | Tl 81 Thallium<br>Low-Temperature Thermometers | Pb 82 Lead<br>Weights | Bi 83 Bismuth<br>Fire Sprinklers | Po 84 Polonium<br>Anti-Static Brushes | At 85 Astatine<br>Radioactive Medicine | Rn 86 Radon<br>Surgical Implants |
| 7 | Fr 87 Francium<br>Laser Atom Traps | Ra 88 Radium<br>Luminous Watches | 89 - 103<br>Actinide Metals | Rf 104 Rutherfordium | Db 105 Dubnium | Sg 106 Seaborgium | Bh 107 Bohrium | Hs 108 Hassium | Mt 109 Meitnerium | Ds 110 Darmstadtium | Rg 111 Roentgenium | Cn 112 Copernicium | 113 | 114 | 115 | 116 | 117 | 118 |

Superheavy Elements: radioactive, never found in nature, no uses except atomic research

| | 6 Rare Earth Metals | | 7 Actinide Metals |
|---|---|---|---|
| La 57 Lanthanum | Telescope Lenses | Ac 89 Actinium | Radioactive Medicine |
| Ce 58 Cerium | Lighter Flints | Th 90 Thorium | Gas Lamp Mantles |
| Pr 59 Praseodymium | Torchworkers' Eyeglasses | Pa 91 Protactinium | Radioactive Waste |
| Nd 60 Neodymium | Electric Motor Magnets | U 92 Uranium | Nuclear Power |
| Pm 61 Promethium | Luminous Dials | Np 93 Neptunium | Radioactive Waste |
| Sm 62 Samarium | Electric Motor Magnets | Pu 94 Plutonium | Nuclear Weapons |
| Eu 63 Europium | Color Televisions | Am 95 Americium | Smoke Detectors |
| Gd 64 Gadolinium | MRI Diagnosis | Cm 96 Curium | Mineral Analyzers |
| Tb 65 Terbium | Fluorescent Lamps | Bk 97 Berkelium | Radioactive Waste |
| Dy 66 Dysprosium | Smart Material Actuators | Cf 98 Californium | Mineral Analyzers |
| Ho 67 Holmium | Laser Surgery | Es 99 Einsteinium | |
| Er 68 Erbium | Optical Fiber Communications | Fm 100 Fermium | |
| Tm 69 Thulium | Laser Surgery | Md 101 Mendelevium | |
| Yb 70 Ytterbium | Scientific Fiber Lasers | No 102 Nobelium | |
| Lu 71 Lutetium | Photodynamic Medicine | Lr 103 Lawrencium | |

radioactive, never found in nature, no uses except atomic research

Both the short and long table contains seven periods arranged horizontally and eight groups arranged vertically.

Out of the seven periods, all the periods started at alkali metal (except first period) and ending with an inert gas.

The first period contains 2 elements (hydrogen and helium), the second and third periods (short periods) contain 8 elements of different properties and valencies arranged in the same order, so that each element in the period resembles that vertically above it in the second. The fourth and fifth periods contain 18, the sixth period contains 32 elements which are placed as row of elements, but in order for the row to fit on a page, part of it appears as the bottom of the table and the seventh period contains 16 elements though not completed also appears as the bottom of the Table 2.5.

**Table 2.5** Period number and number of elements present

| Period number | Number of elements present |
|---|---|
| I | 2 |
| II & III | 8 |
| IV & V | 18 |
| VI | 32 |
| VII | 16 (Current) |

The first period contains two identical elements hydrogen and helium. In the 2[nd] and 3[rd] periods, the s and p orbitals are filled in normal fashion. These groups are called as "typical elements". The 2[nd] period starts with lithium (Li) and ending with Neon (Ne). These are designated as A groups.

In the 4[th] and successive periods, d orbital is filled between s and p orbital. The filling of these "low–lying" orbital with one or two electrons in the "overlying" s-orbital causes the properties of these elements to differ somewhat from their A-group counter parts. These are designated as B groups. The periods 4, 5 and 6 are the centre part of the periodic table.

The fourth period starts with two closely similar elements, present in the groups I and II, but differs from the short period from the next ten elements, which are all metal and are called transitional elements.

The fifth period is similar to the fourth one, each element resembling the analogue element in that period.

The sixth period is the very long period with 32 elements but is same like that of fourth and fifth, except that the fourteen elements which are started from lanthanum having close resemblance with other elements and all are assigned to one position and present below the periodic table. These are called as rare earth metals or lanthanones. These are formed by the filling of very low lying f-orbitals.

The seventh period, all the elements are radioactive, incomplete, repetition of sixth period, analogues of sixth period, so it is called as actinones.

Each of the long periods is divided into even and odd series.

The even series begins with an alkali metal and ends with a group of three transitional elements (Group VIII). These belong to subgroup "A".

The odd series starts with metals (copper, silver etc.) and ends with inert gases, contains eight elements which belong to subgroup "B".

The groups in the periodic table are started numbering from I to VII, ending with the inert gas group '0' as suggested by IUPAC. Some of periodic table models some "A and B" letters are mentioned along with Roman numerals.

The "A" indicates main group elements and "B" indicates transition elements. The two rows of elements at the bottom of the table are called as inner-transition elements.

The elements present in the same group have a common valency equal to the group number and elements in the same subgroup shows close resemblance to each other in physical and chemical properties though differing in these respects from the elements in the other subgroup despite the common valency. (Subgroup of the group-I where a = alkali metal with high reactivity and b = unreactive coinage metals).

Some of the elements in the periodic table are possesses characteristics between metals and non-metals and these are called as metalloids. For example, silicon, germanium. These are usually good semiconductors.

### 2.8.1 General Properties of the Elements in the Periodic Table

1. **Electropositivity:** (Tendency to form cations)

   In the periodic table, the electropositivity of the elements increases from the top to bottom of the table and decreases from left to right.

   Example: Cesium – Most or high electropositivity
   Fluorine – Least one.

2. **Diagonal relationship:** The electropositivity of an element may be same as that of the element in the following period and group as a result of the two effects of compensating one another. This property is called as "Diagonal Relationship".

   Example: Lithium and Magnesium
   Beryllium and Aluminium
   Boron and Silicon

3. **Metallic properties:** Metallic properties of elements generally decrease in given periods as the atomic number increases.

4. **Electro negativity:** It is defined as the relative tendency of the atom in a molecule to attract the shared pair of electrons towards itself. In a period, electronegativity increases on moving from left to right due to that the nuclear charges increases whereas atomic radius decreases. In a group, electronegativity decreases on moving down the group due to the effect of increased atomic radius.

5. **Electron affinity:** Electron affinity or electron gain enthalpy is defined as the amount of energy released when an isolated gaseous atom accepts an electron to form a monovalent gaseous anion. In periodic table, this property is generally increase from left to right in a period and decreases on moving down the group.
6. **Ionization potential:** The energy required to remove the loosely bound electrons from isolated atom in a gaseous state is called as ionization energy. In period, the value of ionization energy increases from left to right with breaks where the atoms have stable configurations. In a group, the ionization potential decreases from top to bottom.

## 2.9 GENERAL TERMS USED IN THE INORGANIC CHEMISTRY

***Accuracy:*** How closely a measured value agrees with the correct value.

***Acid (Arrhenius):*** A substance that yields hydrogen or hydronium ion in an aqueous solution.

***Acid (Bronsted-lowry):*** A substance that donates a proton.

***Acid (Lewis):*** A substance that accepts a pair of electrons.

***Acidimeter:*** An instrument used in acidimetry.

***Acidimetry:*** Determination of the amount of free acid in solution.

***Activation energy:*** Amount of energy that must be absorbed by reactants in their ground state to reach the transition state.

***Active metal:*** Metal with low ionization energy that loses electrons readily to form cations.

***Adhesive forces:*** Force of attraction between a liquid and another surface.

***Adjuvant:*** A substance that used to increase the bulk of the formulations.

***Adsorption:*** Adhesion of a substance on to surfaces of particles.

***Alkalimetry:*** Determination of alkali in any substance.

***Allotropism:*** The existence of an element in two or more distinct forms.

***Alum:*** Hydrated Sulphate [$KAl(SO_4).12H_2O$].

***Amorphous solid:*** A non crystalline solid with no well defined ordered structure.

***Amphoterism:*** Ability to react with acids and bases. Ability of substance to act as either an acid or a base.

***Anion:*** A negatively charged atom or group of atoms.

***Aqueous solution:*** A solution in which water is a solvent.

***Assay:*** It is a chemical analysis to determine the amount of the active ingredient or the amount of the impurity present in formulations.

***Atomic Mass Unit (AMU):*** One twelfth mass of an atom of carbon-12 isotope. A unit used for stating atomic and formula weights also called Dalton.

***Base (Arrhenius):*** A substance that yields hydroxide ions in aqueous solution.

***Base (Bronsted-lowry):*** A substance that accepts a proton.

***Base (Lewis):*** A substance that donates a pair of electrons.

***Beta particle:*** Electron emitted from the nucleus when a neutron decays to a proton and an electron.

***Boiling point:*** The temperature at which the vapour pressure of a liquid is equal to applied pressure. Liquid boils at this temperature.

***Buffers:*** A substance in a solution capable of neutralizing within the limits of both acids and bases and maintaining the original or constant pH of the solution.

***Catalyst:*** A substance that changes the rate of chemical reaction, but no net change itself during the reaction.

***Cation:*** A positively charged atom or group of atoms.

***Celsius temperature:*** It is a measure of temperature. Freezing point of water is 0 °C and its boiling point is 100 °C at atmosphere of pressure.

***Chelate:*** A stable complex of a metal with one or more polydentate ligands.

***Chemical equilibrium:*** A states of dynamic balance in which rate of forward and reverse reactions are equal.

***Chemical properties:*** A characteristic that can be observed when a substance is interacting with other substances resulting in a change in chemical composition.

***Clay:*** A class of silicate and aluminosilicate minerals with sheet like structures that have enormous surface areas that can absorb large amount of water.

***Cohesive forces:*** All the forces of attraction among particles of a liquid.

***Colloid:*** A solution in which solute particles is between 1 and 100 nanometers. Particles of solute pass through filter but not membranes.

***Compound:*** A substance consisting of two or more atoms, combined chemically in definite proportions by mass.

***Concentrated solution:*** A solution containing a relatively large amount of solute.

***Concentration:*** Ratio of mass or volume of solute to mass or volume of solution or solvent.

***Condensation:*** A change of state of matter from a gas to a liquid.

***Coordination number:*** Number of donor atoms coordinated to a metal.

***Crystalline solid:*** A solid characterized by a regular, ordered arrangement of particles.

***Crystallization:*** The process by which a substance is given definite form.

***Dehydration:*** Removal of water molecule.

***Deliquescent:*** Substances that absorbs moisture from the atmosphere and becomes liquid.

***Demasking agent:*** It is substance which releases the masked metal ions.

***Density:*** The ratio of mass of substance to its volume.

***Diffusion:*** The movement of molecules or other particles in a solution from an area of greater concentration to an area of lesser concentration until equal concentration is reached.

***Dilute solution:*** A solution containing a relatively small amount of solute.

***Dimer:*** Molecule formed by combination of two smaller (identical) molecules.

***Dipole:*** Separation of charge between two covalently bonded atoms.

***Dissociation constant:*** Equilibrium constant that applies to dissociation of complex ions into simple ions and coordinating species (ligands).

***Dissociation:*** In aqueous solution, the process in which a solid ionic compound separates into ions.

***Distillate:*** The material in a distillation apparatus that is collected in the receiver.

***Distillation:*** Separation of liquid mixture into its components on the basis of differences in boiling points.

***Dye:*** Natural or synthetic substance that is used to impart colour to another material.

***Effervescence:*** Bubbling of a solution due to liberation of a gas. Gas may be formed in a chemical reaction as in a carbonated or fermenting liquid.

***Efflorescence:*** Loss of water of crystallization from a hydrated substance to the atmosphere on exposure to air.

***Electronegativity:*** A measure of relative tendency of an atom to attract electrons to itself when chemically combined with another atom.

***Electrodes:*** Surfaces upon which oxidation and reduction half reactions occurs in electrochemical cells.

***Electrolysis:*** Process occurs in electrolytic cells.

***Electrolyte:*** A substance whose aqueous solution conduct electricity.

***Electrophile:*** Positively charged or electron deficient species.

***Element:*** A simple substance which cannot be decomposed by ordinary chemical reaction.

***End point:*** The point at which an indicator changes color and titrations completed.

***Endothermic reaction:*** A chemical reaction that absorbs or requires heat from its surroundings.

***Equivalence point:*** The point at which chemically equivalent amounts of reactants have reacted.

***Exothermic reaction:*** A chemical reaction that releases or gives off heat.

***Fluffy:*** Light and soft solid.

***Fluorescence:*** Absorption of high energy radiation by a substance and subsequent emission of visible light.

***Fractional distillation:*** The process in which a fractioning column is used in distillation apparatus to separate components of a liquid mixture with different boiling point.

***Freezing:*** A change of state of matter from a liquid to a solid.

***Galvanization:*** Placing a thin layer of zinc on ferrous material to protect the underlying surface from corrosion.

***Geiger counter:*** A gas filled tube which discharges electrically when ionizing radiation passes through it.

***Granules:*** A small compact particles of a substance between 2 and 4 millimeters in diameter.

***Half life:*** The time required for half of given sample to undergo radioactive decay or the time required for half of a reactant to be converted into product.

***Half reactions:*** Either the oxidation part or reduction part of a redox reaction.

***Halogens:*** Group VIIA elements. Example: F, Cl, Br, I.

***Hardness of water:*** Condition of water which results from dissolved minerals and metallic ions such as calcium and magnesium.

***Heavy water:*** Water containing deuterium, a heavy isotope of hydrogen.

***Hybridization:*** Mixing a set of atomic orbitals to form a new set of atomic orbitals with same total electron capacity and with properties and energies intermediate between those of original unhybridized orbitals.

***Hydrolysis:*** A chemical reaction in which molecules breakdown by water.

***Hygroscopic:*** It is a property of substance to absorb or adsorb water from the air.

***Hypertonic solution:*** A solution having a greater concentration of dissolved solute than solution to which it is compared.

***Hypotonic solution:*** A solution having a lesser concentration of dissolved solute than solution to which it is compared.

***Incineration:*** It is the process to burn up the compounds completely and converts to ashes.

***Insoluble compound:*** A compound not soluble in solvent.

***Intermolecular forces:*** Forces between individual particles.

***Ion:*** An atomic or molecular species with a positive or negative electrical charge.

***Ionic product of water:*** Equilibrium constant for ionization of water.

***Ionization:*** In an aqueous solution, the process in which molecular compound reacts with water and forms ions.

***Isotonic solution:*** A solution having an equal concentration of dissolved solute as the solution to which it is compared. Example, 0.9% w/v sodium chloride solution.

***Ligand:*** A molecule or ion that binds to a metal and not shared a complex.

***Liquification:*** Conversion of a solid or gas into liquid form.

***Loan pair:*** Pair of electrons residing on one atom and not shared by other atoms.

***Loss on drying:*** It is a test determines the amount of water and volatile matter in a sample, when sample is dried under specified conditions.

***Loss on ignition:*** It is a test determines the amount of moisture or impurities lost when sample is ignited under specified conditions.

***Luster:*** Radiance or brilliance of light; reflecting light.

***Masking agent/complexing agent/auxillary chelating agent:*** It is a substance that will form complex more strongly with the metal than titrant under the conditions of titration.

***Melting point:*** The temperature at which the solid melts and converted to liquid.

***Metal:*** An element marked by luster, malleability, ductility and conductivity of electricity and heat.

***Molecule:*** An aggregation of two or more atoms.

***Neutralization:*** Reaction of an acid with base to form a salt and water.

***Neutron:*** A neutral subatomic particle having a mass of 1.0087 amu.

***Noble gases (Rare gases):*** Elements of periodic group 0. They are inert in nature.

***Opalescence:*** Exhibiting a milky brightness.

***Opaque:*** Impenetrable by light; not transparent.

***Oxidation number:*** A number used to represent number of electrons lost, gained or shared in a chemical change.

***Oxidation:*** A combination of a substance with oxygen; an increase in oxidation number; loss of electrons.

***Periodic table:*** The tabular arrangement of elements in the order of increasing atomic number so that the columns of elements represent periodic recurrence of elements with similar properties.

***pH:*** Measure of hydrogen ion concentration of a solution, indicating the nature of the solution that is acidic or basic or neutral.

***Physical change:*** A change in the form or state of matter without any change in chemical composition.

***Physical properties:*** Properties of a substance that are observed without a change in chemical composition, which include color, odor, taste, solubility, density, hardness, melting point and boiling point.

***Polymer:*** A large molecule made by linking together a number of monomers or basic chemical units.

***Polymerization:*** The linking together of monomers or basic chemical units to form polymer.

***Potential energy:*** Energy that is stored.

***Precipitate:*** A deposit of an insoluble or very slightly soluble substance in solution.

***Primary standard:*** A substance of a known high degree of purity that undergoes one invariable reaction with other reactant of interest.

***Proton:*** A subatomic particle normally found in nucleus of an atom. It has a relative mass of 1 and electrical charge of +1.

***Radiation:*** High energy particles or rays emitted during the nuclear decay process.

***Radioactivity:*** The spontaneous disintegration of atomic nuclei.

***Rate determining step:*** The slowest step in mechanism, the step that determines the overall rate of reaction.

***Rate of reaction:*** Change in concentration of a reactant or product per unit time.

***Reactants:*** Substance consumed in chemical reaction.

***Recrystallization:*** It is a technique used to purify the chemical compounds. In this method dissolving both impurities and a compound in an appropriate solvent, compound become precipitated as a crystal.

***Reducing agent:*** The substance that reduces another substance and the reducing agent itself get oxidized.

***Reduction:*** A decrease in oxidation number; A gain of electrons; The combination of a substance with hydrogen.

***Residue:*** A small amount of substance remains after process has been completed.

***Reverse osmosis:*** Forcing solvent molecule to flow through a semipermeable membrane from a concentrated solution into a dilute solution by application of greater hydrostatic pressure on concentration side than the osmotic pressure.

***Reversible reaction:*** Reaction that does not go to completion and occurs in both forward and reverse direction.

***Salt:*** Any group of substances that result from the reaction between acids and bases other than water which undergoes ionization in solution and produce anion and cation.

***Saturated solution:*** Solution in which no more solute can be dissolved.

***Solid:*** Condensed state of matter having a definite shape and volume.

***Solidification:*** Conversion of a liquid or a gas into a solid form.

***Solubility:*** The measure of how well a substance goes into solution in the given solvent.

***Solute:*** A substance dissolved in a solvent to form a solution; component of a solution present in lesser amount.

***Solution:*** A homogenous mixture of one or two substances (solutes) dissolved in a sufficient quantity of solvent.

***Solvation:*** The process of dissolving a solute in an appropriate solvent.

***Solvent:*** A substance that the dissolves solutes in a solution or a component of a solution present in a greater amount.

***Specific gravity:*** The ratio of density of substance to the density of water.

Standard electrodes: ***Half cell in which the oxidized and reduced forms of a species are present at unit activity.***

***Stoichiometry:*** Description of quantitative relationships among elements and compounds as they undergo chemical changes.

***Sublimation:*** A physical change of state during which a substance changes directly from a solid to a gas.

***Substrate:*** The material upon which an enzyme works.

***Super saturated solution:*** A solution that contain higher than saturation concentration of solute.

***Surface tension:*** The force that acts on the surface of a liquid and tends to minimize surface area.

***Temperature:*** A measure of intensity of heat.

***Theoretical yield:*** Maximum amount of specified product that could be obtained from specified amount of reactants, assuming complete consumption of reactants according to only reaction and complete recovery of product.

***Titrant:*** A substance such as a solution of known concentration used in titration; solution in a titration that is added from a burette to a measured quantity of another solution present in conical flask.

***Titrate:*** Substance whose concentration is to be determined by titration.

***Titration:*** A process in which one solution added to another solution until chemical reaction between the two is complete.

***Trace elements:*** Any of various chemical elements such as iron, manganese, zinc, copper and iodine that occur in very small amounts in organism and are essential for many physiological and biochemical processes.

***Unctuous:*** Having the characteristic of oil or ointment; slippery.

***Unsaturated solution:*** A solution containing less of the solute than can be held in solution by solvent.

***Valance electrons:*** Outermost electron of atoms, which forms bonding with other atoms.

***Vaporization:*** The physical change from a liquid to a gas.

***Vapour:*** A gas, especially the gaseous form of a substance that at ordinary temperature in a liquid or solid.

***Volatile:*** Conversion of liquid to gaseous state.

## PROBABLE QUESTIONS

1. What are atomic symbols, explain with examples.
2. Define stoichiometric equations and briefly explain with one example.
3. What is mean by balanced equation?
4. Explain about the inspection method of balancing equation with one example.
5. Write the steps for balancing redox reactions.
6. Define oxidation with one example.
7. Define reduction with one example.
8. Write briefly about oxidizing agents and reducing agents.
9. What is meant by oxidation number and write rules for calculating it.
10. Explain about balancing redox equation by inspection method in acidic medium with one example.
11. Explain about balancing redox equation by inspection method in basic medium with one example.
12. Balance the following neutralization equations:

$$NaOH + HNO_3 \longrightarrow$$

$$HCl + Ba(OH)_2 \longrightarrow$$

13. In the following reactions, label the oxidizing agent and reducing agent.

$$P_4 + 5O_2 \longrightarrow P_4O_{10}$$

$$Hg + NO_2 + H_2O \longrightarrow Hg + 2H^+ + NO_3^-$$

$$ZnO + C \longrightarrow Zn + CO$$

14. Balance the following oxidation reduction reactions, occur in acidic medium.

$$H_3PO_2 + KMnO_4 + H_2SO_4 \longrightarrow K_2SO_4 + MnSO_4 + H_3PO_4 + H_2O$$

$$H_3PO_2 + H_2SO_4 \longrightarrow SO_2 + S_2 + H_3PO4 + H_3PO_3 + H_2O$$

$$KMnO_4 + H_2SO_4 + H_2O_2 \longrightarrow K_2SO_4 + MnSO_4 + H_2O + O_2\uparrow$$

15. Balance the following oxidation reduction reactions, occur in acidic medium.

$$Mn + H_2SO_3 \longrightarrow Mn^{2+} + SO_4^{2-}$$

$$Mn^{2+} + BiO_3 \longrightarrow MnO_4 + Bi^{3+}$$

16. Define empirical formula and write the steps for calculating it with example.
17. What is mean by molecular formula and write the steps for calculating it with example.

CHAPTER 3

# ACIDS, BASES AND BUFFERS

## 3.1 INTRODUCTION

Majority of the chemical substances can be classified under acids, bases and neutral substances. But the concept of acids and bases are various, apart from historical aspects that one interpretation may be better than the other one, depends upon the type of reaction.

According to the old concept, acid is defined as any substance which has sour taste and base is defined as any substance which has bitter taste and is present in plants. Both acids and bases change the colour of litmus paper (blue litmus to red and red litmus to blue respectively).

## 3.2 VARIOUS CONCEPTS OF ACIDS AND BASES

Various concepts of acids and bases are described as follows

1. Arrhenius concept
2. Bronsted Lowry's concept
3. Lewis concept

1. **Arrhenius concept:** According to Arrhenius concept "Acid means, any substance which is capable of producing or providing hydrogen ions ($H^+$ ions) in aqueous solution".

$$HCl \xrightleftharpoons{H_2O} H^+ + Cl^-$$

According to Arrhenius concept strong acid is a substance that is completely dissociates in aqueous solution to give $H_3O^+$ and an anion.

For example: $H_2SO_4 + H_2O \longrightarrow H_3O^+ + HSO_4^-$

Other examples of acid are $HClO_4$, HI, HBr, HCl and $HNO_3$.

Base is defined as "any substance containing hydroxyl group and / or capable of producing or providing hydroxide ion ($OH^-$) in aqueous solution".

$$NaOH \xrightleftharpoons{H_2O} Na^+ + OH^-$$

According to this concept, a neutralization reaction takes place by combination of the acid and base to yield salt and water.

The neutralization can be illustrated by the following general equation between an acid (HA) and a base (BOH).

$$\underset{\text{Acid}}{HA} + \underset{\text{Base}}{BOH} \rightleftharpoons \underset{\text{Salt}}{B^+A^-} + H_2O$$

***Limitations of Arrhenius concept***

(a) Non hydroxide containing compounds which function as a basic ion in aqueous solutions are not included in this definition. Example, many organic substances like aniline does not contain hydroxide ion but acts as a base.

(b) This concept is not able to explain about acidic/basic properties of substances in non aqueous systems. Example: $NH_4NO_3$ in $NH_3$ acts as an acid but never gives $H^+$ ion.

(c) The neutralization property of an acid and base in the absence of solvent was not explained.

2. **Bronsted Lowry's Concept (Protonoic concept of acid-base character):** This theory was developed by J.N. Bronsted and J.M. Lowry in 1923. They discovered that the acid base reactions are taken place by proton-transfer reactions. So that the acids and bases are defined in terms of the proton ($H^+$) transfer. According to this theory an acid is a "substance, capable of donating a proton in a chemical reaction". This definition is same as that Arrhenius concept. But a base is defined as "any substance capable of accepting a proton in a chemical reaction". This definition is neither excluded hydroxide ion as a base nor a base to $OH^-$ producing substances.

According to the above definition, the acid and bases are summarized as follows

An acid is a proton donor and a base is a proton acceptor.

For example, the reaction between hydrochloric acid and ammonia.

$$HCl + NH_3 \longrightarrow NH_4Cl$$

The ionic equation of the reaction is mentioned as follows

$$H_3O^+ + \not{C}l^- + NH_3 \longrightarrow H_2O + NH_4^+ + \not{C}l^-$$

Then the net ionic equation is

$$H_3O^+ + NH_3 \longrightarrow H_2O + NH_4^+$$

Here, in aqueous solution, the proton ($H^+$) transfer from $H_3O^+$ to $NH_3$ gives water and ammonium ion. Here $H_3O^+$ acts as a proton donor or acid, $NH_3$ is the proton acceptor or base.

Some other examples for acids are as follows

$$HCl \rightleftharpoons H^+ + Cl^-$$

$$H_2CO_3 \rightleftharpoons H^+ + HCO_3^-$$

$$NH_4^+ \rightleftharpoons H^+ + NH_3$$

$$CH_3COOH \rightleftharpoons H^+ + CH_3COO^-$$

Some examples for bases are as follows

$$H_2O + H^+ \rightleftharpoons \underset{\text{Hydronium ion}}{H_3O^+}$$

$$OH^- + H^+ \rightleftharpoons H_2O$$

$$HCO_3^- + H^+ \rightleftharpoons H_2CO_3$$

From the Bronsted Lowry's concept, the bronsted acid liberates the acid and its conjugate base. This is explained by as follows.

$$HA \rightleftharpoons H^+ + \underset{\text{Conjugate Base}}{A^-}$$

$$HCl \rightleftharpoons H^+ + Cl^-$$

$$HCl + H_2O \rightleftharpoons \underset{\text{Hydronium ion}}{H_3O^+} + Cl^-$$

In the above forward reaction, hydrochloric acid donates one hydrogen ion or one proton to the water molecule, forms hydronium ion. So it acts as an acid or the water molecule accepts one hydrogen atom from the hydrochloric acid and acts as a base.

In the above equation consider the backward or reverse reaction, the $H_3O^+$ ions gives one proton to the $Cl^-$ ion , so it acts as an acid or $Cl^-$ accept one proton from the $H_3O^+$ ion, and acts as a base. In equilibrium, the rate of both forward and backward reaction is same. The acid base pairs, the members of which can be formed from each other mutually by the gain or loss of the proton are called conjugate acid base pair.

In the above reaction, hydrochloric acid is called an acid; $Cl^-$ is called as a conjugate base of hydrochloric acid

In the above reverse reaction, $H_3O^+$ $acid_2$ and $H_2O$ is a $base_2$.

$$Acid_1 + Base_2 \longrightarrow Acid_2 + Base_1$$

Some other examples of conjugate acid base pairs.

$$H_2SO_4 \rightleftharpoons H^+ + HSO_4^-$$

$$H_2CO_3 \rightleftharpoons H^+ + HCO_3^-$$

$$H_3PO_4 \rightleftharpoons H^+ + H_2PO_4^-$$

Some other examples of conjugate base acid pairs are as follows.

$$OH^- + H^+ \rightleftharpoons H_2O$$

$$NH_3 + H^+ \rightleftharpoons NH_4^+$$

$$H_2O + H^+ \rightleftharpoons H_3O^+$$

$$HCO_3^- + H^+ \rightleftharpoons H_2CO_3$$

In some cases example: $HSO_4^-$ and $H_2PO_4^-$ may react as acid or base, the acidity or basicity of this species is determined by the conditions of the chemical reactions.

***Amphoteric nature of water:*** Here water is very interesting solvent which acts as both acid and base. In the presence of an acid, it behaves as a proton acceptor (base), but in the presence of strong base it behaves as a proton donor (acid).

$$\underset{\text{acid}}{H_2O} + \underset{\text{base}}{NH_3} \rightleftharpoons \underset{\text{base}}{OH^-} + \underset{\text{acid}}{NH_4^+}$$

$$\underset{\text{base}}{H_2O} + \underset{\text{acid}}{HCl} \rightleftharpoons \underset{\text{acid}}{H_3O^+} + \underset{\text{base}}{Cl^-}$$

In the above first equation, water donates one proton to the ammonia ($NH_3$) and forms hydroxide ion, so it acts as an acid.

But in the above second equation, it accepts one proton from HCl, it acts as a base. **When any substance or species which can donate as well as accept a proton, it is called as amphoteric or amphiprotic.**

From all the above points, it can be explained about the relative strength of acid, bases and their conjugate species.

According to the definition, a strong acid is one which readily donates its proton to a base. Therefore, the conjugate base of such an acid must be weak. So generally, "Strong acids have weak conjugate base and strong bases have weak conjugate acids".

***Limitations***

(a) The Bronsted Lowry's concept mainly based on the proton transfer phenomenon, there are many common acids which are protonic in nature, but they do not act as an acid.

(b) It does not explain about the acid base reactions in non protonic solvent such as $SO_2$, $N_2O_4$ etc.

(c) Many of the acid base reactions do not takes place by proton transfer, the theory failed to explain this type of reaction.

3. **Lewis acid base concept (electron donor-acceptor concept or electronic concept of acid base character):** This concept was introduced by Lewis at about the same time of Bronsted Lowry's concept. This theory is very important to the general understanding of all acid base chemical reactions.

According to this theory "an acid is defined as any substance which is an electron deficient or electrophilic species or accepts an electron pair to form a coordinate bond and a base is defined as any substance which is electron rich or nucleophile or donate an electron pair to form a coordinate bond".

Thus, the Lewis concept of an acid is an electron acceptor and a base is an electron donor.

According to the Lewis concept, the neutralization reaction is explained as follows.

$$\underset{\substack{\text{Nucleophile}\\\text{(electron}\\\text{donor, Base)}}}{NH_3:} + \underset{\substack{\text{Electrophile}\\\text{(electron}\\\text{acceptor, Acid)}}}{H^+} \longrightarrow \underset{\text{Adduct}}{H \leftarrow NH_3}$$

(Coordinate bond: $H \leftarrow NH_3$)

The neutralization reaction takes place between an acid and base due to the formation of coordination bond.

***Example for Lewis acid:*** $BF_3$, $AlCl_3$, $FeCl_3$, $Ag^+$, $Fe^{2+}$, $Zn^{2+}$

***Example for Lewis base:*** $NH_3$, $H_2O$, $Cl^-$, $CN^-$

**Some other examples of Lewis acid-base reactions (neutralization reaction)**

1. ***Formation of boron tetraflouride***

$$\underset{\text{Acid}}{\mathrm{F{:}\overset{\overset{F}{\cdot\cdot}}{\underset{\underset{F}{\cdot\cdot}}{B}}}} + \underset{\text{Base}}{:\ddot{\underset{\cdot\cdot}{F}}:} \longrightarrow \underset{\text{Adduct}}{\left[\mathrm{F{:}\overset{\overset{F}{\cdot\cdot}}{\underset{\underset{F}{\cdot\cdot}}{B}}{:}F}\right]}$$

2. ***Formation of zinc tetrachloride***

$$\mathrm{Cl{:}Zn{:}Cl} + 2\,:\ddot{\underset{\cdot\cdot}{Cl}}: \longrightarrow \left[\mathrm{Cl{:}\overset{\overset{Cl}{\cdot\cdot}}{\underset{\underset{Cl}{\cdot\cdot}}{Zn}}{:}Cl}\right]^{-2}$$

***Applications***

(a) This concept is used to describe the mechanism of many organic and inorganic reactions.

(b) By this concept, the complexation and solubility principles are also explained.

***Limitations***

(a) It is failure to arrange the relative strength of Lewis acids and bases.

(b) The Lewis acid base neutralization reaction involves the transfer of electrons, actually the reaction rate should be fast, but practically this reaction rate is slow.

### 3.2.1 Hard and Soft Acid-base Concept (HSAB concept)

This concept was developed by R.G. Pearson, so it is otherwise called as Pearson principle of hard and soft acids and bases or Pearson HSAB principle.

According to this concept, acids and bases are further classified according to the properties of charge, size (ionic radius) and polarizability etc.

| S. No. | Hard acids | Soft acids |
|---|---|---|
| 1. | These are electron acceptors with high positive charges. | These are electron acceptors with low positive charges. |
| 2. | It is small in size. | It is large in size. |
| 3. | It is having unfilled valence shell orbital. | It is having filled valence shell orbital. |
| 4. | These are having the properties impart high electronegativities (electron seeking) and low polarizabilities.<br>Examples: $Na^+$, $K^+$, $Mg^+$, $Ca^+$, $I^{7+}$, $H^+$, $Sr^{2+}$, $Li^+$, HX (Hydrogen bonding molecules). | These are having the properties impart low electronegativities (electron seeking) and high polarizabilities.<br>Examples: $Cu^{2+}$, $Ag^+$, $Au^+$, Hg, $I^+$, $Br^+$, $I_2$, $OH^+$, O, Cl, Br, I. |

Some of the hard or soft acids are not having all characteristics and these are called as Borderline category acids and bases.

Examples for Borderline acids: $Fe^{2+}$, $Cu^{2+}$, $Zn^{2+}$, $Pb^{2+}$, $Sn^{2+}$, $Sb^{2+}$, $Bi^{2+}$.

| Hard bases | Soft bases |
|---|---|
| These are electron donors, easily reducible with stable shell structure. Examples: $H_2O$, $OH^-$, $F^-$, $PO_4^{3-}$, $SO_4^{2-}$, $CO_3^{2-}$, ROH, $NO_3^-$, $R_2O$, $Cl^-$. | These are having low electronegatives, easily oxidized, low lying orbitals, high polarizabilities. Examples: $I^-$, $H^-$, RSH, $R_2AS$, $CN^-$ |

Borderline bases: $Br^-$, $SO_3^{-2}$, aromatic amines, pyridine.

From this above HSAB concept, a general rule or description may be explained as follows.

The most stable complexes or adducts are formed between hard acids and hard bases and/or between soft bases and soft acids. The relative stabilities of these adducts also depends upon the relative hardness or softness of the acids and bases participated in the neutralisation reaction. In periodic table, the softness would be expected to decrease from left to right, in any substituted elements.

**Applications**

It is used to explain about the relative acidity-basicity of acids and bases.

For example the reaction between hard acid with water leads to the formation of relatively undissociated complex.

$$H^+ + H_2O \rightleftharpoons \underset{\text{Weaker acid}}{H_3O^+}$$

The hydronium ion, $H_3O^+$ should be much weaker acid than the combination of proton with iodide ion.

### 3.2.2 Relative Strength or Specification of Acidity and Basicity

The reactivity of acids and bases are depends upon their strength and the conditions of the particular chemical reaction. These conditions sometimes may increase or decrease the donor-acceptor properties of acids and bases in aqueous solution. This topic explain about the relative strength of acids and bases via taking reaction of water molecules as an example, because it is commonly used as a vehicle for all liquid pharmaceutical preparations and it has amphoteric nature. It is explained as follows.

### 3.2.3 Dissociation Constants

When the acid is dissolved in water, the strength of an acid depends upon the degree of dissociation. This is explained by the following equation.

$$\underset{\text{(Acid)}}{HA} + H_2O \rightleftharpoons H_3O^+ + A^-$$

Then the degree of dissociation or ionization is expressed in the equilibrium constant.

$$Keq = \frac{[H_3O^+][A^-]}{[HA][H_2O]} \longrightarrow (1)$$

Where $K_{eq}$ = Equilibrium constant

$$K_a = Keq\,[H_2O] = \frac{[H_3O^+][A^-]}{[HA]} \longrightarrow (2)$$

$K_a$ = ionization constant for the acid

According to the strength, there are two general types of acids, they are strong and weak.

### 3.2.4 Strong Acids and Bases

These are almost completely ionized in dilute aqueous solution with large ionization constant ($K_a > 1$). Example: HCl, NaOH.

### 3.2.5 Weak Acids and Bases

These are only partially ionized in dilute aqueous solution with smaller ionization constants.

Example: $CH_3COOH$, $NH_4OH$.

Most of the biochemicals containing the functional groups are weakly acidic or basic.

Example: Amino group, carboxyl group present in all proteins.

### 3.2.6 Ionization Constant of Weak Acids

Consider the dissociation reaction of acetic acid in water.

$$\underset{\text{Acetic acid}}{CH_3COOH} + H_2O \rightleftharpoons \underset{\text{Acetate ion}}{CH_3COO^-} + H_3O^+$$

Then the equilibrium constant is written as follows.

$$Keq = \frac{[CH_3COO^-][H_3O^+]}{[CH_3COOH][H_2O]}$$

The brackets represent the stoichiometric molar concentration of acetic acid in dilute solution. In dilute solution, the concentration of water is excess. So it is considered as constant. Then the equation is

$$K \times H_2O = \frac{[CH_3COO^-][H_3O^+]}{[CH_3COOH]}$$

$$K_a = \frac{[H_3O^+][CH_3COO^-]}{[CH_3COOH]}$$

The concentration of hydronium ion in solution is expressed as moles/L or gram ions/L.

## 3.3 HYDROGEN ION CONCENTRATION, pH AND pOH

Another way for expressing the strength of an acid is hydrogen ions concentration. If the strength of an acid increases, it would be expected to give more number of hydrogen atoms.

The ionization of purified water is illustrated as follows.

$$H_2O \rightleftharpoons H^+ + OH^-$$

$$K = \frac{[H^+][OH^-]}{[H_2O]}$$

$$K[H_2O] = [H^+][OH^-]$$

$$K_w = [H^+][OH^-] = 1 \text{x} 10^{-14}$$

Where $K_w$ = Ionic product of water, the value of it is $1\text{x}10^{-14}$, so

$$1\text{x}10^{-14} = [H^+][OH^-]$$

Pure water contains equal consent ratio of $[H^+]$ and $[OH^-]$ ions and each having the value of $1 \times 10^{-7}$.

$$[H^+] = [OH^-] = 1 \text{ x } 10^{-7} \longrightarrow (3)$$

$$[H^+] = 10^{-7}$$

The scientist Sorenson introduced a practical concept of expressing acidity of an acid. It is defined as follows.

"The acidity of an acid is a negative logarithm to the base 10 of the hydrogen ions concentration. This is defined as pH (in German word p= power (potenz) and H= hydrogen)".

$$pH = -\log[H^+] = -\log[H_3O^+] \longrightarrow (4)$$

$$= \log\frac{1}{[H^+]} = \log\frac{1}{[H_3O^+]}$$

The pH scale values ranges from 0 to 14 which includes all the hydrogen ion concentration.

**Relationship between pH and Hydrogen Ion Concentration**

It should be noted that the concentration of hydrogen ion increases, the acidity and pH decreases.

### 3.3.1 pH and pOH Relationship

| [H+] Moles / L | or | $[H_3O+]$ g-equiv / L | pH | | pOH |
|---|---|---|---|---|---|
| 1.0 | | $1 X 10^{0}$ | 0 | Increasing acidity ↑ | 14 |
| 0.1 | | $1 X 10^{-1}$ | 1 | | 13 |
| 0.01 | | $1 X 10^{-2}$ | 2 | | 12 |
| 0.001 | | $1 X 10^{-3}$ | 3 | | 11 |
| 0.0001 | | $1 X 10^{-4}$ | 4 | | 10 |
| 0.00001 | | $1 X 10^{-5}$ | 5 | | 9 |
| 0.000001 | | $1 X 10^{-6}$ | 6 | | 8 |
| 0.0000001 | | $1 X 10^{-7}$ | 7 | Neutral | 7 |
| 0.00000001 | | $1 X 10^{-8}$ | 8 | Increasing alkalinity ↓ | 6 |
| 0.000000001 | | $1 X 10^{-9}$ | 9 | | 5 |
| 0.0000000001 | | $1 X 10^{-10}$ | 10 | | 4 |
| 0.00000000001 | | $1 X 10^{-11}$ | 11 | | 3 |
| 0.000000000001 | | $1 X 10^{-12}$ | 12 | | 2 |
| 0.0000000000001 | | $1 X 10^{-13}$ | 13 | | 1 |
| 0.00000000000001 | | $1 X 10^{-14}$ | 14 | | 0 |

The determination of pH involves the potentiometric methods using a pH meter.

### 3.3.2 Relationship between Dissociation Constants and pH

The equilibrium constant can also be written according to equation (1)

$$K_a = [H_3O^+] \frac{[A^-]}{[HA]}$$

Taking negative logarithm of both sides of equation

$$-\log K_a = -\log [H_3O^+] - \log \frac{[A^-]}{[HA]} \longrightarrow (5)$$

According to the equation (4)

$$-\log Ka = pKa \longrightarrow (6)$$

The equation (5) may be written as

$$pKa = pH - \log \frac{[A^-]}{[HA]} \longrightarrow (7)$$

or

$$pKa = pH + \log \frac{[HA]}{[A^-]} \longrightarrow (8)$$

Equations (7) and (8) are called as Henderson-Hasselbalch equation.

### 3.3.3 Henderson-Hasselbalch Equation

The following points are explained from the above two equations (7 and 8)

(a) According to the concept of pH, the lower the pKa value, the stronger the acid (the more ionized acid in the water).

(b) Very strong acids (100%) are having negative pKa values and weak acids having positive pKa values (between 5 to 10).

### 3.3.4 Dissociation Constant of bases and pOH

For general base, consider the following equilibrium reaction.

$$B: + H_2O \rightleftharpoons B{:}H^+ + OH^- \longrightarrow (9)$$

The dissociation constant can be written as follows

$$Keq = \frac{[B{:}H^+]\,[OH^-]}{[B:]\,[H_2O]} \longrightarrow (9a)$$

$$K_b = Keq[H_2O] = \frac{[B{:}H^+]\,[OH^-]}{[B:]} \longrightarrow (9b)$$

Where, $K_b$ = ionization of neutral base

The stronger the base, the more equilibrium lies toward the right and larger is the $K_b$.

Similar to the hydrogen ion concentration, the hydroxyl ion concentration is a measure of basicity of a compound in water.

According to the definition,

$$-\log[OH^-] = pOH \longrightarrow (10)$$

Equation (10) expresses the basicity of a solution.

Relationship between $K_a$ and $K_b$, pH and pOH can be easily explained by the ionic product concept of water $K_w$.

$$B:H^+ + H_2O \rightleftharpoons B: + H_3O^+ \longrightarrow (11)$$

Assume that the bases and conjugate acid in equation (9) and (11) are similar, multiply equation (9a) and (11) together gives the following equation.

$$K_a = \frac{[B:]\,[H_3O^+]}{[BH^+]} \longrightarrow (12)$$

$$K_a \cdot K_b = \frac{[B:]\,[H_3O^+]}{[B:H^+]} \; \frac{[B:H^+]\,[OH^-]}{[B:]} \longrightarrow (13)$$

$$= [H_3O^+]\,[OH^-] \longrightarrow (14)$$

$$= K_w$$

$$K_a \cdot K_b = K_w = 1\text{x}10^{-14}$$

$$pK_a + pK_b = pK_w = 14 = pH + pOH \longrightarrow (15)$$

**The relationship between pH and hydrogen ion concentration**

| $[H^+]$ *moles / L* | | *pH* |
|---|---|---|
| 0.00001 | ..................... | 5.0 |
| 0.00002 | ..................... | 4.69 |
| 0.00003 | ..................... | 4.52 |
| 0.00004 | .............. .... | 4.39 |
| 0.00005 | ..................... | 4.30 |
| 0.00006 | ..................... | 4.22 |
| 0.00007 | ..................... | 4.15 |
| 0.00008 | ..................... | 4.09 |
| 0.00009 | ..................... | 4.04 |
| 0.0001 | ..................... | 4.0 |

## 3.4 BUFFERS

The control of pH of the pharmaceutical liquid preparations is very important for stability of them in long storage purpose. For patient comfort, solubility and stability of the pharmaceutical products, the control of pH is necessary.

For example, a solution of hydrochloric acid have a pH equal to 4, but the value is slightly changed because this solution is extremely sensitive to alkali from glass container and ammonia from air, likewise a solution of sodium hydroxide is sensitive to atmospheric carbondioxide. The stabilization of the pH of the above solution can be attributed by buffer solutions.

### 3.4.1 Definition

The resistance capacity of a solution to change in hydrogen ion concentration (pH) upon the addition of small amounts of acids or alkalis is called buffer action. A solution which exhibit buffer action is called as buffer solution. The composition of buffer solution is a combination of weak acid and its conjugate base (its salt) or a weak base and its conjugate acid (ammonium hydroxide and ammonium chloride).

### 3.4.2 Types of Buffer Solution

Two types of buffer solutions are there

Acidic buffer solution

Basic buffer solution

### 3.4.3 Characteristics of Buffer Solution

1. It has the definite pH value.
2. The pH of the buffer solution is not changed until longtime storage or dilution.
3. After addition of small amount of acids and bases to the buffer solution, the pH remains constant.

### 3.4.4 Mechanism of Buffer Action

The two components of the buffer system will complement each other. When a small amount of hydrogen ions are introduced into the medium, they will combine with the conjugate base present in the buffer system, which form a weak acid, will be slightly ionized. When a small amount of hydroxide ion is added to the medium, they will combine with the conjugate acid, to form conjugate base and water. By this way it prevents major changes in the pH of the solution.

For example phosphate buffer system, it consists of sodium dihydrogen phosphate $NaH_2PO_4$ as the acidic member and disodium hydrogen phosphate as the basic member $Na_2HPO_4$.

If a small amount of hydrochloric acid is added to a non buffered solution, a complete ionization will takes place and it forms hydronium ion, leads to significant reduction in the pH.

$$HCl + H_2O \longrightarrow H_3O^+ + Cl^-$$

In a solution having phosphate buffer, the basic member of the buffer pair ($HPO_4^-$) reacts with the hydronium ion, the equilibrium shifted to right.

$$HPO_4^{-2} + H_3O^+ \rightleftharpoons H_2PO_4^- + H_2O$$

Similarly, a small amount of NaOH is added to the solution, a complete ionization will takes place, and it form hydroxide ions, which will decrease the $H_3O^+$ ion concentration.

$$NaOH \rightleftharpoons Na^+ + OH^-$$

$$OH^- + H_3O^+ \rightleftharpoons 2\,H_2O$$

If the solution is buffered with phosphate buffer, disodium hydrogen phosphate (acidic pair) reacts with hydroxide ion and forms water and conjugate base.

$$H_2PO_4^- + OH^- \rightleftharpoons HPO_4^{-2} + H_2O$$

This buffer action is started when a small amount of acid or base is added, so buffer action is not limited.

### 3.4.5 Henderson-Hasselbalch Equation

The pH of a buffer solution is depending upon the $pK_a$ of acidic member of the buffer and the log ratio of buffering species.

This relationship is described by *Henderson Hasselbalch* equation or buffer equation. Two separate equations are there for each type of buffer.

$$pH = pka + \log\frac{[salt]}{[acid]}$$

$$pH = pk_w - pk_b + \log\frac{[base]}{[salt]}$$

### 3.4.6 Buffer Capacity

It is also known as buffer index, buffer efficiency and buffer value. Koppel, Spiro and Van slyke introduced the concept of buffer capacity which is defined as the ratio of increment of strong acid or base to small changes in pH brought about by this addition.

Buffer capacity is mathematically expressed by the following equation.

$$\beta = \frac{\Delta B}{\Delta pH}$$

According to the equation, the buffer capacity of a solution has a value of 1, when an addition of 1 gm equivalent of strong base to 1 litre of buffer solution leads to a change of 1 pH unit.

## 3.5 SELECTION OF PHARMACEUTICAL BUFFER SYSTEM

The selection of buffers for pharmaceutical purposes is based on two factors

1. Chemical factors
2. Pharmacological factors

1. ***Chemical factors:*** According to the chemical aspects
   1. The buffer pair should not reacts with the active ingredients.
   2. It should not alter the solubility of other components.
   3. It should not involve in the oxidation-reduction reaction.
   4. It should not involve in the acid base reaction except their buffer action.
   5. It must possess the chemical stability and it should not contain any volatile impurities.
2. ***Pharmacological factors***
   1. The buffer should neither contribute nor decrease the pharmacological properties of the active ingredients.
   2. Some of the buffers are toxic in nature, care should be taken for selection of this buffers. For example, borate buffers (used in ophthalmic preparations) are toxic in nature when administered systematically, so care should be taken.
   3. A buffer system containing common biochemical acids and conjugate bases is having the ability to support the microbial growth because they can serve as nutrient media for certain microbes particularly when the pH is neutral, nor too basic or too acidic. Since too acidic or too basic pH solutions are acts as germicides. These types of buffer solutions are preserved by low concentrations of quaternary ammonium antimicrobial agents [0.002% benzalkonium chloride].

## 3.6 PHARMACEUTICAL BUFFER SYSTEMS

Buffer system used in pharmacy can be classified in two categories.

1. Standard buffer system
2. Actual pharmaceutical buffer system.

1. **Standard buffer system:** These are solutions of standard pH values, mainly used for reference purposes in measurements and carryout many pharmacopoeial tests.

   IP 2010 describes the following standard buffer solutions. Refer Table 3.1.

**Table 3.1** Standard buffer solutions

| S. No. | Buffer name | pH range |
|---|---|---|
| 1 | Hydrochloric acid buffer | 1.2-2.2 with 0.1 intervals |
| 2 | Acid phthalate buffer | 2.2-4.0 with 0.2 intervals |
| 3 | Neutralized phthalate buffer, phthalate buffer | 4.2-5.8 with 0.2 intervals |
| 4 | Phosphate buffer | 5.8-8.0 with 0.2 intervals |
| 5 | Alkaline borate buffer | 8.0-10.0 with 0.2 intervals |

**Other buffer solutions:** Among the all inorganic buffers phosphate and borate buffers are very important buffers for pharmaceutical preparations Table 3.2.

**Table 3.2** Buffer solutions

| S. No. | Buffer solution name | pH |
|---|---|---|
| 1. | Acetate buffer | 2.8, 3.4, 3.5, 3.7, 4, 4.4, 4.6, 4.7, 5.0, 5.5, 6.0 |
| 2. | Acetate-EDTA Buffer | 5.5 |
| 3. | Acetic acid-ammonium acetate buffer | 5.5 |
| 4. | Acetic ammonia buffer | 3.7 |
| 5. | Albumin- phosphate | 7.2 |
| 6. | Ammonia-ammonium chloride | 10.0 |
| 7. | Ammonia buffer | 9.5, 10, 10.9 |
| 8. | Barbitone buffer | 7.4, 8.6 |
| 9. | Boric or borate buffer | 9 |
| 10. | Buffer solution | 2.5 |
| 11. | HEPES buffer solution | 7.5 |
| 12. | Carbonate buffer solution | 9.7 |
| 13. | Chloride buffer solution | 2.0 |
| 14. | Citro-Phosphate buffer | 5, 6, 7, 7.2, 7.6 |
| 15. | Cupric sulphate solution, buffered | 2, 4, 5.2 |
| 16. | Diethanolamine buffer | 10 |
| 17. | Glycine buffer | 11.3 |
| 18. | Imidazole buffer | 6.5, 7.4 |
| 19. | Phosphate-albumin saline buffer | 7.2 |
| 20. | Phosphate buffer | 2, 2.5, 3, 3.6, 4, 4.9, 5, 5.5, 6.5 |
| 21. | Tris-acetate buffer | 8.5 |
| 22. | Tris-chloride buffer | 7.4 |
| 23. | Tris-amino methane buffer | 7.4-8.1 |

### 3.6.1 Phosphate Buffer System

**Advantages of phosphate buffer system**

The phosphate buffer contains dihydrogen and monohydrogen anions, similar to that of buffer system in the body (lacrimal fluid, pH=7.4).

**Disadvantages of phosphate buffer system**

1. Insolubility of phosphate in metals like Ag, Al and Zn. So it cannot be used along with these metal preparations (gargles, collyria). When it is taken internally, it precipitates all the metal ions in the intestine.
2. It permits or supports the growth of microbes at room temperature. So 0.002% of benzalkonium chloride is added which acts as an antimicrobial agent.

Modified phosphate buffer system to include the addition of sodium chloride to make it isotonic with body fluid is called as "Sorensen phosphate buffer" with a pH ranges from 5.9 to 8.0.

### 3.6.2 Borate Buffer System

Borate buffer systems have been used in many pharmaceutical preparations containing metals that would otherwise precipitate in the presence of phosphates. There are three types of primary borate buffer system are available

(i) Feldman's buffer system pH 7-8.2

(ii) Atkins and Pantin buffer system pH 7.6-11.0

(iii) Gifford's buffer system pH 6 -7.8

**Disadvantages**

1. Boric acid is toxic in nature, so it should not be used for internal preparations and injectables.
2. The $pK_a$ value of boric acid is 9.2, makes borate buffers inefficient to physiological pH, but it can be used in alkaline pH ranges but it leads to incompatibility.
3. Borate buffer system is weak bacteriostatic, it allows the growth of microbes when it stored for a month or two months at room temperature.
4. Borate buffers are suitable for ophthalamic, nasal external preparations but contraindicated for parentral preparations.

The buffer pair in each of these is tetra borate anion and boric acid, but in the later two sodium tetra borate is formed *in situ*.

Other buffer systems used in the pharmaceutical preparations are organic acids and their conjugate base. Example: Citrate buffer, acetic acid-ammonium acetate buffer.

These are having low toxicity because they are normal body metabolites and these are not supporting the microbial growth. These are highly soluble in water, administered internally, also used in parentrals or injectables.

## 3.7 PHYSIOLOGICAL BUFFERS

The maintenance of acid base balance in our body is very important for proper cellular function. The principal buffer systems of the body fluids are three types.

1. Protein buffer system
2. Carbonic acid - Bicarbonate buffer system
3. Phosphate buffer system

1. **Protein buffer system:** It is the most abundant buffer system in intracellular fluid and blood plasma. Proteins are made up of amino acids, that contain at least one carboxyl group at one end and at least one amino group ($-NH_2$) at another end. The free carboxyl group present at the one end acts as an acid by the release of $H^+$ ion.

The dissociation reaction is illustrated as follows

$$H_2N-\underset{H}{\overset{R}{C}}-COOH \xrightarrow[-H^+]{\text{Raise in pH}} H_2N-\underset{H}{\overset{R}{C}}-COO^-$$

The liberated $H^+$ ion reacts with any excess $OH^-$ ions in the fluid and forms water.

The amino group present at the another end of the amino acid acts as a base, and it accept any $H^+$ ions, when pH falls.

$$COOH-\underset{H}{\overset{R}{C}}-NH_2 + H^+ \xrightleftharpoons{\text{pH falls}} COOH-\underset{H}{\overset{R}{C}}-NH_3^+$$

Like this way proteins acts as buffer due to both acidic and basic property.

Another important protein buffer system in the blood is haemoglobin buffer system, which is the important buffer in RBC.

When blood flows through the capillaries, $CO_2$ gas is transported from the tissues to RBC cells, where it combines with water and form carbonic acid.

$$\underset{\text{(entering RBC)}}{CO_2 + H_2O} \rightleftharpoons \underset{\text{carbonic acid}}{H_2CO_3}$$

At the same time, $O_2$ present in the oxyhaemoglobin is transferred to the tissue cells. This reduced hemoglobin catches the most of the $H^+$ ions. So it can be always written as Hb-H.

$$H_2CO_3 \rightleftharpoons H^+ + HCO_3^-$$

$$\underset{\substack{\text{Oxy haemo}\\\text{globin}\\\text{(in RBC's)}}}{Hb\text{-}O_2} + \underset{\substack{\text{From}\\\text{Carbonic acid}}}{H^+} \rightleftharpoons \underset{\substack{\text{Reducing}\\\text{haemoglobin}}}{Hb\text{-}H} + \underset{\substack{\text{(Released to the}\\\text{tissue cells)}}}{O_2}$$

2. **Carbonic acid- Bicarbonate buffer system:** This buffer system is based upon the bicarbonate ion ($HCO_3^-$) which can acts as a weak base and carbonic acid ($H_2CO_3$) which can act as a weak acid. This buffer system is present in kidney and plasma.

   $HCO_3^-$ ion is important anion present in intracellular and extracellular fluids. Kidney also synthesizes $HCO_3^-$ and reabsorbs it.

   $HCO_3^-$ acts as an weak base and remove the excess $H^+$ ions, when $H^+$ ions excessively present.

$$\underset{\text{Hydrogen ion}}{\text{Excess } H^+} + \underset{\substack{\text{Bicarbonic}\\\text{acid}}}{HCO_3^-} \longrightarrow \underset{\text{Carbonic acid}}{H_2CO_3}$$

This carbonic acid gets dissociated into water (excreted in urine) and carbon dioxide (exhaled from lungs).

$$H_2CO_3 \longrightarrow H_2O + CO_2\uparrow$$

Conversely if lack of $H^+$ ions occurs, the $H_2CO_3$ function as a weak acid and liberate $H^+$ ions.

$$H_2CO_3 \longrightarrow H^+ + HCO_3^-$$

3. **Phosphate buffer system:** The components of phosphate buffer system are dihydrogen phosphate ($H_2PO_4^-$) and monohydrogen phosphate ($HPO_4^-$). Major amount of phosphate ions are present in intracellular fluids and less in extracellular fluid.

   ***Mechanism of action:*** The dihydrogen phosphate acts as a weak acid and it buffering the strong bases such as $OH^-$ ions.

$$\underset{\text{Strong base}}{OH^-} + \underset{\text{Weak acid}}{H_2PO_4^-} \longrightarrow H_2O + \underset{\text{Weak base}}{HPO_4^{2-}}$$

   The monohydrogen phosphate acts as a weak base by accepting $H^+$ ions from strong acid (HCl).

$$\underset{\text{Strong acid}}{H^+} + \underset{\text{Weak base}}{H_2PO_4^-} \longrightarrow \underset{\text{Weak base}}{H_3PO_4}$$

   It is an important buffer system which regulates the pH in cytosol. This buffer system also used to maintain the pH of the blood through kidney by excreting $H^+$ in urine.

## 3.8 ROLE OF BUFFERS IN PHARMACY

1. ***Enhancing or increasing the solubility:*** If the pH of the solution is not adjusted properly, the active ingredients may get precipitated. For example sodium salicylate gets precipitated as salicylic acid, when acidified. So the optimum pH should be adjusted by using buffer for attaining maximum solubility.
2. ***Increasing the stability:*** Many of the drugs are getting dissociated in aqueous solutions, buffers are added to these drugs to increase or getting the optimal stability of drugs. Example: Vitamin, thiamine hydrochloride is maintained at the pH range of 3.5-4.5 (not <5).

## PROBABLE QUESTIONS

1. Define an acid and base according to the Arrehenius concept. Give an example for each.
2. Define an acid and base according to the Bronsted- Lowrey concept.
3. Explain hard and soft acid base concept with one example.
4. What is meant by the conjugate acid of the base?

5. Describe the four ways in which the Bronsted- Lowrey concept enlarges on the Arrehenius concept.
6. Define an acid and base according to the Lewis concept. Give a chemical equation to illustrate.
7. Write two important factors that determine the strength of an acid. How does an increase in each factor affect the acid strength?
8. Explain about the followings
   (a) Relative strength of an acid and base (b) Dual character of water.
9. What is mean by pH of a solution and explain about Henderson- Hasselbach equation.
10. Write in brief about the importance of pH in pharmaceuticals.
11. Explain about the ionic product of water.
12. Calculate the molarity of a solution obtained by dissolving 0.3M sulphuric acid and 200 ml of 1.5M sulphuric acid.
13. Calculate the molality of a solution obtained by mixing 0.85gm ammonia in 100 gm of water.
14. 0.548 gm of the metal reacts with dilute acid and liberates 0.0918 gm of hydrogen at S.T.P. Calculate the equivalent mass of the metal.
15. Define buffers with examples.
16. Briefly describe the methods for determining the $pk_a$ value for a weak acid.
17. Describe briefly about the degree of ionization of a weak acid changes as a concentration increases.
18. What is meant by the capacity of buffer? Describe the buffer with low capacity and same buffer with greater capacity.
19. Explain about the ideal characteristics of buffer solution.
20. Write briefly about the physiological buffer system.
21. Explain about the factors to be considered while selecting pharmaceutical buffer system.
22. Enumerate the role of buffer system in pharmacy.
23. Explain about the mechanism of buffer action.

CHAPTER 4

# QUANTITATIVE ANALYSIS (VOLUMETRIC AND GRAVIMETRIC ANALYSIS)

## 4.1 INTRODUCTION

Analytical chemistry is the branch of chemistry which deals about the analysis of chemicals or pharmaceuticals. Analysis is of two types, i.e., Qualitative analysis and Quantitative analysis.

Qualitative analysis deals with the identification of the chemical constituents present in a mixture of chemical substances. Quantitative analysis deals with the actual amount of the chemical constituent present in a mixture of chemical substance or in a pharmaceutical dosage form. The methods used are called as assay methods. It is used to find out the purity of chemical substances or to determine the amount of active drug present in the given dosage form. The different methods of quantitative analysis are volumetric analysis, gravimetric analysis, photometry, electrochemical methods, refractometry, polarimetry, fluorimetry, chromatographic methods and biological methods.

### 4.1.1 Volumetric Analysis

Volumetric analysis is also called as **titrimetric analysis**. It is performed in a simple manner and hence used routinely. In this, the volume of a solution of known concentration (standard) required to react completely with a solution of the substance to be analyzed is determined.

The substance to be analyzed is called titrate. A known concentration of substance which is added to the solution of the substance to be analyzed is called titrant.

In volumetric analysis, two solutions (titrate and titrant) are always made to react in a conical flask known as titration flask. One of these solutions is taken in a burette (titrant) and other in the titration flask. From burette, titrant is added to the titration flask until the titrate react completely (this point is called as end point i.e., point at which a reaction is completed during titration).

This process of finding out the volume of titrant required to react completely with the substance (as solution) under study is known as titration. To recognise the end point of the titration, indicators are added which shows a distinct colour change at the completion of the chemical reaction. In volumetric analysis standard solutions are used as titrant which may be expressed as molar (M) (or its fraction) or normal (N) (or its fraction) concentration.

**Conditions for volumetric analysis**

Estimation by volumetric analysis is only feasible if the reaction involved fulfils the following conditions:

1. The reaction should be instantaneous under the experimental conditions.
2. The reaction should take place and complete under the study conditions.
3. The chemical reaction must be simple and should take place completely to form known products.
4. The end point should be well defined.

**Terms in volumetric analysis**

Some of the terms used in volumetric analysis are listed below.

***Titrate*:** The chemical substance under study to determine is called as titrate.

***Titrant*:** The substance of known concentration used to react is called as titrant.

***Titration*:** The process of finding out the volume of the titrant required to react completely with the test substance.

***End point*:** The point at which the reaction completed is called as the end point.

***Indicator*:** Chemical substance used to detect the end point of the titration is called as the indicator.

***Standard solution*:** The solution of known concentration is called as the standard solution.

***Primary standard*:** The substance having known purity which yields standard solution by dissolving a definite weight of a substance in a definite volume is called as primary standard. This solution can be used as a titrant. Only few of the substances can be used as primary standard. Examples: Oxalic acid, sodium carbonate, potassium hydrogen phthalate.

***Secondary standard*:** It is a standard which is prepared in the laboratory for a specific analysis. It is standardized against a primary standard. Example: Solutions of sodium hydroxide.

**Methods of expressing concentrations in volumetric analysis**

Various terms used for expressing the concentration are described below. Normality and molarity are the two terms used frequently. Sometimes percent strengths are also used.

***Normality:*** Defined as the number of gram equivalents of solute present in one litre of the solution. It is expressed as "N".

$$\text{Normality} = \frac{\text{Number of gram equivalent of solute}}{\text{Volume of solution in litre}}$$

***Weight percent*:** It specifies the number of grams of solute per 100 grams of solution.

***Molarity*:** Defined as the number of moles of solute present in one litre of the solution. It is represented by "**M**".

$$\text{Molarity} = \frac{\text{Number of moles of solute}}{\text{Volume of solution in litres}}$$

***Molality*:** Defined as the number of gram moles of solute dissolved in 1000 gm or 1 kg of a solvent. It is expressed as "**M**".

$$\text{Molality} = \frac{\text{Number of moles of solute}}{\text{Mass of solvent in kilograms}}$$

***Equivalent weight*:** Defined as the weight of the substance that reacts or contains 1.008 gm of hydrogen or 16.0 gm of oxygen or 35.5 gm of chlorine. E.g., hydrochloric acid contains equivalent of 1.008 gm of hydrogen and its equivalent is 36.5 gm of HCl. Hence equivalent weight of it is 36.5 similarly equivalent weight of NaOH is 40.

***Molar solution*:** If the given solution contains 1 mole of a titrant in one litre it is termed as one molar (M) solution. From this, solutions of lower strengths (M/2, M/4, M/5, M/10, M/20, M/50, and M/1000) are prepared.

***Normal solution*:** When the solution contains 1 gram equivalent weight of the substance in one litre, it is called one normal (N) solution. From this, solutions of lower strengths (N/2, N/4, N/5, N/10, N/20, N/50, and N/1000) are prepared. Mathematically the normality of a solution may be expressed as follows:

***Normality of a solution*:** Concentration (or strength) in grams per litre/Equivalent weight.

***Strength*:** The amount of solute in grams present in one litre of the solution. It is expressed in gm/litre.

$$\text{Strength} = \frac{\text{Mass of solute in grams}}{\text{Volume of solution in litres}}$$

***Equivalent mass of acid and base*:** Equivalent mass of an acid is the number of parts by mass of the acid which contains 1.008 parts by mass of replaceable hydrogen atom.

$$\text{Equivalent mass of an acid} = \frac{\text{Molar mass of the acid}}{\text{Number of replaceble hydrogen atom (Basicity)}}$$

Equivalent mass of a base is the number of parts by mass of the base which contains one replaceable hydroxyl ion or which completely neutralizes one gram equivalent of an acid.

$$\text{Equivalent mass of a base} = \frac{\text{Molar mass of the base}}{\text{Acidity of the acid}}$$

**Introduction to Statistical Analysis**

By using quantitative analysis numerical data results are determined. In this area, the question arises for the analyst what is the correctness of the measured quality? What is the reliability of the method used, whether they followed proper sampling procedure or not and how efficiently they carried out the work? The answers for all the above questions provoke the statistical methods by which the analyst describes the accuracy, precision, deciding proper sampling and designing of the experiment. In fact, the next question arises i.e. how to estimate or determine the absolute or true value of a quantity. It is not at all possible to find out the absolute or true value of a quantity. why and what for means "Because of the presence of defects in the mechanical apparatus, presence of inherent impurities in the chemicals for which it is not at possible on the part of even an expert analyst to determine the exact value of quantity. Hence, the numerical value or results so obtained deviates from the absolute or true value.

**Errors:** From the preceding paragraph or introduction of this chapter indicates that the observed value of quantity may differ from the most probable value. The magnitude of difference between these two values is a measure of deviation which may be positive or negative. This duration accounts for the errors in the experimental results. Accordingly error may be defined as a deviation of observed value (i.e. the true average number of results) of a large number of results.

**Classification of errors:** Errors are classified in to two major types.

1. Systematic, determinate or constant errors.
2. Random, indeterminate or accidental errors.

1. **Systematic, determinate or constant errors:** The errors that magnitude can be determined and corrected or which can be avoided are known as systematic, determinate or constant errors. Generally these errors are present in each measurement and affect the result of series of determination to the same extent. The main reason for arising these errors are usage of faulty methods and wrong operation of the measuring instruments.

**Types:** Systematic errors are classified into 6 types.

1. Operational errors.
2. Personal errors.
3. Instrumental errors.
4. Reagent errors.
5. Errors due to methods followed.
6. Additive and proportional errors.

1. **Operational errors:** These are physical in nature and arise when proper analytical technique is not followed. For example;
   - Impurities present in chemicals.

- Mechanical loss of the material in various steps of analysis such as ignition of precipitate at incorrect temperatures, absorption of moisture by hygroscopic materials before or during weighing.

2. **Personal errors:** These errors are occurs by the individual analyst but not connected with method or procedure used. *For example*:
   - Reading a meniscus of burettes or pipettes.
   - Pouring and mixing of liquids.
   - Wrong observation of the swing of a balance pointer during weighing the chemicals.
   - Matching colours.

3. **Instrumental errors:** This is mainly due to the faulty construction of instruments. *For example*:
   - Uses of uncalibrated or improperly calibrated weights.
   - Unequal lengths of balanced arms.
   - Improperly calibrated volumetric apparatus or other instruments.

   The instrumental errors can be avoided by using calibrated weights and glass wares.

4. **Reagent errors:** This type of error is brought out in an experiment by the usage of reagents with impurities, attack of reagents on glass wares etc.. These can be prevented by using pyrex glass wares and pure reagents.

5. **Errors due to methods followed or applied:** These errors are arise due to incorrect sampling and incompleteness of reaction. *For example*: In Gravimetric analysis, error occurs due to coprecipitation, post precipitation, volatilization or decomposition of the precipitate etc.

   In titrations, errors may occurs by incompletion of reaction, possibility of chain reactions, chemical reaction of the substance other than the desired components and the difference between the observed end point and stiochiometric end point of reaction concerned . These all types of errors are minimized by using suitable techniques.

6. **Additive and proportional errors:** The absolute value of an additive error does not depend on the amount of component present in the determination. For example; the loss in weight of crucible in which precipitate is ignited increases or adds errors to the weight. These types of errors can be known by taking the samples of different weight.

   **Proportional errors:** This error arises from the impurity present in standard substances that gives a wrong value for the normality of standard solution in titration.

**II Random, Indeterminate or Accidental Errors**

These are occurs by chance or accidentally so, they called random, indeterminate or accidental errors. These are mainly due to arising of small variations taking place in successive measurements made by the same analyst. These can't be allowed for or corrected due to the natural fluctuations occurring in all measurements.

**Types**

(a) Erratic errors.

(b) Variable determinate errors.

**(a) Erratic errors:** These types of errors occur due to

(i) Accidental loss of material during analysis.

(ii) Variations involved in reading instruments. These are otherwise known as pseudo accidental or variable determinate errors.

The measurements varies from one to another, the analyst cannot control over such error. The random error occurs in filling number of capsules with a drug.

**True indeterminate error:** The error that occurs from true random fluctuations in nature is known as true indeterminate error.

**Minimization of errors:** The errors that occur from random fluctuations in nature can't be minimized. But the error occurred from the use of uncalibrated glass wares, temperature difference should be minimized by using any one of the following methods.

1. **Calibration of apparatus:** All types of burettes, pipettes and glass ware should be calibrated before determination and corrections to be made to the original measurements.

2. **Use of independent method of analysis:** Different methods of analysis of the sample in order to check the accuracy.

   For example; Normality of HCl solution may be determined by titration it with standard NaOH solution, and also by precipitating and weighing as AgCl.

3. **Performing a blank determination:** Error occurs due to the presence of impurities in the reagent and reacting with vessels can be eliminated by performing the experiment without taking the sample under exactly the same experimental procedure as followed in the actual analysis of sample.

4. **Standard addition method:** The amount of particular component in a sample is determined by using appropriate analytical methods, a known amount of said component is added to another lot of sample and the total component present in the sample is determined by the same method. The difference between the results for the sample with and without component gives the recovery of the quantity of the added component. If the recovery is good, it indicates the accuracy of the method. This method is used in spectrophotometric analysis.

5. **Carryout parallel measurements:** It involves the same determination which is carried out simultaneously by a number of analysts. The values obtained should not vary more than three parts per thousand or parts per hundred (i.e.0.3%)

6. **Isotopic dilution:** A known quantity of a pure component contain a radioactive isotope is mixed with the sample, and the component to be determined is isolated in pure from a compound. The radio activity of the isolated compound is measured and

compared with that of added component from which the weighing the component in the unknown sample is calculated.

7. **By using internal standards:** A fixed amount of a standard substance (internal standard) is added to series of known amount of the sample to be measured. This method is used in spectroscopic, polarographic and chromatographic measurements. A straight line obtained by plotting the measured values against concentration and any unknown concentration can be calculated.

8. **Performing a control measurement:** An amount of particular component present in the unknown sample is obtained from the standard substance containing the same component under identical experimental conditions.

*The weight of the desired component is calculated by the following formula.*

$$\frac{\text{Result obtained for the standard}}{\text{Result obtained for the sample}} = \frac{\text{Weight of the component in the standard}}{\text{Weight of desired component}}$$

**Mean:** The arithmetic mean is the best measure of central value of a frequency distribution curve. The theoretical means for sufficiently large number of measurements is known as universe (or) population mean and indicated by a symbol M.

Arithmetic mean $\overline{X} = \sum x_i/N$

where

$x_i$ = 'i'$^{th}$ the individual measurement

N = Number of measured values.

**Median:** It is used as a measure of the centrally distribution of the values. It is a value about which all other values equally distributed.

For odd numbers of observations

$$\text{Median} = 1/2(n+1)$$

For even number of observations

$$\text{Median} = 1/2\ n\ \text{(or)}\ 1/2\ (n+1)$$

Mean and median may or may not be the same.

**Standard deviation (Root mean square deviation):** A small number of the measured values are used, the mean deviation gives greater precision, then standard deviation ($\sigma$) is considered.

Standard deviation is defined as "The Square root of the mean of squares of deviations."
$\sigma = (\Sigma(x_i\text{-}x)^2 / N)^{1/2}$

The spread of the values can be determined by S.D.

$$S = \left[\frac{\Sigma(x-\overline{x})^2}{N-1}\right]^{1/2}$$

where N–1= numbers of degrees of freedom.

The square root of S.D is known as Variance.

**Relative Standard Deviation (R.S.D):** A more accurate measure of the precision is known as relative standard deviation.

$$RSD = \frac{S}{X}$$

The value of RSD is expressed as percentage, known as coefficient of variation (CV)

$$CV = \frac{S}{\overline{X}} \times 100$$

**Accuracy and Precision:** The absolute error of a determination is "The difference between the measured value (X) and the true (or) most probable value (T) of the quantity measured.

Absolute error "e" = X–T

where,

"e" is the measure of the accuracy of the measurement. So accuracy is defined as "The concordance between the observed and the true or most probable value."

**Precision:** It is defined as "The concordance of a series of determinations of the same quantity. The precision is a function of random errors. Both are inversely related. i.e., Random error values are small; the precision of the measurement is high and vice versa. The mean deviation or the relative mean deviation is a measure of precision.

In quantitative analysis, the precision of measurements exceeds rarely one or two parts per thousand.

## 4.2 TYPES OF TITRATIONS

Titrations can be carried out by adopting any one of the following three methods.

1. ***Direct titration***: In this method, the substance is dissolved in a solvent to make as solution of the substance, which is then determined quantitatively by titrating directly with a suitable titrant using an appropriate indicator or suitable instrument to find out the end point. Example: Assay of hydrochloric acid or sulphuric acid with sodium hydroxide using phenolphthalein as indicator.
2. ***Back titration***: When the test substance is not able to assay by direct titration this method is followed. Substances which are not water soluble or weak acids or bases are assayed by this method. Example: Assay of magnesium hydroxide. In this assay the substance is treated with Known Excess Standard (KES) 1N sulphuric acid and the excess unreacted (EUR) sulphuric acid is determined by titrating with 1N sodium hydroxide using methyl red as an indicator. End point is the yellow colour. A blank determination (without substances) should be performed. From the difference in value, the volume of titrant required for the substance is calculated.

3. ***Indirect Titration***: If the test substance not undergoing suitable chemical reaction, then by employing some chemical reaction it can be precipitated or removed from the reaction and the product thus formed is assayed or measured.

**Classification of Volumetric or Titrimetric Methods**

Based on the chemical reaction involved these methods can be classified into various types.

1. ***Acid base titrations:*** When the acid and base reacts neutralization reaction takes place, it is called as acid-base or neutralization titration. Example: Assay of hydrochloric acid.
2. ***Non aqueous titration:*** When the test substance is very weakly acidic or basic or salts of weakly acidic or basic it cannot be titrated in aqueous media, the strength of such substances can be increased by dissolving them in an appropriate non aqueous solvents. Hence these substances are titrated in a non aqueous media. Example: Assay of sodium acetate.
3. ***Redox titrations***: When the titrant and titrate reacts and the oxidation and reduction takes place in the assay it is called as Redox titrations. Example: Assay of hydrogen peroxide.
4. ***Precipitation titrations:*** When the titrant and titrate reacts and the formation of the precipitate occurs it is called as Precipitation titrations. Example: Assay of sodium chloride.
5. ***Complexometric titrations:*** When the titrant and titrate reacts and the formation of complex occurs it is called as Complexometric titrations. Example: Assay of magnesium sulphate.
6. ***Diazotization Titrations:*** When the diazotization reaction occurs during the assay it is called as diazotization titrations. Test compounds having aromatic primary amines are assayed by this method. Example: Assay of sulpha drugs.

These methods are described in detail below.

### 4.2.1 Acid Base Titrations

The reactions between acids and bases are termed as neutralization reactions. These reactions take place rapidly. In acidimetry-alkalimetry, the reactions occur with neutralization along with the formation of salt and water. It can be divided into two types, i.e., Acidimetry and alkalimetry.

(i) *Acidimetry method:* The titrations between base and the acid which is used as titrant is called acidimetry.

In this a known volume of an alkaline substance is taken in a conical flask, added suitable indicator and titrated against a standard solution of an acid taken in burette until the end point.

**Example:** ***Assay of sodium bicarbonate:*** In this assay the substance is dissolved in water and titrated with 0.5N hydrochloric acid, using methyl orange as an indicator. End point is the orange colour. In this assay the sodium bicarbonate (the base) reacts with hydrochloric acid and neutralization takes place during the titration. The indicator is yellow colour in alkali medium and it changes to orange colour in acidic medium which is the end point.

As the acid and alkali involved in this assay, it is called as acidimetry-alkalimetry method of titration and the neutralization takes place in this assay during titration hence this assay is also called as Neutralization method. The chemical reactions of this assay are shown below.

$$NaHCO_3 + HCl \longrightarrow NaCl + H_2O + CO_2$$

(ii) ***Alkalimetry method:*** The titrations between acid and the base which is used as titrant is called as alkalimetry.

In this a known volume of an acidic substance is taken in a conical flask, added suitable indicator and titrated against a standard solution of an alkali taken in burette until the end point.

**Example:** ***Assay of hydrochloric acid:*** In this assay the substance is diluted with water and titrated with sodium hydroxide, using phenolphthalein as an indicator.

In this assay the sodium hydroxide (the base) reacts with hydrochloric acid and neutralization takes place during the titration. The indicator is colourless in acidic and it changes to pink colour upon reaching basic which is the end point.

As the acid and alkali involved in this assay, it is called as acidimetry-alkalimetry method of titration and the neutralization takes place in this assay during titration hence this assay is also called as Neutralization method. The chemical reactions of this assay are shown below.

$$HCl + NaOH \longrightarrow NaCl + H_2O$$

***Acid base indicators:*** The indicators used in acid base titrations to locate their end point are called acid base indicators. These indicators have one colour in acid solution while an altogether different colour in alkaline solution. The colour change usually takes place in small range of pH value (usually 2). This is called the pH range of an indicator. The pH ranges of various acid base indicators are shown in the Table 4.1.

**Table 4.1** pH range of acid base indicators

| Indicator | pH range | Colour in acid | Colour in alkali |
|---|---|---|---|
| Methyl orange | 2.9 - 4.6 | Orange | Yellow |
| Methyl red | 4.5 - 6.5 | Red | Yellow |
| Phenolphthalein | 8.3 - 10.5 | Colour less | Pink |

## Neutralisation Curves

The curve obtained by plotting pH against the amount of acid neutralized in percentage or the number of milliliters of alkali added is known as neutralisation curve or titration curve. This may be determined experimentally by measuring the pH at various stages during the titration using potentiometric method or theoretical principles.

**1. Strong acid Vs strong base**

The reaction between a strong acid and a strong base is represented by as follows.

$$H + OH \rightleftharpoons H_2O$$

This reaction is a reversible reaction of ionization of water. Consider the titration of 100 ml of HCl with 1 N NaOH solution.

After the addition of 1 ml of NaOH solution, the volume of solution becomes 101 ml and it contains 1X100 milli equivalence of acid(m.eq=NxV)and 1x1 milli equivalence of base.

Hence the amount of HCl present in the solution

= 100 – 1 = 99 milli equivalence of an acid

= 101 ml

(H) = 99/101 = pH = 0.008

Similarly if 50 ml of base is added, there will be 50 ml of unneutralised acid in 150 ml.

$$[H^+] = \frac{50}{150} = 0.33$$

pH = 0.58.

Like this the following calculations are made

If 75 ml of base is added means

$$[H^+] = 21.43 \times 10^{-1}$$

pH = 0.94

If 90 ml base is added means

$$[H^+] = 5.27 \times 10^{-2} = pH = 1.3$$

If 99 ml base is added means

$$[H^+] = 5.03 \times 10^{-3}, pH = 2.3$$

If 99.9 ml base is added means

$$[H^+] = 5.01 \times 10^{-4}, pH = 3.3$$

Further addition of 100 ml of base, the pH of the solution sharply changes to 7, the equivalence point is obtained. (sharp change of pH from 3.3 to 7)

In quantitative analysis, changing the pH near to the equivalence point that they are of practically special interest. So the graph shown in large scale of Fig.(4.1) which indicates the colour change of some indicators.

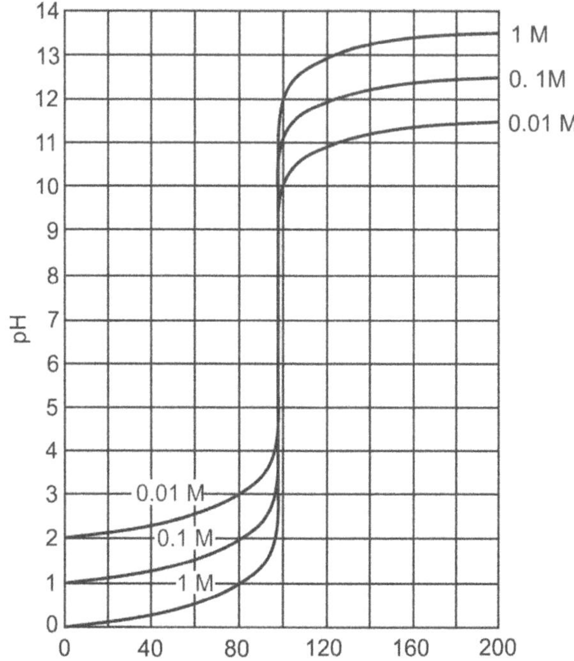


**Fig. 4.1** Calculated curves for strong acid (100 ml 1M HCl) Vs strong base (1M NaOH). In graph X axis = amount of alkali added (ml), Y axis = pH

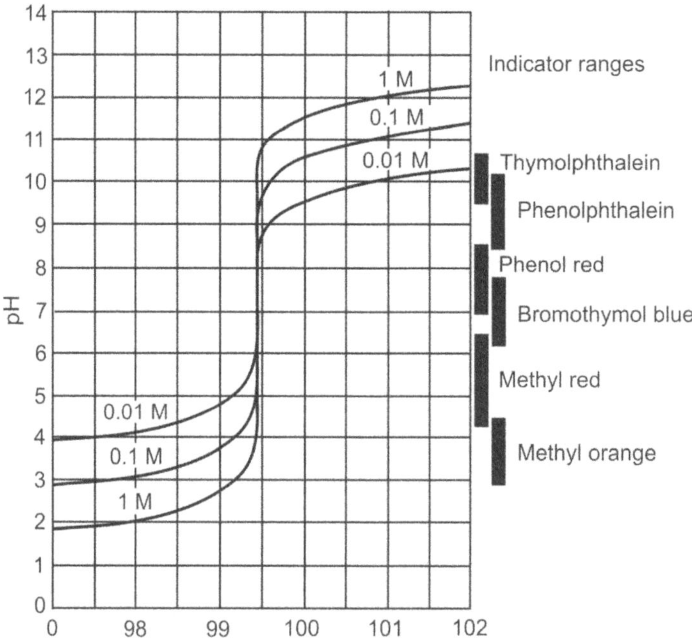


**Fig. 4.2** Equivalence point of Fig.4.2 with range of indicators. In graph X axis = amount of alkali added (ml), Y axis = pH

For 1 M solution, the use of any possible indicators having an effective pH range between 3and 10.5, the color change will be sharp and titration error is negligible.

For 0.1 M solutions, the use of possible indicator is methyl orange because it will exist in alkaline form when 99.8 ml of alkali is added and the titration error will be 0.2%, which is negligible error, so it is important to add NaOH solution until the indicator is present completely in the alkaline form. The other indicator used is phenolphthalein with a pH range of 5.5 to 8.5.

For 0.01M solutions, the indicators used are methyl red, bromothymol blue or phenol red.

All the above factors are considered when the reaction takes place in the absence of carbon dioxide. But practically a small quantity of $CO_2$ is present in the solution due to the presence of small amount of carbonate in sodium hydroxide or from atmosphere. This will present equilibrium with carbonic acid and weakens the both side of ionization. It produces a small error when high pH range of indicators are used (pH = more than 5) *For e.g*; phenolphthalein or thymolphthalein. This type of error is eliminated by selecting indicator with a pH range below 5 or boils the acid solution to complete removal of $CO_2$ and continue the titration in cool condition.

2. **Weak acid Vs strong base:** Consider the neutralization of 0.1ml acetic acid with 0.1ml NaOH solution. The pH of the solution at equivalence point is calculated by using the following equation.

$$pH = 1/2\ pKw + \frac{1}{2}\ pKa\ \frac{-1}{2}\ pc$$

$$= 7 + 2.37 - 1/2(1.3) = 8.72$$

For other concentration, we should use the mass equation.

$$K_a = \frac{[H^+][CH_3COO^-]}{[CH_3COOH]} \quad \rightarrow (1)$$

$$pH = \log\frac{(\text{salt})}{(\text{acid})} + pKa \quad \rightarrow (2)$$

The concentration of salt is calculated at any point by using the volume of alkali added. The initial pH of 0.1m acetic acid is calculated from the equation (1) the dissociation of the acid is very small, so it may be neglected.

$$1.82 \times 10^{-5} = [H^+]\ [CH3COO^-]/[CH_3COOH]$$

$$= 1.82 \times 10^{-5} = [H^+]^2 /0.1$$

$$[H^+] = \sqrt{1.82 \times 10^{-6}} = 1.35 \times 10^{-3}$$

$$pH = 2.87.$$

When 50 ml of 0.1ml NaOH solution is added

$$[\text{salt}] = 50 \times 0.1/150 = 3.33 \times 10^{-2}$$

$$[acid] = 50 \times 0.1/150 = 3.33 \times 10^{-2}$$

$$pH = \log(3.33 \times 10^{-2}/3.33 \times 10^{-2}) + 4.74 = 4.74$$

The pH of the other portions of the curve can be calculated similarly. After the equivalence point, the concentration of $[OH^-]$ excess which indicates, the pH of the solution is due to the presence of excess of base. So this region the titration curve will almost coincide with the curve for 0.1M HCl. All the results are indicated in table should attach.

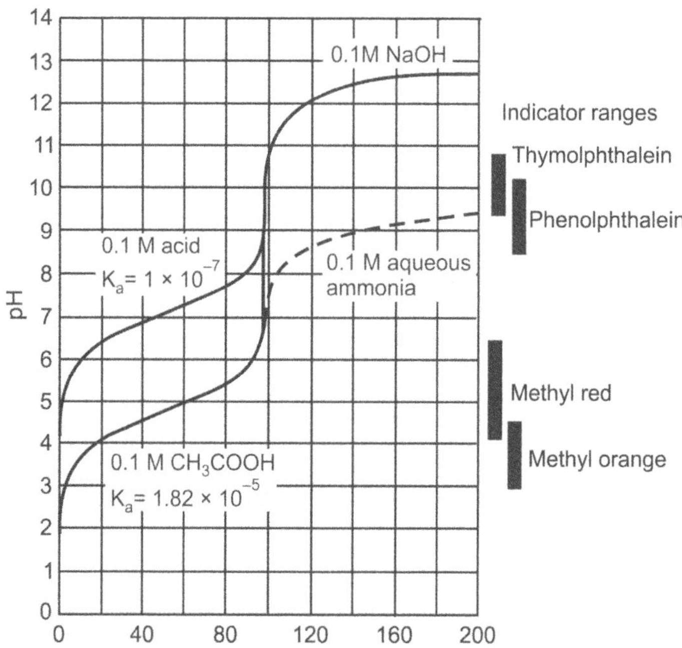


**Fig. 4.3** Calculated curves for weak acid (100 ml 0.1M $CH_3COOH$) Vs strong base (0. 1M NaOH) with range of indicators.
In graph X axis = amount of alkali added (ml), Y axis = pH

The titration indicates that neither methyl orange nor methyl red can be used as an indicator. Phenolphthalein also used but the color change of it takes place from after addition of 92ml of alkali, so it does not produce sharp endpoint, but in thymolphthalein the color change occurs at the pH 9.3-10.5, so it can be used.

3. **Weak base Vs strong acid**: Consider the titration of 0.1M aqueous ammonia with 0.1M HCl. The pH of the solution at the equivalence point is calculated by

$$pH = 1/2pKw - 1/2pKb + 1/2pc.$$

$$= 7 - 2.37 + 1/2(1.3)$$

$$= 5.28$$

For other concentrations the pH may be calculated by using the following equation

$$K_b = [NH_4]^+ [OH]/[NH_3] \qquad \rightarrow(3)$$

$$pOH = \log [salt]/[base] + pK_b \qquad \rightarrow(4)$$

$$pH = pKw - pKb - \log[salt]/[base] \qquad \rightarrow(5)$$

After the equivalence point reached, the solution contains excess of $H^+$ions and hydrolysis of the salt is suppressed, the subsequent pH changes may be assumed with sufficient accuracy due to the excess of acid present .

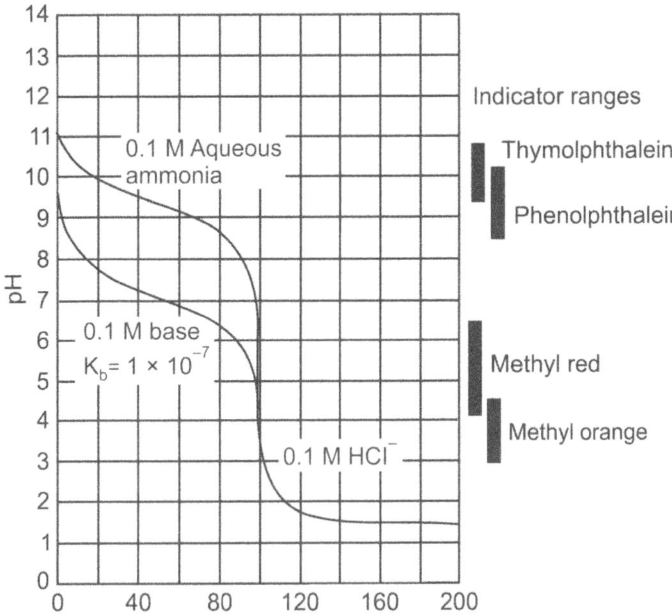


Fig. 4.4 Calculated curves for weak base (100 ml 0.1 M aqueous ammonia) Vs strong acid (0.1 M HCl).
In graph X axis = amount of acid added (ml), Y axis = pH

The indicator used in the titration is neither thymolphthalein nor phenolphthalein. The equivalence point at pH 5-5.3, so the pH indicator used must possess the slight acidic pH (pH = 3 to 6.5) *e.g*: methyl red, methyl orange, bromophenol blue or bromo phenol green.

4. **Weak acid Vs weak base:** Consider the following example. The titration of 0.1M acetic acid Vs 0.M $NH_3$.

   The pH of the solution at equivalence point is calculated by

   $$pH = 1/2pK_w + 1/2pK_a - \tfrac{1}{2}pK_b$$

   $$= 7 + 2.38 - 2.37$$

   $$= 7.1$$

The neutralization curve up to the equivalence point is identical with that using 0.1M NaOH as the base.

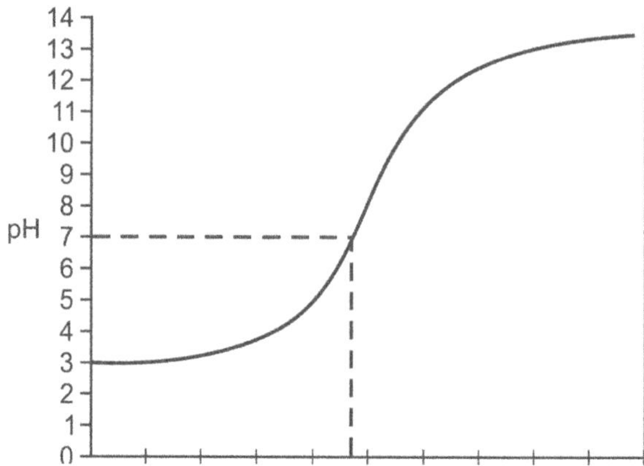


Fig. 4.5 Calculated curves for weak acid (100 ml 0.1M $CH_3COOH$) with Vs weak base (0.1 M aqueous ammonia).
In graph X axis = amount of alkali added (ml), Y axis = pH

For titrations of acetic acid with ammonia solutions, neutral red-methylene blue mixed indicator may be used, but on the whole, it is best to avoid the use of indicators, between titration of weak acid and weak base

## 4.2.2 Non-aqueous Titrations

When the test substance is very weakly acidic or basic or salts of weakly acidic or basic it cannot be titrated in aqueous media, the strength of such substances can be increased by dissolving them in an appropriate non aqueous solvents. Hence these substances are titrated in a non aqueous media. The end point is located by the colour change of the indicator or by potentiometric method.

Non-aqueous titrations are similar to acid base titration in aqueous medium. In aqueous medium acid base neutralization may be regarded as reaction between proton donors (acid) and proton acceptors (base). Whereas in non aqueous medium, it is a reaction between weakly protophilic substances which accept a pair of electrons and highly protophilic substances which provide a pair of electrons in the formation of covalent bonds.

***Applications:*** This method is mainly used for analysis of very weak acids and bases and the salts of weakly acidic or basic substances. Organic acids or bases which are insoluble in water can be made to dissolve in non aqueous solvents and titrated. Many of the organic medicinal agents are either poorly soluble in water or very weakly reactive in water these agents are assayed by this method.

***Types of solvents*:** The solvent used in non-aqueous titrations plays a major role. It should be non toxic in nature. Solvents used in non aqueous titration are classified in to four types according to their self dissociation capacity, dielectric constant and acid base character of solvent.

1. Aprotic solvent
2. Protogenic solvents

3. Protophillic solvent
4. Amphiprotic solvent

1. **Aprotic solvents:** Aprotic solvents are in inert in nature and they have low dielectric constant and do not favour ionization.

   *Example*: Benzene and chloroform

2. **Protogenic solvents:** These are acidic in nature and produces protons. These are having high dielectric constant. They get ionised. The ionic product is less than the ionic product of water.

   *Example*: Acetic acid, Formic acid, Sulphuric acid etc.

3. **Protophillic solvents:** These are basic in nature and accept protons from acids to give solvated protons.

$$\text{Solvent} + \text{HB (acid)} \rightarrow \text{Solvent } H^+ + B^-$$

***Types***: Two types

1. Strongly basic solvent - Stronger ability to accept protons
2. Weakly basic solvent- Weaker ability to accept protons

***Levelling solvent***: A strongly basic solvent accepts the protons from any acid either strong acid or weak acid. This type of solvents are known as levelling solvent and the effect is known as levelling effect, Since it does not differentiate between strong acid or weak acid.

***Differentiating solvents***: A weakly basic solvent accept protons from strong acid only and not from weak acids. These types of solvents are known as differentiating solvents and this effect is known as differentiating effect. These are not used in non aqueous titrations.

Similary, strongly acidic solvents are used as levelling solvents for strong bases and weak bases (they donate protons to strong bases and weak bases equally). So, strongly acidic solvent such as perchloric acid in acetic acid is used in non aqueous titration of weak bases.

***Acidimetry in non aqueous medium:*** The commonly used titrant is standard N/10 perchloric acid solution. Weakly basic substances such as alkali salts of organic acids, amines, amine salts, and heterocyclic nitrogen compounds are analysed. Indicators used are crystal violet, thymol blue, methyl rosaniline chloride. Example: Ephedrine hydrochloride is assayed by this method.

Titrant reacts with the solvent and gets protonated as follows.

$$B + CH_3COOH \rightleftharpoons \underset{\text{Conjugate acid of base}}{BH^+} + \underset{\text{Conjugate base}}{CH_3COO^-}$$

Titration reaction with conjugate base anion may be shown as follows.

$$HClO_4 + CH_3COOH \rightleftharpoons CH_3COOH_2^+ + ClO_4^-$$

So overall reaction may be put follows.

$$CH_3COO^- + CH_3COOH_2^+ \rightleftharpoons 2\ CH_3COOH$$

$$B + HClO_4 \longrightarrow BH^+ + ClO_4^-$$

### Titrants for Titration of Weakly Basic Substances

### Preparation of 0.1 M Perchloric Acid Solutions

Mix 8.5 ml of perchloric acid with 500 ml of anhydrous glacial acetic acid and 25 ml of acetic acid anhydride, cool and add anhydrous glacial acetic acid to produce 1000 ml. Allow the prepared solution to stand for 1day for the excess anhydride to be combined and carry out the determination of water. If the water content exceeds 0.5 percent, add more acetic anhydride. If the solution contains no titratable water, add sufficient water to obtain a content of water between 0.02 percent and 0.5 percent. Allow the solution to stand for 1 day and again titrate the water content. The solution obtained should contain between 0.02 percent and 0.5 percent of water. Standardise the solution in the following manner.

Weigh accurately about 0.35g of potassium hydrogen phthalate, previously powdered lightly and dried 120°C for 2 hours and dissolve it in 50 ml of anhydrous glacial acetic acid. Add 0.1 ml of crystal violet solution and titrate with the perchloric acid solution until the violet colour changes to emerald-green. Perform a blank determination and make any necessary correction.

1 ml of 0.1 M perchloric acid is equivalent to 0.0204042 g of $C_8H_5KO_4$.

### Indicators

| S.No | Indicator | Color change |
|---|---|---|
| 1 | 0.5% Crystal violet in glacial acetic acid | violet to blue |
| 2. | 0.1% Quinaldine red | Pink to color less |
| 3. | 0.2% Alpha-naphthol benzene in glacial acetic acid | Blue green to orange |
| 4. | 0.5% Oracet blue in glacial acetic acid | Blue to purple |

***Alkalimetry in non aqueous medium:*** Commonly used titrant is sodium methoxide or lithium methoxide. Other titrants are sodium amino methoxide (which is the strongest base) and sodium triphenylmethane which is used for weakly acidic compounds like phenol and pyrroles. Indicators used are azo violet, *ortho* nitroaniline and thymol blue (Table 4.2). Example: Assay of benzoic acid.

Titrant reacts with the acid as follows.

$$C_6H_5COOH + CH_3ONa \longrightarrow C_6H_5COONa + CH_3OH$$

$$\underset{\text{Dimethyl formamide (DMF)}}{C_6H_5COOH + HCON(CH_3)_2} \rightleftharpoons \underset{\text{Protonated DMF}}{HCO\overset{+}{N}H(CH_3)_2} + C_6H_5COO^-$$

Reaction between solvated proton and methoxy ion may be shown as follows.

$$HCO\overset{+}{N}H(CH_3)_2 + CH_3O^- \rightarrow HCON(CH_3)_2 + CH_3OH$$

### Preparation of 0.1 m Lithium Methoxide Solution

Dissolve in small portions of 0.7 g of freshly cut lithium in 150 ml of anhydrous methanol, cooling the flask during the addition of the metal. When reaction is complete add sufficient toluene to produce 1000 ml. If cloudiness of precipitation occurs, add sufficient anhydrous methanol to clarify the solution. Standardise the solution immediately before use in the following manner.

Weigh accurately about 0.25 g of benzoic acid; dissolve in 25 ml of dimethylformamide. Titrate with lithium methoxide solution, using quinaldine red solution as an indicator and protecting the solution form atmospheric carbon dioxide throughout the titration. Perform a blank determination and make any necessary correction.

1 ml of 0.1 M lithium methoxide is equivalent to 0.01221 g of $C_7 H_6 O_2$

### Preparation of 0.1 M Sodum Methoxide Solution

Cool 150 ml of anhydrous methanol in ice water and add, in small portions, about 2.5 g of freshly cut sodium. When the metal has dissolved, add sufficient toluene, previously dried over sodium wire, to produce 1000 ml. Standardise the solution in the following manner immediately before use.

Weigh accurately about 0.4 g of benzoic acid, dissolve in 80 ml of dimethylformamide, add 0.15 ml of thymolphthalein solution and titrate with sodium methoxide solution to a blue end-point. Protect the solution from atmospheric carbon dioxide throughout the titration. Perform a blank determination and make any necessary correction.

1 ml of 0.1 M sodium methoxide is equivalent to 0.01221 g of $C_7 H_6O_2$.

### Preparation of 0.1m Tetrabutyl Ammonioum Hydroxide Solution

Dissolve 40 g of tetrabutylammonium iodide in 90 ml of dehydrated methanol in glass – stoppered flask. Place in an ice bath, add 20 g of powered sliver oxide, insert the stopper and agitate vigoursly for 1hours. Centrifuge a few ml, and test the supernatant liquid for iodides, if the test is positive, 30 minutes with intermittent agitation. When all of the iodide has reacted, filter through fine sintered – glass filter. Rinse the flask and filter three quantities, each of 50 ml of anhydrous toluene. Flush the solution for 10 minutes with dry, carbon dioxide- free nitrogen. Stored and protected from carbon dioxide and moisture, and discard after 60 days. Standardise the solution in the following manner immediately before use.

Weigh accurately about 0.4 g of benzoic acid, dissolve in 80 ml of dimethylformamide, add a few drops of a 1 percent w/v solution of thymol blue in dimethylforamamide and titrate with the tetrabutyl ammonium hydroxide solution to a blue end point. Protect the solution from atmospheric carbon dioxide throughout the titration. Perform a blank titration also.1 ml of 0.1 M tetrabutyl ammonium hydroxide is equivqlent to 0.01221 g of $C_7H_6O_2$.

Table 4.2 Indicators for non-aqueous titrations

| S.No | Indicator | Colour change |
|---|---|---|
| 1. | 0.1% Quinaldine red in methanol | Pink to colorless |
| 2. | Thymol blue-1% solution in dimethyl formamide | Yellow to blue |
| 3. | 0.2% Azoviolet in benzene | Orange via pink to blue. |

*Example*: Following pharmaceutical preparations are assayed by non-aqueous method.

| S.No | Name of drug | Solvent used | Indicator |
|---|---|---|---|
| 1. | Adrenaline | Glacial acetic acid | crystal violet |
| 2. | Bisacodyl | Glacial acetic acid | 1 -Naphthol benzene solution. |
| 3. | Chlorpheniramine Maleate | Glacial acetic acid | - |
| 4. | Codeine phosphate | Glacial acetic acid | crystal violet |
| 5. | Metformin | anhydride HCOOH | crystal violet |
| 6. | Verapamil | Glacial acetic acid+mercuric acetate | crystal violet |

### 4.2.3 Oxidation Reduction (Redox) Titrations

Oxidation refers to the process in which loss of one or more electrons and reduction refers process in which gain of one or more electrons by atoms or ions.

In oxidation reduction (called as redox) reactions, electrons are transferred from reducing agent to the oxidizing agent. The oxidizing agent gains electrons and gets reduced and the reducing agent loses electrons and is oxidized to oxidation state. Oxidation of reducing agent and reduction of an oxidizing agent happens simultaneously.

The commonly used titrants in these oxidizing and reducing titrations are as follows:

- ✓ Potassium permanganate
- ✓ Iodine
- ✓ Potassium iodate
- ✓ Ceric ammonium sulphate
- ✓ Sodium thiosulphate
- ✓ Titanous sulphate or chloride.
- ✓ Potassium dichromate etc.

Redox titrations involve the following methods.

**(i)** ***Iodimetry and iodometry method:*** Estimation of reducing substances by using standard iodine is called iodimetry. Iodine is an oxidizing agent. Strong reducing agents such as sodium thiosulphate, stannous chloride react with iodine even in acidic solutions.

$$I_2 + 2\,Na_2S_2O_3 \longrightarrow 2\,NaI + Na_2S_4O_6$$

Sodium thiosulphate — Sodium tetrathionate

The above reaction is used for estimating an oxidizing agent which reacts with KI to set free an equivalent quantity of iodine. This indirect estimation of oxidizing agent which liberate iodine and determination of the liberated iodine is called as iodometry. Example: Assay of chlorinated lime and copper sulphate.

The indicator used in titrating iodine solution with sodium thiosulphate is starch solution. It produces blue coloured adsorption complex with free iodine.

**Example:** ***Assay of Chlorinated lime:*** It is assayed by **Iodometry method** of titration (also called **Redox titration**) to find out the "available chlorine".

In this assay the substance is treated with acetic acid in presence of excess of potassium iodide and titrated with sodium thiosulphate, using starch mucilage as an indicator. End point is the disappearance of blue colour.

In this assay when the substance is reacted with acetic acid in presence of excess of potassium iodide, available chlorine is liberated from chlorinated lime and it displaces equal amount of iodine from potassium iodide. The liberated iodine is determined by titrating with N/10 sodium thiosulphate using starch mucilage as an indicator. End point is the disappearance of blue colour. During this titration iodine is reduced to sodium iodide and sodium thiosulphate is oxidized to sodium tetrathionate. As the oxidation and reduction takes place simultaneously this is called Redox titration. The chemical reactions of this assay are shown below.

$$Ca(OCl)Cl + 2\,CH_3COOH \longrightarrow (CH_3COO)_2Ca + HOCl + HCl$$

(Chlorinated lime)

$$HOCl + HCl \rightleftharpoons Cl_2 + H_2O$$

$$Cl_2 + 2KI \longrightarrow I_2 +_2 KCl$$

$$I_2 +_2 Na_2S_2O_3 \longrightarrow 2\,NaI + Na_2S_4O_6$$

Sodium thiosulphate — Sodium tetrathionate

**(ii)** ***Permanganometry method:*** It is a type of redox titration in this assay, the test sample is diluted with 1M sulphuric acid and the solution is titrated against potassium permanganate. Potassium permanganate is acting as a self indicator. End point is the appearance of permanent pale pink colour.

During this assay, sulphuric acid first reacts with potassium permanganate and liberate nascent oxygen. Thus the liberated nascent oxygen oxidizes the test substance. After the completion of this reaction, addition of potassium permanganate remains in the flask and its colour is retained i.e., permanent pale pink colour. As the oxidation and reduction takes place simultaneously this is called Redox titration.

**Example:** ***Assay of hydrogen peroxide:*** In this assay the substance is diluted with 1M sulphuric acid and the solution is titrated against potassium permanganate. Potassium permanganate is acting as a self indicator. End point is the appearance of permanent pale pink colour.

During this assay, sulphuric acid first reacts with potassium permanganate and liberate nascent oxygen. Thus the liberated nascent oxygen oxidizes the hydrogen peroxide to water and oxygen. After the completion of this reaction, addition of potassium permanganate remains in the flask and its colour is retained i.e., permanent pale pink colour. As the oxidation and reduction takes place simultaneously this is called Redox titration. The chemical reactions of this assay are shown below.

$$2\,KMnO_4 + 3\,H_2SO_4 \longrightarrow K_2SO_4 + 2\,MnSO_4 + 3\,H_2O + 5(O)$$

$$5\,H_2O_2 + 5(O) \longrightarrow 5\,H_2O + 5\,O_2$$

The reaction can also be written as follows

$$2\,KMnO_4 + 3\,H_2SO_4 + 5\,H_2O_2 \longrightarrow K_2SO_4 + 2\,MnSO_4 + 8\,H_2O + 5\,O_2$$

**(iii)** ***Ceriometry method:*** It is type of Redox titration, in this assay sample is dissolved in water and 1M sulphuric acid and titrated with 0.1M ceric ammonium nitrate or sulphate using suitable indicator (Table 4.3).

## Redox Titrations

### Titration involving Ceric Ammonium Sulphate

### Advantages of Ceric Ammonium Sulphate

1. In acidic solution, reduction of ceric ion takes place as follows.

$$Ce^{4+} + e^- \rightleftharpoons Ce^{3+}$$

   So, the equivalent weight is equal to molecular weight.
2. Ceric ammonium sulphate solutions are more stable for long time and not affected by heat and light.
3. This is a versatile oxidizing agent and can be used for all types of determinations.

### Preparation of 0.1M Ceric Ammonium Sulphate

Dissolve 65 g of Ceric ammonium sulphate, with gentle heat, in a mixture of 30 ml of $H_2SO_4$ and 500 ml of water. Cool, filter the solution if turbid and dilute to 1000 ml with water.

### Standardisation:

Weigh accurately about 0.2 g of arsenic trioxide previously dried at 105 °C for 1 hr and transfer into a conical flask. Wash the inner walls of the flask with 25 ml of 8% w/v solution of sodium hydroxide, add 100 ml of water and mix. Add 30 ml of dilute $H_2SO_4$, 0.15 ml of arsenic acid solution. Titrate the resulting solution slowly with ceric ammonium sulphate solution using ferroin sulphate solution as an indicator. End point is the color change from pink to pale blue.

1 ml of 0.1M ceric ammonium sulphate is equivalent to 0.004946 g of $AS_2O_3$.

**Applications of Redox Titrations using Ceric Ammonium Sulphate**

1. Assay of paracetamol tablet, ascorbic acid tablet, ferrous sulphate tablet, iron-dextran injection etc.

***Redox Titration using Titanous Chloride as Titrant*:** Titanous chloride is a strong or powerful reducing agent. The choice of indicator used is depend on the $E^o$ value i.e., $Ti^{4+}/Ti^{3+}$ 0.06v).

***Preparation and Standardization of 0.1M Titanous Chloride Solution***: Add 103 ml of titanous chloride solution to 100ml of HCl and dilute to 1000ml with recently boiled and cooled water, mix well. Standardize the solution immediately before use.

***Standardization of 0.1N Titanous Chloride Solution*:** Place an accurately measured volume of about 30 ml of standardized 0.1M ferric ammonium sulphate in a conical flask and pass in a rapid stream of $CO_2$ until all the air has been removed. Add the titanous chloride solution from a burette and in an atmosphere of $CO_2$ until near the calculated endpoint, then add 5ml of ammonium thiocyanate solution and continue the titration until the solution is colorless. Each ml of 0.1N Ferric ammonium sulphate is equivalent to 0.01543gm of titanous chloride.

**Types of titanus chloride titrations**:

1. Direct titrations
2. Back titrations.

1. **Direct titrations:** Azodyes, Ferric salts and quinones can be assayed by this method.
2. **Back titrations:** A know excess standard (KES) of 0.1N $TiCl_3$ is added and the excess unreacted reagent (EUR) is back titrated with ferric ammonium sulphate using ammonium thiocyanate as an indicator.

This method is used when the compounds which are not easily reduced. *Example*: Drugs with $NO_2$ groups and NO (Assay of chloramphenicol, metronidazole) compounds are assayed by this method.

***Redoxindicators*:** Indicators which are used to detect the endpoint in redox titration is known as redox indicators. There are two types of redox indicators.

1. General redox indicators.
2. Specific redox indicators.

### Selected Oxidation/Reduction Indicators

| S.No | Indicators | Color oxidized | Reduced | $E_0$ | Conditions |
|---|---|---|---|---|---|
| 1 | 5-Nitro-1,10 phenanthroline iron (II) complex. | Pale-blue | Red-violet | +1.25 | 1M $H_2SO_4$. |
| 2 | 2,3'-Diphenylamine dicarboxylic acid | Blue- violet | Colorless | +1.12 | 7-10M $H_2SO_4$. |
| 3 | Erioglamin A | Blue red | Yellow green | +0.98 | 0.5M $H_2SO_4$ |
| 4 | Diphenylamine sulphonic acid | Violet | Colorless | +0.76 | Dilute acid |
| 5 | Phenosafranine | Red | Colorless | +0.28 | 1M acid |
| 6 | *p*-Ethoxy chrysoidine | Yellow | Red | +0.76 | Dilute acid |
| 7 | 1,10-Phenanthroline iron(II) complex | Pale blue | Red | +1.11 | 1M $H_2SO_4$ |

**Example:** ***Assay of ferrous sulphate*:** In this assay sample is dissolved in water and 1M sulphuric acid and titrated with a 0.1M ceric ammonium nitrate using ferroin sulphate as indicator. End point is the disappearance of red colour.

**Table 4.3** Indicators for oxidation-reduction titrations

| Indicator | Color change | |
|---|---|---|
| | Oxidized form | Reduced form |
| Ferroin | Pale blue | Red |
| Methylene blue | Blue | Colour less |

**(iv)** ***Dichromate titrations:*** It is a type of Redox titration, in this assay sample is dissolved in water and 1M sulphuric acid and titrated with 0.1M potassium dichromate solution using suitable indicator.

### 4.2.4 Precipitation Titrations

Titrations involving precipitation of compounds are known as precipitation titrations. Metallic halides generally assayed by this method by titrating with sliver nitrate. These titrations are also termed as argentometric processes.

**Example:** ***Assay of sodium chloride:*** It is assayed by **Precipitation method** of (Back) titration by modified Volhard's method.

In this assay the substance is dissolved in water and acidified with nitric acid and to this a Known Excess Standard solution of (KES) silver nitrate added and silver chloride is precipitated. To this nitrobenzene added and the excess unreacted silver nitrate is back titrated against 0.1N ammonium thiocyanate. Ferric ammonium sulphate (Ferric alum) is used as an indicator. End point is the appearance of brick red colour.

During this assay, sodium chloride reacts with silver nitrate and silver chloride is formed. After completion of this reaction, the Excess Unreacted silver nitrate is determined by titrating against ammonium thiocyanate. After the completion of this reaction, further addition of ammonium thiocyanate reacts with the indicator ferric ammonium sulphate and yield brick red colour ferric thiocyanate, which is the end point. Nitrobenzene used in this assay prevent interaction of silver chloride with ferric thiocyanate. As the test substance is converted to a precipitate during this assay this is called precipitation method. The chemical reactions of this assay are shown below.

$$NaCl + AgNO_3 \longrightarrow AgCl\downarrow + NaNO_3$$

$$AgNO_3 + NH_4SCN \longrightarrow AgSCN\downarrow + NH_4NO_3$$

Three different methods are used to detect end point in argentometric titration using different visual indicators.

1. ***Mohr's method:*** It is developed by Mohr in 1856 using potassium chromate as an indicator. This method involves the titration of silver nitrate against halides (like sodium chloride) by using 2 percent solution of potassium chromate indicator. End point is the appearances of a brick red precipitate or colour due to the formation of silver chromate.

$$2\,Ag^+ \quad CrO_4^{2-} \longrightarrow \underset{\text{(Brick Red)}}{Ag_2CrO_4\downarrow}$$

***Limitations of this method:***

1. Solution to be titrated should be neutral because silver chromate is soluble in acid.
2. The barium sulphate is more insoluble than silver chromate and will be precipitated earlier hence for titration of chlorides and bromides of barium the solution is treated with a slight excess of potassium sulphate.
3. This method is also not suitable for iodides because of adsorption difficulties and also difficulty in detecting the end point.

2. ***Volhard's method:*** It was designed by Volhard's in 1874 for the estimation of silver by titrating with ammonium thiocyanate solution in the presence of ferric salt as indicator. Later it was used for chlorides, bromides and other analysis. In this assay the substance is dissolved in water and acidified with nitric acid and to this a Known Excess Standard (KES) silver nitrate added and the precipitated silver chloride is filtered. The filtrate and washings are combined, ferric alum added as an indicator and the excess unreacted (EUR) silver nitrate is back titrated against 0.1N ammonium thiocyanate. During this assay, chloride reacts with silver nitrate and forms silver chloride. After completion of this reaction, the Excess Unreacted silver nitrate is determined by titrating against ammonium thiocyanate. After the completion of this reaction, further addition of ammonium thiocyanate reacts with the indicator ferric ammonium sulphate and yield brick red colour ferric thiocyanate, which is the end point.

***Modified Volhard's method:*** In this method, nitrobenzene is used which does not allow the interaction of a silver chloride with ferric thiocyanate and hence avoids the need for filtration of silver chloride.

3. ***Fajan's method:*** Method was introduced by Fajan in 1923, adsorption indicators used for the detection of end point. At end point the indicator gets adsorbed by the precipitate and during the process of adsorption a change in colour of the indicator takes place results in a substance of different colour. Hence they are termed as adsorption indicators.

   Commonly used adsorption indicators are mentioned below (Table 4.4).

   1. Fluorescein - It gives sudden change of white precipitate in greenish yellow medium to distinctly red at the end point.
   2. Dichloro fluorescein - Yellowish green to red at the end point.

**Table 4.4** Indicators for precipitation titrations

| Indicators | Color change | Use |
|---|---|---|
| Fluorescein | Yellow green to pink | $Cl^-$, $Br^-$ with $Ag^+$ |
| Dichloro fluorescein | Yellow green to red | $Cl^-$, $Br^-$ with $Ag^+$ |

### 4.2.5 Complexometric Titrations

Titrations involving metal ions forming complex with some of the reagents are called Complexometric titrations and are stable.

In this titration, metal ion accepts electrons and the ligand (species which donates electrons are called ligand) donates electrons. Most of metals form complexes with ligands. The ligand molecule has at least one lone pair of electrons (oxygen, nitrogen or sulphur) by which co-ordinate linkage with metal ions happens. The number of ligand molecules which can be associated with a metal ion is called the co-ordination number of the metal.

Ligands can be classified according to the number of sites present in them through which co-ordination linkage with metal ion occurs. If a single site is present in a ligand it is called unidentate (e.g., cyanide ion ($CN^-$)), if more than 2 or 3 sites are present it is called multidentate ligand (e.g., Ethylene Diamine Tetra Acetic Acid (EDTA) or disodium EDTA).

***Complexometric titrations using EDTA:*** Ethylene Diamine Tetra Acetic Acid (EDTA) and its disodium salt form complex with versatile metal ions. EDTA is hexadentate ligand, the complexes formed are of chelate type.

The structure of disodium EDTA and the complex metal ion (zinc) are shown below.

$Zn^{2+}$ + $NaOOCH_2C$ / $HOOCH_2C$ > N–$CH_2$–$CH_2$–N < $CH_2COONa$ / $CH_2COOH$

Disodium EDTA

↓

$NaOOCH_2C$, $H_2C$, N, N, $CH_2COONa$, $CH_2$, $Zn^{2+}$, O=C, O, O, C=O

Zinc-EDTA Complex

**Types of EDTA Titrations**

The most important procedures used for the titrations of metal with EDTA are as follows:

**(i) Direct titrations:** To the solution of the metal ion to be determined, added buffer and titrated directly with standard EDTA solution using suitable indicator.

**Example:** ***Assay of magnesium oxide heavy:*** In this assay the substance is dissolved in hydrochloric acid, to this ammonia-ammonium chloride solution is added as buffer solution and it is then titrated against 0.05M disodium Ethylene Diamine Tetra Acetate (EDTA) using mordant black II mixture as an indicator. End point is the disappearance of pink colour.

In this assay magnesium ions of heavy magnesium oxide reacts with disodium EDTA, whereby the complexation takes place. As the magnesium ions forms complex with disodium EDTA in this assay, it is called as complexometry method of titration. The chemical reactions of this assay are shown above.

**(ii) Back titration:** Many times direct titration may not be possible due to any of the following reason:

(a) It may not be possible to keep the metal in solution because of too high pH.

(b) The rate of formation of the EDTA complex of the metal may be too slow.

(c) There may be no indicator available which gives a suitable colour reaction.

(d) The metal ion may not form a sufficiently stable complex with the indicator.

In the back titration, a Known Excess Standard (KES) of EDTA is added. Then the excess unreacted EDTA is determined by titrating with a suitable salt (zinc sulphate or lead nitrate) solution.

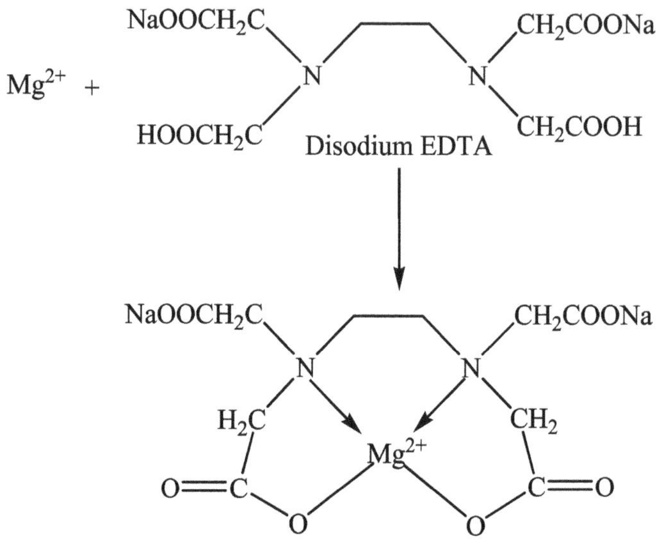

$Mg^{2+}$ + Disodium EDTA ($NaOOCH_2C$, $HOOCH_2C$ on one N; $CH_2COONa$, $CH_2COOH$ on the other N) → Magnesium-EDTA Complex

Magnesium-EDTA Complex

**Example:** ***Assay of aluminium hydroxide gel:*** In this assay the substance is dissolved in hydrochloric acid by warming, to this Known Excess Standard (KES) 0.05N disodium Ethylene Diamine Tetra Acetate (EDTA) added and the solution is neutralized with 1N sodium hydroxide using methyl red as an indicator (colour change from red to yellow). To this solution hexamine added as a buffer and xylenol orange as an indicator and titrated against 0.05M lead nitrate. End point is the appearance of violet colour due to the formation of lead-xylenol orange complex.

In this assay aluminium ions of aluminium hydroxide reacts with disodium EDTA, whereby the complexation takes place, after this reaction, the excess unreacted (EUR) disodium EDTA is determined by titrating with lead nitrate. The indicator is colour less before complexation and change into violet colour due to the formation of lead-xylenol orange complex. As the aluminium ions forms complex with disodium EDTA in this assay, it is called as complexometry method of titration. The chemical reactions of this assay are shown above.

**(iii) Displacement or substitution titrations:** Adopted for metal ions that do not react (or react unsatisfactorily) with a metal indicator or for metal ions which form EDTA complexes that are more stable than those of other metals such as magnesium and calcium.

**Example:** To the solution of calcium salt ammonia-ammonium chloride buffer is added. Now to this a standard known volume of magnesium salt is added. In the reaction stable calcium EDTA complex is formed and magnesium ions are liberated which may be titrated with a standard EDTA solution.

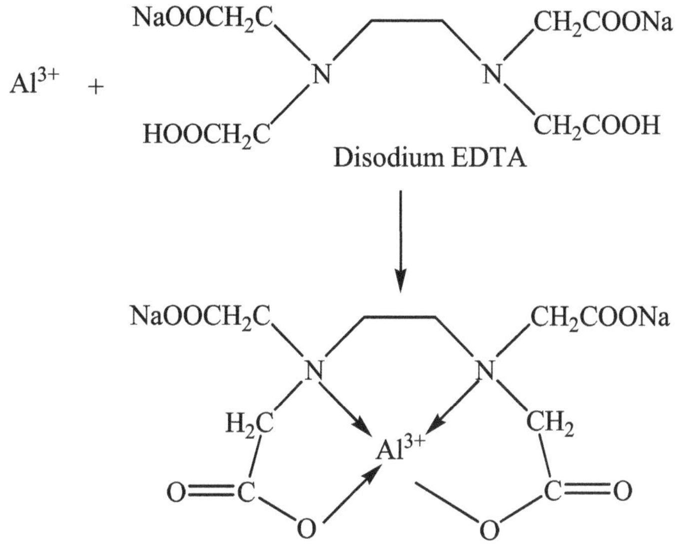

$Al^{3+}$ + Disodium EDTA ($NaOOCH_2C$, $HOOCH_2C$, $CH_2COONa$, $CH_2COOH$) → Aluminium-EDTA Complex

Disodium EDTA

Aluminium-EDTA Complex

***Indirect or residual titrations:*** In the residual titration method excess of standard solution of EDTA is added to the sample then pH is adjusted for back titration with metal ion solution (zinc sulphate) using an indicator which is sensitive to titrant. The metal under analysis remains complexed with EDTA and does not interfere with EDTA complexation.

**(iv)** ***Alkalimetric titration:*** When a solution of disodium EDTA is added to a solution containing metallic ion complexes are formed with liberation of two equivalents of hydrogen. The hydrogen ions thus set free can be titrated with a standard solution of a base using an acid base indicator.

**(v)** ***Miscellaneous methods:*** A number of anions have been determined indirectly with EDTA by reactions based upon precipitation and complex formation with selected cations. Halogens are determined by precipitating as the silver halide, the latter dissolves in a solution of nickel cyanide to form an equivalent amount of free nickel ions which are then titrated rapidly with standard EDTA solution using murexide indicator.

***Metal ion indicators:*** They give one colour in the presence of metal ions and a different colour in the absence of metal ions or in a free state. Solochorme black T, mordant black T, variamine blue, murexide etc., are some metal indicators which are used in titrations (Table 4.5).

**Table 4.5** Indicators for complexometric titrations

| Indicators | pH range | Color change |
|---|---|---|
| Murexide | 10-11 | Yellow to blue (Ni, Co)<br>Red to blue violet (Ca) |
| Eriochrome black T | 10 | Red to blue |
| Xylenol orange | 1-2<br>4-6 | Red to lemon (Zn)<br>Red to yellow (Pb, Mn, Ni) |

### 4.2.6 Diazotization Titrations

Aromatic primary amino group containing compounds are assayed by this method, based on its reaction with nitrous acid (generated *in situ* by the reaction of sodium nitrite and hydrochloric/sulphuric acid) to form diazonium salt. Many of the simple aromatic primary amino compounds are determined quantitatively by titrating with sodium nitrite solution which is required to bring about their conversion into diazonium salts quantitatively.

In this method, a weighed amount of a substance (aromatic amino compound) is dissolved in dilute hydrochloric acid and solution is cooled below 15 °C and the solution is titrated against standard sodium nitrite. After the completion of the diazotization reaction with the sample the excess addition of the sodium nitrite is determined by removing the drops of the titrating solution and spotting them on a starch iodide paper. The immediate appearance of a blue colour on the paper indicates the end point. Determination of the end point by using starch iodide paper has some difficulty, which can be overcome by adopting potentiometric end point determination.

## 4.3 GRAVIMETRIC ANALYSIS

In this method, the test sample is converted in the form of insoluble compound of known composition. Then it is filtered, washed to make it free from bye products, dried and weighed as such or ignited to leave a residue of some other compound which is then weighed.

Gravimetric analysis involves the following experimental steps, 1. Precipitation, 2. Filtration and Washing, 3. Drying or ignition, 4.Weighing.

Gravimetric analysis is useful in the estimation of aluminium from alum, magnesium sulphate, sodium sulphate, silver nitrate, lead acetate, zinc sulphate.

**Various important steps involved in Gravimetric Analysis**

1. Sampling
2. Preparation of solution or dissolution
3. Precipitation and testing the completeness of precipitation
4. Digestion or ageing of precipitate
5. Filtration

6. Washing
7. Drying or ignition of precipitate
8. Weighing
9. Calculations

1. **Sampling:** It is important one to take a representative sample correctly to ensure that the results obtained are accurate. The amount of the sample needed for quantitative analysis also small in size.
2. **Dissolution:** Transfer the required amount of sample in to a beaker and add sufficient water to the sample to get a clear solution. Proper adjustment of solution conditions before precipitation may prevent the interferences. If the sample is soluble in acids or alkalis, the reaction proceeds with evolution gases. The reaction is allowed to continue to ceases the complete evolution of gases. Heating is needed for dissolution, heat the solution on water bath or heating mantles.
3. **Precipitation:** It is generally carried out in resistant glass beaker with slow addition of precipitant with continuous stirring. The reaction should be carried out in hot solution. A small excess of precipitant is added, if large excess of precipitant is added results in increase the solubility of the precipitate. Boiling solution of the sample should not be used in order to avoid the losses due to spattering.

   **Selection of precipitant or precipitating agent:** Selection of proper precipitant depends upon the specificity of the reagent.

   **Ideal characteristics of Precipitants**

   (a) It should be easily react with the sample.
   (b) The precipitate obtained is easily filtered and washable one.
   (c) It should be free from impurities.
   (d) The precipitate should have the proper and known composition after drying.

   **Testing of completeness of precipitation:** Before filtration, it is always necessary to check the completeness of precipitation. It is done by adding a few drops of precipitants through the sides of the beaker wall carefully to the solution with settled precipitate. If no turbidity is produced on the edge, indicates that the complete precipitation occurred.
4. **Digestion or ageing of precipitate:** Digestion is used to increase the purity as well as the rate of filtration of precipitate. It is generally carried out at higher temperature to increase the rate of reaction but some cases it is done at room temperature.
5. **Filtration:** By using this process the formed precipitate is separated from the mother liquor. Several kinds of filtering media are used for this purpose. They are

   (a) Filter paper.
   (b) Filter pulp.
   (c) Filter mats.
   (d) Permanent porous filter discs.

**(a) Filter paper:** In gravimetric analysis, filter paper with low ash content is used. These are available in different degree of porosities, generally in three degree of porosities.

- for coarse and gelatinous particles
- for medium particles
- for very fine particles

Rate of filtration depends upon the degree of porosities. In the above, speed of filtration is fast in the first one, second one is medium and third one is slow. Whatmaan filter paper is normally used for filtration. They are available in different grades and different pore sizes.

Whatmaan filter paper No: 30, 31, 32 and 52, 54 is used normally and cheap and No.42 filter paper is used for very fine particles and No. 41 is used for gelatinous precipitate.

**(b) Filter Pulp:** Filtration of gelatinous precipitate by using quantitative filter paper is not effective because the pores are clogged by the precipitate. So in this case, filter pulp is used which is prepared by macerating the filter paper pieces with hot distilled water. Sometime Whatmaan filter clipping are also used.

**(c) Filter mats:** Examples for filter mats are as follows .

- **Gooch crucibles**: These are made up of asbestos, porcelain and silica. It is commonly used for precipitate that needs heating up to 250 °C

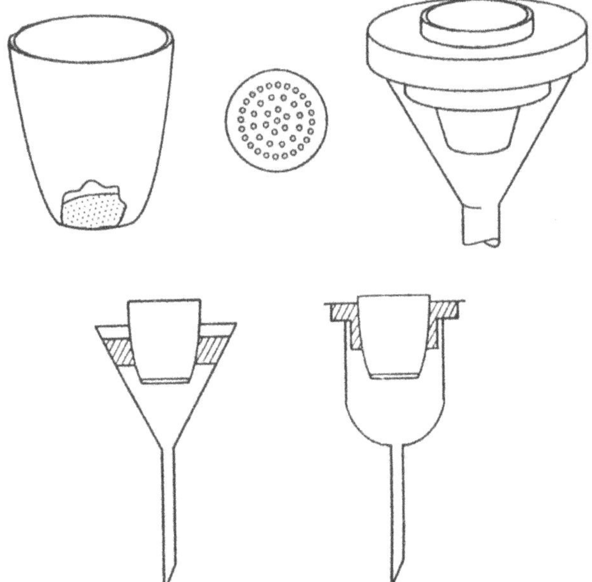

Fig. 4.6 Gooch crucible

- **Munroe Crucibles:** These are made up of platinum.The main advantages are

  1. Resistance to chemicals.

2. Filtration of very finest particles.
3. Heating at very high temperature.
4. Rapid filtration rate.

- **Glass fibre discs:** These are made up of fine borosilicate glass fibres. These are having excellent retention property with increased filtration rate and heating at high temperature up to 500 °C.

**(d)** ***Permanent porous filter discs*:** Examples for this type of filter discs are

- Sintered glass crucibles.
- Silica crucibles.
- Porcelain crucibles.
- **Sintered glass crucibles:** These are made up of resistant glass with porous disc of sintered ground glass fused in the body of the crucible .These can be heated up to 200 °C.

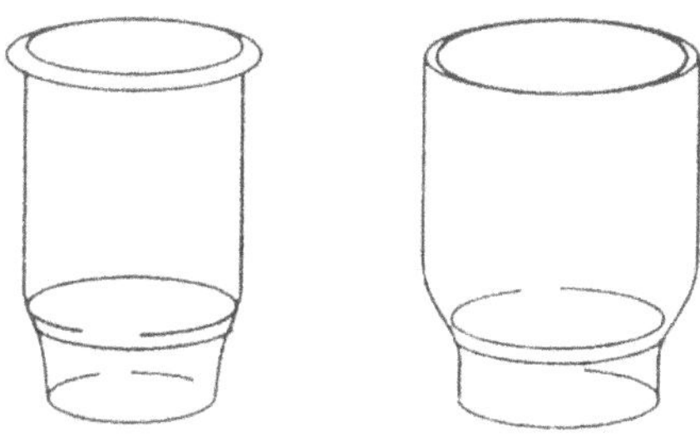

Fig. 4.7 Sintered glass crucible

- **Silica Crucibles:** These are made up of vitriol and used for drying of precipitate upto 1000 °C. These are resistant to chemicals but affected by strong acids, alkalis and phosphate.
- **Porcelain crucibles:** These are glazed in both inside and outside and available in different sizes. They can withstand relatively high temperature. They should not be directly heated in the flame.

**6.** ***Washing*:** After filtration, the impurities and the mother liquor present along with the precipitate should be removed by washing. Many of the precipitates are not washed with water but with ideal washing solution that does not have solvent action on the precipitate but it should dissolve any impurity easily.

**Types of washing solution:**

- **Washing with water:** If the precipitate is more stable, then it should be washed with water.

  *Example*: Washing of $BaSo_4$ with water.

- **Washing with the solution of precipitant:** In this, the precipitate is washed with dilute solution of precipitant.

*Example*: Lead sulphate precipitate is washed by dilute $H_2SO_4$.

- **Washing with electrolyte solution:** The precipitate is converted in to colloidal state by washing with electrolyte solution.

  *Example*: AgCl precipitate is washed with Dilute $HNO_3$.

- **Washing with substances which decreases the hydrolysis of precipitate:** Sometimes, during washing, precipitate undergoes hydrolysis and increases the solubility of the precipitate. It can be prevented by washing the precipitate with the solution which decreases or prevents the hydrolysis.

  *Example*: Washing of magnesium ammonium phosphate with dilute ammonia solution.

7. **Drying and Ignition of the precipitate:** The main purpose of drying a precipitate is to convert it in to possess constant weight of composition. Heating or igniting the precipitate is removing waste and other dissolved electrolytes from washing solution.

   "Heating to constant weight" is an important aspect in gravimetry.

8. **Weighing and calculations:** After drying, the sample is cooled to room temperature by using dessicator and weighed in analytical balance.

   Generally, the calculations are made in terms of percentage

$$\% \text{ A} = \frac{\text{gA (weight of analyte)}}{\text{(g) sample}} \times 100$$

where, gA = weight of residue in gram.

g sample = Amount of sample taken for analysis.

**Pharmaceutical Applications Gravimetric Analysis**

1. Assay of $BaSO_4$
2. Assay of piperazine tablets.
3. Assay of Thioacetazone.
4. Determination of nicotine in pesticides, lactose in milk, cholesterol in cereals and benzaldehyde in almond extract.

**Advantages of Gravimetric Analysis**

1. Gravimetry does not require any standardization or calibration, because the results are directly calculated from the atomic masses and experimental data.
2. It requires less time and less effort since one or two samples can be analysed.

**The gravimetric analysis has the following limitations:**

1. This method is complicated, tedious, time consuming and less precise.
2. The test substance is quantitatively converted to an insoluble product, but still small amount of the sample is dissolved or some colloidal form of the precipitate may pass through the filter.

3. Some of the impurities in the test sample also converted into an insoluble form which may give wrong results.
4. During the final step of heating for removing moisture loss of some precipitate by spurting or cracking may occur.
5. The filter paper used during recovery or other process may sometime add weight which gives wrong results.
6. The method is applicable to few substances, because few of the substance only quantitatively insoluble.

**Example: Assay of barium sulphate:** In this assay, barium sulphate is first reacted with sodium carbonate and potassium carbonate whereby all the barium is converted in to barium carbonate. To the barium carbonate is then added ammonium acetate solution as a buffer and treated with potassium dichromate followed by urea (Urea is added in this assay to avoid the formation of fine diffusible precipitate; the medium must be made alkaline and buffered to complete precipitation of barium chromate). Now all the barium is precipitated as barium chromate. The precipitate of barium chromate is dried and ignited to a constant weight. From the weight of barium chromate the amount of barium sulphate is calculated. As the test substance is converted to a precipitate and sedimented which is used for calculating the actual amount of barium sulphate present this is called Gravimetric assay.

$$2\,BaSO_4 + Na_2CO_3 + K_2CO_3 \longrightarrow 2BaCO_3\downarrow + Na_2SO_4 + K_2SO_4$$

$$2\,BaCO_3 + 4\,HCl \longrightarrow 2\,BaCl_2 + 2\,H_2O + 2\,CO_2\uparrow$$

$$2\,BaCl_2 + K_2Cr_2O_7 + 2\,NH_4OH \longrightarrow 2\,KCl + 2\,NH_4Cl + H_2O + 2BaCrO_4\downarrow$$

## 4.4 INDICATORS

An indicator is any of several chemical species that point out the presence, absence or concentration of another substance or the level of reaction between two or more substances by means of a characteristic colour change in particular point. The common indicators used are litmus paper or phenolphthalein. These are used to determine whether the solution is acidic, basic or neutral. Blue litmus turns red in acid and red litmus turns blue in base.

**Theories of indicators**: There are two types of theories which explain the colour change of indicators according to the pH change.

1. Ostwald's theory
2. Quinonoid theory

**Ostwald's theory:** This theory was first suggested by W. Ostwald. According to this, indicators are very weak acid or weak bases. The color changes of the indicators are due to their structural changes leads to the formation of resonance. This concept is explained by using phenolphthalein indicator and all phthalein indicators. In the presence of acidic solution phenolphthalein is colorless but in the presence of dilute alkali, the lactone ring of

(A) opens to give the triphenyl carbinol (B) which further undergo loss of water molecule to produce the resonating ion (C) which is red in color. If phenolphthalein is treated with excess of concentrated alcoholic alkali the red color disappears due to the formation of the structure (D).

**Quinonoid theory:** This theory was introduced by Bernthsen, Friedlander and Witt. The colour of the indicators are mainly associated with the presence of some unsaturated chromophores like C=C, C=O, N=O and N=N. Further the colour is intensed by auxochromes such as $NH_4$ and OH. Due to the presence of this auxochromes, the colour changes of the indicators are resulting from the transformation of benzenoid form into quinonoid form or vice versa, due to the changes in the hydrogen ion concentration of the solution.

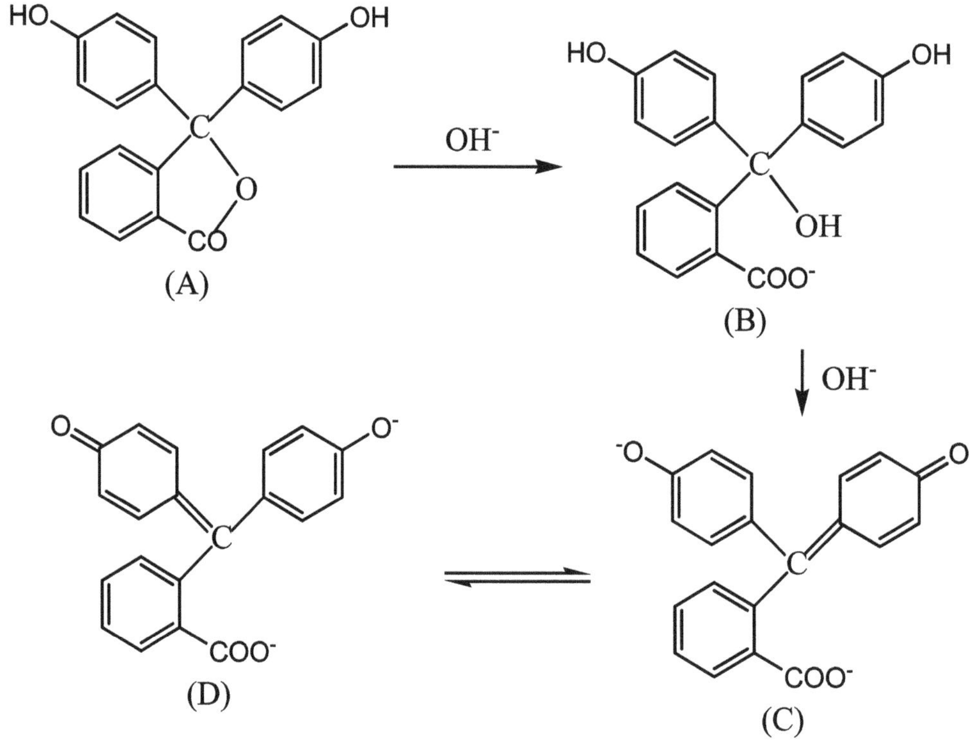

HO OH C O CO (A) $OH^-$ HO OH C OH $COO^-$ (B) $OH^-$

O $O^-$ C $COO^-$ (D) $^-O$ O C $COO^-$ (C)

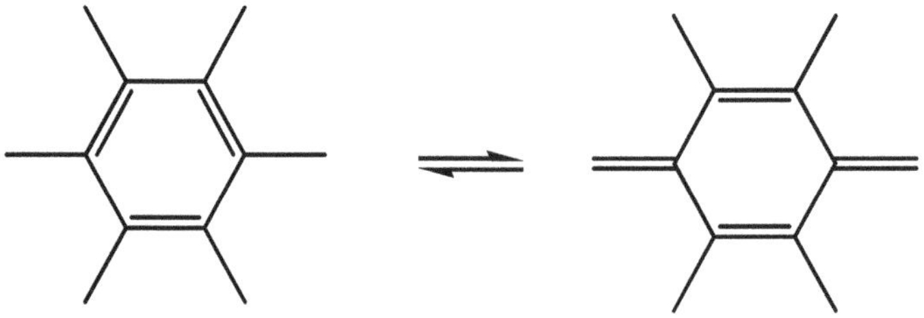

Benzenoid form (colourless) Quinonoid form (coloured)

**Example 1: *p*-Nitro phenol:** In acid solution the color of *p*-nitro phenol is almost colorless due to its benzenoid structure but in alkaline medium the benzenoid structure is converted in to quinonoid form which imparts deep yellow color.

**Example 2: Methyl orange :** In alkaline solution the color of methyl orange is almost yellow color due to the presence of N=N group but in acid medium the azoid structure is converted in to quinonoid form which imparts orange color.

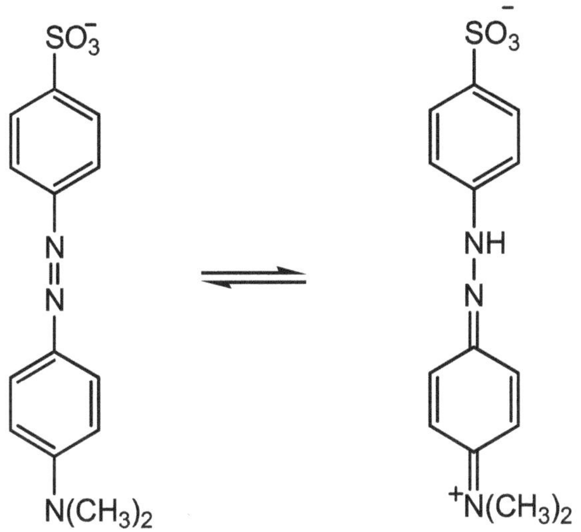

$SO_3^-$ ... $N=N$ ... $N(CH_3)_2$ ⇌ $SO_3^-$ ... $NH-N=$ ... $=N^+(CH_3)_2$

Azoid form, yellow in alkali/neutral solution

Quinonoid form, orange in acid solution

### Types of Indicators

Various types of indicators are used in various type of titrimetric analysis. Table No.4.1 to 4.5 shows the list of indicators suitable for titrimetric analysis and the colorimetric determination of pH.

## PROBABLE QUESTIONS

1. Define the following terms.
   (a) Quantitative analysis (b) Qualitative analysis
   (c) Analytical chemistry
2. What is mean by volumetric analysis and write the importance of it.
3. Explain about the various terms used in volumetric analysis.
4. Define the following terms.
   (a) Primary standard (b) Secondary standard.

5. From the definition of molar concentration, show that moles of solute equal to the molar concentration times the volume of solution in details.
6. Write the terms used to describe the expression of concentration of solute in solutions.
7. Define titrimetric analysis and explain the various terms used.
8. Explain about the different type of titrations.
9. Explain about the acid base titrations with suitable examples.
10. Explain about the complexometry titrations with suitable examples.
11. Write about the significance of titrations.
12. Write about the important conditions needed for the titrimetric analysis.
13. What is mean by back titration and explain with one example.
14. Define the following terms.

    (a) Redox titration (b) End point

    (c) Indicator (d) Equivalence point.
15. What is the principle involved in precipitation method of titration. Briefly explain it with one example.
16. Explain about the followings.

    (a) Volhard's method. (b) Modified Volhard's method.

    (c) Mohr's method. (d) Fajan's method.
17. Write in detail about redox titrations and explain about the different type of redox titrations.
18. Define permanganometry titrations and explain with one example.
19. Explain about ceriometry and dichromate titrations with one example.
20. Explain about the various types of complexometric titrations.
21. Define gravimetric analysis. Write the importance of it.
22. Explain about the principle involved in the gravimetric analysis with one example.
23. Write about the theory of indicators with suitable examples.
24. Explain about the various indicators used in various types of titration.
25. Enumerate the different steps in gravimetric analysis and explain.
26. Define diazotization titrations. What type of drugs determined by this method.
27. Explain about adsorption indicators.

28. Define non-aqueous titrations. Explain about the important conditions of non aqueous titrations.
29. Highlight the importance of iodimetry and iodometry with appropriate official compounds in I.P.
30. What are the limitations of gravimetric analysis?
31. Define errors. Explain the various types of error with example?

CHAPTER 5

# QUALITY CONTROL AND TEST FOR PURITY

## 5.1 INTRODUCTION

When a substance contains an impurity, it is said to be impure. Impurity may be defined as any foreign matter present in the active substance. It is impossible to prepare a substance without any impurity, but can be obtained as maximum as possible pure if we take utmost care in the manufacturing. Some of the substances even though prepared purely, become impure upon storage due to the degradation.

Purity of a chemical or pharmaceutical indicates that the substance is free from any of the foreign matter. It depends upon many of the factors like method of manufacture, type of purification etc. Absolute pure formulations are impossible to obtain, the impurity may arise in the synthesis or in the formulation stage during the process of mixing active ingredient along with other additives or during storage.

The quality of pharmaceutical substance is important in order to obtain the expected therapeutic efficacy. Hence the quality control tests of pharmaceuticals i.e., raw materials and finished products (formulations) are performed as required to ascertain the purity of the pharmaceuticals.

The word **pure,** is a relative term. Hence the Pharmacopoeia prescribed various tests to test the purity of the official drugs and the limit for impurity. The standards required for the chemicals/pharmaceuticals are determined by various factors like method of manufacture, method of formulation of a dosage form, additives used and storage etc. While fixing the standards we must consider the required potency of the drug and accidental contamination or adulteration etc.

### 5.1.1 Impurities found in Drugs and Formulations (Pharmaceuticals)

The following type of impurities may present in the drugs and formulations

1. The impurities which reduce the quality of the active substance.
2. The impurities when present in more than the prescribed limits produce undesired effects. E.g., Lead and Arsenic.

3. The impurity which may be less strength than the active substance, but affect the commercial profit of the product.
4. The impurities which produce technical difficulty in producing formulations.
5. The impurities which affect the colour, odour, taste, appearance etc.
6. The impurities, which make incompatibility with the other substances of the formulation.

## 5.2 SOURCES OF IMPURITIES IN PHARMACEUTICALS

The impurities which occur generally in a particular product are known by batch analysis. For a new substance one should be able to deduce the likely impurities present in the final product. The possible impurities in pharmaceutical products can be easily assumed based on the raw materials used, the method of manufacture and the stability of the product.

The type and intensity of impurity depends upon several factors as mentioned below.

1. **Raw materials used in manufacture:** If the impurities present in the raw materials are not tested and removed, it will be carried through the process and present in the final product. For example small amount of calcium sulphate and magnesium chloride are present in rock salt. Hence sodium chloride prepared by using this source will contain traces of calcium and magnesium.

   Method employed in the manufacture of substances also determines the nature of impurities which may present in it. For example, by the action of sulphuric acid on copper turnings copper sulphate is prepared. Copper turnings contain iron and arsenic as impurities. Hence these impurities may present in negligible or appreciable amount in the final product, if the copper turnings enter as impurity.
2. **Reagents used in the manufacturing process:** During the preparation of pharmaceuticals/chemicals some of the reagents are used. If these reagents are not removed by washing from the product, they may enter into final product. For example, Magnesium hydroxide mixture is prepared by adding sodium hydroxide to magnesium sulphate. The precipitated magnesium hydroxide should be washed well with water to remove the unreacted magnesium sulphate otherwise the magnesium sulphate may present as impurity in the magnesium hydroxide mixture.
3. **Method or process used in manufacture:** Some of the impurities are incorporated by the process of manufacturing. The type and intensity of impurity varies according to the method adopted. For example, some of the drugs are synthesized by a multiple steps through various intermediates. If these intermediates are not removed stage by stage, they react with the reagents or solvents used and produce new types of impurity at the final products.
   (i) ***Reagents used in the process:*** Calcium carbonate is prepared by the reaction of soluble calcium salt and soluble carbonate; hence the product is liable to possess soluble alkali as an impurity.
   (ii) ***Reagents used to remove other impurity:*** In the manufacture of potassium bromide, barium is added to remove the excess sulphate. Hence the product potassium bromide is liable to possess barium as impurity.

(iii) ***Solvents:*** Water is used as a solvent wherever possible, because of cheapest cost. But it contains the ions like $Na^{+}$, $Cl^{-}$, $Mg^{+2}$, $Ca^{+2}$, $SO_4^{-2}$ and $CO_3^{-2}$ which may present in trace amount in final product. These trace amount of ions can be eliminated by using distilled water but the cost effect is more.

(iv) ***Solvents and reagents effect in reaction vessels:*** Most of the organic compounds are prepared by using metallic reaction vessels. Hence the product is liable to have metallic ions as impurity in the final product. By using hard glass containers this problem can be eliminated but the cost effect is heavy.

4. **Chemical process used in the manufacture:** In the process of synthesizing drugs, many of the chemical reactions like nitration, oxidation, reduction, halogenation etc. are performed using various chemicals. These chemicals may also interact with metallic ions present in the water used in the process and hence IP has recommended the permissible limits for the impurities. For example, Potassium iodide is prepared from iodine, which is obtained by the burning of sea weed 'kelp', cyanides are liable to form, when the nitrogenous organic matter is burnt with alkalies. Hence the limit of cyanide in potassium iodide is prescribed.

5. **Contamination during the manufacturing by atmosphere:** Dust particles and some gases like carbon dioxide, sulphur dioxide and hydrogen sulphide are present in the industrial area. Some of the drugs are contaminated with these atmospheric gases and dust particles. For example, Sodium hydroxide when exposed to carbon dioxide, it is converted to sodium carbonate. Hence IP has prescribed the permissible limits for the sodium carbonate in sodium hydroxide as 3%.

6. **Intermediate products in the manufacturing process:** Some of the impurities formed during the preparation of drugs/chemicals. Some of these impurities may be carried into the final product also. Example: Potassium iodide is prepared from iodine and potassium hydroxide. Potassium iodate formed in the first step is liable to present in the final product of potassium iodide. Hence IP has prescribed the test for iodate in potassium iodide.

7. **Defects in the manufacturing process:** Due to the defects in the manufacturing process like incompleteness, imperfect mixing, not maintaining proper temperature and pressure, pH or reaction conditions impurities may arise in the product. For example, calcium chloride is prepared by mixing calcium carbonate to the dilute hydrochloric acid. If the hydrochloric acid is not mixed well with calcium carbonate, some amount of hydrochloric acid remains as impurity in final product. Hence IP has prescribed a test for acidity in calcium chloride.

8. **Manufacturing hazards:** Presence of hazards in a well manufacturing industry also gives rise to impurities. Quality control on manufacturing with adequate analytical techniques can only assures the standards of the product. Manufacturing house should be established in such a way to avoid contamination due to accidental or microbial.

   (i) ***Particulate contamination:*** By a number of ways particulate matters can arise in the product, like accidental inclusion of dirt, glass, metal, porcelain and plastic fragments from the machines used. This type of contamination comes from the raw materials used in the product manufacturing. This is dangerous especially in sterile dosage forms and it can be eliminated by performing clarity test.

(ii) ***Process errors:*** It is serious especially in the manufacture of potent medicaments. It can be analyzed by normal analytical control procedures. Another example is that mixing of granules or powder in solid dosage form is important in the low dosage forms. If it is not mixed well, the medicament in each unit varies drastically and severe toxic effects may be elicited.

(iii) ***Cross contamination:*** The handling of powders and granules in bulk industries creates air borne dust which leads to cross contamination. If it is not controlled, it is dangerous in case of manufacturing units of steroidal and other synthetic hormones.

(iv) ***Microbial contamination:*** Microbial contamination is a serious issue to be considered in ophthalmics and injections. Sterility test should be performed for the materials used and the end product to avoid any untoward effect. Some of the raw materials used are prone to particular microbial contamination (example, Acacia and tragacanth are susceptible for *Salmonellae* contamination). Hence they should be sterilized to prevent the contamination of final product.

(v) ***Packing errors:*** In the packing and labelling section when there is two or more similar size tablets are done. There is a chance of mislabelling of either or both. Handling of such a similar size products in a one place should be avoided and the control procedures be used to guard the possibility of such misshapes.

9. **Storage conditions:** The chemicals/drugs should be stored in different types of containers according to the nature of chemical substance. Some of the containers may react with the chemicals and undergo physical or chemical changes. For example:

   1. Ferrous sulphate is oxidized to insoluble ferric oxide by air and moisture, if it is not stored well and exposed to air.
   2. Chloroform if exposed to air and light, it is decomposed into a poisonous substance called "Phosgene". To avoid the deterioration, all chemicals should be stored in air tight containers made-up of metal or dark glass, avoiding extreme temperatures. If the products are not stored well the following effects may occur.

      (i) ***Filth:*** During the storage some of the products especially products derived from vegetable source may be contaminated with insects, dust etc. hence suitable tests must be performed for filth.

      (ii) ***Chemical instability:*** During the storage, due to the chemical incompatibility impurity may arise in the product. This type decomposition catalyzed by light, air, oxygen, water vapour, carbon dioxide etc. Hence storage should be designed based on the knowledge of chemical nature of the products. For example if a substance affected by light it should be stored in an opaque container. If the product is susceptible for oxidation, suitable anti oxidants like Butylated Hydroxy Anisole (BHA), Butylated Hydroxy Toluene (BHT) etc are added before packing into the product.

(iii) ***Reaction with container:*** The reaction between contents and container liable to produce hazard metal surface used for creams and ointments tend to react. Example, Metal tubes must not be used for packing salicylic acid ointment. Hence the container or closure used to pack the product must be free from any reaction to avoid the creation of any impurity.

(iv) ***Physical change:*** It can be observed without any tests. Physical changes like agglomeration, cracking of emulsion, caking of suspension particles may affect availability of active medicament and in turn the potency. It happens due to light, heat or any chemical change.

(v) ***Temperature:*** The physical or chemical change of the drug is influenced by the temperature. The ointments, pastes and creams etc must be prepared in the containers which maintain its consistency in this temperature condition.

10. **Decomposition of the product during storage:** During storage the products may undergo decomposition. In presence of air, light, or oxygen the effect will be more. The decomposed product become impure and affects the potency, sometimes produces toxicity. Decomposition can avoided based on the chemical knowledge of the chemistry of the products and its possible predicted reactions. Some of the chemical reactions occur during storage are hydrolysis, oxidation, racemization etc.

11. **Accidental substitution or deliberate adulteration with spurious or useless materials:** Accidental substitution happens due to storage or mixing of more toxic products with the usual products. Deliberate mixing of low standard products to the products performed for the better profit to the company. For example, Potassium bromide is expensive it may be adulterated by mixing low cost sodium bromide.

    To identify the possible impurities in drugs, one should have through knowledge of the raw material, the process by which it is manufactured, the chemical properties and its behavior in natural and abnormal conditions. All the chemicals/drugs cannot be tested for all impurities.

## 5.3 EFFECT OF IMPURITIES

Manufacturing of pure chemical compounds are very difficult and that contain small quantity or traces of impurities which are always remains in the final products. The impurities present in the final product may exert the following effects.

1. Toxic impurities like lead and arsenic salts can be injurious to health when they present above the prescribed limits.
2. Some of the impurities decrease the shelf life of a medicinal compound.
3. Impurities may lead to change the color or flavor of the active substances (unhygienic compound). Example: Sodium chloride becomes damp due to the presence of magnesium salts. If the phenolic compounds present, the sodium salicylate gets decolorization.
4. Impurities which alters the physical and chemical properties of the compounds and make them to unfit for medicinal purposes.

5. Impurities may decrease the activity of the active compounds. Example: Presence of water in hard soap.
6. Due to the presence of impurities the active substance becomes incompatible with other substances.
7. Impurities cause technical difficulties in the use of the substance. For example: Carbonate in ammonia solution, Potassium iodate in potassium iodide.
8. Impurities with harmless effect also decrease the therapeutic efficacy and the active strength of the substances, when they are present in large proportions.
9. Traces of impurities may produce a cumulative toxic effect after a certain period of time. In some cases, the trace amount of impurities may add the therapeutical value of the active substances. Example: Traces of copper increase the medicinal value of iron preparations which induces the formation of haemoglobin due to its catalytic action.

### 5.3.1 Permissible Impurities

Medicinal compounds should be pure in order to achieve the maximum therapeutic effect, but it is not practically possible to prepare a medicinal compound without any impurity. By keeping this in mind pharmacopoeial committee has accepted some of the impurities, which are called as permissible impurities. But it should present in the accepted limit. While fixing the permissible impurities, the following aspects are considered by the pharmacopoeial committee.

(a) Sometimes the pure substance can be produced at the high production cost, due to several purification processes, but it will results in the increased cost of medicine, which may affect the commercial aspect of pharma industry.

(b) The impurities (like lead and arsenic) which cause deleterious effects should not be present in the level which causes harmful biological effects.

(c) Some of the impurities, even though it is not harmful (harmless impurities), should not be present in heavy amount which will reduce the content of active ingredient and ultimately produce sub standard therapeutic effect.

(d) Adulteration of pharmaceuticals with similar quality products also done sometimes. Even though the adulterant may also yield similar therapeutic effect, it is called as an impurity. Due to commercial reasons this type of impurity arises in pharmaceuticals.

## 5.4 METHODS USED TO PURIFY THE INORGANIC SUBSTANCES

The most commonly used solvent for washing and purifying the inorganic compounds is water. The following are simplest methods used for the purification of inorganic compounds.

1. Washing
2. Drying
3. Recrystallization
4. Sublimation

**Washing:** This method is used when the final product is water insoluble. Here the impurities are water soluble in nature, they are washed away with water and the final product is water insoluble and it is retained.

**Drying:** Drying is also an important unit operation for removal of volatile impurities at normal temperature and pressure. But it needs care and precaution to prevent the entry of dust, deterioration of chemicals due to oxidation, light, bacterial growth and caking. When anhydrous chemicals or expensive chemicals are manufactured on small scale, drying process is performed under vacuum.

**Recrystallization:** This method is commonly used for purification of solid substances. Very less number of inorganic substances only crystallized from non aqueous solvents. Here the impure solid is dissolved in minimum volume of solvent. The water soluble impurities pass into solution and insoluble one left behind. Then they are filtered and allowed for crystallizing which are highly purified. Many of the substances are purified by this method.

**Sublimation:** Heating of some inorganic substances, directly converted in to vapour state without melting. The vapours when cooled give back the solid substance. This phenomenon is known as sublimation which is very useful for separating volatile substances from non volatile substances. Example: Purification of ammonium chloride and arsenic trioxide etc.

**Procedure for sublimation:** The substance to be purified is placed in a large beaker. The beaker is covered with a glass lid or watch glass. The beaker is heated gently and the resulting vapours condense at the watch glass as crystals. The watch glass can be removed after some time and the crystals are collected. Substances with very less vapour pressure are sublimated under reduced pressure.

## 5.5 TEST FOR PURITY

Test for impurity or test for purity are actually performed to check and fix the presence and limit the amount of impurities present in the chemical substances and pharmaceuticals. The major guiding factor for fixing a limit of tolerance for certain impurity is toxicity. For example, arsenic and lead are very toxic even if ingested in very trace amounts. Therefore, very small limits (parts per million) is prescribed. The tests for purity refer to few of the impurities to ensure that drugs do not have any adverse effect due to the presence of these impurities.

**Determination of Test for Purity:** Determination of impurities are depends upon some analytical tests which are described in pharmacopoeias. Some of these tests are described below.

***Clarity of solution*:** The following terms are used to define the degree of clarity or opalescence of a solution in various pharmacopeias.

(a) Clear,

(b) Very slightly opalescent,

(c) Opalescent,

(d) Very opalescent

The determination of clarity of the solution is done by direct comparison with a reference solution either with the help of light or by viewing through the solution in diffused light against black background. The clarity of the solution is similar to that of water or the solvent used. Example: In limit test for chloride by comparing with the opalescence produced in the standard sodium chloride solution and silver nitrate. The following aspects are to be tested to ascertain the purity of the pharmaceuticals.

1. **Particulate matter:** Clarity of injectables indicates freedom from particulate matter. It is determined by viewing the injection by eye against black back ground in upright vertical and horizontal positions under a screened light with specified intensity.
2. **Color, odour and taste:** These tests are performed for the substances when other tests for purity are not available. These are used to determine purity and hygenicity of the substance up to some extent. A solution may be described as colorless, if it has the similar appearance of water when examine under specified conditions. Varying degrees of colors are permissible by direct comparison with specified standard solutions.
3. **Insoluble matter:** This test is used to control small amounts of solvent insoluble impurity or readily soluble materials. For example: Presence of borax in boric acid is determined by its solubility in ethanol.
4. **Soluble matter:** This test is used to detect or control the water soluble impurities in official substances which are completely insoluble in a particular solvent. Example: Determination of soluble barium salts in barium sulphate required for X-ray determinations (Radio opaque contrast media).

   **Acid soluble matter:** It is used to detect the presence of oxides, hydroxides and carbonates in purified talc and other substances. A water soluble acid in undecenoic acid is also determined by using this test.
5. **Non volatile matter:** This test is used for both type of inorganic substances which are readily volatile and volatile only when strong ignition. This limit is used to control the contamination by other salts and dirt. Example, Hydrogen peroxide solution, ammonium bicarbonate, water for injections, ethanol etc are examined by this way.
6. **Residue on ignition:** Limits or tests for residue on ignition are commonly used to substance which easily undergoes decomposition leaving a residue of definite composition. It is a non specific method of assay. Example: Detect the limit of zinc oxide in zinc cream.
7. **Loss on ignition:** This limit is applied to thermostable substances which contains more quantity of tightly bound water (magnesium trisilicate) or determine the thermolabile impurities like carbonate in light magnesium oxide.
8. **Ash values:** These are mainly used to detect or limit impurities in crude drugs. The ash content of a crude drug is the inorganic residue left after incineration. The official ash values are used for examining the powdered drugs.

*Applications of ash values*

(i) To confirm the absence of extraneous minerals in crude drugs which are added accidentally or on further treatment. For example: Sand, earth etc.

(ii) To detect the adulteration of crude drugs, with exhausted drugs or stone cell or starch.

(iii) To detect and ensure the absence of other parts of plants.

There are four types of ash values mentioned in British Pharmacopoeia.

They are

(a) *Ash content:* It is mainly used to limit the amount of calcium oxalate in ginger.

(b) *Acid insoluble ash:* It is one of the important tests to detect and limit the excess soil present in the crude drug.

(c) *Water soluble ash and water soluble extractives:* This test is only specified for one official drug ginger and also used to identify samples which are extracted by using water.

(d) *Sulphated ash:* It is mainly used to detect the impurities in unorganized drugs and the limit of non volatile inorganic impurities in organic substances. Example: Asprin, Benzyl benzoate etc.

9. **Acidity, alkalinity and pH:** Many of the pharmacopoeial compounds contain acidic and alkaline impurities. They are themselves gives acidic and basic reaction, when dissolved in water. The tests for acidity or alkali include the titration of specific quantity of sample or its solution with standard alkali or acidic solution. This is used to detect the extent of impurity.

   *pH:* Some of the compounds are having definite pH value at a particular concentration. The pH values are changed when it contains impurities. Example: Sodium aurothiomalate, ferrous sulphate etc.

10. **Physicochemical requirements:** The physicochemical determination includes the solubility criteria of the substance in various solvents. It includes boiling point, melting point, optical rotation for optically active compound, refractive index and viscosity for liquids, specific gravity or weight per ml, freezing point.

    *Chromatographic concern:* $R_f$ values, retention time and $R_m$ values.

    *Photometric determination:* Colorimetry, Nephelometry and Flame photometry.

    *Spectrophotometry:* Ultra violet spectroscopy, IR, NMR, Mass and ESR spectroscopy.

    *Quantitative Determination:* The following tests are used to detect the quality of vegetable oils.

    (a) Acid value.

    (b) Esterification value.

    (c) Hydroxyl value.

    (d) Acetyl, ester, iodine and saponification values.

11. **Other parameters**: The other parameters used to determines the purity are swelling power of bentonite, adsorption power of kaolin, coarser particles (light kaolin) and fine particles, setting properties of plaster of paris, stability of solution (Sodium antimony gluconate).
12. **Moisture content:** It is determined by the estimation of amount of water of crystallization present. This test is used for drugs those looses their therapeutic potency in the presence of water due to hydrolysis. Example: Digitalis leaves.
13. **Anions and cations:** Certain anions and cations are incorporated to the active substance during the processing of the substance by absorption and co-precipitation. Such as chloride, sulphate, lead, arsenic, heavy metal etc. General qualitative tests or limit tests are prescribed by pharmacopoeias with necessary variation to check the presence of these impurities.
14. **Assay:** It is the quantitative chemical analysis of a compound to confirm whether it confirms to the prescribed standard or not. The common assay methods used are 1. Gravimetric analysis, 2. Volumetric analysis, 3. Photometric analysis, 4. Precipitation method, 5. Radioimmuno assay etc.
15. **Arsenic:** The arsenic content in the substance can be expressed as parts per million. Monographs on many substances do not contain any test for arsenic because of advanced method of preparation. It should be tested only for substances those are commercially contaminated with arsenic. The permissible limit of the arsenic in substance depends upon
    (a) Size and frequency of the dose.
    (b) Difficult in removing it from the compound.
16. **Precipitation methods:** These tests are used to test the moderate amount of impurities such as aluminium, iron and silica etc. Example: Test the limit of iron, aluminium and phosphate in calcium hydroxide.

## 5.6 COMMON TESTS FOR PERMISSIBLE IMPURITIES

1. **Test for free chlorine:** To the required quantity of sample, add carbon dioxide free water (Boiling water), 10% w/v potassium iodide solution and add one to two drops of starch solution, allowed to stand at the dark for 2 min. Then add 0.01M sodium thiosulphate solution. If the sample contains chlorine, it oxidizes the potassium iodide to iodine which reacts with starch solution to produce blue color. Upon addition of sodium thiosulphate solution, the blue colour disappears due to the removal of iodine by the reaction with sodium thiosulphate.
2. **Test for sulphates:** To the sample solution, add dilute hydrochloric acid and barium sulphate reagent and then make up it to 50 ml with water in Nessler's cylinder. The opalescence or turbidity produced in the test is compared with the standard opalescence or turbidity which is prepared as per the individual monograph. If the sample contains sulphate ion as an impurity, it reacts with barium sulphate reagent and produce opalescence. The opalescence produced in the test solution is compared with

that of standard solution. If the test opalescence is less than that of standard opalescence, the given sample complies with the standards of Pharmacopoeia.

3. **Test for chlorides:** To the sample solution, add dilute nitric acid and silver nitrate solution (1 ml, 0.1M) dilute to 50 ml with water. Stir immediately with glass rod and allowed to stand for 5 min, protected from light. The opalescence or turbidity produced in the test solution is compared with the standard solution which is prepared as per the individual monograph. If the chloride is present as an impurity, it reacts with silver nitrate reagent and produce opalescence. The opalescence produced in the test solution is compared with that of standard solution. If the opalescence produced in the test solution is less than that of standard opalescence; the given sample complies with the standards of Pharmacopoeia.
4. **Test for bromides:** To the small amount of sample solution, add 1 ml of chloroform and chlorinated lime with constant shaking. The chloroform layer does not show brown color if bromide not present. If bromide is present in the sample as an impurity, it reacts with chlorinated lime and produce brown color. The color produced in the test solution is compared with that of standard solution. If the colour produced in the test solution is less than that of standard, the given sample complies with the standards of Pharmacopoeia.
5. **Test for iodides:**

   ***Method* 1:** To the small amount of sample solution, add 1 ml of chloroform and chlorinated lime with constant shaking. The chloroform layer does not show color if iodide is not present. If iodide is present in the sample as an impurity, it reacts with chlorinated lime to produce color. The color produced in the test solution is compared with that of standard solution. If the color produced in the test sample is less than that of standard sample, the given sample complies with the standards of Pharmacopoeia.

   ***Method* 2:** To the sample solution, add iodide free starch solution, 0.5M sulphuric acid, one or two drops of sodium nitrate solution and make up to 25 ml with water. Keep the above solution (stand) for 5 min and examine the mixture in day light. No blue colour is produced after 5 min if iodides are not present. If color is produced in the test solution, then it is compared with that of standard solution. If the color produced in the test sample is less than that of standard sample, the given sample complies with the standards of Pharmacopoeia.
6. **Test for heavy metals:**

   ***Method* 1:** To the sample solution, add 10 ml of freshly prepared hydrogen sulphide solution, mix, dilute to 50 ml with water, allow to stand for 5 minutes and view downwards over a white surface. The color produced in the test solution is compared with that of standard solution which was prepared as per monograph. If the color produced in the test sample is less than that of standard sample, the given sample complies with the standards of Pharmacopoeia. This method is used for the substance which gives a clear colorless solution under specified conditions.

   ***Method* 2:** This method is used for the substance which does not give a clear colorless solution under specified conditions. Refer the procedure under limit test for heavy metals.

*Method* **3:** In this method the substance to be determined is dissolved in sodium hydroxide and remaining procedure is similar to that of method A.

7. **Test for iron:** To the sample solution, add 2 ml of 20% w/v solution of iron free citric acid and 0.1 ml or one to two drops of thioglycolic acid, mix well, make alkaline with iron free ammonia solution, dilute to 50 ml with water and allow to stand for 5 minutes. The pink color produced in the test solution is compared with that of standard solution. If the color produced in the test sample is less than that of standard sample, the given sample complies with the standards of Pharmacopoeia.
8. **Test for arsenic:** If the sample contains arsenic as an impurity, it is converted in to arsine gas which reacts with mercuric chloride paper, and produces yellow to brown color stain. The intensity and length of the stain depends upon the amount of arsenic present in the sample. The intensity of the stain produced in the test solution is compared with that of standard solution. If the intensity of the stain produced in the test sample is less than that of standard sample, the given sample, complies with the standards of Pharmacopoeia.
9. **Test for magnesium:** To the sample solution add small amount of strong ammonia solution, shake well. The resulting solution should be clear and colorless. If magnesium is present as an impurity it gives turbid solution. The turbidity produced in the test solution is compared with that of standard solution. If the turbidity produced in the test sample is less than that of standard sample, the given sample complies with the standards of Pharmacopoeia.
10. **Test for acidity:** To the one portion of sample add 10 portion of water, add one to two drops of methyl red or phenolphthalein indicator and titrated with standard sodium hydroxide solution. If the titer value is not be more than 0.5 ml, the given sample complies with the standards of Pharmacopoeia.
11. **Test for alkalinity:** To the one portion of sample, add required quantity of water, add methyl orange indicator and titrated against 0.01M hydrochloric acid. If the titer value is not be more than 0.5 ml, the given sample complies with the standards of Pharmacopoeia.
12. **Test for loss on ignition:** It is the loss in weight in percent w/w results from any part of the test material that is volatilized under specified conditions. This test is only applied for finely powdered materials.

    ***Method:*** Weigh the silica or platinum crucible with lid which is previously ignited for one hour at specified temperature and cooled. Transfer the required amount of sample in to the crucible. Then take the weight of the crucible along with lid and the substance. Place the uncovered crucible in a covered muffle furnace or in an oven that is capable of maintaining the temperature needed for the test. Ignite the crucible for particular time and temperature which is prescribed as per the monograph. Ignition is repeated for every one hour until constant weight is obtained. After completion of each ignition, cover the crucible, allowed to cool to room temperature before taking the weight. The weight of test sample is compared with that of standard. If the weight of the test sample is within the limit, the given sample complies with the standards of Pharmacopoeia.

13. **Test for loss on drying:** It is the weight loss of the substance expressed as percentage w/w results from the loss of water or any other volatile substances under specified conditions. It is determined by two methods.

    ***Method A*:** Accurately weigh the weighing bottle under the specified condition which is used for the determination. Transfer the required quantity of the sample, cover it and accurately weigh the bottle and its contents with lid. Dry the bottle along with the contents in the drying chamber without lid as per in the monograph. Dry the sample to a constant weight at a particular time and temperature as per the monograph. After drying is completed remove the bottle from the drying chamber, place the lid and allowed to cool to room temperature. Weigh the bottle and its contents with lid. Drying of the sample is done by any one of the following methods.

    1. ***By using desiccator:*** Dry over at phosphorous pentoxide at room temperature and pressure. Care should be taken to keep the desiccant fully effective by frequent replacement.
    2. ***Drying by "in vacuo":*** Dry over at phosphorous pentoxide, at a pressure of 1.5 kPa to 2.5 kPa at room temperature.
    3. ***Drying by "in vacuo within a specified temperature range":*** Dry over at phosphorous pentoxide, at a pressure of 1.5 kPa to 2.5 kPa within a particular temperature as per the monograph.
    4. ***Drying in an oven within a specified temperature range:*** Dry in an oven within the range mentioned in the given monograph. The drying temperature is mentioned by a single value, dry at the temperature ± 2 °C.
    5. ***Drying at high vacuum:*** Dry over at phosphorous pentoxide, at a pressure not more than 0.1 kPa, at the temperature mentioned in the monograph.

    **Method B:** In this method loss of drying is determined by thermogravimetry method. In this technique the weight of the sample is recorded as the function of temperature under a controlled temperature program by using thermobalance.

14. **Test for barium:** To the small amount of sample, add required quantity of distilled water, small volume of dilute sulphuric acid and allowed to stand for 5 minutes. No opalescence is produced which examined against the light if barium is absent. If barium is present as an impurity, it gives opalescence. The opalescence produced in the test solution is compared with that of standard solution. If the opalescence produced in the test solution is less than that of standard opalescence, the given sample complies with the standards of Pharmacopoeia.
15. **Test for ferric ion:** To the sample solution add small amount of hydrochloric acid, boil and cool it. To this add required amount of potassium iodide, allowed to stand in dark for 15 minutes. The liberated iodine is titrated with standard sodium thiosulphate solution using starch solution as an indicator. Blank determination also done. The volume of sodium thiosulphate consumed should not be more than that of prescribed value.
16. **Microbial contamination:** It is determined by plate count method.

17. **Appearance of solution:** The required quantity of substance is dissolved in appropriate solvent (depends upon the solubility nature). The solution should be clear and colorless.
18. **Test for aluminium:** The sample solution is treated with hydrochloric acid, boil the solution, and add ammonia. If aluminium is present as an impurity it gives precipitate due the formation of aluminium hydroxide. The above solution is filtered, washed and added ammonium chloride solution. The opalescence produced in the test solution is compared with that of standard solution. If the opalescence produced in the test solution is less than that of standard opalescence, the given sample complies with the standards of Pharmacopoeia.
19. **Test for copper, lead, mercury and tin:** To the sample solution add hydrogen sulphide solution, if no precipitate is obtained, the given sample complies with the standards of Pharmacopoeia.
20. **Test of carbonates and bicarbonates:** Mix small quantity of sample with required quantity of hydrochloric acid, if no brisk effervescence is produced, the given sample complies with the standards of Pharmacopoeia.
21. **Test for acid soluble substances:** Digest small amount of sample with required amount of dilute hydrochloric acid for 15 minutes, filter it and evaporate the filtrate. To the residue add one to two drops of sulphuric acid and ignite to a constant weight. If the weight of the residue within a limit prescribed as per the monograph, the given sample complies with the standards of Pharmacopoeia.
22. **Test for water soluble substances:** To the required quantity of sample add small amount of water, filter, and evaporate the filtrate to constant weight. If the weight of residue should be within the limit prescribed as per the monograph, the given sample complies with the standards of Pharmacopoeia.
23. **Test for organic compounds:** The color of the residue after loss on drying should not be slight yellow or grey colour or the color of the test residue is compared with that of standard residue. If the color produced in the test residue is less than that of standard residue, the given sample complies with the standards of Pharmacopoeia.
24. **Test for copper:** Dissolve small quantity of sample in water, boil and add dilute ammonia solution. If copper is present as an impurity it gives blue colour. The blue color produced in the test solution is compared with that of standard solution. If the color produced in the test solution is less than that of standard color, the given sample complies with the standards of Pharmacopoeia.
25. **Test for calcium:** To the small amount of sample solution add ammonium oxalate solution, dilute acetic acid and diluted with water. Stir well. Keep it aside for 5 min. The opalescence produced in the test solution is compared with that of standard solution. If the opalescence produced in the test solution is less than that of standard opalescence, the given sample complies with the standards of Pharmacopoeia.
26. **Test for acid neutralizing capacity:** To the required quantity of sample, add required quantity of 0.1M hydrochloric acid previously heated to 37 °C. Measure the pH of the solution at this temperature after 10, 15, 20 min time interval. The pH of the solution should be 1.8, 2.3 and 3 respectively. Then add 10 ml of 0.5M hydrochloric acid and

titrate with 0.1N sodium hydroxide solution. If the burette reading is within the limit, the given sample complies with the standards of Pharmacopoeia.

27. **Test for ferrocyanide:** To the small amount of sample, add water and add a mixture of 1% w/v solution of ferric ammonium sulphate (FAS) and 0.25% w/v of sulphuric acid and add required amount of 1% w/v ferrous sulphate solution. If ferrocyanide is present as impurity it gives blue color. The blue color produced in the test solution is compared with that of standard solution. If the color produced in the test solution is less than that of standard color; the given sample complies with the standards of Pharmacopoeia.
28. **Test for cyanide:** Warm the sample solution, add one drop of ferrous sulphate solution and add very little quantity of sodium hydroxide solution and acidify the solution with hydrochloric acid. If cyanide is present as an impurity blue color is produced. The blue color produced in the test solution is compared with that of standard solution. If the color produced in the test solution is less than that of standard color, the given sample complies with the standards of Pharmacopoeia.
29. **Water insoluble matter:** Dissolve required amount of sample in 50 ml water, boil and filter it. Wash the filtrate with water until get a clear colorless filtrate. The weight of the residue after drying at 105 °C should be within the limit.
30. **Test for sulphated ash:** Heat a silica or platinum crucible to redness for 10 minutes. Allow to cool in a desiccator and weigh it. 1 gm of the sample is taken in a crucible and weighs it. Ignite the crucible until the substances is charred. Cool and moisten the residue with small amount of sulphuric acid, heat slowly until the white fumes are evolved, and ignite at 800 ± 25 °C until black color disappeared. Allow the crucible to cool, add a few drops of sulphuric acid and heat it. Continue the operation until two successive weighing does not differ by more than 0.5 mg.
31. **Test for total ash:** Heat a silica or platinum crucible to redness for 30 minutes. Allow to cool in a desiccator and weigh it. Transfer 1 gm of the substance to the crucible and dry the crucible at 100 to 105 °C for one hour and ignite to a constant weight in a muffle furnace 600 ± 25 °C. Cool it and calculate. Calculate the percentage of ash content which should be within the limit.
32. **Test for reducing substances:** To the sample solution add sulphuric acid and 0.02M potassium permanganate and heat it on a water bath for 5 minutes. If any reducing substances are present in the sample as impurity produces red color. The red color produced in the test solution is compared with that of standard solution. If the color produced in the test solution is less than that of standard color, the given sample complies with the standards of Pharmacopoeia.
33. **Test for water content**: It is determined by Karl Fischer's titration.
34. **Test for pH:** It is determined by potentiometric titrations.
35. **Test for thiocyanate:** To the acidic or basic solution of sample, add two to four drops acidic ferric chloride solution. If the sample contains thiocyanate as an impurity, produces red colour. The red color produced in the test solution is compared with that

of standard solution. If the color produced in the test solution is less than that of standard color, the given sample complies with the standards of Pharmacopoeia.

36. **Test for microbial contamination:**

*Medium used:* Soya bean digest broth.

Inoculate the required amount (1 ml or 1 gm) of sample to the above medium and incubate at 30-35 °C for 18-24 hr. After incubation, 1 ml of the broth is transferred to Macconkey broth and incubates at 42-44 °C for 2 days. Once again inoculate the broth in Macconkey agar medium for 3 days, if no pink color colonies are produced.

37. **Test for oxalate:** To a small amount of sample add hydrochloric acid and zinc granules and warm it. Allow to stand, collect the supernatant by adding one drop of 1% w/v phenyl hydrazine hydrochloride solution and heated to boil. Cool immediately, add equal volume of hydrochloric acid and potassium ferricyanide solution, shake and allow to stand for half an hour. If oxalate is present as an impurity gives pink color. The pink color produced in the test solution is compared with that of standard solution. If the color produced in the test solution is less than that of standard color, the given sample complies with the standards of Pharmacopoeia.

## 5.7 LIMIT TEST

**Definition:** Limit tests are quantitative or semi-quantitative test designed to identify and control small amounts of impurity which is likely to be in the pharmaceuticals. Generally it is carried out to identify the impurities present in the pharmaceutical substances and compare it with the standard. The error of these tests depends upon different operators. So designs of these tests include some of the following factors.

1. Sensitivity
2. Specificity
3. Control of personal error.

### 5.7.1 Importance of Limit Tests

1. It is used to find out the amount of avoidable or unavoidable amounts of impurities present in the substances.
2. It is used to find out harmful amount of impurities.

The limit of impurity is provided in terms of parts per million (ppm = 1 μg = $10^{-6}$ gm). In these tests, the test opalescence/turbidity/colour/stain produced by the reaction of specified amount of impurity in the test sample with the reagent is compared with the standard opalescence/turbidity/colour/stain produced by the reaction of known amount of impurity with the reagent. So limit tests are comparative tests in which both must be prepared simultaneously at the similar conditions. In case of the limit test for chloride, sulphate, iron and heavy metals, Nesseler's cylinders of 50 ml capacity are used which are matched glass tubes with uniform internal diameter and a flat, transparent base. The overall height is about 150 mm, the thickness of the wall is 1 to 1.5 mm and the thickness of the base is 1 to 1.5 mm. The external height to the 50 ml mark of the cylinders used for a test must not vary by more than 1 mm.

The pharmacopoeia gives no numerical values for the limits in these tests. It would not be practicable to do so, since the amount of impurity necessary to cause a certain opalescence, turbidity or color is influenced to a large extent by the relatively large quantities of other substances are present.

In general, the limit tests are performed by using distilled water, but sometimes the solution is prepared by a special method. They are as follows.

1. Alkaline substances are first neutralized with hydrochloric acid or nitric acid.
2. Water insoluble substances are dissolved in acid or an aqueous extracts of the substances are used, because if insoluble substances sometimes modifies the opalescence/turbidity and color of the tests.
3. Organic acid salts are liberated the water soluble free organic acid during acidification which is filtered off, the filtrate is used for the test.
4. Colored substances are carbonized, the ash obtained is extracted with water and the aqueous extract is used for the limit test.
5. Deeply colored substances are decolorized before test. For example potassium permanganate is decolorized by boiling with ethanol, filter it and the filtrate is used for the test.
6. Reducing substances should be oxidized before carrying the test.

### 5.7.2 Limit Test for Chlorides

**Principle:** Limit test for chloride is based upon the reaction of chloride impurities with silver nitrate in the presence of dilute nitric acid. The turbidity/opalescence produced in the test solution is compared with the standard turbidity/opalescence produced or obtained by the reaction of known quantity of chloride with silver nitrate.

$$Cl^- + AgNO_3 \xrightarrow{\text{Dilute } HNO_3} \underset{\text{Opalescence/ Turbidity}}{AgCl\downarrow} + NO_3^-$$

The silver chloride precipitate formed is insoluble in dilute nitric acid which gives turbidity/opalescence.

**Reasons: 1.** Dilute nitric acid is used to dissolve other impurities if present.

***Procedure:***

| S. No. | Test solution | Standard solution |
|---|---|---|
| 1. | Dissolve the given sample in 20 ml of water and transfer to a Nessler's cylinder. | Transfer 10 ml of standard chloride solution (25 ppm) in to a Nessler's cylinder and add 5 ml water. |
| 2. | Add 10 ml of dilute nitric acid, dilute to 50 ml with water. | Add 10 ml of dilute nitric acid, dilute to 50 ml with water. |
| 3. | Add 1 ml of 0.1M silver nitrate solution. | Add 1 ml of 0.1M silver nitrate solution. |
| 4. | Stir immediately with a glass rod and allowed to stand for 5 mins, protected from light and viewed transversely against a black background. | Stir immediately with a glass rod and allowed to stand for 5 mins, protected from light and viewed transversely against a black background. |

**Observation and inference:** If the opalescence /turbidity produced in the test solution is less than that of the standard solution, then the given sample complies with the standards of Pharmacopoeia.

### 5.7.3 Limit Test for Sulphates

**Principle:** Limit test for sulphate is based upon the the reaction of sulphate impurities with barium chloride in the presence of dilute acetic acid. The turbidity/opalescence produced in the test solution is compared with the standard turbidity/opalescence produced or obtained by the reaction of known quantity of sulphate with barium chloride.

$$SO_4^{2-} + BaCl_2 \xrightarrow[]{\text{dilute acetic acid}} \underset{\text{Turbidity/opalescence}}{BaSO_4\downarrow} + 2\,Cl^-$$

In the earliest edition of I.P., the barium chloride reagent is replaced by barium sulphate reagent which contains barium chloride, sulphate free alcohol and small amount of potassium sulphate. The dilute acetic acid also replaced by dilute hydrochloric acid.

**Reasons:**

1. The barium sulphate precipitate formed is insoluble in dilute acetic acid which gives opalescence/turbidity.
2. Potassium sulphate is used as a seeding agent to increase sensitivity of the test by rapid and complete precipitation.
3. Ethanol is used to prevent supersaturation and thus produce uniform turbidity/opalescence.

The change in the reagent does not affect the objective of the test.

***Procedure:***

| S. No. | Test solution | Standard solution |
|---|---|---|
| 1. | Transfer 1 ml of a 25 % w/v solution of barium chloride in to Nessler's cylinder. | Transfer 1 ml of a 25 % w/v solution of barium chloride in to Nessler's cylinder. |
| 2. | Add 1 ml of ethanolic sulphate standard solution (10 ppm $SO_4$), mix and allow to stand for 1 min. | Add 1 ml of ethanolic sulphate standard solution (10 ppm $SO_4$), mix and allow to stand for 1 min. |
| 3. | Dissolve the given sample in 15 ml of water and add 0.15 ml of 5M acetic acid and pour the solution into a Nessler's cylinder. | Add 15 ml of standard sulphate solution (10 ppm $SO_4$) and 0.15 ml of 5M acetic acid to the Nessler's cylinder. |
| 4. | Add sufficient water to make up 50ml. | Add sufficient water to make up 50ml. |
| 5. | Stir immediately with a glass rod and allowed to stand for 5 min and viewed transversely against a black background. | Stir immediately with a glass rod and allowed to stand for 5 min and viewed transversely against a black background. |

**Observation and inference:** If the opalescence/turbidity produced in the test solution is less than that of the standard solution, then the given sample complies with the standards of Pharmacopoeia.

## 5.7.4 Limit Test for Iron

**Principle:** The limit test for iron is based upon the reaction between iron in ammoniacal solution with thioglycolic acid (mercaptoacetic acid) in the presence of iron free citric acid to produce iron thioglycollate complex which is pale pink to deep reddish purple in color. The color produced in the test solution is compared with the standard solution.

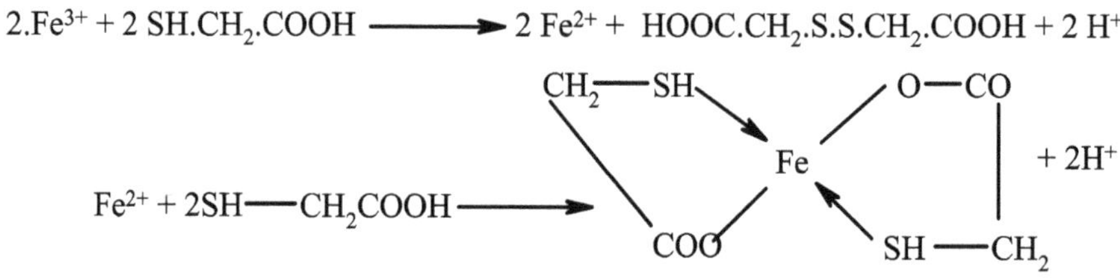


Ferrous thioglycollate complex
(pale pink to deep reddish color)

**Reasons:**

1. Iron free citric acid is used to complex metal cations other than iron if any present.
2. Thioglycolic acid acts as a reducing agent and it converts ferric ion ($Fe^{3+}$) to ferrous ion ($Fe^{2+}$) if any present.
3. The complex formed gives purple color in the presence of alkaline medium only.
4. Citric acid forms ammonium citrate buffer when ammonia is added to make alkaline, which in turn stabilizes the complex formed.

***Procedure:***

| S. No. | Test solution | Standard solution |
|---|---|---|
| 1. | Dissolve the given sample in 20 ml water and transfer into Nessler's cylinder. | Transfer 2 ml of iron standard solution (20 ppm Fe) to a Nessler's cylinder. |
| 2. | Add 2 ml of 20% w/v of iron free citric acid. | Add 2 ml of 20% w/v of iron free citric acid. |
| 3. | Add 0.1 ml of thioglycolic acid. | Add 0.1 ml of thioglycolic acid. |
| 4. | Then make the solution to alkaline with iron free ammonia solution. | Then make the solution to alkaline with iron free ammonia solution. |
| 5. | Dilute to 50 ml with water and allow stand for 5 minutes and observe the color transversely. | Dilute to 50 ml with water and allow stand for 5 minutes and observe the color transversely. |

**Observation and inference:** If the color produced in the test solution is less than that of the standard solution. Then the sample complies with the standards of Pharmacopoeia.

**Note:** All the reagents used for the test should be free from iron.

### 5.7.5 Limit Test for Heavy Metals

**Principle:** The limit test for heavy metals is based on the test color (brownish color) produced by the reaction between heavy metal impurities and standard solution of hydrogen sulphide and comparing with the standard color produced by the reaction between known quantity of lead with saturated solution of hydrogen sulphide.

$$Pb + H_2S \longrightarrow \underset{\substack{\text{Lead sulphide} \\ \text{(brown color)}}}{PbS\downarrow} + 2H^+$$

Metals that response to this test is lead, bismuth, mercury, arsenic, antimony, tin, cadmium, copper, molybdenum and bismuth.

The limits of metallic impurities are expressed as parts per million (ppm). The usual limits for heavy metals as per I.P. is 20 ppm.

In this test dilute ammonia, acetic acid, hydrochloric acid, nitric acid, potassium cyanide and sulphuric acid are used as reagents.

Dilute acetic acid and ammonia are used to maintain pH between 3 and 4, so that the precipitate formed is colloidal and uniform. The saturated solution of hydrogen sulphide needed for this test should be freshly prepared.

IP adopted three methods for the limit test for heavy metals depends upon the solubility nature of the substance.

**Method I:** It is used for the substance which gives a clear, colorless solution under specified conditions.

**Method II:** It is used for the substance which do not gives a clear, colorless solution.

**Method III:** It is used for the substance which gives a clear, colorless solution in sodium hydroxide medium.

Let us discuss each method in detail.

**Method I:** It is used for the substance which gives a clear, colorless solution under specified conditions.

| S. No. | Test solution | Standard solution |
|---|---|---|
| 1. | The sample solution is prepared as per the monograph and 25 ml of solution is transferred into a Nessler's cylinder. | Transfer 2 ml of standard lead solution into Nessler's cylinder and dilute to 25 ml with water. |
| 2. | Add dilute ammonia or acetic acid solution to adjust the pH between 3 to 4. | Add dilute ammonia or acetic acid solution to adjust the pH between 3 to 4. |
| 3. | Dilute to 35 ml with distilled water and mix well. | Dilute to 35 ml with distilled water and mix well. |
| 4. | Add 10 ml of freshly prepared hydrogen sulphide solution, mix, dilute to 50 ml with water. | Add 10 ml of freshly prepared hydrogen sulphide solution, mix, dilute to 50 ml with water. |
| 5. | Allow to stand for 5 min and view downwards over a white background. | Allow to stand for 5 min and view downwards over a white background. |

**Observation and inference:** If the color produced in the test solution is not more intense than that of standard solution, the sample complies with the IP standard or vice versa.

**Method II:** It is used for the substance which does not give a clear, colorless solution.

| S. No. | Test solution | Standard solution |
|---|---|---|
| 1. | Transfer the prescribed quantity of sample into a crucible. | Transfer 2 ml of standard lead solution and dilute to 25 ml with water. |
| 2. | Moisten the sample with sulphuric acid and ignite on a low flame until complete charring of the sample. | Add dilute ammonia or acetic acid solution to adjust the pH between 3 to 4 |
| 3. | Add 2 to 3 drops of nitric acid and heated to 500 °C and cool it. | Dilute to 35 ml with distilled water and mix well. |
| 4. | Then add 4 ml of dilute hydrochloric acid and digest for 2 min and evaporate to dryness. Then add 10 ml of dilute hydrochloric acid and digest the residue for two min. | Add 10ml of freshly prepared hydrogen sulphide solution, mix, dilute to 50 ml with water. |
| 5. | Neutralize with dilute ammonia solution and just acidified with acetic acid. | Allow to stand for 5 min and view downwards over a white background. |
| 6. | Adjust the pH between 3 to 4, filter if necessary. Dilute to 35 ml with water. | |
| 7. | Add 10 ml of freshly prepared hydrogen sulphide solution. Dilute to 50 ml with water. | |
| 8. | Allow to stand for 5 minutes and view downwards over a white background. | |

**Observation and inference:** If the color produced in the test solution is not more intense than that of standard solution, the sample complies with the standards of Pharmacopoeia.

**Method III:** It is used for the substance which gives a clear, colorless solution in sodium hydroxide medium.

| S. No. | Test solution | Standard solution |
|---|---|---|
| 1. | The required quantity of sample is dissolved in 20 ml of water; add 5 ml of sodium hydroxide solution or the sample solution is prepared as per monograph. | The standard solution is prepared by using 2 ml of standard lead solution; add 5 ml of sodium hydroxide solution. |
| 2. | Make up to 50 ml with water. | Make up to 50 ml with water. |
| 3. | Add 5 drops of sodium sulphide solution mix well and kept aside for 5 minutes. | Add 5 drops of sodium sulphide solution mix well and kept aside for 5 minutes. |

**Observation:** If the color produced in the test solution is not more intense than that of standard solution, the sample complies with the standards of Pharmacopoeia vice versa.

Heavy metals present in the volatile oils are determined by the following method. In this test instead of Nesseler's cylinder, 25 ml glass stoppered test tubes are used.

The required volume of oil sample (10 ml) is shaken with an equal volume of water, add one drop of hydrochloric acid. Hydrogen sulphide gas is passed through this mixture, until it gets saturation.

If no dark color is produced either in the oil or water layer, then the given oil sample complies with standards of Pharmacopoeia.

### 5.7.6 Limit Test for Lead

Lead is the one of the most important undesirable impurities in medicinal substances. The main source of lead impurity is as follows.

1. Use of sulphuric acid.
2. Use of lead lined apparatus.
3. Storage of some chemicals in glass bottles.

**Principle:** It is based upon the reaction between lead and diphenyl thiocarbazone (dithizone). The color produced by the test solution in chloroform layer is compared with the color of the standard solution in chloroform. Dithizone in chloroform is able to extract lead from alkaline aqueous solution as lead dithizone complex (violet in color).

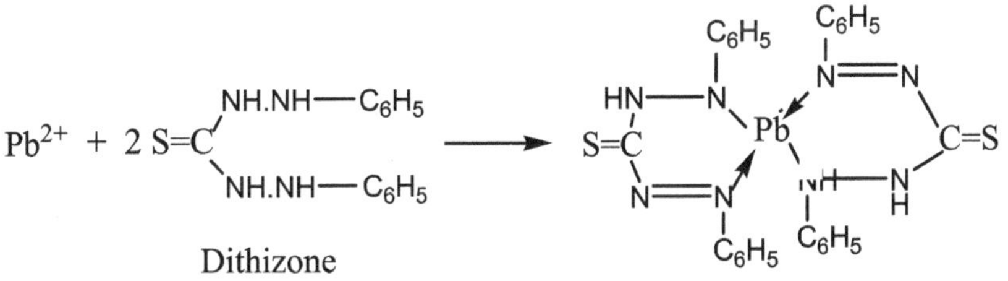

$$Pb^{2+} + 2\, S{=}C(NH.NH{-}C_6H_5)_2 \longrightarrow \text{Lead-dithizone complex}$$

Dithizone

Lead-dithizone complex

**Method:**

| S. No. | Test solution | Standard solution |
|---|---|---|
| 1. | The required quantity of sample is dissolved in water and transferred into a separating funnel. | Transfer a required amount of lead standard solution (1 ppm lead) equivalent to the amount of lead permitted in the substance being examined into a separating funnel. |
| 2. | Add 6 ml of ammonium citrate solution (Sp). | Add 6 ml of ammonium citrate solution (Sp). |

*Contd...*

| S. No. | Test solution | Standard solution |
|---|---|---|
| 3. | Add 2 ml of hydroxylamine hydrochloride solution (Sp). Add two drops of phenol red solution. | Add 2 ml of hydroxylamine hydrochloride solution (Sp). Add two drops of phenol red solution. |
| 4. | Make the solution just alkaline (red colour) by the addition of strong ammonia solution, cool it if necessary. | Make the solution just alkaline (red colour) by the addition of strong ammonia solution, cool it if necessary |
| 5. | Add 2 ml of potassium cyanide solution (Sp). | Add 2 ml of potassium cyanide solution (Sp). |
| 6. | Extract immediately with several quantities, each of 5 ml of dithizone extraction solution until it becomes green and draining of each extract into another separating funnel. | Extract immediately with several quantities, each of 5 ml of dithizone extraction solution until it becomes green and draining of each extract into another separating funnel. |
| 7. | Combine the dithizone extracts and shaken for 30 seconds with 30 ml of 1% v/v solution of nitric acid and discard the chloroform layer. (dithizone remains in chloroform layer, lead nitrate in aqueous layer). | Combine the dithizone extracts and shaken for 30 seconds with 30 ml of 1% v/v solution of nitric acid and discard the chloroform layer (dithizone remains in chloroform layer, lead nitrate in aqueous layer). |
| 8. | To this acid solution add 5 ml of standard dithizone solution. | To this acid solution add 5 ml of standard dithizone solution. |
| 9. | Shake well for 30 minutes and observe the color of chloroform layer. | Shake well for 30 minutes and observe the color of chloroform layer. |

**Observation:** A lead dithizone complex is violet color in the chloroform layer. This color is compared with the standard color. If the color produced in the test solution is not more than that of standard solution, then the given sample complies with the standards of Pharmacopoeia.

**Reasons:**

1. All the reagents used in this test should be free from lead and labeled as Sp.
2. The glasswares used also must be made up of borosilicate only and must be free from lead.
3. Glasswares should be rinsed thoroughly with dilute nitric acid followed by water.

### 5.7.7 Limit Test for Arsenic

The limit test for arsenic is a standardized test by using special type of apparatus. The basic principle of this test is a modification of the Gutzeit test.

The capacities and the dimensions of the apparatus used in this test and the conditions of the test are precisely described.

The original Gutzeit test was quantitative one and the liberated arsine gas is detected by covering the mouth of the flask with filter paper, on which small amount of silver nitrate crystals were placed. The liberated arsine turns silver nitrate complex black.

In the modified test, filter paper dipped in mercuric chloride solution is used, which yields a yellow colored complex. It produces a stain in the filter paper.

**Principle:** It is based upon the comparison of the intensity and length of the test stain obtained by the reaction of arsenic impurities with mercuric chloride paper with the intensity and length of the standard stain obtained by the reaction of known quantity of arsenic with mercuric chloride paper.

Here, the arsenic impurity present in the sample is first converted into arsenious acid by the action of reducing agents like potassium iodide, zinc, hydrochloric acid and stannous chloride.

$$\underset{\text{Arsenic acid in sample}}{H_3AsO_4} \longrightarrow \underset{\text{Arsenious acid}}{H_3AsO_3}$$

The arsenious acid is then reduced to arsine by the action of nascent hydrogen which is produced by the reaction between zinc and hydrochloric acid.

$$H_3AsO_3 + 3\,H_2 \longrightarrow \underset{\text{Arsine (gas)}}{AsH_3} + 3\,H_2O$$

The liberated arsine gas reacts with mercuric chloride paper and forms yellow stain.

$$2AsH_3 + HgCl_2 \longrightarrow Hg\begin{matrix} / AsH_2 \\ \backslash AsH_2 \end{matrix} + 2\,HCl$$

The length and the intensity of the stain in the mercuric chloride paper depends upon the amount of arsenic present in the sample.

The test includes four stages

1. Preparation of test solution
2. Description of apparatus
3. Procedure or method
4. Observation and inference.

1. **Preparation of test solution:** Preparation of test solution is not uniform for all substances. During preparation, the removal of the sample substance is important, if it

infers in the final test. Similarly, the removal of other interfering substances also essential one.

2. **Apparatus:**

- It consists of a wide mouthed bottle with a capacity of 100 ml with stopper as shown in Fig 5.1.
- The stopper assembly is prepared by selecting a rubber stopper with central hole through which a glass tube is passes.
- The external diameter of the tube is 8 mm and the internal diameter is 6.5 mm and the length of the tube is 200 mm.
- The upper end of the tube is fire polished, flat and flush with the top of a rubber bung.

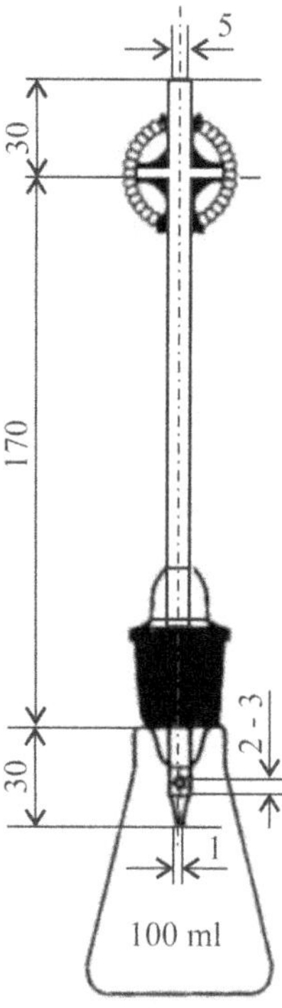


Fig 5.1 Apparatus for Arsenic limit test

- The lower end is slightly drawn to a narrow opening (1 mm in diameter) and with a side hole (2 mm in diameter).

- The drawn end the side hole should be below the lower edge of the stopper but above the 70 ml of final liquid level.
- The drawn end is used to allow the condensed vapours to drop in the bottle without block the side hole through which the vapours are enter rise in the tube.
- In side of the  tube, about 25 mm below the top end a cotton wool dipped in lead acetate solution is inserted gently through this the vapours are must passes.
- On the top of the rubber bung, a small piece of dried filter paper which is dipped in mercuric chloride solution is placed and sandwiched by placing another one inverted rubber bung.
- The upper rubber bung also with the hole of 6.5 mm diameter, exactly corresponding in position with the glass tube fitted in to the lower bung.
- The two rubber bung assemblies are held in position by using spring clips as shown in the Fig 5.2.
- Due to this assembly the liberated gas rises from the wide mouthed bottle to the filter paper through the filter paper, cotton wool in that order.

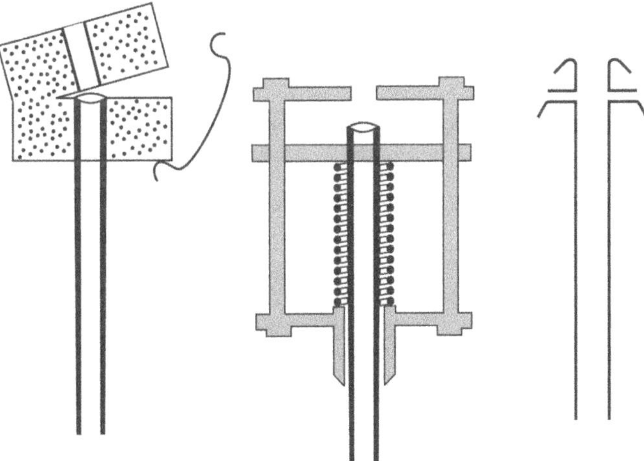

Fig 5.2 Stopper assembly in the apparatus

**3. Method or procedure (Preparation of test stain):**

- The required amount of sample solution is placed in the wide mouthed bottle.
- To this add 1 gm of potassium iodide and 10 gm of granulated zinc AsT.
- Immediately close the bottle with stopper assembly.

- The acid present in the test solution and zinc reacts, produces nascent hydrogen which reacts with arsenious acid present in the sample and liberates arsine gas which passes through the tube and reacts with mercuric chloride paper and produces yellow stain.
- The reaction is maintained for 40 minutes to ensure complete conversion of arsenious acid to arsine gas. Some heat, pressure are produced during the reaction due to the increased amount of gas in the inside of the apparatus.
- The rate of the reaction is increased by placing the total assembly on a warm surface.

***Preparation of standard stain:***

- Standard stain is prepared by using dilute arsenic solution (0.132 gm of arsenic in 100 ml).
- One ml of the above solution is diluted to 100 ml. This solution is transferred in to a wide mouthed bottle and remaining procedure is similar to that of test.

The comparison of the stain is done after the completion of the test immediately, so the test and standard should be carried out simultaneously.

4. **Observation and inference:** The stain produced in the filter paper fades quickly, so the comparison is done quickly.

- If the intensity of stain produced in the test is less than that of the standard, the test sample complies with the limit test for arsenic.
- If the stain present in the filter paper becomes dark, the test should be repeated by using pure reagents.

**Notes:**

1. The most suitable temperature for carry out this test is 40 °C.
2. Cotton wool dipped in lead acetate solution is used to trap any hydrogen sulphide gas liberated with arsine gas.
3. Care must be taken that the filter paper remains quite dry during the reaction.
4. During succeeding tests the tube must be washed with hydrochloric acid AsT, rinsed with water and dried.
5. All the reagents used for this test should be free from arsenic and mentioned as AsT.

## 5.8 IDENTIFICATION TESTS FOR CATIONS AND ANIONS

### 5.8.1 Tests for Cations

| Procedure | Observation | Inference |
|---|---|---|
| **1. Aluminium ($Al^{3+}$):**<br>(i) The amount of sample equivalent to 20 mg of aluminium ion is dissolved in water or prescribed volume of sample solution is taken in a test tube. To this add one drop of 2N hydrochloric acid and one drop of thioacetamide reagent. | No precipitate is formed. | Aluminium ion is confirmed. |
| To the above solution add dilute sodium hydroxide solution drop wise.<br>$AlCl_3 + 3\ NaOH \longrightarrow Al(OH)_3 + 3\ NaCl$<br>$Al(OH)_3 + NaOH \rightleftharpoons NaAlO_2 + 2\ H_2O$ | White precipitate is obtained which dissolves in excess of sodium hydroxide solution. | Aluminium ion is confirmed. |
| Then to this add ammonium chloride solution drop wise.<br>$NaAlO_2 + 2\ H_2O + NH_4Cl \longrightarrow Al(OH)_3\downarrow + NH_4OH + NaCl$ | A white gelatinous precipitate is formed. | Aluminium ion is confirmed. |
| (ii) A solution of aluminium compound is acidified with dilute hydrochloric acid, partially neutralized with ammonium acetate solution and add 5 drops of mordant blue 3 solution. (Excess addition of ammonium acetate leads to the formation of basic white aluminium acetate).<br>$AlCl_3 + CH_3COONH_4 + \text{Mordant Blue 3} \longrightarrow \text{Intense purple color}$ | An intense purple colour compound is produced. | Aluminium ion is confirmed. |
| (iii) An acidified solution of sample is treated with dilute ammonia solution. To this add freshly prepared quinalizarin solution, heated to boil, cooled and acidified with excess of acetic acid.<br>$AlCl_3 + 3\ NH_3 + 3\ H_2O \longrightarrow Al(OH)_3 + 3\ NH_4Cl$ | A faint precipitate is produced. A reddish violet colour is formed (due to the quinalizarin in alkali). | Aluminium ion is confirmed. |

*Contd...*

| Procedure | Observation | Inference |
|---|---|---|
| $Al(OH)_3 + \text{Quinalizarin} + NaOH \xrightarrow[\text{Excess acetic acid}]{\text{Boil, Cool}}$ Reddish violet color (Aluminium-quinalizarin complex) | Further addition of acetic acid reproduces the color of the solution or colored precipitate, which is stable and may increase intensity on standing. Color or turbidity or precipitate depends upon the concentration of aluminium ion. | Aluminium ion is confirmed. |
| **2. Ammonium ion ($NH_4^+$):**<br>(i) A prescribed quantity of dry ammonium salt is heated with sodium hydroxide solution.<br>$NH_4Cl + NaOH \longrightarrow NaCl + NH_3\uparrow + H_2O$ | Ammonia gas is evolved which is observed by its characteristic odour, it converts moist red litmus to blue. | Ammonium ion is confirmed. |
| (ii) To the required quantity of sample solution, add magnesium oxide. Then a current of air passes through the solution. The liberated gas is passed through the methyl red solution, which changes the color of the solution to yellow. To this add a small amount of sodium cobalt nitrite solution.<br>**Note:** In this test, volatile ammonia is collected in acid, before treating with cobalt nitrite, because potassium also gives a yellow precipitate with cobalt nitrite. But potassium ions are non-volatile and not liberated by magnesium oxide.<br>$3\ NH_4Cl + Na_3[CO(NO_2)_6] \longrightarrow (NH_4)_3[CO(NO_2)_6]\downarrow + 3\ NaCl$<br>Ammonium cobalt nitrate (Yellow precipitate) | A yellow precipitate is obtained (formation of ammonium cobalt nitrite). | Ammonium ion is confirmed. |
| **3. Antimony ($Sb^{3+}$):** To the required quantity of neutralized sample solution, add sodium sulphide solution drop wise.<br>$2\ Sb^{3+} + 3\ Na_2S \longrightarrow Sb_2S_3\downarrow + 6\ Na^+$<br>(Orange red precipitate) | Orange red or reddish brown precipitate is produced, which is soluble in sodium hydroxide solution. | Antimony ion is confirmed. |

*Contd...*

| Procedure | Observation | Inference |
|---|---|---|
| **4. Arsenic ($As^{3+}$):**<br>(i) A small amount of sample solution is heated with an equal volume of hypo phosphorous reagent. | A brown precipitate is formed. | Arsenic ion is confirmed. |
| (ii) To a small amount of sample solution add hydrochloric acid and hydrogen sulphide.<br>$2\,AsCl_3 + 3\,S^{2-} \longrightarrow As_2S_3\downarrow + 6\,Cl^-$<br>$As_2S_3 + 6OH^- \longrightarrow AsO_3^{3-} + AsS_3^{3-} + 3H_2O$ (Solution)<br>$As_2S_3 + 3\,CO_3^{2-} \longrightarrow AsO_3^{3-} + AsS_3^{3-} + 3\,CO_2$ | A yellow precipitate is obtained which is soluble in NaOH and ammonium carbonate. | Arsenous ion is confirmed. |
| **5. Barium ($Ba^{2+}$):**<br>**(i) Flame test:** Small amount of sample is taken in a watch glass. To this add hydrochloric acid to make a paste which is introduced in to the non-luminous part of the flame by using platinum wire. | Blue colour flame is produced when viewed through green colored glass. The flame appears green or apple green to the naked eye. | Barium ion is confirmed. |
| (ii) The required quantity of sample is dissolved in small amount of dilute hydrochloric acid, to this add dilute sulphuric acid.<br>$BaCl_2 + H_2SO_4 \longrightarrow BaSO_4\downarrow + 2\,HCl$<br>(White precipitate)<br>**Note:** The only barium compound official in I.P is barium sulphate which is insoluble in water and acids. In order to test, it is first fused with sodium carbonate to convert barium carbonate which is soluble in dilute hydrochloric acid. The solution is used for the above test. | A white precipitate is obtained (barium sulphate). | Barium ion is confirmed. |

*Contd...*

| Procedure | Observation | Inference |
|---|---|---|
| **6. Bismuth ($Bi^{3+}$):**<br>(i) The small amount of sample solution is boiled with dilute hydrochloric acid.<br>$Bi^{3+} + 3\,HCl \longrightarrow \underset{\text{Bismuth chloride}}{BiCl_3} + 3\,H^+$ | A white precipitate is formed (bismuth chloride). | Bismuth ion is confirmed. |
| To the above solution add water.<br>$BiCl_3 + H_2O \longrightarrow \underset{\substack{\text{Bismuth oxychloride}\\\text{(White precipitate)}}}{BiOCl} + 2\,HCl$ | A white precipitate is obtained (bismuth oxy chloride). | Bismuth ion is confirmed. |
| To this add few drops of sodium sulphide.<br>$2Bi^{3+} + 3S^{2-} \longrightarrow Bi_2S_3$ | A brown precipitate is obtained which is insoluble in excess alkali sulphide or ammonium sulphide solution. | Bismuth ion is confirmed. |
| (ii) To the small amount of sample solution add dilute nitric acid, boil it. Allow to cool, filter if necessary. To the solution add thiourea.<br>$Bi^{3+} + 3\,HNO_3 \longrightarrow Bi(NO_3)_3 + 3\,H^+$<br>$Bi(NO_3)_3 + \underset{\text{(Thiourea)}}{NH_2CSNH_2} \longrightarrow$ Orange yellow precipitate<br>To the above solution or precipitate add sodium fluoride, stand for half an hour.<br>**Note:** These tests appear to be redundant as there are no bismuth compounds official in the pharmacopeias for which these tests are usually prescribed. | An orange yellow color or an orange precipitate is produced.<br>No decolorization of the precipitate occurs. | Bismuth ion is confirmed. |
| **7. Calcium ($Ca^{2+}$):**<br>(i) A small amount of sample is dissolved in acetic acid. To this add potassium ferrocyanide.<br>$2\,CaCl_2 + K_4Fe(CN)_6 \longrightarrow \underset{\text{Soluble}}{Ca_2Fe(CN)_6} + 4\,KCl$ | No precipitate is formed. | Calcium ion is confirmed. |

*Contd...*

| Procedure | Observation | Inference |
|---|---|---|
| To the above clear solution add required amount of ammonium chloride.<br>$Ca_2Fe(CN)_6 + 2\,NH_4Cl \longrightarrow \underset{\text{Ammonium ferrocyanide (White precitate)}}{Ca(NH_4)_2[Fe(CN)_6]\downarrow} + CaCl_2$<br>In this test magnesium ions interfere | A white crystalline precipitate is formed. | Calcium ion is confirmed. |
| (ii) A solution of sample is treated with few drops ammonium oxalate solution.<br>$CaCl_2 + (COONH_4)_2 \longrightarrow Ca(COO)_2 + 2\,NH_4Cl$<br>$Ca(COO)_2 + 2HCl \longrightarrow CaCl_2 + 2\begin{array}{c}COOH\\ \vert \\ COOH\end{array}$ | A white precipitate of calcium oxalate is obtained which is sparingly soluble in dilute acetic acid and completely soluble in dilute hydrochloric acid and oxalic acid. | Calcium ion is confirmed. |
| (iii) Small volume of sample is dissolved in dilute hydrochloric acid, neutralize the solution by adding dilute sodium hydroxide solution. To the above solution, ammonium carbonate is added.<br>$CaCl_2 + (NH_4)_2CO_3 \longrightarrow 2\,NH_4Cl + \underset{\text{White precitate}}{CaCO_3\downarrow}$ | A white precipitate is formed. | Calcium ion is confirmed. |
| **8. Ferric salt ($Fe^{3+}$):**<br>(i) A small quantity of sample solution is treated with potassium ferrocyanide solution.<br>$FeCl_3 + K_4[Fe^{2+}(CN)_6] \longrightarrow KFe^{3+}[Fe^{2+}(CN)_6]\downarrow + 3\,KCl$ | An intense blue (prussian blue) precipitate is obtained which is insoluble in dilute HCl. | Ferric ion is confirmed. |

*Contd...*

| Procedure | Observation | Inference |
|---|---|---|
| (ii) To the small amount of sample add dilute hydrochloric acid, and small amount of ammonium thiocyanate solution. The solution becomes blood red color. This is divided into two portions<br>$Fe^{3+} + NH_4SCN \longrightarrow [Fe(SCN)]^{2+} + NH_4^+$ To the first portion add small amount of solvent ether. | Ether layer becomes pink or blood red color. | Ferric ion is confirmed. |
| To the second portion, add small amount of mercuric chloride solution.<br>$2\,[Fe(SCN)^{2+}] + HgCl_2 \rightleftharpoons \underset{\text{Mercuric thiocyanate (Colorless)}}{Hg(SCN)_2} + 2Fe^{3+} + 2\,Cl^-$ | Red color disappears. | Ferric ion is confirmed. |
| (iii) Small amount of sample solution, is strongly acidified with acetic acid solution. To this add small amount of 8-hydroxy-7-iodoquinoline-5-sulphonic acid (Ferron reagent) 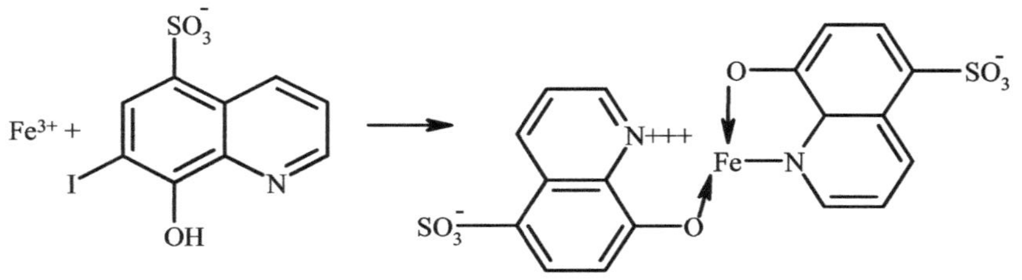<br>$Fe^{3+}$ + [8-hydroxy-7-iodoquinoline-5-sulphonate ($SO_3^-$, I, OH, N)] → [Fe complex: two quinoline-5-sulphonate ($SO_3^-$) ligands bound through O and N; N+++] | A permanent green color is formed. | Ferric ion is confirmed. |
| **9. Ferrous salt ($Fe^{2+}$):**<br>(i) To the small amount of sample solution, add dilute sulphuric acid, small amount of 1, 10-phenanthroline. 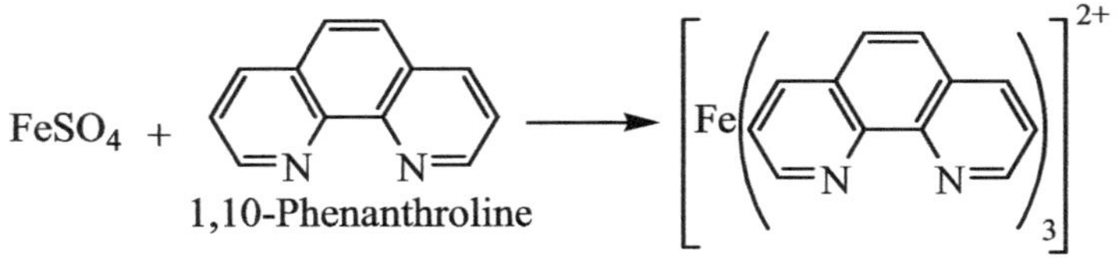<br>$FeSO_4$ + 1,10-Phenanthroline → $[Fe(\text{phen})_3]^{2+}$ | An intense blue color is produced, which is decolorized by the addition of slight excess of 0.1N ceric ammonium sulphate.<br>Decolorization is due to the oxidation of ferrous to ferric. | Ferrous ion is confirmed. |

*Contd...*

| Procedure | Observation | Inference |
|---|---|---|
| (ii) To the prescribed amount of sample solution, add small amount of potassium ferri-cyanide.<br>$FeSO_4 + K_3[Fe(CN)_6] \longrightarrow KFe[Fe(CN)_6]\downarrow + K_2SO_4$<br>($K_3[Fe(CN)_6]$: Potassium ferri cyanide; $KFe[Fe(CN)_6]$: Ferrous ferric cyanide (Dark blue precipitate)) | A dark blue precipitate (turnbull's blue) is formed which is insoluble in dilute hydrochloric acid but decomposed by sodium hydroxide solution. | Ferrous ion is confirmed. |
| (iii) The small amount of sample solution is treated with potassium ferrocyanide solution.<br>$FeSO_4 + K_4Fe(CN)_6 \xrightarrow[-K_2SO_4]{} K_2Fe[Fe(CN)_6]^+ \xrightarrow[\text{air}]{[O]} KFe[Fe(CN)_6]$<br>($K_4Fe(CN)_6$: Potassium ferrocyanide; $K_2Fe[Fe(CN)_6]^+$: White precipitate; $KFe[Fe(CN)_6]$: (Prussian blue)) | A white precipitate is obtained which becomes blue due to atmospheric oxidation, insoluble in dilute hydrochloric acid. | Ferrous ion is confirmed. |
| **10. Lead ($Pb^{2+}$):**<br>(i) To the sample solution add small amount of dilute acetic acid, small amount of potassium chromate solution.<br>$PbCl_2 + K_2CrO_4 \longrightarrow PbCrO_4\downarrow + 2\,KCl$<br>($K_2CrO_4$: Potassium chromate; $PbCrO_4$: Lead chromate (Yellow precipitate)) | A yellow precipitate is obtained which is insoluble in sodium hydroxide solution. | Lead is confirmed. |
| (ii) To a small amount of sample solution, in dilute acetic acid or appropriate solvent, add required quantity of water, one drop of potassium iodide. Heated to boil and then cooled.<br>$Pb(NO_3)_2 + 2\,KI \longrightarrow PbI_2\downarrow + 2\,KNO_3$<br>($PbI_2$: Yellow precipitate) | A yellow precipitate is obtained. The precipitate becomes glistering plates. | Lead is confirmed. |

*Contd...*

| Procedure | Observation | Inference |
|---|---|---|
| (iii) A small amount of sample solution is treated with potassium cyanide solution and made alkaline with ammonia.<br>The above solution is mixed with lead free dithizone solution, the lead dithizone complex is formed which dissolves in chloroform. 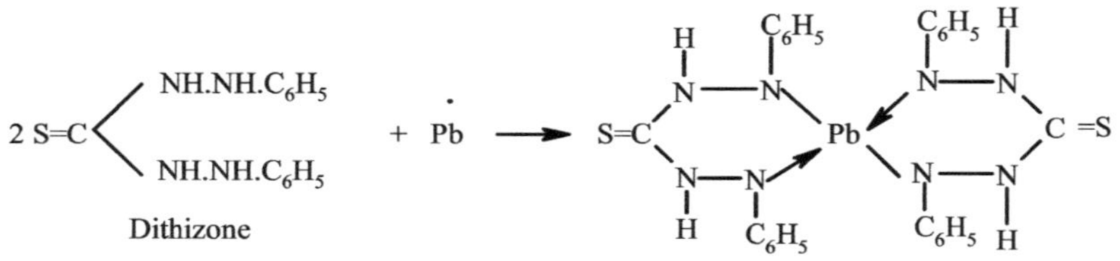<br>$2\ S{=}C(NH.NH.C_6H_5)_2 + Pb \longrightarrow$ Lead-dithizone complex<br>Dithizone<br>Lead-dithizone complex<br>(Brick red color) | A brick red solution is formed.<br><br>The chloroform layer shows brick red color | Lead is confirmed. |
| **11. Lithium ($Li^+$):**<br>(i) A small amount of lithium carbonate or the given sample to be examined is dissolved in small amount of hydrochloric acid. The carbon dioxide formed is removed by boiling and the solution is made alkaline by adding sodium hydroxide solution. To this add disodium hydrogen phosphate solution and boil if needed.<br>$3\ LiCl + Na_2HPO_4 \longrightarrow Li_3PO_4 + HCl + 2\ NaCl$<br>**Note:** The formation of sodium hydroxide interferes with the reaction, so the reaction rate is enhanced by adding small amount of hydrochloric acid. | A white precipitate is formed (formation of lithium phosphate). | Lithium ion is confirmed. |
| **(ii) Flame test:** The small amount of sample is solution taken in a watch glass. To this add small amount of dilute hydrochloric acid and make a paste and introduced into a non-luminous flame. | A red color is formed. | Lithium ion is confirmed. |

*Contd...*

| Procedure | Observation | Inference |
|---|---|---|
| **12. Magnesium ($Mg^{2+}$) :**<br>(i) To the small amount of sample, add dilute ammonia solution and dilute ammonium chloride solution.<br>To this solution add disodium hydrogen phosphate.<br>$Mg(NO_3)_2 + 2\,NH_4OH \longrightarrow 2\,NH_4NO_3 + \underset{\text{(White precipitate)}}{Mg(OH)_2}$<br>$Mg(OH)_2 + 2\,NH_4Cl \longrightarrow MgCl_2 + 2\,NH_4OH$ (Excess $NH_4Cl$)<br>$MgCl_2 + Na_2HPO_4 + NH_4OH \longrightarrow 2NaCl + Mg(NH_4)PO_4 + H_2O$<br>Magnesium ammonium phosphate (White crystalline precipitate) | A white precipitate is formed which is soluble in ammonium chloride solution (due to common ion effect)<br><br>A white crystalline precipitate is obtained. | Magnesium ion is confirmed. |
| (ii) To a small amount of acidic sample solution or neutral solution add few drops of titan yellow solution and few drops of sodium hydroxide solution. | A bright red turbidity or precipitate is produced ($Mg(OH)_2$ forms complex with titan yellow). | Magnesium ion is confirmed. |
| **13. Mercury ($Hg^{+2}$):**<br>(i) A small amount of sample to be examined is placed on a well scrapped copper foil. A dark grey stain appears slowly (spot). This on rubbing becomes shining, now dried copper foil is heated in a test tube.<br>$HgCl_2 + Cu^{2+} \longrightarrow Hg^{2+} + CuCl_2$ | The spot disappears. | Mercury ion is confirmed. |
| (ii) To a sample solution, add potassium iodide solution<br>$\underset{\text{Mercuric chloride}}{HgCl_2} + 2\,KI \longrightarrow \underset{\text{Mercuric iodide}}{HgI_2}\downarrow + 2\,KCl$<br>(iii) If sample contains mercurous salt, it reacts with potassium iodide solution.<br>$\underset{\text{Mercurous chloride}}{HgI_2} + 2\,KI \longrightarrow K_2[HgI_4]$ | A bright red precipitate is formed (mercuric iodide) it is soluble in excess of potassium iodide solution (test for mercuric iodide). | Mercuric ion is confirmed. |

*Contd...*

| Procedure | Observation | Inference |
|---|---|---|
| (iv) A small amount of sample solution is treated with strong sodium hydroxide until the solution strongly alkaline.<br>$Hg_2(NO_3)_2 + 2\,NaOH \longrightarrow Hg_2O + 2\,NaNO_3 + H_2O$ | Yellow precipitate is produced which changes to green on standing (test for mercurous salt). | Mercurous ion is confirmed. |
| (v) A small amount of sample is treated with dilute hydrochloric acid.<br>$Hg_2(NO_3)_2 + 2\,HCl \longrightarrow \underset{\text{Mercurous chloride (White precipitate)}}{Hg_2Cl_2\downarrow} + 2\,HNO_3$ | A dense yellow precipitate is produced. | Mercuric ion is confirmed. |
| To the above precipitate add dilute ammonia solution.<br>$Hg_2Cl_2 + 2\,NH_3 \longrightarrow \underset{\text{(White precipitate)}}{Hg(NH_2)Cl\downarrow} + \underset{\text{(Black precipitate)}}{Hg} + NH_4Cl$<br>**Note:** None of the mercury compound is official in I.P. | A white precipitate is obtained.<br>The white precipitate becomes black. | Mercurous ion is confirmed. |
| **14. Potassium ($K^+$):** Most of the potassium salts are water soluble.<br>(i) To a small volume of sample solution add small amount of dilute acetic acid and freshly prepared sodium cobalt nitrite solution<br>$3\,KCl + Na_3[CO(NO_2)_6] \longrightarrow \underset{\text{Potassium cobaltnitrite (Orange yellow precipitate)}}{K_3[CO(NO_2)_6]} + 3\,NaCl$ | A yellow or orange yellow precipitate is formed immediately. | Potassium ion is confirmed. |
| (ii) The small amount of sample solution is heated | No precipitate is obtained. | Potassium ion is confirmed. |

*Contd...*

| Procedure | Observation | Inference |
|---|---|---|
| To this add one drop of sodium sulphide solution. Now the solution is cooled in ice water, and then adds tartaric acid solution. Then solution is allowed to cool.<br>$KCl + H_2C_4H_4O_6 \longrightarrow KHC_4H_4O_6 + HCl$<br>Potassium bitartarate<br>(White precipitate) | A white crystalline precipitate is obtained. | Potassium ion is confirmed. |
| (iii) To a few mg of ignited sample, cool the residue and dissolve in water. To this solution, add little amount of platinic chloride and hydrochloric acid solution.<br>$2\,KCl + H_2PtCl_6^{2-} \longrightarrow K_2[PtCl_6] + 2\,HCl$<br>(Yellow precipitate) | A yellow crystalline precipitate is obtained which on ignition leaves a residue of potassium chloride and platinum. | Potassium ion is confirmed. |
| **15. Silver ($Ag^+$):**<br>(i) A small amount of sample solution is treated with dilute hydrochloric acid solution.<br>$AgNO_3 + HCl \longrightarrow AgCl + HNO_3$<br>$AgCl + 2\,NH_4OH \longrightarrow [Ag(NH_3)_2]^+ + Cl^- + 2\,H_2O$ | A curdy white precipitate is obtained which is soluble in dilute ammonia solution. | Silver ion is confirmed. |
| To the above alkaline solution, potassium iodide solution is added<br>$AgCl + KI + 2H_2O \longrightarrow AgI + KCl + 2NH_4OH$ | A yellow precipitate is obtained which is in soluble in excess ammonia. | Silver ion is confirmed. |
| (ii) A solution of silver salt is treated with small amount of potassium chromate solution.<br>$2\,AgNO_3 + K_2CrO_4 \longrightarrow 2\,KNO_3 + Ag_2CrO_4$<br>Silver chromate<br>(Red precipitate)<br>$Ag_2CrO_4 + 2\,HNO_3 \longrightarrow 2\,AgNO_3 + H_2CrO_4$ | A red precipitate is obtained which is soluble in nitric acid and also in ammonia. | Silver ion is confirmed. |
| The above precipitate is treated with sodium hydroxide solution it get decomposed.<br>$Ag_2CrO_4 + 2\,NaOH \longrightarrow Na_2CrO_4 + Ag_2O + H_2O$<br>(Black precipitate) | Brownish black color precipitate is obtained. | Silver ion is confirmed. |

***Contd...***

| Procedure | Observation | Inference |
|---|---|---|
| **16. Sodium ($Na^+$):** | | |
| (i) To a small amount of sample solution, add little quantity of potassium carbonate solution. Then add freshly prepared potassium antimonite solution. Boil it, cooled in water, if necessary the inner wall of the test tube is rubbed with glass rod.<br>$NaCl + \underset{\text{Potassium antimonate}}{KH_2SbO_4} \longrightarrow \underset{\text{Sodium pyro antimonate (White precipitate)}}{NaH_2SbO_4 \downarrow} + KCl$ | A dense white precipitate is obtained. | Sodium ion is confirmed. |
| (ii) The sample solution is acidified with dilute acetic acid, add excess of magnesium uranyl acetate solution.<br>$NaCl + \underset{\text{Magnesium uranyl acetate}}{3\,UO_2(CH_3COO)_2 + Mg(CH_3COOH)_2} + CH_3COOH \downarrow$<br>$\underset{\text{Sodium magnesium uranyl acetate (Yellow precipitate)}}{NaMg(UO_2)_3(CH_3COO)_9 \downarrow} + HCl$ | A yellow crystalline precipitate is obtained. | Sodium ion is confirmed. |
| **17. Zinc ($Zn^{2+}$):** | | |
| (i) A small amount of sample is treated with one or two drops of sodium hydroxide solution. To the precipitate add excess sodium hydroxide solution. The precipitate is dissolved. To this add ammonium chloride solution.<br>$Zn(OH)_2 + 2\,NaOH \longrightarrow \underset{\text{Sodium zincate}}{Na_2ZnO_2} + 2\,H_2O$ | A white precipitate is formed due to sodium zincate. | Zinc ion is confirmed. |
| To the above clear solution add sodium sulphide solution.<br>$Na_2ZnO_2 + Na_2S + 2\,H_2O \longrightarrow \underset{\text{Zinc sulphide (White flocculent precipitate)}}{ZnS} + 4\,NaOH$<br>$ZnCl_2 + 2\,NaOH \longrightarrow 2\,NaCl + \underset{\text{Zinc hydroxide}}{Zn(OH)_2}$ | A white flocculent precipitate is obtained (zinc sulphide). | Zinc ion is confirmed. |

*Contd...*

| Procedure | Observation | Inference |
|---|---|---|
| (ii) A required amount of sample solution is acidified with dilute sulphuric acid solution, then add one drop of copper sulphate solution and add little amount of ammonium mercuric thiocyanate solution.<br>$Zn^{2+} + [Hg(SCN)_4]^{2-} \longrightarrow Zn[Hg(SCN)_4]$<br>Zinc mercuric thiocyanate<br>(Violet precipitate)<br>**Note:** If copper ions are present alone, they do not form a precipitate. If zinc ions are present alone, they form white precipitate. | A violet precipitate is formed. | Zinc ion is confirmed. |
| (iii) Small amount of sample solution is treated with excess of potassium ferrocyanide solution.<br>$2\ ZnSO_4 + K_4[Fe(CN)_6] \longrightarrow Zn_2[Fe(CN)_6]\downarrow + 2\ K_2SO_4$<br>Zinc ferrocyanide<br>$3\ Zn_2[Fe(CN)_6] + K_4[Fe(CN)_6]$ (excess) $\longrightarrow 2\ Zn_3K_2[Fe(CN)_6]$<br>Zinc potassium ferrocyanide<br>(White precipitate) | A white precipitate is formed, which is insoluble in dilute hydrochloric acid. | Zinc ion is confirmed. |

## 5.8.2 Tests for Anions

| Procedure | Observation | Inference |
|---|---|---|
| **1. Acetates ($CH_3COO^-$):** | | |
| (i) Small quantity of sample is warmed with an equal quantity of oxalic acid.<br>$2\,CH_3COONa$ (Sodium acetate) + $(COOH)_2$ (Oxalic acid) $\longrightarrow$ $2\,CH_3COOH$ (Acetic acid) + $(COONa)_2$ (Sodium oxalate) | White acid vapours are liberated with characteristic odour of acetic acid (vinegar smell). | Acetate ion is confirmed. |
| (ii) Small quantity of sample is warmed with 1 ml of sulphuric acid and alcohol.<br>$2\,CH_3COONa$ (Sodium acetate) + $2\,C_2H_5OH$ (Ethanol) + $H_2SO_4$ $\longrightarrow$ $2\,CH_3COOC_2H_5$ (Ethyl acetate) + $Na_2SO_4$ (Sodium sulphate) + $H_2O$ | Fruity smell is evolved, due to the formation of ester. | Acetate ion is confirmed. |
| (iii) To the sample, add one drop of lanthanum nitrate solution followed by one drop of 0.1N iodine solution and one drop of dilute ammonia solution. Heat to boil. | Intense blue color precipitate or solution is produced (due to the adsorption of iodine by lanthanum acetate). | Acetate ion is confirmed. |
| **2. Benzoates ($C_6H_5COO^-$):** | | |
| (i) The dilute (10% w/v) neutral solution of sample is treated with ferric chloride solution. Mix well.<br>$3\,C_6H_5COONa$ (Sodium benzoate) + $2\,FeCl_3$ (Ferric chloride) + $3\,H_2O$ $\longrightarrow$ $Fe(C_6H_5COO)_3 . Fe(OH)_3$ (Slight yellow precipitate) + $3NaCl$ | Slight yellow precipitate is obtained. | Benzoate ion is confirmed. |
| (ii) A small amount of substance to be examined is moistened with one drop of sulphuric acid, warm the test tube gently.<br>$2\,C_6H_5COONa$ (Sodium benzoate) + $H_2SO_4$ $\xrightarrow{Warm}$ $2\,C_6H_5COOH$ (Benzoic acid) + $Na_2SO_4$ | A white sublimate is formed which is deposited on the inner walls of the test tube. Melting point of the sublimate is 121 °C. | Benzoate ion is confirmed. |

| Procedure | Observation | Inference |
|---|---|---|
| (iii) To the aqueous solution of sample or sample solution in appropriate solvent, is added one ml of hydrochloric acid.<br>$\underset{\text{Sodium benzoate}}{C_6H_5COONa} + HCl \longrightarrow \underset{\text{Benzoic acid}}{C_6H_5COOH} + NaCl$ | A white color precipitate is obtained. Melting point is 121 °C (benzoic acid). | Benzoate ion is confirmed. |
| **3. Bicarbonates ($HCO_3^-$):**<br>(i) The sample solution to be examined is boiled in a test tube.<br>$\underset{\text{Sodium bicarbonate}}{2\,NaHCO_3} \xrightarrow[\text{(Boil)}]{\Delta} \underset{\text{Sodium carbonate}}{Na_2CO_3} + CO_2\uparrow + H_2O$ | A brisk effervescence is produced (carbon dioxide gas is evolved). | Bicarbonate ion is confirmed. |
| (ii) To the sample solution add magnesium sulphate.<br>$NaHCO_3 + MgSO_4 \xrightarrow{\text{Cold}} \text{No reaction}$ | No precipitate is formed. (If carbonate is present gives result) | Bicarbonate ion is confirmed. |
| If the mixture is boiled.<br>$2\,NaHCO_3 + MgSO_4 \xrightarrow{\text{Boil}} \underset{\text{White precipitate}}{Mg(OH)_2} + Na_2SO_4 + 2CO_2$<br>While heating,<br>$2\,NaHCO_3 \longrightarrow Na_2CO_3 + CO_2\uparrow + H_2O$<br>$Na_2CO_3 + H_2O \rightleftharpoons 2\,Na^+ + 2\,OH^- + CO_2$<br>$MgSO_4 + 2\,OH^- + 2\,Na^+ \longrightarrow \underset{\text{White precipitate}}{Mg(OH)_2} + Na_2SO_4$ | A white precipitate is formed. | Presence of bicarbonate ion is confirmed. |
| (iii) The required quantity of sample solution or a pinch of sample to be examined is taken in a test tube. To this add small amount of 2N acetic acid. The tube is closed with two way bent tubes immediately. Heat the tube gently and the liberated gas is collected in barium hydroxide solution.<br>$NaHCO_3 + \underset{\text{Acetic acid}}{CH_3COOH} \longrightarrow \underset{\text{Sodium acetate}}{CH_3COONa} + CO_2\uparrow + H_2O$ | A white precipitate (barium carbonate) is formed which is dissolved in excess of dilute hydrochloric acid. | Bicarbonate ion is confirmed. |

*Contd...*

| Procedure | Observation | Inference |
|---|---|---|
| $CO_2 + \underset{\text{Barium hydroxide}}{Ba(OH)_2} \longrightarrow \underset{\text{White precipitate}}{BaCO_3\downarrow} + H_2O$<br>$BaCO_3 + 2\,HCl \longrightarrow \underset{\text{Barium chloride}}{BaCl_2} + CO_2 + H_2O$ | | |
| (iv) The aqueous solution of bicarbonate is treated with mercuric chloride solution.<br>$2\,NaHCO_3 + \underset{\text{Mercuric chloride}}{HgCl_2} \longrightarrow \underset{\text{Mercuric bicarbonate}}{Hg(HCO_3)_2} + 2\,NaCl$ | A yellow color precipitate is obtained (formation of mercuric bicarbonate). | Bicarbonate ion is confirmed. |
| $Hg(HCO_3)_2 \xrightarrow{\text{Hydrolysis}} \underset{\text{Mercuric hydroxide}}{Hg(OH)_2} + 2\,CO_2\uparrow$<br>$Hg(OH)_2 \xrightarrow{\text{Decomposition}} \underset{\text{Mercuric oxide (Red precipitate)}}{HgO\downarrow} + H_2O$ | The intensity of the yellow color of the precipitate is decreased due to hydrolysis, finally gives red color precipitate (due to formation of mercuric oxide decomposition) | Bicarbonate ion is confirmed. |

**Note:** In the test (iii) acetic acid is used instead of mineral acids because if mineral acid is used means the impurities like thiosulphates and sulphites are present, which yield sulphur dioxide. The liberated sulphur dioxide reacts with barium hydroxide gives a white color precipitate of barium sulphite. So the reaction gives positive result. (Barium sulphite also completely soluble in dilute hydrochloric acid). But acetic acid does not liberate sulphur dioxide, so interference is prevented.

*Contd...*

| Procedure | Observation | Inference |
|---|---|---|
| **4. Bromides ($Br^-$):** | | |
| (i) Take the sample being examined is equivalent to 3 mg of bromide or the sample solution is acidified with 2N nitric acid, one drop of silver nitrate solution is added. The solution is allowed to stand. <br> $\underset{\text{Sodium bromide}}{NaBr} + \underset{\text{Silver nitrate}}{AgNO_3} \xrightarrow{HNO_3} \underset{\text{Silver bromide}}{AgBr\downarrow} + \underset{\text{Sodium nitrate}}{NaNO_3}$ <br> (Pale yellow precipitate) | A curdy pale yellow precipitate is formed (formation of silver bromide). | Bromide ion is confirmed. |
| The above solution is centrifuged, and the precipitate is repeatedly washed with water. To the resulting precipitate add 2 to 3 water drops of dilute ammonia solution. <br> $AgBr + 2\,NH_3 \longrightarrow \underset{\text{Silver ammonium bromide}}{Ag(NH_3)_2^+Br}$ | The precipitate obtained is insoluble in dilute ammonia solution and it is also insoluble in nitric acid. | Bromide ion is confirmed. |
| (ii) To the required amount of sample solution, small amount of chlorine solution is added. <br> $2\,NaBr + Cl_2 \longrightarrow 2\,NaCl + Br_2\uparrow$ <br> (soluble in $CHCl_3$) | Bromine gas is evolved as red vapours which is soluble in chloroform and gives reddish color solution. | Bromide ion is confirmed. |
| To the above reddish colored solution containing liberated bromine is treated with phenol solution. <br> $3\,Br_2$ + phenol (OH) ⟶ 2,4,6-tribromophenol (OH; Br, Br, Br) + $3\,HBr$ <br> 2,4,6-Tribromo phenol (White precipitate) <br> In order to prevent the interference of iodide in this test, it is performed by boiling aqueous solution of sample with excess of lead dioxide before doing the test. | A white precipitate is obtained. (formation of tribromo phenol) | Bromide ion is confirmed. |

*Contd...*

| Procedure | Observation | Inference |
|---|---|---|
| **5. Carbonates ($CO_3^{2-}$):** | | |
| (i) The required quantity of sample solution to be examined is taken in a test tube and boil the solution. To this add small amount of 2N acetic acid. The tube is closed with two way bent tubes immediately. Heat the tube gently and the liberated gas is collected in barium hydroxide solution.<br>$\underset{\text{Acetic acid}}{Na_2CO_3 + 2\,CH_3COOH} \longrightarrow \underset{\text{Sodium acetate}}{2\,CH_3COONa} + CO_2\uparrow + H_2O$<br>$CO_2 + \underset{\text{Barium hydroxide}}{Ba(OH)_2} \longrightarrow \underset{\text{White precipitate}}{BaCO_3\downarrow} + H_2O$ | A brisk effervescence is liberated.<br>A white precipitate is formed that dissolves on addition of excess of dilute hydrochloric acid. | Carbonate ion is confirmed. |
| (ii) The required quantity of sample solution is treated with mercuric chloride solution.<br>$4\,Na_2CO_3 + 4\,HgCl_2 \xrightarrow{H_2O} \underset{\text{Reddish brown precipitate}}{HgCO_3 . 3\,HgO\downarrow} + 3\,CO_2 + 8\,NaCl$ | A reddish brown precipitate is obtained (formation of basic mercuric carbonate). | Carbonate ion is confirmed. |
| (iii) To the neutral solution of sample, barium chloride solution is added. | No precipitate is formed. | Carbonate ion is confirmed. |
| (iv) The neutral solution of sample is taken in two test tubes. The lead acetate solution is added to one test tube, another one test tube silver nitrate solution is added.<br>$Na_2CO_3 + Pb(CH_3COO)_2 \longrightarrow \underset{\text{White precipitate, Soluble in acid}}{PbCO_3\downarrow} + 2\,CH_3COONa$<br>$Na_2CO_3 + 2\,AgNO_3 \longrightarrow \underset{\text{Silver carbonate (soluble in acid and ammonia)}}{Ag_2CO_3} + 2NaNO_3$ | A white precipitate is formed in both test tubes which is soluble in acid and ammonia solution. | Carbonate ion is confirmed. |

*Contd...*

| Procedure | Observation | Inference |
|---|---|---|
| **6. Chlorides ($Cl^-$):** | | |
| (i) A quantity of sample being tested equivalent to 2 mg of chloride ion or required quantity of sample in appropriate solvent is taken in a test tube. The solution is acidified with dilute nitric acid and add 1 to 3 drops of silver nitrate solution. The tube is shaken well and allowed to stand for some time.<br>$\underset{\text{Sodium chloride}}{NaCl} + AgNO_3 \longrightarrow \underset{\text{Silver chloride (Curdy white precipitate)}}{AgCl\downarrow} + NaNO_3$<br>$AgCl + 2\,NH_3 \longrightarrow \underset{\text{(Soluble)}}{Ag(NH_3)_2Cl}$<br>$Ag(NH_3)_2Cl + 2\,HNO_3 \longrightarrow AgCl + 2\,NH_4NO_3$ | A curdy white precipitate is formed which is insoluble in nitric acid but soluble in dilute ammonia solution. It is once again reprecipitated by the addition of nitric acid. | Chloride ion is confirmed. |
| (ii) To the required amount of sample solution, potassium dichromate and 2 to 3 drops of sulphuric acid is added. A filter paper is moistened with diphenyl carbazide solution is placed over the mouth of the test tube.<br>$4\,NaCl + \underset{\text{Potassium dichromate}}{K_2Cr_2O_7} + 6\,H_2SO_4 \longrightarrow \underset{\text{Chromyl chloride}}{2\,CrO_2Cl_2} + 2\,KHSO_4 + 4\,NaHSO_4 + 3\,H_2O$<br>$CrO_2Cl_2 + H_2O + \underset{\text{(Filter paper)}}{\text{Diphenyl carbazide}} \longrightarrow \text{Violet red color}$ | The paper turns to violet red color. | Chloride ion is confirmed. |
| **7. Citrates ( $C_6H_5O_7^{3-}$):** | | |
| (i) To the neutralized solution of sample under examination, add calcium chloride solution.<br>Boil the solution.<br>$2\,\underset{\text{Sodium citrate}}{HO{-}C(CH_2COONa)_2{-}COOH} + \underset{\text{Calcium chloride}}{3\,CaCl_2} \xrightarrow{\text{Boil}} \underset{\text{Calcium citrate}}{\left(HO{-}C(CH_2COO)_2{-}COO\right)_2 3Ca^{2+}} + 4NaCl + 2HCl$ | No precipitate is obtained.<br>White precipitate is obtained (formation of calcium citrate) which is soluble in acetic acid. | Citrate ion is confirmed. |

*Contd...*

| Procedure | Observation | Inference |
|---|---|---|
| (ii) The required quantity of sample is taken in a test tube. To this one drop of sulphuric acid and 3 ml of potassium permanganate solution are added. Just warm the solution. | The pink color of potassium permanganate gets decolorized. | Citrate ion is confirmed. |
| Now to the above solution, add one drop of 10% w/v sodium nitroprusside solution in 1M sulphuric acid and small quantity of sulphamic acid. The solution is made alkaline with strong ammonia solution until get a clear solution. Add excess ammonia solution. | A violet color solution is obtained which turns blue. | Citrate ion is confirmed |
| (iii) To the neutral solution of sample to be examined is treated with excess of silver nitrate solution.<br>$2\,HO-C(CH_2COONa)_2-COOH$ (Sodium citrate) $+ 3AgNO_3$ (Silver nitrate) $\xrightarrow{Boil}$ $(HO-C(CH_2COO)_2-COO)_2\,3Ag^{2+}$ (Silver citrate) $+ 4NaNO_3 + 2HNO_3$ | A white precipitate is obtained (formation of silver citrate which is soluble in nitric acid and dilute ammonia solution. | Citrate ion is confirmed. |
| (iv) To the alkaline solution of sample, add mercuric sulphate and heat it. Then add potassium permanganate solution. | The pink color of the solution is decolorized and a white precipitate is obtained. | Citrate ion is confirmed. |
| **8. Fluorides (F⁻):**<br>(i) To the sample solution, add barium chloride or lead acetate solution.<br>$2NaF + BaCl_2 \longrightarrow 2NaCl + BaF_2$<br>$2NaF + (CH_3COO)_2Pb$ (Lead acetate) $\longrightarrow PbF_2\downarrow$ (White precipitate) $+ 2CH_3COONa$ (Sodium acetate) | A white precipitate is obtained (formation of barium fluoride or lead fluoride). The precipitate is soluble in nitric acid. | Fluoride ion is confirmed. |

*Contd…*

| Procedure | Observation | Inference |
|---|---|---|
| (ii) To the sample solution, add silver nitrate solution. <br> $NaF + AgNO_3 \longrightarrow$ No reaction | No precipitate is obtained. | Fluoride ion is confirmed. |
| (iii) The required quantity of sample is treated with calcium chloride solution. <br> $2\,NaF + CaCl_2 \longrightarrow 2\,NaCl + CaF_2$ <br> Calcium fluoride (white gelatinous precipitate) | A white gelatinous precipitate is obtained. | Fluoride ion is confirmed. |
| (iv) The required quantity of sample is taken in a dry test tube, add concentrated sulphuric acid. Heat it. <br> $2NaF + H_2SO_4 \longrightarrow Na_2SO_4 + 2HF$ | The white vapours are evolved (HF), which is identified by etching the upper part of the glass wall of the test tube. | Fluoride ion is confirmed. |
| **9. Iodides ($I^-$):** <br> (i) To the required quantity of sample solution or the amount of sample equivalent to about 4 mg of iodide is acidified with nitric acid, add one drop of silver nitrate solution. The solution is mixed well and allowed to stand. <br> $NaI + AgNO_3 \xrightarrow{HNO_3} AgI\downarrow + NaNO_3$ | A curdy, pale yellow precipitate is obtained which is insoluble in dilute ammonia solution. | Iodide ion is confirmed. |
| (ii) To the required quantity of sample solution, add one drop of 2N sulphuric acid, one to two drops of potassium dichromate solution. Equal amount of water and chloroform are added. Shake the mixture well for few seconds, allowed to stand for 5 minutes. <br> $6I^- + Cr_2O_7^{2-} + 14\,H \longrightarrow 2\,Cr^{3+} + 7\,H_2O + 3\,I_2$ | Chloroform layer shows violet or violet red color. | Iodide ion is confirmed. |

*Contd...*

| Procedure | Observation | Inference |
|---|---|---|
| (iii) To the small amount of sample, add mercuric chloride solution.<br>$2\,KI + HgCl_2 \longrightarrow HgI_2\downarrow + 2\,KCl$ Mercuric iodide (Dark red precipitate)<br>$HgI_2 + 2\,KI$ (excess) $\longrightarrow K_2HgI_4$ Potassium mercuric iodide or Vaslers reagent<br>$NaI + AgNO_3 \xrightarrow{dil.HNO_3} AgI + NaNO_3$ Silver iodide (Curdy pale yellow precipitate) | A dark red precipitate is obtained which is completely soluble in excess of potassium iodide solution. | Iodide ion is confirmed. |
| **10. Lactates ($CH_3CH(OH)COO^-$):** A required quantity of sample solution is taken in a test tube. To this add 1 ml of bromine solution and one drop of sulphuric acid. Heat it on a water bath until the color is discharged. To this ammonium sulphate is added and mixed. Then add one drop of 10% w/v solution of sodium nitroprusside in sulphuric acid drop wise and also added strong ammonia solution without mixing. Allowed to stand for 30 minutes. | A green ring is formed between the interfaces of the two liquids. | Lactate ion is confirmed. |
| **11. Metabisulphite ($S_2O_4^{2-}$):** To the sample solution, add iodine solution, similar to that of thiosulphates. But the resulting mixture gives tests for sulphate (Not given by thiosulphates). | Iodine gets decolorized. | Metabisulphite is confirmed. |
| **12. Nitrates ($NO_3^-$):** | | |
| (i) The required quantity of sample solution is prepared by dissolving the sample in water, add 1 ml of sulphuric acid, mix and cool it. To this add 1-2 drops of freshly prepared ferrous sulphate solution through the sides of the test tube.<br>$NaNO_3 + H_2SO_4 \longrightarrow NaHSO_4 + HNO_3$<br>$6\,FeSO_4 + 2\,HNO_3 + 3\,H_2SO_4 \longrightarrow 3\,Fe_2(SO_4)_3 + 2\,NO + 4\,H_2O$<br>$FeSO_4 + NO \longrightarrow FeSO_4.NO$ (Brown-ring) | A brown color ring is formed at the interface of the two liquids. | Nitrate ion is confirmed. |
| (ii) A small amount of sample to be examined is added to the mixture of nitrobenzene and one drop of sulphuric acid. Allowed to stand for 5 minutes and cooled in ice water. Add 5 ml of water and 5 ml of sodium hydroxide solution with stirring slowly. Add 5 ml of acetone, shake and allow to stand. | The acetone layer gets intense violet color | Nitrate ion is confirmed. |

*Contd...*

| Procedure | Observation | Inference |
| --- | --- | --- |
| **13. Phosphates, orthophosphates ($PO_4^{3-}$):** | | |
| (i) The required quantity of neutralized sample solution is added to 5 ml of silver nitrate solution.<br>$2\,HPO_4^{2-} + 3\,Ag^+ \longrightarrow \underset{\text{Silver phosphate}}{Ag_3PO_4\downarrow} + H_2PO_4^-$<br>$Na_2HPO_4 + 3\,AgNO_3 \longrightarrow Ag_3PO_4\downarrow + HNO_3 + 2\,NaNO_3$ | A pale yellow precipitate is formed which is not disappeared by boiling, soluble in dilute ammonia and dilute nitric acid. | Phosphate or orthophosphate ion is confirmed. |
| (ii) To the small amount of sample solution, add five drops of ammoniacal magnesium sulphate solution.<br>$Na_2HPO_4 + MgSO_4 + NH_3 + 6\,H_2O \longrightarrow \underset{\text{Magnesium ammonium phosphate (White crystalline precipitate)}}{MgNH_4PO_4.\,6H_2O} + Na_2SO_4$ | A white crystalline precipitate is obtained. | Phosphate or orthophosphate ion is confirmed. |
| (iii) To the required quantity of sample solution, add dilute nitric acid, ammonium molybdate solution and warm the solution.<br>$H_3PO_4 + 12(NH_4)_2MoO_4 + 21\,HNO_3 \longrightarrow$<br>$\underset{\text{Canary yellow precipitate}}{(NH_4)_3PO_4.\,12MoO_3} + 21NH_4NO_3 + 12H_2O$ | A bright canary yellow precipitate is obtained. | Phosphate or orthophosphate ion is confirmed. |
| **14. Salicylates ($C_7H_5O_3^-$):** | | |
| (i) To the small amount of sample solution to be examined is treated with one drop of ferric chloride solution.<br>$\underset{\text{Sodium salicylate}}{3\,C_6H_4(OH)COONa} + FeCl_3 \longrightarrow \underset{\text{Ferric salicylate (Violet color)}}{[C_6H_4(OH)COO]_3Fe} + 3\,NaCl$ | Violet color is produced, which does not disappear by the addition of one drop of dilute acetic acid. | Salicylate ion is confirmed. |

***Contd…***

| Procedure | Observation | Inference |
|---|---|---|
| (ii) To the required amount of sample in water, added one drop of hydrochloric acid.<br>$C_6H_4(OH)COONa + HCl \longrightarrow \underset{\text{Salicylic acid}}{C_6H_4(OH)COOH\downarrow} + NaCl$<br>(iii) To the prescribed volume of sample solution, add small amount of bromine solution.<br>$\underset{\text{Salicylic acid}}{C_6H_4(OH)COOH} + 3\,Br_2 \longrightarrow \underset{\text{Tribromo phenol (Cream color precipitate)}}{C_6H_2Br_3OH} + 3\,HBr + CO_2$ | White precipitate is obtained (melting point is 159 °C).<br>A cream colored precipitate is obtained. | Salicylate ion is confirmed.<br>Salicylate ion is confirmed. |
| **15. Silicates ($Si_2O_7^-$):** The required quantity of the sample solution is taken in a platinum crucible or lead crucible. To this add required amount (10 mg) of sodium fluoride and one drop of sulphuric acid. The crucible is covered with a thin plastic plate under which a drop of water is suspended. Warm it gently. | White ring formed around the water droplet. | Salicylate ion is confirmed. |
| **16. Sulphates: ($SO_4^{2-}$)**<br>(i) To the required amount of sample, add 1 ml of dilute hydrochloric acid and add 1 ml of barium chloride solution.<br>$Na_2SO_4 + BaCl_2 \xrightarrow{\text{dil.HCl}} BaSO_4\downarrow + 2\,NaCl$ | A white precipitate is formed. | Sulphate ion is confirmed. |
| (ii) To the required amount of sample solution, add 2 ml of lead acetate solution.<br>$K_2SO_4 + (CH_3COO)_2Pb \longrightarrow \underset{\text{(White precipitate)}}{PbSO_4\downarrow} + \underset{\text{Potassium acetate}}{2\,CH_3COOK}$ | A white color precipitate is obtained which is soluble in ammonium acetate solution and sodium hydroxide solution. | Sulphate ion is confirmed. |

*Contd...*

| Procedure | Observation | Inference |
|---|---|---|
| (iii) A suspension or precipitate obtained from the above test (i) is treated with one drop of iodine solution. | Yellow color is formed (distinction from sulphates and di thionites).The yellow color disappears. | Sulphate ion is confirmed. |
| To the above yellow suspension or precipitate, add stannous chloride solution drop wise (distinction from iodates).<br>Boil the mixture. | No colored precipitate is obtained (distinction from selenates and tungstates) | Sulphate ion is confirmed. |
| **17. Tartrates ($C_4H_4O_6^{2-}$):**<br>(i) To the required quantity of sample is warmed with sulphuric acid, charring occurs.<br>$H_2C_4H_4O_6 \longrightarrow CO_2\uparrow + CO\uparrow + 2\,C + 3\,H_2O$<br>$C + 2\,H_2SO_4 \longrightarrow 2\,SO_2 + CO_2\uparrow + 2\,H_2O$<br>$2\,CO + O_2 \xrightarrow[\text{as blue flame}]{\text{Combustion}} 2\,CO_2$<br>$\underset{\text{Tartaric acid}}{\begin{array}{l}CH\text{-}(OH)\text{-}COOH\\ \vert\\ CH\text{-}(OH)\text{-}COOH\end{array}} + 2\,H_2SO_4 \longrightarrow 2\,SO_2 + CO_2 + 3\,CO + 5\,H_2O$ | Carbon monoxide is evolved, which burns with blue flame when ignited. | Tartarate ion is confirmed |
| (ii) To the 5 ml of sample solution in water add one drop of 1% w/v ferrous sulphate solution and one drop of hydrogen peroxide solution.<br>To the colorless solution, add 2M sodium hydroxide solution drop wise.<br>$\begin{array}{l}CH\text{-}(OH)\text{-}COOH\\ \vert\\ CH\text{-}(OH)\text{-}COOH\end{array} + H_2O_2 \longrightarrow \underset{\text{Dihydroxy malic acid (Intense blue color)}}{\begin{array}{l}C\text{-}(OH)\text{-}COOH\\ \Vert\\ C\text{-}(OH)\text{-}COOH\end{array}} + 2\,H_2O$ | A transient yellow color is produced which disappears within 5 min.<br>An intense blue color appears | Tartarate ion is confirmed |

*Contd...*

| Procedure | Observation | Inference |
|---|---|---|
| (iii) To the prescribed volume of sample taken in a test tube, add one drop of 10% w/v potassium bromide solution, one drop of 2% w/v resorcinol solution and add 3 ml of sulphuric acid. | A dark blue colour is produced that changes to red when cooled and poured into water. (The condensation of product of resorcinol and glycolic acid anhydride. The complex is $CH_2.OH.CH[C_6H_3(OH_2)]_2$ ) | Tartarate ion is conformed. |
| **18. Thiosulphates ($S_2O_3^{2-}$):** <br> (i) To the prescribed quantity of sample solution, add dilute HCl. <br> $Na_2S_2O_3 + 2\,HCl \longrightarrow 2\,NaCl + H_2S_2O_3$ <br> $H_2S_2O_3 \longrightarrow \underset{\text{Yellow precipitate}}{S\downarrow} + SO_2 + H_2O$ | A white precipitate is formed which turns yellow and $SO_2$ is evolved with characteristic odour. | Thiosulphate is confirmed. |
| (ii) To the sample solution add ferric chloride solution. <br> $2\,FeCl_3 + Na_2S_2O_3 + H_2O \xrightarrow[\text{Acid}]{H_3O+} 2\,FeCl_2 + 2\,NaCl + H_2SO_4 + S$ <br> $Na_2S_2O_3 + 2\,HCl \rightleftharpoons 2\,NaCl + H_2S_2O_3$ <br> $3\,H_2SO_3 + 2\,FeCl_3 \rightleftharpoons \underset{\text{Ferric thiosulphate (Transient violet color)}}{Fe_2(SO_3)_3} + 6\,HCl$ <br> $Fe_2(SO_3)_3 \longrightarrow FeSO_3 + FeS_2O_6$ | Dark violet color is produced which quickly disappears. | Thiosulphate is confirmed. |
| (iii) To the sample solution, add iodine solution which does not give the reactions of sulphates. <br> $2\,Na_2S_2O_3 + I_2 \longrightarrow 2\,NaI + Na_2S_4O_6$ | The iodine gets decolorized. | Thiosulphate is confirmed. |
| (iv) To the sample solution, add bromine solution which gives the reactions of sulphates. | The bromine gets decolorized. | Thiosulphate is confirmed. |

## PROBABLE QUESTIONS

1. Define the terms Purity and Impurity.
2. Explain about the various types of impurities present in the formulations.
3. Write a note on sources of impurities in pharmaceuticals.
4. Explain briefly about the importance of quality control of pharmaceutical substances.
5. Write a short note on effect of impurities.
6. What are the various methods used to purify the inorganic substances and briefly explain it.
7. Define, test for purity and standards and write the important criteria which decide the choice of tests prescribed in Pharmacopoeia.
8. Define limit test and write the importance of limit tests.
9. Why the pharmacopoeia does not prescribe 'Numerical Value" for the limits of impurities likely to be present in pharmaceutical compounds?
10. Explain the principle and procedure involved in the following limit tests.
    (a) Limit test for sulphate. (b) Limit test for chloride.
    (c) Limit test for iron.
11. Explain about the factors which are to be considered while fixing the limit.
12. Write the reasons of the followings.
    (a) Uses of dilute nitric acid in the limit test for chloride.
    (b) Use of barium sulphate reagent in the limit test for sulphate.
    (c) Use of citric acid, thioglycolic acid and dilute ammonia solution in the limit test for iron.
13. Explain about the limit test for heavy metals.
14. Write about the modified Gutzeit method for the limit test for arsenic.
15. Explain about the principle and procedure underlying the limit test for lead in I.P.
16. Write the two characteristic reactions of sodium, potassium and calcium.
17. Write the confirmatory tests for chloride and sulphate with balanced chemical equations.
18. How do you differentiate between anions and cations?
19. What is mean by loss on drying and loss on ignition? Write about the significance of it and explain the method.
20. Explain how the limit test for lead is different from the limit test for heavy metals.
21. How the ferrous ions and ferric ions are identified and differentiated by chemical tests.
22. Enumerate the two identification tests for nitrate and phosphate.
23. Explain about the identification test for carbonates and bicarbonates.
24. Write note on indicators.
25. What are indicators, explain their importance in analytical chemistry.
26. Define the term impurity. How do they get incorporated in pharmaceutical substances?

CHAPTER 6

# INORGANIC PHARMACEUTICALS (INORGANIC COMPOUNDS USED IN PHARMACY)

## 6.1 GASTROINTESTINAL AGENTS AND RELATED COMPOUNDS

### 6.1.1 Digestive System

**Introduction**

Food we eat plays an important role in our life because it is the main source of chemical energy needed to our body. However, most of the food consists of large size of molecules and that are too large to be used by the cells of our body. Hence it must be broken into smaller size to enter in to the cells.

***Digestion:*** It is the mechanical and chemical process that occurs in our body to break down the ingested food in to smaller molecules.

***Digestive system:*** The organs used to break down the food in to smaller molecules which can be easily absorbed and enters into body cells are collectively known as Digestive system. It also absorb minerals, vitamins and water. It is a tubular system, starts from the buccal cavity (mouth) to the anus, forms an extensive surface area in contact with the external environment and close association with blood vessels.

***Various organs of alimentary canal or Gastro intestinal tract (GIT) or Digestive system:*** The various parts of digestive system are oral cavity (mouth), pharynx, esophagus, stomach, small intestine, large intestine, rectum and anal canal. The other accessory digestive organs are teeth, tongue, three pairs of salivary glands, liver, gallbladder and pancreas.

**Functions of the Digestive system**

***Mouth:*** Secretion of saliva, mastication, size reduction of food particles and swallowing.

***Pharynx and Esophagus:*** Deglutition, relaxation and secretion of mucus.

***Stomach:*** Secretion of gastric juice, digestion of proteins, secretion of enzymes (gastrin, pepsin), formation of chyme by mixing of food with gastric juice and regulates the passage of chyme from stomach to duodenum. It serves as a food reservoir of food, before releasing in to the small intestine.

***Small intestine:*** Mixing of chyme with digestive juice, digestion of lipids, proteins, nucleic acids and absorption.

***Large intestine:*** Haustral churning, peristalsis and movement of colon contents in to rectum; absorption of some amount of water, vitamins and ions, finally excretion or defecation of unabsorbed waste products.

Various processes of digestion are as follows.

1. Ingestion.
2. Secretion.
3. Mixing and propulsion.
4. Digestion.
5. Absorption.
6. Defecation.

The medical specialty that deals with the function, diagnosis and treatment of diseases of the digestive system is called as **Gastroenterology.**

**Disorders of Digestive system:** Whenever the above functions are not happening in a normal manner, there occur diseases or undesirable conditions as mentioned below:

1. ***Vomiting:*** Vomiting or emesis is the forceful expulsion of the contents of the upper GIT, through the mouth due to strongest stimuli.
2. ***Dysphagia:*** Difficulty in swallowing due to inflammation.
3. ***Nausea:*** Loss of appetite and vomiting sensation due to local irritation of the GIT.
4. ***Diarrhoea:*** Due to indigestion, inadequate absorption of fluids and minerals from large intestine leads to loose, urgent bowel movements and dehydration.
5. ***Traveler's Diarrhoea:*** Infectious disease of GIT leads to loose, urgent bowel movements, abdominal pain, nausea and dehydration due to the ingestion of contaminated water or contaminated food.
6. ***Constipation:*** Lack of peristaltic movements of large intestine.
7. ***Gastroenteritis:*** Inflammation of the layers of small intestine and stomach due to bacterial or viral infection
8. ***Achlorhydria or hypochlorhydria:*** Inadequate secretion of gastric juice (hydrochloric acid) in stomach leads to increase in the stomach pH. The symptoms are mild diarrhoea and epigastric pain.
9. ***Heart burn:*** A burning sensation in a region near to the heart due to the esophagus irritation by gastric acid (improper closing of esophageal sphincter).
10. ***Hyperacidity or Ulcers:*** Excessive gastric acid secretion in stomach leads to imbalance of hydrochloric acid and pepsin ratio. It ranges from gastric ulcer to peptic ulcer with pain and sometimes hemorrhages.

The above diseases of GIT can be treated by the administration of inorganic or organic drugs. Several inorganic drugs used for treating the above diseases are described in this chapter.

## 6.1.2 Acidifiers and Alkalinising Agents

**Introduction**

***Acidifiers:*** These are inorganic chemicals which produce or become acid. They increase the level of gastric acid in the stomach when ingested, and hence decreasing the pH of stomach. Patients suffering from achlorhydria are having deficient secretion of hydrochloric acid in stomach. In such cases acidifiers provide the necessary acidity to ascertain proper digestion of food. Systemic acidifiers when given by injection reduces the alkali reserve in the body and also useful in reducing metabolic alkalosis.

Among the many types of acidifiers, three are main type:

- Gastric acidifiers, used in controlling pH of stomach.
- Urinary acidifiers, used in controlling pH of urine.
- Systemic acidifiers, used in controlling pH of all the parts of body.

***Alkalinizers:*** These are substances (example sodium bicarbonate) boost the alkali reserve artificially in the body and also useful in reducing metabolic acidosis.

### Dilute Hydrochloric Acid B.P.

**Mol. Formula:** HCl **Mol. Weight:** 36.5

Dilute hydrochloric acid contains not less than 9.5% w/w and not more than 10.5% w/w of hydrochloric acid.

***Preparation:*** It is prepared by adding 274 gm of concentrated hydrochloric acid slowly in to 726 gm of purified water.

***Physical properties:*** A clear colorless liquid with pungent odour and fuming in nature. It is miscible with water and alcohol. Specific gravity at 25 °C is 1.04 to 1.05, very strongly acidic in nature

***Chemical properties:*** It is reacts with metals but at slower rates and evolves hydrogen gas.

$$2HCl + 2Na \longrightarrow 2NaCl + H_2\uparrow$$

***Test for identification:*** The sample solution gives the characteristic reactions of chloride ion.

***Test for purity:*** It should be tested for arsenic, heavy metals, free chlorine, residue on evaporation and sulphates.

***Test for arsenic:*** Mix a small quantity of sample with water and stannous chloride AsT. The resulting solution complies with the limit tests for arsenic (0.05 ppm).

***Test for residue on evaporation:*** It should not be more than 0.01%.

***Test for heavy metals:*** Dissolve the residue obtained from the above test by adding 2M hydrochloric acid and dilute to 25 ml with water. Take 2 ml of the above solution. Add small amount of dilute acetic acid and make up to 25 ml with water. The resulting solution complies with the limit test for heavy metals (2 ppm).

***Test for sulphate:*** The sulphate impurity should be within the range of 5 ppm. To the small quantity of sample solution add sodium bicarbonate and evaporate to dryness and dissolve the residue with water. The resulting solution complies with limit test for sulphate (5 ppm).

**Assay**

***Principle:*** It is assayed by **acidimetry-alkalimetry method** of titration (also called **neutralization method**).

In this assay the substance is diluted suitably with water and titrated with sodium hydroxide, using methyl red as an indicator. End point is the Red colour. In this assay the sodium hydroxide (the base) reacts with hydrochloric acid and neutralization takes place during the titration. The indicator is yellow colour in alkali medium and it changes to red colour upon neutralization which is the end point.

As the acid and alkali are involved in this assay, it is called as acidimetry-alkalimetry method of titration and the neutralization takes place in this assay during titration hence this assay is also called as Neutralization method. The chemical reactions of this assay are shown below.

$$HCl + NaOH \longrightarrow NaCl + H_2O$$

***Procedure:*** Weigh accurately about 6 gm, add 30 ml of water, mix and titrate with 1M sodium hydroxide using methyl red solution as indicator.

***Uses:*** It is used as an acidifier.

***Dose:*** 0.6 to 8 ml.

***Storage:*** It should be stored in a well closed glass or inert container at a temperature of not exceeding 30 °C.

## Dilute Phosphoric Acid I.P., B.P., U.S.P.

**Mol. Formula:** $H_3PO_4$. **Mol. Weight:** 98

It contains 10% w/w of phosphoric acid (limits 9.5% to 10.5%)

***Preparation:*** It is prepared by mixing 112 gm of phosphoric acid with 888 gm of purified water to get the desired strength.

***Physical properties:*** It is a clear, colorless liquid having specific gravity of 1.057. It is miscible with water and alcohol.

***Test for identification, Test for purity and Storage:*** Similar to phosphoric acid.

**Assay**

***Principle:*** It is assayed by **acidimetry-alkalimetry method** of titration (also called **neutralization method**).

In this assay the substance is dissolved in water and sodium chloride solution is added and titrated with 1N sodium hydroxide, using phenolphthalein as an indicator. End point is the appearance of permanent pale pink colour. In this assay the sodium hydroxide (the base) reacts with phosphoric acid and neutralization takes place during the titration. The indicator is colourless in acid medium and it changes its colour to pink in alkali medium which is the end point.

As the acid and alkali involved in this assay, it is called as acidimetry-alkalimetry method of titration and the neutralization takes place in this assay during titration hence this assay is also called as neutralization method. The chemical reactions of this assay are shown below.

$$2\,NaOH + H_3PO_4 \longrightarrow Na_2HPO_4 + 2\,H_2O$$

***Procedure:*** To 8.6 gm add a solution of 10 gm of sodium chloride in 30 ml of water. Titrate with 1M sodium hydroxide, using phenolphthalein solution as indicator.

***Uses:***

1. It is used as a pharmaceutical aid (acidifying agent).
2. It is also used in dental ailment and in the treatment of lead poisoning.

***Dose:*** 0.3 to 4 ml.

## Sodium Phosphate I.P., B.P., U.S.P.

**(Synonym: Disodium hydrogen phosphate, Disodium hydrogen ortho phosphate dodeca hydrate)**

**Mol. Formula:** $Na_2HPO_4.12H_2O$ **Mol. Weight:** 358.1

It contains not less than 98% and not more than 101% of $Na_2HPO_4$, calculated on the anhydrous basis or with the anhydrous standard.

***Preparation:***

1. *From Sodium carbonate:* Sodium carbonate when added to a hot solution of phosphoric acid, it gives disodium hydrogen phosphate solution. The solution is neutralized, concentrated and the crystals are separated by centrifugation, washed and dried.

$$Na_2CO_3 + H_3PO_4 \longrightarrow Na_2HPO_4 + H_2O + CO_2$$

2. *From Calcium phosphate:* The correct proportions of calcium phosphate and sulphuric acid are reacted to yield mono basic calcium phosphate and calcium sulphate.

$$Ca_3(PO_4)_2 + 2H_2SO_4 \longrightarrow Ca(H_2PO_4)_2 + 2CaSO_4\downarrow$$

To the above mixture add boiling water and filtered. To the filtrate add sodium carbonate to yield the sodium phosphate solution and the dibasic calcium phosphate gets deposited.

The solution is filtered off and the sodium phosphate crystals obtained from this by concentrating the solution and crystallization.

$$Ca(H_2PO_4)_2 + Na_2CO_3 \longrightarrow CaHPO_4 + Na_2HPO_4 + CO_2 + H_2O$$

***Physical properties:*** It is a colorless or white, transparent crystals with saline taste. It is soluble in water and insoluble in alcohol. It effloresces in air.

***Chemical properties:*** When it is heated at 300 °C loses one molecule of water and converted into sodium pyrophosphate.

$$2\,Na_2HPO_4 \xrightarrow[300\ ^\circ C]{\Delta} Na_4P_2O_7 + H_2O$$

***Test for identification:*** The 10% w/v solution of sodium phosphate gives the characteristic reactions of sodium and phosphate.

***Test for purity:*** It should be tested for appearance of solution, arsenic, heavy metals, iron, chlorides, and sulphates, reducing substances, sodium dihydrogen phosphate and water.

***Test for appearance of solution:*** A 10% w/v solution in distilled water should be clear and colorless.

***Test for arsenic*** (**Limit range:** 2 ppm): To the sample solution add required amount of stannated hydrochloric acid AsT. The resulting solution complies with the limit test for arsenic.

***Test for heavy metals*** (**Limit range:** 10 ppm): Prepare the sample solution by using water and acetic acid, the resulting solution complies with the limit test for heavy metals (Refer Method A).

***Test for iron:*** (**Limit Range:** 20 ppm).

***Test for chloride:*** (**Limit range:** 250 ppm).

***Test for sulphate:*** (**Limit range:** 600 ppm).

***Test for sodium dihydrogen phosphate:*** The value of expression is $(n_2\text{-}25)/(25\text{-}n_1)$

where $n_1$, $n_2$ = Volume of 0.1M sodium hydroxide consumed which is obtained from assay. The above value should not exceed 0.025.

**Assay**

***Principle:*** It is assayed by **acidimetry-alkalimetry method** of titration (also called **neutralization method**).

In this assay the substance is dissolved in water and titrated with 0.5N sulphuric acid, using bromocresol green as an indicator. End point is the appearance of yellow colour. (For better end point bromocresol green and methyl red mixture used, which gives the end point greenish-grey colour). In this assay the sodium phosphate (the base) reacts with sulphuric acid and neutralization takes place during the titration. The indicator is blue colour in alkali medium and it changes to yellow colour upon neutralization which is the end point.

As the acid and alkali involved in this assay, it is called as acidimetry-alkalimetry method of titration and the neutralization takes place in this assay during titration hence this assay is also called as neutralization method. The chemical reactions of this assay are shown below.

$$Na_2HPO_4 + H_2SO_4 \longrightarrow Na_2SO_4 + H_3PO_4$$

***Uses:*** It is used as a laxative, catharatic, buffering agent and pharmaceutical aid.

***Dose:*** 2 to 16 gm.

***Storage:*** It should be stored in airtight container and protected from moisture.

## Dried Sodium Phosphate B.P.

**(Synonym: Anhydrous sodium phosphate)**

**Mol. Formula:** $Na_2HPO_4$ **Mol. Weight:** 142

It contains not less than 99% of $Na_2HPO_4$ calculated on the anhydrous basis or with the anhydrous standard.

***Physical properties:*** It is white or colorless powder with saline taste. It is soluble in water and insoluble in alcohol.

***Test for identification:*** It gives the characteristic reactions of sodium and phosphate.

***Test for purity:*** It should be tested for appearance of solution, arsenic, heavy metals, iron, chlorides, and sulphates, reducing substances, sodium dihydrogen phosphate and water.

**Assay**

***Principle:*** It is assayed by **acidimetry-alkalimetry method** of titration (also called **neutralization method**).

In this assay the substance is dissolved in water and titrated with 0.5N sulphuric acid, using bromocresol green as an indicator. End point is the appearance of yellow colour. (For better end point bromocresol green and methyl red mixture used, which gives the end point greenish-grey colour). In this assay dried sodium phosphate (the base) reacts with sulphuric acid and neutralization takes place during the titration. The indicator is blue colour in alkali medium and it changes to yellow colour upon neutralization which is the end point.

As the acid and alkali involved in this assay, it is called as acidimetry-alkalimetry method of titration and the neutralization takes place in this assay during titration hence this assay is also called as neutralization method. The chemical reactions of this assay are shown below.

$$Na_2HPO_4 + H_2SO_4 \longrightarrow Na_2SO_4 + H_3PO_4$$

***Uses:*** It is used as saline catharatic.

***Storage:*** It should be stored in airtight container and protected from moisture.

## Sodium Acid Phosphate I.P.

**(Synonym: Sodium dihydrogen phosphate dihydrate)**

**Mol. Formula:** $NaH_2PO_4 . 2H_2O$ **Mol. Weight:** 156

It contains not less than 98.0% and not more than 100.5% of $NaH_2PO_4$ calculated on the basis of dried substance.

***Preparation***

1. *From Sodium phosphate:* Sodium acid phosphate is prepared by adding the correct proportion of sodium phosphate to phosphoric acid and crystallizes the product.

$$\underset{\text{Sodium phosphate}}{Na_2HPO_4} + \underset{\text{Phosphoric acid}}{H_3PO_4} \longrightarrow \underset{\text{Sodium acid phosphate}}{2NaH_2PO_4}$$

2. *Laboratory preparation:* Sodium acid phosphate is prepared by the gradual addition of sodium carbonate to a measured quantity of boiled, diluted solution of phosphoric acid until the solution is just alkaline to litmus. A further amount phosphoric acid equal to that originally used, is then added to form the sodium dihydrogen salt. The solution is then evaporated to dryness and the crystals are collected and dried.

$$Na_2CO_3 + 2\,H_3PO_4 \longrightarrow 2NaH_2PO_4 + CO_2 + H_2O$$

***Physical properties:*** It is a clear white powder or colorless crystals, odorless, soluble in boiling water, insoluble in alcohol and it is slowly effloresces in air.

***Test for identification:***

(a) The 10% w/v solution should be faintly acidic in nature.

(b) The above solution is neutralized with 10% w/v potassium hydroxide which gives the characteristic reactions of sodium salts.

(c) The solution of sample gives the characteristic reactions of phosphate.

***Test for purity:*** It should be tested for appearance of solution, pH, heavy metals, arsenic, iron, chlorides, sulphates, reducing substances, disodium phosphate and loss on drying.

***Test for appearance of solution:*** The 10% w/v solution of sample in carbon dioxide free water should be clear and colorless.

***Test for pH of the solution:*** The pH of the solution should be 4.2 to 4.5.

***Test for heavy metals:*** (Limit is 10 ppm): The sample solution in boiling water should comply with the limit test for heavy metals which is determined by method D.

***Test for iron:*** Limit is 20 ppm.

***Test for chlorides:*** Limit is 250 ppm.

***Test for sulphates:*** Limit is 300 ppm.

***Test for disodium phosphate:*** Dilute one part of sample solution with 50 parts of water and titrate with 0.05M sulphuric acid using bromocresol green solution as an indicator. The volume of sulphuric acid required should not be more than 1 ml.

***Test for loss on drying:*** It should be 21.5 to 24%. It is determined by heating or drying a required quantity of sample in an oven at 130 °C.

**Assay**

***Principle:*** It is assayed by **acidimetry-alkalimetry method** of titration (also called **neutralization method**).

In this assay the substance is dissolved in water and titrated with 0.5N sodium hydroxide, using bromocresol green as an indicator. End point is the appearance of yellow colour. The end point can also be determined potentiometrically. In this assay the sodium acid phosphate (the base) reacts with sodium hydroxide and neutralization takes place during the titration. The indicator is blue colour in alkali medium and it changes to yellow colour upon neutralization which is the end point.

As the acid and alkali involved in this assay, it is called as acidimetry-alkalimetry method of titration and the neutralization takes place in this assay during titration hence this assay is also called as neutralization method. The chemical reactions of this assay are shown below.

$$NaH_2PO_4 + NaOH \longrightarrow Na_2HPO_4 + H_2O$$

***Procedure:*** Weigh accurately about 2.5 gm, dissolve in 40 ml of water and titrate with carbonate-free 1M sodium hydroxide, determining the end-point potentiometrically.

***Uses:*** It is used as an urinary acidifier.

***Dose:*** 2 to 4 gm

***Storage:*** It should be stored in well closed container and protected from moisture.

## Dilute Ammonia Solution B.P.

**Mol. Formula:** $NH_3$ **Mol. Weight:** 17

It contains 10% w/w of ammonia.

***Preparation:*** It is prepared by diluting strong ammonia solution with freshly boiled and cooled purified water.

***Physical Properties:*** It is a colorless liquid with ammonical odour.

***Test for purity:*** It should be tested for relative density.

**Assay**

***Principle:*** It is assayed by **acidimetry-alkalimetry method** of (Back) titration (also called **neutralization method**).

In this assay the substance is dissolved in Known Excess Standard (KES) 1N sulphuric acid and the excess unreacted (EUR) sulphuric acid is titrated with 1N sodium hydroxide using methyl red as an indicator. End point is the yellow colour.

In this assay the ammonia (the base) reacts with sulphuric acid and neutralization takes place, after this reaction the excess unreacted sulphuric acid is titrated with sodium hydroxide. The indicator is red colour in acid medium and it changes to yellow colour upon neutralization which is the end point.

As the acid and alkali involved in this assay, it is called as acidimetry-alkalimetry method of titration and the neutralization takes place in this assay during titration hence this assay is also called as Neutralization method. The chemical reactions of this assay are shown below.

$$2\,NH_4OH + H_2SO_4 \longrightarrow (NH_4)_2SO_4 + 2\,H_2O$$

$$H_2SO_4 + 2\,NaOH \longrightarrow Na_2SO_4 + 2\,H_2O$$

***Uses:***

1. Dilute ammonia solution is mainly used as a respiratory stimulant (smelling salts).
2. It is also used as a reflux stimulant for fainted persons. It stimulates the respiration and increases heart rate.
3. It is used as a rubefacient and vasoconstrictor, particularly when applied locally to insect stings.

***Caution:*** Care should be taken to inhale dilute ammonia solution since it is highly irritant and gives asphyxia and pulmonary edema.

***Storage:*** It should be stored in tightly closed containers in a cool place, otherwise ammonia will slowly escape.

***Labelling:*** The label should state that

1. The storage conditions.
2. The expiry date of the solution.

---

## Ammonium Chloride I.P., B.P.

**(Synonym: Sal ammoniac)**

**Mol. Formula:** $NH_4Cl$ **Mol. Weight:** 53.5

It contains not less than 99.5% and not more 100.5% of $NH_4Cl$ which is calculated with reference to substance dried over silica gel for 4 hours.

***Preparation:***

1. *Commercial preparation:* Ammonium chloride is commercially prepared by neutralizing hydrochloric acid with ammonia and evaporating the resulting solution to dryness.

$$HCl + NH_3 \longrightarrow NH_4Cl$$

   The purification of the product is done by sublimation from iron pans or crystallization.

2. *From ammonium sulphate:* Ammonium chloride is also prepared by heating ammonium sulphate with sodium chloride.

$$(NH_4)_2SO_4 + 2NaCl \longrightarrow 2NH_3 + 2HCl + Na_2SO_4$$

$$NH_3 + HCl \longrightarrow NH_4Cl$$

3. *Preparation of crude ammonium chloride (Sal ammoniac):* By using this method ammonical gas liquors are treated with lime. During this process the ammonia gas is liberated which is passed in to hydrochloric acid solution. The crude ammonium chloride obtained is commercially known as "Sal ammoniac".

$$NH_3 + HCl \longrightarrow NH_4Cl$$

***Physical properties:*** It is a colorless or white, fine or coarse crystalline powder with cooling saline taste. It is partially soluble in water, carbon dioxide free water, completely soluble in glycerin and slightly soluble in alcohol. It is slightly hygroscopic in nature.

A 0.8% w/v solution of ammonium chloride is isotonic with serum. The sal ammoniac forms fibrous, tough crystalline masses.

***Chemical properties:*** The freshly prepared solution of ammonium chloride is neutral in nature. It becomes quickly acidic on standing because of hydrolysis. Ammonium chloride is soluble in water; the ammonium ion combines with the hydroxyl ion of water leads to the formation of partially undissociated ammonium hydroxide. Due to this effect the hydrogen ion concentration of the solution is slight excess which lowers the pH of the solution to acidic.

$$NH_4Cl + 2H_2O \longrightarrow NH_4OH + H_3O^+ + Cl^-$$

***Test for identification:*** The sample solution gives the characteristic reactions of ammonium ion and chloride ion.

***Test for purity:*** It should be tested for pH, sulphate, iron, arsenic, lead, barium, heavy metals, loss on drying, non volatile matter and thiocyanate.

***Test for non-volatile matter:*** It is determined by drying the substance in vacuum desiccators over phosphorous pentoxide at room temperature. The value should not be more than that of 0.5% w/w.

**Assay**

***Principle:***

***1st method (old method):*** It is assayed by **precipitation method of (Back) titration (Modified Volhard's method).**

In this assay the substance is dissolved in water and acidified with nitric acid and to this a Known Excess Standard (KES) silver nitrate and nitrobenzene added and the Excess Unreacted (EUR) silver nitrate is back titrated against 0.1N ammonium thiocyanate. Ferric ammonium sulphate (Ferric alum) is used as an indicator. End point is the appearance of brick red colour.

During this assay, ammonium chloride reacts with silver nitrate and forms silver chloride. After completion of this reaction, the Excess Unreacted silver nitrate is determined by titrating against ammonium thiocyanate. After the completion of this reaction, further addition of ammonium thiocyanate reacts with the indicator ferric ammonium sulphate and yield brick red colour ferric thiocyanate, which is the end point. As the test substance is converted to a precipitate during this assay, it is called precipitation method. The chemical reactions of this assay are shown below.

$$NH_4Cl + AgNO_3 \longrightarrow NH_4NO_3 + AgCl\downarrow$$

$$AgNO_3 + NH_4SCN \longrightarrow AgSCN\downarrow + NH_4NO_3$$

***2nd method (New method):*** It is assayed by **acidimetry-alkalimetry method** of titration (also called **neutralization method**).

In this assay the substance is dissolved in water and to it previously neutralized formaldehyde (formaldehyde may have small amount of formic aid, which must be neutralised before with sodium hydroxide using phenolphthalein) added and titrated against sodium hydroxide using phenolphthalein as an indicator. End point is the appearance of permanent pale pink colour.

In this assay ammonium chloride undergoes hydrolysis and yield ammonium hydroxide and hydrochloric acid. This reaction is facilitated by formaldehyde, by fixing ammonia as hexamine. The acid formed is now titrated against sodium hydroxide without any interference. The indicator is colourless in acid medium and it changes its colour to pink in alkali medium which is the end point.

As the acid and alkali involved in this assay, it is called as acidimetry-alkalimetry method of titration and the neutralization takes place in this assay during titration hence this assay is also called as Neutralization method. The chemical reactions of this assay are shown below.

$$NH_4Cl + H_2O \longrightarrow NH_4OH + HCl$$

$$4\,NH_4OH + 6\,HCHO \longrightarrow \underset{\text{Hexamine}}{(CH_2)_6N_4} + 10\,H_2O$$

$$HCl + NaOH \longrightarrow NaCl + H_2O$$

***Procedure:*** Dissolve 1 gm in 20 ml of water and add a mixture of 5 ml of formaldehyde solution previously neutralised to phenolphthalein solution and 20 ml of water. After 1-2 min, titrate slowly with 1M sodium hydroxide, using a further 0.2 ml of the same indicator.

***Uses:***

1. It is used as a systemic acidifier and diuretic.
2. It is also used as an expectorant and diaphoretic.
3. It increases the local irritation which leads to increasing the respiratory tract secretions and makes the less viscous mucus. So ammonium chloride and ammonium carbonate are used in cough preparations.

***Dose:*** 1 to 2 gm four times a day as systemic acidifier, 0.3 to 0.5 gm as an expectorant.

***Storage:*** It should be stored in well closed container.

***Official formulations:*** Ammonium chloride injection B.P. Ammonium chloride tablet B.P.

## Aromatic Spirit of Ammonia

**(Synonym: Spirit of sal volatile)**

It contains 1.12- 1.3% w/v of free ammonia and 2.76-3.24% w/v ammonium carbonate and 64-70% w/v alcohol along with lemon oil, nutmeg oil which are used as flavouring agents.

***Composition:***

| | | |
|---|---|---|
| Ammonium bicarbonate | = | 25 gm |
| Strong ammonia solution | = | 75 ml |
| Lemon oil | = | 5 ml |
| Nutmeg oil | = | 3 ml |
| Alcohol (90%) | = | 750 ml |
| Purified water (q.s) | = | 1000 ml |

***Preparation:*** It is prepared by distilling the all oils with water, collect the distillate, add ammonia and ammonium bicarbonate solution. Then they are warmed gently on a water bath at 60 °C with occasional stirring, filter it. Sufficient amount of water is added to it to make up the volume.

***Physical properties:*** It occurs as a colorless, odorless liquid with pungent odour.

**Assay**

***Principle:*** It is assayed for both ammonia and ammonium carbonate.

***Test for ammonia:*** It is assayed by **acidimetry-alkalimetry method** of (Back) titration (also called **neutralization method**).

***For $NH_3$:*** In this assay the substance is treated with Known Excess Standard (KES) 1N sulphuric acid and the Excess Unreacted (EUR) sulphuric acid is titrated with 1N sodium hydroxide using methyl red as an indicator. End point is the yellow colour.

In this assay ammonia (the base) reacts with sulphuric acid and neutralization takes place, after this reaction the excess unreacted sulphuric acid is titrated with sodium hydroxide. The indicator is red colour in acid medium and it changes to yellow colour upon neutralization which is the end point.

As the acid and alkali involved in this assay, it is called as acidimetry-alkalimetry method of titration and the neutralization takes place in this assay during titration hence this assay is also called as Neutralization method. The chemical reactions of this assay are shown below.

$$2\,NH_4OH + H_2SO_4 \longrightarrow (NH_4)_2SO_4 + 2\,H_2O$$

$$H_2SO_4 + 2\,NaOH \longrightarrow Na_2SO_4 + 2\,H_2O$$

***For $NH_4CO_3$:*** It is assayed by **acidimetry-alkalimetry method** of (Back) titration (also called **neutralization method**).

In this assay the substance is treated with sodium hydroxide, boil the mixture and cool. It is then titrated with sulphuric acid using methyl orange as an indicator. End point is the change of colour from yellow to orange.

***Procedure:***

*For total ammonia:* Transfer 10 ml of sample to a 250 ml conical flask containing 50 ml of water. Add 30 ml of 0.5N sulphuric acid, and boil until the solution becomes clear. Cool, add methyl red, and titrate the excess acid with 0.5N sodium hydroxide. Perform a blank determination.

*For ammonium carbonate:* Transfer 10 ml to a flask of about 300 ml capacity. Add 30 ml of 0.5N sodium hydroxide, and boil the mixture, replacing the water lost by evaporation, until the vapors no longer turn moistened red litmus paper blue. Cool, dilute with 100 ml of cold, boiling water, add about 6 drops of phenolphthalein and then add just enough 0.5N sulphuric acid to discharge the color of the phenolphthalein. Add methyl orange and titrate with 0.5N sulphuric acid. Perform a blank determination also.

***Uses:***

1. It is used as a respiratory stimulant by inhalation.
2. It is also used as a flavouring agent.

***Storage:*** It should be stored in small, well closed container. Rubber stoppers are not used because it absorbs ammonia.

## 6.1.3 Acids and Bases used as Pharmaceutical Aids

**Introduction:** Acids and bases are encountered very frequently both in chemistry and in everyday life. They have opposite properties and have the ability to neutralize each other. Acids and bases are carefully regulated in the body by the lungs, blood, and kidneys through equilibrium processes.

To determine whether a substance is an acid or a base, count the hydrogen ions on each substance before and after the reaction. If the number of hydrogen ions has reduced that substance is the acid (donates hydrogen ions). If the number of hydrogen ions has risen that substance is the base (accepts hydrogen ions). Hence acids and bases can be defined in short as follows.

Acid is a substance which when added to water produces hydrogen ions [$H^+$]. Base is a substance which when added to water produces hydroxide ions [$OH^-$].

## Hydrochloric Acid I.P., B.P., U.S.P.

**(Synonym: Concentrated hydrochloric acid, Spirit of salt, Muriatic acid, Acidum hydrochloricum)**

**Mol. Formula:** HCl **Mol. Weight:** 36.5

It contains not less than 35% w/w and not more than 38% w/w of HCl. It is also known as "spirit of salt" because first of all it was prepared by the distillation of sea salt with concentrated sulphuric acid.

***Preparation:***

1. *Leblanc Soda Process:* Hydrochloric acid is manufactured by the action of concentrated sulphuric acid on sodium chloride.

The equal amount of acid is run to the equal quantity of sodium chloride salt in the cast-iron pan of a cake-salt furnace, the hydrochloride gas is evolved, and the reaction is completed by gentle heating.

$$NaCl + H_2SO_4 \longrightarrow NaHSO_4 + HCl\uparrow$$

The pasty mass of sodium bisulphate with the excess of sodium chloride is then raked out into the muffle furnace and heated to dull redness to get more hydrogen chloride gas and leaves a residue of anhydrous sodium sulphate (salt-cake).

$$NaCl + NaHSO_4 \longrightarrow \underset{\text{Sodium Sulphate}}{Na_2SO_4} + HCl\uparrow$$

The hydrogen chloride obtained from the above method is passed through the pipeline towards the container containing lumps of coke, down which water trickles. By this way crude concentrated hydrochloric acid obtained is contaminated with iron, sulphuric acid, arsenic acid, sulphur dioxide, ferric chloride, chlorine and other impurities.

*Purification process:* The impure hydrochloric acid obtained by the above process is treated with barium chloride which removes sulphuric acid as barium sulphate. Volatile impurities ($SO_4^{2-}$, $Cl_2$) come out first and are rejected. Ferric chloride is left behind as residue. Arsenic impurity is removed by heating the commercial acid with stannous chloride as perchloro stannane.

$$2\,AsCl_3 + 3\,SnCl_2 \longrightarrow 2\,As + 3\,SnCl_4$$

2. *By electrolysis:* The commercial hydrochloric acid obtained by the above process is difficult to purify, so the large amount of pure acid is synthesized from hydrogen and chlorine which are obtained as byproducts in the electrolytic caustic soda manufacture method.

$$H_2 + Cl_2 \longrightarrow 2HCl$$

The chlorine is burned in hydrogen in large diameter silica tubes; the hydrogen chloride so formed is absorbed in water to get hydrochloric acid.

***Physical properties:*** It is a clear, colorless, fuming liquid, with pungent odour. It is miscible with water and alcohol. The weight per ml of the liquid is 1.18. It is a strong acid attacks metals, forming their metal hydrochlorides with the evolution of hydrogen gas. Even in high diluted form, it is highly acidic. A non fuming solution can be prepared by diluting one volume of hydrochloric acid with two volumes of water.

***Chemical properties:***

1. It turns moist blue litmus to red.
2. *Reaction with metals:* It reacts with metals and their oxides and carbonates, forms metal chlorides with the evolution of hydrogen gas and carbon dioxide respectively.

$$2Na + 2\,HCl \longrightarrow 2NaCl + H_2$$

$$Mg + 2HCl \longrightarrow MgCl_2 + H_2$$

$$KOH + HCl \longrightarrow KCl + H_2O$$

$$Na_2CO_3 + 2HCl \longrightarrow 2NaCl + CO_2\uparrow + H_2O$$

3. *Reaction with silver nitrate:* Hydrochloric acid reacts with silver nitrate solution and forms a white dense precipitate of silver chloride which is soluble in ammonium hydroxide and insoluble in nitric acid.

$$HCl + AgNO_3 \longrightarrow \underset{\text{White dense precipitate}}{AgCl\downarrow} + HNO_3$$

$$AgCl + 2NH_4OH \longrightarrow \underset{\text{silver ammonium chloride (soluble)}}{Ag(NH_3)_2Cl} + 2H_2O$$

4. *Reaction with lead acetate:* Hydrochloric acid reacts with lead acetate solution and yields a white precipitate of lead chloride

$$2HCl + (CH_3COO)_2Pb \longrightarrow \underset{\text{White precipitate}}{PbCl_2\downarrow} + 2CH_3COOH$$

5. *Reaction with fluorine:* Hydrochloric acid get decomposes with fluorine to form chlorine.

$$2\,HCl + F_2 \longrightarrow 2\,HF + Cl_2$$

6. *Reaction with bicarbonates, sulphides, sulphites, nitrites and thio sulphates:* Hydrochloric acid decomposes the weaker acid salts.

$$NaHCO_3 + HCl \longrightarrow NaCl + CO_2 + H_2O$$

$$2NaNO_2 + 2HCl \longrightarrow 2NaCl + NO + NO_2 + H_2O$$

$$NaNO_2 + HCl \longrightarrow NaCl + HNO_2$$

$$Na_2SO_3 + 2HCl \longrightarrow 2NaCl + SO_2 + H_2O$$

7. *Reaction with ammonia:* Hydrochloric acid reacts with ammonia, and forms white dense fumes of ammonium chloride.

$$HCl + NH_3 \longrightarrow NH_4Cl$$

8. A mixture of 3 parts of concentrated hydrochloric acid and 1 part of concentrated nitric acid is called as "aqua regia" which is used for dissolving noble metals like gold, platinum and their chlorides.

***Test for identification:***

1. When hydrochloric acid is added to potassium permanganate, chlorine gas is evolved.

$$2KMnO_4 + 16HCl \longrightarrow 2MnCl_2 + 5Cl_2 + 2KCl + 8H_2O$$

2. The neutral solution of the sample gives the characteristic reactions of chloride ions.

***Test for purity:*** It should be tested for arsenic, heavy metals, bromide, iodide, free chlorine, sulphite, sulphates and loss on evaporation etc.

**Assay**

***Principle:*** It is assayed by **acidimetry-alkalimetry method** of titration (also called **neutralization method**).

In this assay the substance is diluted with water and titrated with sodium hydroxide, using methyl red as an indicator. End point is the yellow colour. In this assay the sodium hydroxide (the base) reacts with hydrochloric acid and neutralization takes place during the titration. The indicator is red colour in acid medium and it changes to yellow colour upon neutralization which is the end point.

As the acid and alkali involved in this assay, it is called as acidimetry-alkalimetry method of titration and the neutralization takes place in this assay during titration hence this assay is also called as neutralization method. The chemical reactions of this assay are shown below.

$$HCl + NaOH \longrightarrow NaCl + H_2O$$

***Procedure:*** Weigh accurately about 2 gm, add 30 ml of water, mix and titrate with 1M sodium hydroxide using methyl red solution as indicator.

***Uses:***

1. It is mainly used as a pharmaceutical aid especially as an acidifier.

2. Dilute hydrochloric acid (10% w/w), when further diluted to 25-50 volumes of water may be used in the treatment of **achlorhydria** (Low levels of hydrochloric acid in stomach).
3. At suitable dilution hydrochloric acid is administered intravenously for the management of metabolic alkalosis (increase in the alkalinity of blood).
4. It is also used to convert water insoluble organic bases like alkaloids into water soluble hydrochloride salts.
5. It is extensively used as a solvent and catalyst in basic pharmaceuticals.

***Adverse effects***

1. Inhalation of hydrochloric acid causes cough, choking and inflammation of upper respiratory tract.
2. Sometimes photo sensitization and dermatitis also occurs.

***Storage:*** It should be stored in stoppered glass containers or any other inert material at a temperature of not exceeding 30 °C.

## Sulphuric Acid B.P., U.S.P.

**Mol. Formula:** $H_2SO_4$ **Mol. Weight:** 98.1

It contains not less than 95% w/w and not more than 100.5% w/w of sulphuric acid. It is one of the most important mineral acids which are used for the preparation of sulphates and sulphonates.

***Preparation:***

It is manufactured in industries by two processes.

1. *Contact process:* It is an industrial method for the manufacture of sulphuric acid. By this method, sulphuric acid is prepared by the reaction between sulfur dioxide and oxygen to give sulphur trioxide by using vanadium pentoxide as a catalyst, followed by the reaction of sulfur trioxide with water (first sulphur trioxide is dissolved in sulphuric acid, which is then diluted with water).

$$2SO_{2(g)} + O_{2(g)} \xrightarrow[V_2O_5]{\Delta} 2SO_{3(g)}$$

$$SO_{3(g)} + H_2O_{(l)} \longrightarrow H_2SO_{4(aq)}$$

2. *Lead chamber process:* This process was introduced by Birmingham, John Roebuck in England 1974 by using lead-lined chambers, which are less expensive and effective.

   In this method, sulfur dioxide with steam and oxides of nitrogen are passed in to the large lead lined chambers (lead sheets) where gases are spray down with water and acid. In the reaction chamber, both oxides are dissolving in the reaction liquor. Nitrogen dioxide is hydrated to give nitrous acid which on further reaction to yield sulphuric acid and nitric oxide. The reaction is highly exothermic and major consideration to design the chambers to provide a way to dissipate the heat formed in the reactions.

The overall reactions are

$$2NO_2 + H_2O \longrightarrow HNO_2 + HNO_3$$

$$\underset{(aq)}{SO_2} + HNO_3 \longrightarrow NOHSO_4$$

$$NOHSO_4 + HNO_2 \longrightarrow H_2SO_4 + NO_2 + NO$$

$$\underset{(aq)}{SO_2} + 2\,HNO_2 \longrightarrow H_2SO_4 + 2NO$$

The presence of nitrogen dioxide is important for preceding the reaction. Nitrogen oxides are absorbed and regenerated in the process, and thus serve as a catalyst for overall reaction.

***Physical properties:*** It is a colorless, highly corrosive liquid with oily consistency. Soluble in water. Specific gravity is 1.84.

***Test for identification:*** The neutral solution of the sample gives the characteristic reactions of sulphates.

***Test for purity:*** It should be tested for wt/ml, nitrate, chloride, arsenic, heavy metals, oxidisable substances and ash content.

***Test for oxidisable impurity:*** To the small amount of cooled and diluted solution of acid add one drop of dilute potassium permanganate solution. No decolorization occurs within five minutes.

***Test for nitrate:*** A small amount acid is mixed with equal amount of water, add one drop of indigo carmine solution. No decolorization occurs within one minute.

**Assay**

***Principle:*** It is assayed by **acidimetry-alkalimetry method** of titration (also called **neutralization method**).

In this assay the substance is diluted with water and titrated with sodium hydroxide using methyl red as an indicator. End point is the yellow colour.

In this assay the sodium hydroxide (the base) reacts with sulphuric acid and neutralization takes place during the titration. The indicator is red colour in acid medium and it changes to yellow colour upon neutralization which is the end point. The end point can also determined potentiometrically.

As the acid and alkali involved in this assay, it is called as acidimetry-alkalimetry method of titration and the neutralization takes place in this assay during titration hence this assay is also called as neutralization method. The chemical reactions of this assay are shown below.

$$H_2SO_4 + 2NaOH \longrightarrow Na_2SO_4 + 2H_2O$$

***Procedure:*** Weigh accurately about 2 gm, add 30 ml of water, mix and titrate with 1M sodium hydroxide using methyl red solution as indicator.

**Uses:**

1. Chemically it is a strong diprotic acid which is used to form salts of basic organic drugs.
2. It is used as a dehydrating agent and diluted form is used as a pharmaceutical aid.

***Official preparations:*** Dilute sulphuric acid, Aromatic sulphuric acid.

## Phosphoric Acid I.P., U.S.P.

**(Synonym: Orthophosphoric acid, concentrated phosphoric acid)**

**Mol. Formula:** $H_3PO_4$. **Mol. Weight:** 98

Phosphoric acid contains not less than 84% w/w and not more than 90% w/w of $H_3PO_4$.

***Preparation:***

I. *Small scale preparation:*

1. By cautiously warming 7 parts of red phosphorous with 50 parts of water and 40 parts concentrated nitric acid in a large flask, pure phosphoric acid can be prepared. Finally it is boiled until all the phosphorus gets oxidized.

$$4P + 10HNO_3 + H_2O \longrightarrow 4H_3PO_4 + 5NO + 5NO_2$$

The liquid obtained is transferred to a dish and evaporated to form syrup.

2. From phosphorous: Phosphoric acid is prepared by oxidation of phosphorous to phosphorus pentoxide in presence of air and treating phosphorus pentoxide with water to form phosphoric acid.

$$4P + 5\,O_2 \xrightarrow[(O)]{\text{Air}} 2P_2O_5$$

$$P_2O_5 + 3H_2O \longrightarrow 2H_3PO_4$$

II. *Large scale preparation*

1. Wet process: Phosphoric acid is prepared from phosphorous or by digesting crushed mineral phosphate rock or bone ash [$Ca_3(PO_4)_2$] with the correct amount of diluted sulphuric acid, separating the solution from calcium sulphate and other undissolved matter, and evaporating it to a syrup.

$$[Ca_3(PO_4)_2] + 3H_2SO_4 \longrightarrow 3CaSO_4 + 2H_3PO_4$$

2. Thermal process: By this process, phosphate rock is mixed with coke and silica then heated at high temperature in an electrical furnace. The elemental phosphorous obtained is burned to produce phosphorous pentoxide which is dissolved in water to produce phosphoric acid.

$$Ca_3(PO_4)_2 + 3SiO_2 + 5C \xrightarrow{\Delta} 3CaSiO_3 + 5CO\uparrow + 2P$$

$$4P + 5O_2 \longrightarrow 2P_2O_5$$

$$P_2O_5 + 3H_2O \longrightarrow 2H_3PO_4$$

The liquid obtained is transferred into a dish and concentrated.

***Physical properties:*** It is a clear, colorless syrupy liquid. When kept at low temperature it may solidify, producing mass of colorless crystals which do not melt until the temperature reaches 28 °C. On heating, it loses water molecule and leaves meta phosphoric acid, which on further cooling gives a mass with a composition of $H_3PO_4.\frac{1}{4}\ H_2O$. The concentrated phosphoric acid attacks porcelain.

***Test for identification***

1. The sample solution in water is strongly acidic in nature.
2. The neutralized solution of sample gives the characteristic reactions of phosphate.

***Test for purity:*** It should be tested for appearance of solution, arsenic, alkali phosphates, aluminium calcium, heavy metals, iron, sulphates, chlorides, hypo phosphorous acid and phosphorous acid.

**Assay**

***Principle:*** It is assayed by **acidimetry-alkalimetry method** of titration (also called **neutralization method**).

In this assay the substance is dissolved in water and sodium chloride solution is added and titrated with 1N sodium hydroxide, using phenolphthalein as an indicator. End point is the appearance of permanent pale pink colour. In this assay the sodium hydroxide (the base) reacts with phosphoric acid and neutralization takes place during the titration. The indicator is colourless in acid medium and it changes its colour to pink in alkali medium which is the end point.

As the acid and alkali involved in this assay, it is called as acidimetry-alkalimetry method of titration and the neutralization takes place in this assay during titration hence this assay is also called as neutralization method. The chemical reactions of this assay are shown below.

$$2\ NaOH + H_3PO_4 \longrightarrow Na_2HPO_4 + 2\ H_2O$$

***Procedure:*** To 1 gm of liquid add a solution of 10 gm of sodium chloride in 30 ml of water. Titrate with 1M sodium hydroxide, using phenolphthalein solution as indicator.

***Uses:***

1. It is used as a pharmaceutical aid (acidifying agent) for the preparation of dilute phosphoric acid.
2. It is also used in dental ailment and in the treatment of lead poisoning.
3. It aids proteolytic enzymes in peptone formation.

***Storage:*** It should be stored in well closed container and protected from moisture.

## Strong Ammonia Solution B.P., U.S.P.

**(Synonym: Ammonia solution strong, Liquor Ammoniae Fortis, Ammonium hydroxide, Stronger Ammonium water)**

It contains not less than 27.0% w/w and not more than 30.0% w/w of $NH_3$.

***Preparation:***

*Method 1: (Haber's Process):* It is prepared from atmospheric nitrogen.

$$N_2 + 3H_2 \rightleftharpoons 2NH_3$$

*Method 2:* It may be prepared from the ammonical liquors, by distillation with slaked lime. Strong ammonia solution is not fully saturated with ammonia gas at room temperature. The most concentrated commercial solution is having about 35% of $NH_3$ with a specific gravity of 0.880 and it is known as eighty-eight ammonia.

***Physical properties:*** It is clear, colorless liquid, strong pungent odour with characteristic taste. It is miscible with water and alcohol; wt/ml is about 0.90. It is strong alkaline to litmus.

***Chemical properties:***

1. *Reaction with metal oxides:* When ammonia gas is passed over the oxides of metals, nitrogen gas is evolved.

$$3CuO + 2NH_3 \longrightarrow 3Cu + 3H_2O + N_2\uparrow$$

2. *Reaction with halogens:* When a current of halogen vapors are allowed to pass through ammonia gas, the halogen catches fire and forms nitrogen gas and hydrochloric acid.

$$2NH_3 + 3Cl_2 \longrightarrow N_2\uparrow + 6HCl$$

3. *Reaction with hydrochloric acid:* When strong ammonia solution reacts with hydrochloric acid gives ammonium chloride.

$$NH_3 + HCl \longrightarrow NH_4Cl$$

4. *Reaction with hypo chlorites:* Ammonia gets oxidized by hypo chlorites and gives nitrogen and water.

$$2NH_3 + 3NaOCl \longrightarrow 3NaCl + 3H_2O + N_2\uparrow$$

5. *Reaction with potassium permanganate:* Ammonia reduces potassium permanganate to manganese oxide.

$$2NH_3 + 2KMnO_4 \longrightarrow 2KOH + 2MnO_2 + 2H_2O + N_2\uparrow$$

6. *Reaction with metals:* When certain metals are heated with ammonia gas, hydrogen gas is evolved and their respective nitrites are formed.

$$2NH_3 + 3Mg \longrightarrow Mg_3N_2 + 3H_2\uparrow$$

$$2Na + 2NH_3 \longrightarrow 2NaNH_2 + H_2\uparrow$$

Ammonia solution readily forms soluble complex ions when treated with cations of silver, copper, gold and their salts.

$$AgCl + 2NH_3 \underset{}{\overset{H_2O}{\rightleftharpoons}} [Ag(NH_3)_2]^+ Cl^-$$

***Test for identification:***

1. When it is diluted freely with water, the solution obtained is alkaline in nature.
2. When a glass rod is dipped in hydrochloric acid and brought near the surface of the solution, dense white fumes are produced.

***Test for purity:*** It should be tested for, specific gravity (at 25 °C, 0.9000-0.915) arsenic, heavy metals, non-volatile residue (0.01% w/v), and tarry matter.

***Test for tarry matter:*** To the sample solution add small amount of citric acid, heated until citric acid dissolves. No tarry or unpleasant odour is evolved.

**Assay**

***Principle:*** It is assayed by **acidimetry-alkalimetry method of (Back) titration** (also called **neutralization method**).

In this assay the substance is dissolved in Known Excess Standard (KES) 1N sulphuric acid and the Excess Unreacted (EUR) sulphuric acid is titrated with 1N sodium hydroxide using methyl red as an indicator. End point is the yellow colour.

In this assay the ammonia (the base) reacts with sulphuric acid and neutralization takes place, after this reaction the excess unreacted sulphuric acid is titrated with sodium hydroxide. The indicator is red colour in acid medium and it changes to yellow colour upon neutralization which is the end point.

As the acid and alkali involved in this assay, it is called as acidimetry-alkalimetry method of titration and the neutralization takes place in this assay during titration hence this assay is also called as Neutralization method. The chemical reactions of this assay are shown below.

$$2\,NH_4OH + H_2SO_4 \longrightarrow (NH_4)_2SO_4 + 2\,H_2O$$

$$H_2SO_4 + 2\,NaOH \longrightarrow Na_2SO_4 + 2\,H_2O$$

***Procedure:*** Weigh accurately a flask with a ground-glass neck containing 50.0 ml of 1M hydrochloric acid/sulphuric acid. Add 2 ml of the substance to be examined and re-weigh. Add 0.1 ml of methyl red solution as indicator. Titrate with 1M sodium hydroxide until the colour changes from red to yellow.

***Uses:***

1. It is mainly used as an antacid, counter irritant and stimulant.
2. It is used to prepare dilute ammonia solution and it is the one of the ingredient of aromatic spirit of ammonia.

***Storage:*** It should be stored in small, well closed container. Rubber stoppers are not used because it absorbs ammonia.

## Dilute Ammonia Solution B.P.

This compound is discussed under the topic **acidifiers and alkalinising agents**.

## Sodium Carbonate I.P., B.P.

**Mol. Formula:** $Na_2CO_3$ **Mol. Weight:** 106

Sodium carbonate is available in two forms one is anhydrous and another is monohydrated form (with one molecule of water). It contains not less than 99.5% and not more than 100.5% of $Na_2CO_3$ with reference to dried standard.

***Preparation:***

1. *Soda ammonia process:* Most of the sodium carbonate is manufactured by ammonia-soda process. The strong brine solution containing high concentration of ammonia is passed through a carbonating tower where it is saturated with carbon dioxide under pressure, which gives sodium bicarbonate. This is converted in to sodium carbonate by simple heating.

$$NH_3 + H_2O + CO_2 \rightleftharpoons NH_4HCO_3$$

$$NH_4HCO_3 + NaCl \rightleftharpoons NH_4Cl + NaHCO_3$$

$$2NaHCO_3 \longrightarrow Na_2CO_3 + H_2O + CO_2$$

2. *From electrolysis of sodium chloride:* By this method, during the electrolysis of sodium chloride, the sodium ion formed which reacts with water and gives sodium hydroxide. Carbon dioxide gas is passed through the sodium hydroxide solution to give sodium carbonate.

$$NaCl \rightleftharpoons Na^+ + Cl^-$$

$$2\,Na^+ + 2\,H_2O \longrightarrow 2\,NaOH + H_2$$

$$2\,NaOH + CO_2 \longrightarrow Na_2CO_3 + H_2O$$

3. *From sodium bicarbonate:* Heating of sodium bicarbonate yields sodium carbonate.

$$2\,NaHCO_3 \longrightarrow Na_2CO_3 + H_2O + CO_2$$

***Physical properties:*** It is an anhydrous, colorless or white, granular powder and slightly hygroscopic in nature.

***Monohydrate:*** A white crystalline powder or colorless crystals, freely soluble in water, insoluble in alcohol. It is otherwise called as soda ash. Both of the above are having alkaline taste. Monohydrate is stable above 35 °C. It is soluble in water but insoluble in alcohol.

***Chemical properties***

*Neutralization Reaction:* Sodium carbonate reacts with hydrochloric acid; neutralization takes place to yield sodium chloride.

$$Na_2CO_3 + 2\,HCl \longrightarrow 2\,NaCl + H_2O + CO_2$$

*Precipitation reaction:* Sodium carbonate reacts with barium sulphate and barium carbonate gets precipitated.

$$Na_2CO_3 + BaSO_4 \longrightarrow BaCO_3\downarrow + Na_2SO_4$$

***Test for identification***

1. The dilute solution of sodium carbonate in water is strongly alkaline (alkaline to litmus).
2. The above solution gives the characteristic reactions of sodium and carbonate ions.

***Test for purity:*** It should be tested for color and clarity of the solution, alkali hydroxides and bicarbonates, heavy metals, iron, chlorides, sulphates and loss on drying.

***Test for alkali hydroxides and bicarbonates:*** To the small amount of sample solution, add barium chloride solution, filter it. To the filtrate add one drop of phenolphthalein solution. No red color is produced. Heat the remaining portion of the filtrate, no color is produced.

**Assay**

***Principle:*** It is assayed by **acidimetry-alkalimetry method** of titration (also called **neutralization method**).

In this assay the substance is dissolved in water and titrated 0.5N hydrochloric acid, using methyl orange as an indicator. End point is the orange colour. In this assay the sodium carbonate (the base) reacts with hydrochloric acid and neutralization takes place during the titration. The indicator is yellow colour in alkali medium and it changes to orange colour upon neutralization which is the end point.

As the acid and alkali involved in this assay, it is called as acidimetry-alkalimetry method of titration and the neutralization takes place in this assay during titration hence this assay is also called as neutralization method. The chemical reactions of this assay are shown below.

$$Na_2CO_3 + 2\,HCl \longrightarrow 2\,NaCl + H_2O + CO_2$$

***Procedure:*** Weigh accurately about 1.0 gm, dissolve in 25 ml of water and titrate with 1M hydrochloric acid using methyl orange solution as indicator.

***Uses:***

1. It is mainly used as pharmaceutical aid (alkalinizing agent).
2. It also used as an antacid.

3. Topically it is used as a mouth wash and vaginal douch and used to prepare sodium salts of many acids.

***Storage:*** It should be stored in tightly closed, non metallic containers.

## Sodium Hydroxide I.P., B.P.

**(Synonym: Caustic soda)**

**Mol. Formula:** NaOH **Mol. Weight:** 40

It contains not less than 97% and not more than 100.5% of total alkali which is calculated as NaOH including not more than 3% of $Na_2CO_3$.

***Preparation:***

1. *Soda lime process:* Sodium hydroxide is prepared by heating sodium carbonate with water and lime ($Ca(OH)_2$) in large iron tanks.

$$Na_2CO_3 + Ca(OH)_2 \rightleftharpoons CaCO_3\downarrow + 2NaOH$$

The reaction is reversible one, hence the correct proportions are used; more than 90% of sodium carbonate is converted in to hydroxide. The liquor obtained is filtered off and evaporated, and the resulting molten product is converted in to sticks, scales, pellets or masses by suitable processes. The scale and pellet forms are more convenient for general use.

2. *From electrolysis of brine solution:* Sodium hydroxide is also manufactured in large quantities by the electrolysis of brine solution. Several types of electrodes are used, but mostly used are carbon anodes and metallic cathodes. In some devices the sodium hydroxide is produced in an isolated, brine free cathode compartment. The process is summarized as follows.

**At Cathode (-):**

$$Na^+ \longrightarrow Na$$

$$2Na + 2H_2O \longrightarrow 2NaOH + H_2$$

**At Anode (+):**

$$Cl^- \longrightarrow Cl + e^-$$

$$Cl + Cl \longrightarrow Cl_2$$

The advantages of this process are simple and economic. It yields hydrogen and chlorine as valuable byproducts. These gases are collected separately or it is converted into hydrogen chloride.

***Physical properties:*** It is a white, crystalline mass supplied as sticks, pellets or slabs. It is very deliquescent, absorb traces of moisture and liquefy. It is freely soluble in water and alcohol; these solutions are very soapy to touch. It is strongly alkaline and corrosive to animal and vegetable tissues and it rapidly destroys organic tissues. Solutions should be filtered through glass wool or asbestos and stored in hard glass bottles with rubber stoppers. If glass stoppered bottles are used, the solution will dissolve the glass and the stopper will stick in the neck of the bottle. It absorbs carbon dioxide and converted into sodium carbonate partially.

$$H_2O + CO_2 \longrightarrow H_2CO_3$$

$$2\,NaOH + H_2CO_3 \longrightarrow Na_2CO_3 + 2H_2O$$

***Chemical properties:***

1. *Sodium hydroxide is a strong alkali:* It neutralizes all acids or acid oxides and produces its salts.

$$NaOH + HCl \longrightarrow NaCl + H_2O$$

2. *Reaction with metals:* It reacts with metals like zinc, aluminium, tin, sulphur and silicon to evolve hydrogen.

$$Zn + NaOH + H_2O \longrightarrow NaHZnO_2 + H_2$$

$$4S + 6\,NaOH \longrightarrow 2Na_2S + Na_2S_2O_3 + 3H_2O$$

$$Si + 2NaOH + H_2O \longrightarrow Na_2SiO_3 + 2H_2$$

3. *Reaction with ammonium salts:* Sodium hydroxide decomposes the ammonium salts and yields ammonia.

$$NaOH + NH_4Cl \longrightarrow NaCl + NH_3\uparrow + H_2O$$

4. *Reaction with metal salts:* Sodium hydroxide reacts with salts of metal solutions and forms metal hydroxides.

$$Fe_2(SO_4)_3 + 6NaOH \longrightarrow \underset{\text{red ppt}}{2Fe(OH)_3\downarrow} + 3\,Na_2SO_4$$

$$Zn(OH)_2 + 2NaOH \longrightarrow Na_2ZnO_2 + 2H_2O$$

$$Al(OH)_3 + NaOH \longrightarrow NaAlO_2 + 2H_2O$$

The hydroxides of aluminium and zinc are soluble in excess of sodium hydroxide.

5. Sodium hydroxide catalyses the ester hydrolysis. It reacts with fats to form glycerin and sodium salts of fatty acids (soap).

$$\begin{array}{l} CH_2\text{-O-CO-}C_{17}H_{35} \\ | \\ CH\text{-OCO-}C_{17}H_{35} \\ | \\ CH_2\text{-OCO-}C_{17}H_{35} \end{array} + 3NaOH \longrightarrow \underset{\text{soap}}{3C_{17}H_{35}COO^-Na^+} + \begin{array}{l} CH_2OH \\ | \\ CHOH \\ | \\ CH_2OH \end{array}$$

***Test for identification***

1. The neutral solution of sodium hydroxide gives the characteristic reactions of sodium salts.
2. The pH of 0.01% w/v solution is not less than 11.

***Test for purity:*** It should be tested for color, clarity of the solution, arsenic, heavy metals, iron, carbonates, potassium, chloride, sulphates and insoluble substances in hydrochloric acid. The test for aluminium, iron and matter insoluble in hydrochloric acid is determined by gravimetric process.

**Assay:** Sodium hydroxide contains small amount of sodium carbonate, hence it should also be estimated in the assay of sodium hydroxide.

***Principle:*** It is assayed by **acidimetry-alkalimetry method of titration** (also called **neutralization method**). In this assay the substance is dissolved in carbon dioxide free water and titrated with 1N sulphuric acid, using phenolphthalein as an indicator. Titration is continued until the disappearance of pink colour (the volume noted is the amount of titrant required to neutralise the sodium hydroxide). To the reaction mixture now add methyl orange indicator and continue the titration until the orange colour persists (the volume noted is the amount of titrant required to neutralise the sodium carbonate).

As the acid and alkali involved in this assay, it is called as acidimetry-alkalimetry method of titration and the neutralization takes place in this assay during titration hence this assay is also called as neutralization method. The chemical reactions of this assay are shown below.

$$2\,NaOH + H_2SO_4 \longrightarrow Na_2SO_4 + 2\,H_2O$$

$$Na_2CO_3 + H_2SO_4 \longrightarrow Na_2SO_4 + H_2O + CO_2$$

***Procedure:*** Weigh accurately about 2 gm, dissolve in about 80 ml of boiling water, add 0.3 ml of phenolphthalein solution and titrate with 1M hydrochloric acid. Add 0.3 ml of methyl orange solution and continue the titration with 1M hydrochloric acid.

***Uses:***

1. Due to its strong alkaline nature, it is not used therapeutically.
2. An escharotics preparation of sodium hydroxide and calcium oxide (London paste) is used for adjusting the pH of solutions.
3. It is used as a reagent in laboratories and industries.
4. It is also used as a disinfectant for veterinary purposes.

***Storage:*** It should be stored in tightly closed container. It is highly destructive to tissue, so great care should be taken while handling.

## Potassium Hydroxide B.P.

**Mol. Formula:** KOH **Mol. Weight:** 56.1

It contains not less than 85% of total alkali which is calculated as KOH and contains not more than 4% of potassium carbonate ($K_2CO_3$).

***Preparation***

*Method 1 (Electrolysis of Potassium chloride):* Potassium hydroxide is manufactured by electrolysis of potassium chloride solution, a method similar to the electrolysis process for the manufactures of sodium hydroxide. The caustic liquor obtained is evaporated and the resulting fused potassium hydroxide is either allowed to solidify and broken up or cast into sticks or made into more pellets.

**At cathode:**

$$K^+ + e^- \longrightarrow K$$

$$2K + 2H_2O \longrightarrow 2KOH + H_2$$

**At anode:**

$$Cl^- \longrightarrow Cl + e^-$$

$$Cl + Cl \longrightarrow Cl_2$$

***Purification:*** Commercial potassium hydroxide contains considerable proportion of carbonate and other impurities. So it is purified by dissolving the substance in alcohol, filtered and the alcohol is recovered by distillation. The product obtained is more pure and it is sold as, potassium hydroxide pure by alcohol.

*Method 2: From potassium carbonate:* It is also obtained from the reaction between potassium carbonate and calcium hydroxide.

$$K_2CO_3 + Ca(OH)_2 \longrightarrow 2KOH + CaCO_3$$

***Physical properties:*** It occurs as dry, hard, brittle, colorless sticks, fused masses, pellets or flakes. It is very deliquescent, strong alkaline and corrosive. It is soluble in water, alcohol and glycerin.

***Test for identification:*** The sample gives the characteristic reactions of potassium.

***Test for purity:*** It should be tested for aluminium, iron, and matter insoluble in hydrochloric acid, heavy metals, chloride, lead and sulphate.

**Assay**

***Principle:*** It contains carbonates also; hence it is assayed by **Modified Winkder method** of titration (also called **neutralization method**).

In this assay the substance is dissolved in water and barium chloride solution is added to this, whereby soluble carbonates precipitated as barium carbonate.

$$K_2CO_3 + BaCl_2 \longrightarrow BaCO_3\downarrow + 2\,KCl$$

The hydroxide present in the solution is determined by titrating with hydrochloric acid using phenolphthalein as indicator. End point is the disappearance of pink colour. This value indicates the amount of potassium hydroxide present.

$$KOH + HCl \longrightarrow KCl + H_2O$$

To the above solution add bromophenol and continue the titration with hydrochloric acid. This titre value represents the amount of potassium carbonate present in the potassium hydroxide. End point is the colour chage from violet-blue to yellow.

***Procedure:*** Dissolve 2 gm in 25 ml of carbon-dioxide free water. Add 25 ml of freshly prepared barium chloride solution and 0.3 ml of phenolphthalein solution. Add slowly while shaking 25.0 ml of 1M hydrochloric acid and continue the titration with 1 M hydrochloric acid until the colour changes from pink to colourless. Add 0.3 ml of bromophenol blue solution and continue the titration with 1 M hydrochloric acid until the colour changes from violet-blue to yellow.

***Uses:***

1. It is mainly used as a pharmaceutical aid.
2. It is also used as caustic in veterinary practice.

***Storage:*** It should be stored in tightly closed container. It is highly destructive to tissue, so great care should be taken while handling.

---

## Potassium Hydroxide Solution B.P., U.S.P.

**(Synonym: Solution of potash)**

It contains not less than 4.9% w/v and not more than 5.1% w/v of KOH.

This is an aqueous solution of potassium hydroxide contains 50% w/v of total alkali.

***Physical Properties:*** It is a clear colorless liquid, strongly alkaline. Specific gravity at 20 °C is 1.42 gm.

***Test for identification, test for purity and assay:*** Similar to that of potassium hydroxide.

***Uses:***

1. It is mainly used as pharmaceutical aid.
2. It is also used as a volumetric reagent for titration of acids.

***Storage:*** It should be stored in lead free glass bottles (Green color bottle) because the alkali has a solvent action on the lead present in certain types of colorless glass. The bottles should be closed by rubber stoppers, since glass stoppers tend to stick.

## Calcium Hydroxide B.P., U.S.P.

**(Synonym: Slaked lime, hydrated lime)**

**Mol. Formula:** $Ca(OH)_2$ **Mol. Weight:** 74.09

It contains not less than 90% w/w of $Ca(OH)_2$.

***Preparation:***

*Slaking process:* It is prepared by spraying water in to quick lime. This process is called as slaking. Quick lime is prepared from heating lime stone. The lumps of quick lime break into powder and heat is evolved.

$$CaCO_3 \rightleftharpoons CaO + CO_2\uparrow$$

$$CaO + H_2O \longrightarrow Ca(OH)_2$$

In the above process, water is absorbed by the calcium oxide with the evolution of excess of heat. The supernatant liquid is decanted and the residue is air dried.

***Physical properties:*** It is white or colorless soft powder, odorless, alkaline and slightly bitter taste. It is sparingly soluble in water, freely soluble in sugar solution and glycerol. When exposed to air it absorbs atmospheric carbon dioxide and forms calcium carbonate.

***Chemical properties:*** When three to four times of its own weight of water has been added, it forms milk of lime which is differing from lime water. A clear saturated solution of calcium hydroxide is called as lime water. The solution of calcium hydroxide is basic in nature.

1. *Reaction with hydrochloric acid:* Calcium hydroxide reacts with hydrochloric acid forms calcium chloride.

$$Ca(OH)_2 + 2\,HCl \longrightarrow CaCl_2 + 2\,H_2O$$

2. *Reaction with carbonic acid:* Calcium hydroxide when treated with carbonic acid it forms calcium carbonate.

$$Ca(OH)_2 + H_2CO_3 \longrightarrow CaCO_3\downarrow + 2\,H_2O$$

3. *Decomposition reaction:* When it is heated strongly it loses water molecule and is converted in to calcium oxide.

$$Ca(OH)_2 \xrightarrow{\Delta} CaO + H_2O$$

4. *Reaction with gases:* Calcium hydroxide reacts with sulphur dioxide and yields calcium sulphite.

$$Ca(OH)_2 + SO_2 \longrightarrow CaSO_3 + H_2O$$

5. *Reaction with chlorine:* Cold lime water reacts with chlorine and forms calcium chlorate.

$$6\,Ca(OH)_2 + 6\,Cl_2 \longrightarrow Ca(ClO_3)_2 + 5\,CaCl_2 + 6\,H_2O$$

***Test for identification:*** The sample solution in acetic acid gives the characteristic reactions of calcium.

***Test for purity:*** It should be tested for aluminium, iron, phosphate and substance insoluble in hydrochloric acid, arsenic, lead, chloride and sulphate.

**Assay**

***Principle:*** It is assayed by **Complexometry method of (Direct) titration**.

In this assay the substance is dissolved in hydrochloric acid, to this 1N sodium hydroxide added until the pH reaches to 12. The solution is then titrated against 0.05M disodium Ethylene Diamine Tetra Acetate (EDTA) using hydroxy naphthol blue as indicator. End point is the appearance of deep blue colour.

In this assay calcium ions of calcium carbonate reacts with disodium EDTA, whereby the complexation takes place. As the calcium ions forms complex with disodium EDTA in this assay, it is called as complexometry method of titration. The chemical reactions of this assay are shown below.

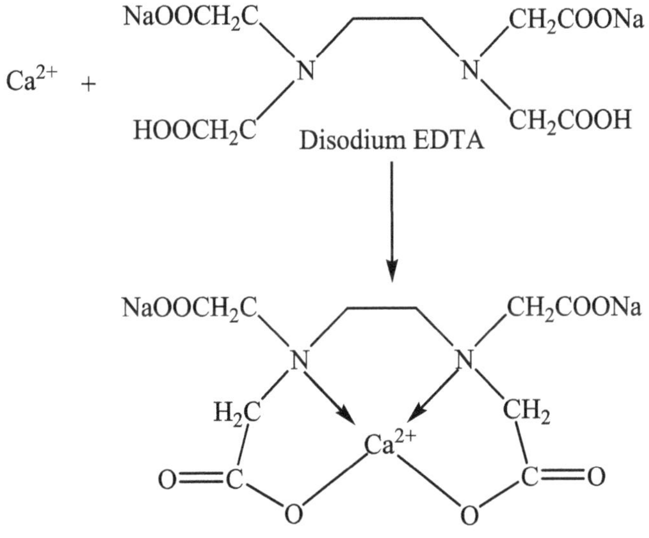

$Ca^{2+}$ + $(NaOOCH_2C)(HOOCH_2C)N-CH_2-CH_2-N(CH_2COONa)(CH_2COOH)$

Disodium EDTA

↓

$NaOOCH_2C$, $CH_2COONa$, N, N, $H_2C$, $CH_2$, $Ca^{2+}$, O=C, C=O, O, O

Calcium-EDTA Complex

***Procedure:*** Transfer about 1.5 gm of calcium hydroxide, accurately weighed, to a beaker, and gradually add 30 ml of 3N hydrochloric acid. When the solution is dissolved, transfer it to a 500 ml volumetric flask, rinse the beaker thoroughly, adding the rinsing to the flask, dilutes with water to volume, and mix. Pipette 50 ml of the solution into a suitable container, add 100 ml of water, 5 ml of 1N sodium hydroxide and 300 mg of hydroxy naphthol blue, and titrate with 0.05M edetate disodium to a blue end point.

***Uses:***

1. The solution of calcium hydroxide is topically used as a protective.

2. It is also used as an antacid.
3. Lime water is used as an astringent in infantile diarrhoea and vomiting.
4. It is used for the preparation of some skin lotions.

***Storage:*** It should be stored in well closed container.

## Dilute Phosphoric Acid B.P., U.S.P.

This compound is discussed under the topic **acidifiers and alkalinising agents**.

## Hypo Phosphorous Acid U.S.P.

**Mol. Formula:** $H_3PO_2$ **Mol. Weight:** 66

It is not official in any pharmacopoeia. It is included in U.S. National Formulary and added in appendix in Indian Pharmacopoeia. It is a monobasic acid and reducing agent.

***Preparation:***

1. *From calcium hypophosphite:* It is prepared by treating a hypophosphite such as calcium hypophosphite with excess of oxalic acid or sulphuric acid.

$$\underset{\text{Calcium hypophosphite}}{Ca(H_2PO_2)_2} + \underset{\text{Oxalic acid}}{\begin{matrix} COOH \\ | \\ COOH \end{matrix}} \longrightarrow \underset{\text{Calcium oxalate}}{\left[\begin{matrix} COO^- \\ | \\ COO^- \end{matrix}\right] Ca^{2+}} + \underset{\text{Hypophosphorous acid}}{2H_3PO_2}$$

The insoluble calcium oxalate formed is filtered and the filtrate is collected and concentrated in vacuum.

$$Ca(H_2PO_2)_2 + H_2SO_4 \longrightarrow 2H_3PO_2 + CaSO_4$$

The insoluble calcium sulphate formed is filtered and the filtrate is collected and concentrated in vacuum.

2. *From potassium hypophosphite:* The pure hypo phosphorous acid is obtained by treating potassium hypophosphite with tartaric acid.

$$KH_2PO_2 + C_4H_6O_6 \longrightarrow H_3PO_2 + KHC_4H_4O_6$$

***Physical properties:*** It is a colorless or yellow color, odorless liquid or slightly acidic odour and taste. It contains 30-32% of phosphoric acid. Specific gravity is 1.14. It is miscible with water and alcohol. It is incompatible with mercury, silver, bismuth and lead salt to form metallic state.

***Chemical properties***

1. *Acidic properties:* It acts as monobasic acid because only one hydrogen atom is ionizable.

$$H_3PO_2 + H_2O \longrightarrow H_3O^+ + PH_2O_2^-$$

2. *Reducing properties:* It is practically never used for its acidic property. The central phosphorous has oxidation number +1, which makes the compound a very powerful reducing agent. It can easily reduce many compounds and forms phosphorous acid ($H_3PO_3$) and an oxidation state of +3, and finally forms phosphoric acid ($H_3PO_4$) with the oxidation state of +5. On reduction it yields phosphine which reacts with mercuric halide papers.
3. *Decomposition reaction:* Reaction with potassium chlorate: It is oxidized to phosphoric acid by reacting with potassium chlorate and hydrochloric acid. The excess of chlorine formed by the interaction of chlorate and hydrochloric acid is removed by boiling and then treatment with stannous chloride.

$$H_3PO_2 + KClO_3 + HCl \longrightarrow H_3PO_4 + Cl_2 + KOH$$

4. *Reaction with iodine:* It reacts with molecular iodine to form iodide ions

$$H_3PO_2 + 2I_2 + 2H_2O \longrightarrow 4HI + H_3PO_4$$

5. *Reaction with potassium permanganate:* Hypophosphorous acid decolorizes potassium permanganate in acidic solution immediately.

$$5H_3PO_2 + 4KMnO_4 + 6H_2SO_4 \longrightarrow 2K_2SO_4 + 4MnSO_4 + 5H_3PO_4 + 6H_2O$$

6. *Reaction with sulphuric acid:* It is oxidized by sulphuric acid to form sulphur dioxide and sulphur.

$$4H_3PO_2 + 3H_2SO_4 \longrightarrow SO_2 + S_2 + 3H_3PO_4 + H_3PO_3 + 3H_2O$$

7. The oxidation reaction between hypophosphorous acid and any oxidizing agent can produce an incompatibility and it can be exploded.
8. *Reaction with carbonates or alkali hydroxides:* The acid can be neutralized with alkali hydroxides or carbonates.

$$2H_3PO_2 + Na_2CO_3 \longrightarrow 2NaH_2PO_2 + H_2O + CO_2$$

***Test for identification:***

1. When a small quantity of sample solution is heated with 5 ml of copper sulphate solution, it gives reddish brown precipitate.
2. The small amount of sample is treated with required quantity of mercuric chloride solution and yields a white precipitate which changes to grey on heating and finally a globule of mercury is deposited.

***Test for purity:*** It should be tested for heavy metals, barium, calcium, iron, chloride, sulphate, phosphoric acid, oxalic acid and weight per ml (specific gravity).

***Test for Phosphoric acid and oxalic acid:*** The solution of calcium chloride and dilute ammonia are added to the dilute solution of hypo phosphorous acid. A slight turbidity is produced.

**Assay**

***Principle:*** It is assayed by **acidimetry-alkalimetry method** of titration (also called **neutralization method**).

In this assay the substance is diluted suitably with water and titrated with sodium hydroxide, using methyl orange as an indicator. End point is the yellow colour.

In this assay the sodium hydroxide (the base) reacts with hypo phosphorous acid and neutralization takes place during the titration. The indicator is orange colour in acid medium and it changes to yellow colour upon neutralization which is the end point.

As the acid and alkali are involved in this assay, it is called as acidimetry-alkalimetry method of titration and the neutralization takes place in this assay during titration hence this assay is also called as neutralization method.

***Procedure:*** Transfer about 7 ml of sample in to tared glass stoppered flask. Dilute with about 25 ml of water, add methyl orange, and titrate with 1N sodium hydroxide.

***Uses:***

1. It is mainly used as an antioxidant in diluted form (0.5-1%).
2. Hypophosphites are source of phosphorous and used as a brain tonic.
3. It is mainly used as a reducing agent in ferrous iodide syrup to prevent the formation of both ferric ion (coloration) and molecular iodide.
4. It prevents the formation of free iodine in hydroiodic acid syrup and in diluted hydroiodic acid.
5. Salts of hypo phosphorous acid such as sodium and ammonium hypophosphite are present as a preservative in certain food preparations.

***Storage:*** It should be stored in well closed containers.

## 6.1.4 Antacids

**Introduction:** In stomach the gastric acid is secreted by the parietal cells of gastric mucosa. These cells contain receptors for the three stimulants of acid secretion. They are

1. Gastrin from G-cells
2. Histamine from Entero Chromaffin Like (ECL) cells
3. Acetylcholine from vagal efferents

The histamine released from the ECL cells binds to the $H_2$ receptors (present in stomach) and increases the intracellular cyclic AMP (cAMP), while gastrin and acetylcholine acts by increasing the cytosolic calcium. Both of the cAMP and cytosolic calcium activates protein kinase and stimulate the HCl secretion *via* $H^+/K^+$ ATPase which is present in the surface of the parietal cells. The secreted $H^+$ ion combines with the $Cl^-$ (from plasma) leads to the formation of HCl.

The carbonic anhydrase enzyme is also catalyses the formation of carbonic acid which in turn undergo dissociation into bicarbonate and $H^+$ ion. These $H^+$ ions also used for the production of HCl by proton pump. Acetylcholine stimulate the acid secretion by directly acting on muscarnic $M_3$ receptors or through $M_1$ receptors and gastrin stimulate the acid secretion from ECL cells which are the major source of histamine release needed for acid secretion. Gastric acid secretion and peptic ulcer formation is depicted in Fig. 6.1

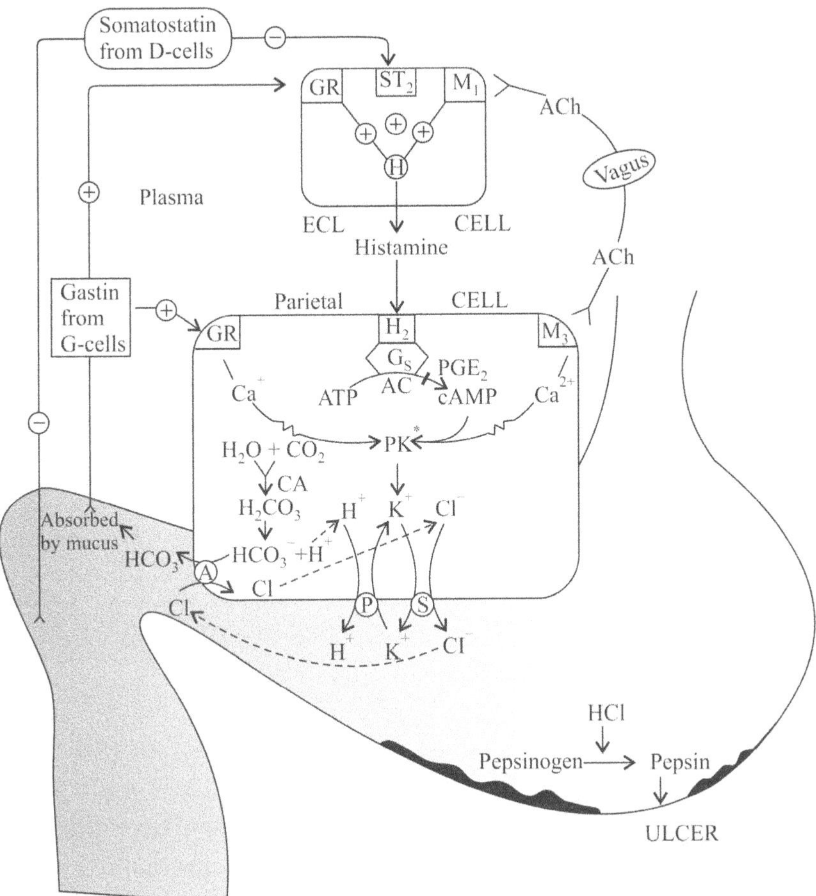


Key: GR–Gastrin receptor; $ST_2$–Somatostain receptor; P–Proton pump ($H^+K^+$-ATPase); S–Symport carrier for $K^+$ and $Cl^-$; A–Antiport carrier for $HCO_3^-$ and $Cl^-$; CA–Carbonic anhydrase; $PK^*$–Protein kinase activated; AC–Adenylate cyclase; H–Histamine (its receptor $H_2$); ECL–Enterochromaffin like cells

**Fig. 6.1** Physiological aspects of gatric acid secretion and peptic ulcer formation

Before the discovery of $H_2$ receptor antagonists and proton pump inhibitors, antacids are primarily used therapeutic agents for the treatment of gastrooesophagul reflux, peptic ulcer and dyspepsia.

Antacids are weak bases that neutralize excess gastric hydrochloric acid there by raising the pH of stomach contents, decreasing the acid load delivered to the duodenum and reduce the pepsin activity. These agents also increase the mucosal defense by the stimulation of prostaglandin production and partly by forming a protective layer against gastric mucosa.

The dose of antacid is meq or mmol of their neutralizing capacity.

Factors which controls the capacity of antacid activity are

1. Formulations (Liquid formulation is most effective than chewable tablet).
2. Gastric emptying.
3. Duration of action (insoluble antacids are relatively longer acting).

***Classification:*** Antacids are usually classified into two types

1. *Systemic antacids:* Sodium bicarbonate
2. *Non- Systemic antacids*:
   (i) Buffer type: Aluminium hydroxide, Magnesium trisilicate, Magaldrate
   (ii) Non buffer type: Magnesium hydroxide
   (iii) Miscellaneous: Alginates, simethicone.

***Buffer type antacids:*** They have slow onset of action but longer duration of action and increase the pH up to 3.5 to 4. Aluminium hydroxide, magnesium trisilicate and magaldrate are acting as buffer type non systemic antacids. These are poorly absorbed from GI tract and do not interfere systemic acid base balance nor do they elevate urinary pH these are two types.

***Mechanism of action:*** Both aluminium hydroxide and magnesium hydroxide reacts with gastric hydrochloric acid to form aluminium chloride and magnesium chloride respectively, further which reacts with intestinal bicarbonates to give aluminium bicarbonate and magnesium bicarbonate. The sodium chloride formed during this process gets reabsorbed to equalize the loss of chloride in during gastric acid neutralization.

$$Al(OH)_3 \xrightarrow[\text{Stomach}]{\text{HCl}} AlCl_3 \xrightarrow[\text{Intestine}]{HCO_3^-,\ PO_4^{3-}} Al_2(CO_3)_3 + AlPO_4 + NaCl$$

***Non buffer type antacids:*** They are powerful type of antacids with fast onset of action, and raises the gastric pH 7. Example: Calcium carbonate and Magnesium hydroxide.

***Mechanism of action:*** Calcium carbonate reacts with gastric hydrochloric acid to neutralize and gives calcium chloride. Which further react with intestinal bicarbonates and stearates to give calcium carbonate and calcium stearate which leads to constipation.

$$CaCO_3 \xrightarrow[\text{Stomach}]{\text{HCl}} CaCl_2 \xrightarrow[\text{Intestine}]{HCO_3^-\text{,Stearates}} \underset{\text{(Constipation)}}{CaCO_3 + \text{Calcium stearate} + NaCl}$$

***Miscellaneous antacids or miscellaneous adjuvant to antacid preparation:*** Simethicone and sodium alginate are the examples for miscellaneous antacids. Simethicone has the water repellent properties, so it acts as an antifoaming agent by this way it reduces gastric flatulence.

Sodium alginate is a colloidal carbohydrate. It is used along with $H_2$ receptor antagonist for the management of heart burn and gastroeasophageal reflux disease (GEPD). Recent antacid preparations contain buffer type antacids with sodium alginate. Antacids should not be used in congestive cardiac failure since it contains sodium ions.

**Qualities of ideal antacids**

The requirements of an antacid to be considered as an ideal antacid are enumerated herein:

- As the antacids are used most widely and chronically, it should be available at cheaper cost.
- It should elicit its effect gradually and should act for long period of time.
- It should not cause the side effects like laxative or constipation which are commonly produced by most antacids.
- It should not cause any other side effects.
- It should be insoluble in water and has fine particle form.
- It should not be absorbable or should not cause systemic alkalosis.
- It should buffer in the pH range 4 to 6.
- It should also inhibit pepsin and other proteolytic enzymes.
- It should be stable and readily available.
- The reaction between antacid and gastric hydrochloric acid should not yield large amount of gas.

None of the compound or antacid preparation meets the above criteria be an ideal antacid, however some of the aluminium, calcium and magnesium compounds are used widely.

**Common drug interactions**

1. Antacids increases the gastric pH due to this property they decrease the absorption of acidic drugs like phenytoin, NSAIDs and barbiturates.
2. Aluminium and magnesium type of antacids decrease the bioavailability, absorption of digoxin.
3. Aluminium, calcium and magnesium type of antacids reduces the absorption of tetracyclines due to the formation of inert complexes. So antacid preparations should not be given within 2 hours of administration of fluoroquinolones, tetracyclines, iron salts.
4. Magnesium containing antacids should be avoided in renal failure patients.

**Common side effects**

1. Long term uses of sodium bicarbonate leads to rebound acidity so it should not be given to patients of hypertensive CHF and renal failure.
2. Excessive dose of calcium carbonate produces metabolic alkalosis when taken along with milk, alkali syndrome constipation.
3. Magnesium salts leads to osmotic diarrhoea and aluminium salts causes constipation hence these two agents are commonly administered together.

In general antacids should be administered in suspension forms but it also available in chewable tablet form and powder forms.

***Acid Neutralizing Capacity:*** The acid neutralizing capacity of antacids is evaluated by the following methods.

*In-vitro test:* A known quantity of an antacid is added to the given amount of standard hydrochloric acid, then at different time intervals pH of this solution/acid is measured to determine the amount of hydrochloric acid consumed by the antacid whose acid neutralizing capacity is under evaluation.

*In-vivo test:* A known quantity of an antacid is administered and at different time intervals by removing aliquots of gastric contents and measuring the pH of the gastric contents the antacid whose acid neutralizing capacity is under evaluation is measured. This is not successful and also not official method.

## Sodium Bicarbonate I.P., B.P., U.S.P.

**(Synonym: Sodium hydrogen carbonate, Baking soda)**

**Mol. Formula:** $NaHCO_3$ **Mol. Weight:** 84

It contains not less than 99% and not more than 101% of $NaHCO_3$.

***Preparation:***

1. *Ammonia soda process or Solvay process (Large scale preparation):* This method was introduced by Brunner and Mond. According to this method strong brine solution (contains high concentration of sodium chloride) is saturated with ammonia which is passed through carbonating water which is saturated with carbon dioxide under pressure. During this process ammonia reacts with carbon dioxide to produce ammonium bicarbonate and this undergoes double decomposition with sodium chloride, leads to the formation of sodium bicarbonate as precipitate which is less soluble in brine solution. All the reactions are reversible.

$$NH_3 + H_2O + CO_2 \rightleftharpoons NH_4HCO_3$$

$$NH_4HCO_3 + NaCl \rightleftharpoons NH_4Cl + NaHCO_3$$

The above sodium bicarbonate obtained is separated by simple filtration and dried at room temperature.

The sodium bicarbonate formed by the above method does not comply with I.P standard so the bicarbonate is heated to get anhydrous sodium carbonate and evolves carbon dioxide.

$$2\,NaHCO_3 \xrightarrow{\Delta} Na_2CO_3 + H_2O + CO_2$$

This sodium carbonate is dissolved in pure water and carbon dioxide is passed through the pure solution up to saturation to yield pure sodium bicarbonate.

$$Na_2CO_3 + H_2O + CO_2 \longrightarrow 2NaHCO_3$$

2. *From Sodium hydroxide:* In this method, sodium bicarbonate is prepared by bubbling carbon dioxide into sodium hydroxide solution. The solution is concentrated and dried.

$$2NaOH + CO_2 \longrightarrow Na_2CO_3 + H_2O$$

$$Na_2CO_3 + H_2O + CO_2 \longrightarrow 2NaHCO_3$$

***Physical properties:*** It is a white crystalline powder or small opaque monoclinic crystals. It is freely soluble in water but insoluble in alcohol. The pH of 1% w/v solution is 8.6.

***Chemical properties:*** When it is heated to 100 °C it forms sesquicarbonate and sodium bicarbonate dihydrate.

$$2NaHCO_3 \xrightarrow{100\ ^\circ C} Na_2CO_3.H_2O + CO_2$$

$$NaHCO_3 \xrightarrow{100\ ^\circ C} NaHCO_3.2H_2O$$

***Test for identification:*** The sample solution gives the characteristic reactions of sodium and bicarbonate ions.

***Test for purity:*** It should be tested for alkalinity, calcium, aluminium, arsenic, lead, iron, chloride, sulphate, carbonate and ammonium compounds (due to the presence of ammonia – soda product).

***Test for ammonium compounds:*** Small quantity of the sample is heated with sodium hydroxide solution; no ammonia gas is evolved (absence of pungent odour).

**Assay**

***Principle:*** It is assayed by **acidimetry-alkalimetry method** of titration (also called **neutralization method**).

In this assay the substance is dissolved in water and titrated with 0.5N hydrochloric acid, using methyl orange as an indicator. End point is the orange colour. In this assay the sodium bicarbonate (the base) reacts with hydrochloric acid and neutralization takes place during the titration. The indicator is yellow colour in alkali medium and it changes to orange colour upon neutralization which is the end point.

As the acid and alkali involved in this assay, it is called as acidimetry-alkalimetry method of titration and the neutralization takes place in this assay during titration hence this assay is also called as neutralization method. The chemical reactions of this assay are shown below.

$$NaHCO_3 + HCl \longrightarrow NaCl + H_2O + CO_2$$

***Procedure:*** Weigh accurately about 1.5 gm, dissolve in 50 ml of carbon dioxide-free water and titrate with 1M hydrochloric acid using 0.2 ml of methyl orange solution as indicator.

***Uses:***

1. It is mainly used for its acid neutralizing property as systemic alkalizers.
2. It is used as an antacid.
3. It is used for preparing buffer solution.

4. The solution of sodium bicarbonate is used in the treatment of burns, insect bites etc.
5. It is the one of the constituent of oral rehydration salt (electrolyte replenisher).

***Dose:*** 1 to 4 gm.

***Storage:*** It should be stored in tightly closed containers and protected from moisture.

***Official preparations:*** Sodium bicarbonate injection I.P, Sodium bicarbonate tablets I.P.

## Sodium Bicarbonate Injection I.P., B.P., U.S.P.

**(Synonym: Sodium bicarbonate intravenous injection)**

Sodium bicarbonate injection is a sterile solution of sodium bicarbonate in water for injection. It contains not less than 94% and not more than 106% of the sodium bicarbonate.

***Physical properties:*** It is a white or color less, clear solution.

***Test for identification:*** Similar to sodium bicarbonate.

***Test for purity:*** Similar to sodium bicarbonate.

***Other requirements:*** It should comply with the requirements for injection (pyrogen test) and for bacterial endotoxin.

**Assay:**

***Principle:*** It is assayed by **acidimetry-alkalimetry method** of titration (also called **neutralization method**).

In this assay, the required volume of sample solution is diluted with water and titrated with 0.5N hydrochloric acid, using methyl orange as an indicator. End point is the orange colour. In this assay the sodium bicarbonate (the base) reacts with hydrochloric acid and neutralization takes place during the titration. The indicator is yellow colour in alkali medium and it changes to orange colour upon neutralization which is the end point.

As the acid and alkali involved in this assay, it is called as acidimetry-alkalimetry method of titration and the neutralization takes place in this assay during titration hence this assay is also called as neutralization method. The chemical reactions of this assay are shown below.

$$NaHCO_3 + HCl \longrightarrow NaCl + H_2O + CO_2$$

***Procedure:*** Titrate a volume containing 1.5 gm of sodium bicarbonate with 1M hydrochloric acid using methyl orange solution as indicator.

***Uses:*** It is used as a systemic alkalizer and electrolyte replenisher.

***Storage:*** It should be stored in single dose containers.

***Labelling:*** The label contains the following.

1. The strength of sodium bicarbonate (percentage of w/v).
2. The approximate concentration of sodium and the bicarbonate ions (mmol/L).
3. The label must indicate that "if the injection containing visible particles in the solution" it should not be used.

## Compound Sodium Bicarbonate Tablets U.S.P.

It contains not less than 0.30 gm and not more than 0.35 gm of sodium bicarbonate. The sodium bicarbonate tablet is prepared from sodium bicarbonate and mentha oil.

**Constituents:**

Sodium bicarbonate = 0.320 gm

Mentha oil = 0.004 ml

***Preparation:*** The sodium bicarbonate tablets are prepared by wet granulation method and mentha oil is added to the tablets.

***Test for identification:*** The powder of sodium bicarbonate tablets should meet the characteristic tests for sodium and bicarbonate. The tablets should comply with the requirements for tablets.

**Assay**

***Principle:*** It is assayed by **acidimetry-alkalimetry method** of titration (also called **neutralization method**).

In this assay twenty tablets are weighed, powdered and the substance is dissolved in solvent and titrated with 0.5N hydrochloric acid, using methyl orange as an indicator. End point is the orange colour. In this assay the sodium bicarbonate (the base) reacts with hydrochloric acid and neutralization takes place during the titration. The indicator is yellow colour in alkali medium and it changes to orange colour upon neutralization which is the end point.

As the acid and alkali involved in this assay, it is called as acidimetry-alkalimetry method of titration and the neutralization takes place in this assay during titration hence this assay is also called as neutralization method. The chemical reactions of this assay are shown below.

$$NaHCO_3 + HCl \longrightarrow NaCl + H_2O + CO_2$$

***Dose:*** 2 to 6 tablets. It must be allowed to dissolve slowly in the mouth.

***Storage:*** It should be stored in tightly closed containers in cool place.

## Potassium Citrate I.P., B.P., U.S.P.

**(Synonym: Potassium cit, kaliicitras, Tripotassium citrate)**

**Mol. Formula:** $C_6H_5K_3O_7 . H_2O$ **Mol. Weight:** 324.4

**Structure:**

$$\begin{array}{c} CH_2COOK \\ | \\ HO-C-COOK . H_2O \\ | \\ CH_2COOK \end{array}$$

Potassium citrate is tripotassium-2-hydroxy propane 1,2,3-tricarboxylate monohydrate.

It contains not less than 99% and not more than 101% of potassium citrate, which is calculated on dried basis.

***Preparation:*** It is prepared by mixing of the hot solutions of citric acid and potassium carbonate or potassium bicarbonate. Then the solution is filtered off and then evaporated to dryness, with constant stirring. A fine powder is obtained by carrying out trituration in a warm mortar.

$$\underset{\text{Potassium bicarbonate}}{3\,KHCO_3} + \underset{\text{Citric acid}}{HO{-}C(CH_2COOH)_2{-}COOH} \longrightarrow HO{-}C(CH_2COOK)_2{-}COOK + 3\,CO_2\uparrow + 3\,H_2O$$

$$\underset{\text{Potassium carbonate}}{3\,K_2CO_3} + 2\,\underset{\text{Citric acid}}{HO{-}C(CH_2COOH)_2{-}COOH} \longrightarrow 2\,HO{-}C(CH_2COOK)_2{-}COOK + 3\,CO_2\uparrow + 3\,H_2O$$

***Physical properties:*** It occurs as a white crystals or granular powder, odorless, with cooling saline taste, hygroscopic in nature. It is soluble in water and glycerin but insoluble in alcohol. At higher temperatures, it carbonizes and evolves inflammable gases which are having pungent acrid odour.

***Test for identification:*** The sample solution gives the characteristic reactions of potassium and citrate ions.

***Test for purity:*** It should be tested for clarity and color of the solution, acidity or alkalinity, arsenic, heavy metals, sodium, chloride, oxalate, sulphate, readily carbonisable substances and water.

**Assay**

***Principle:***

*Method 1:* It is assayed by **acidimetry-alkalimetry method** of (Back) titration (also called **neutralization method**).

In this assay the substance is heated in a crucible until carbonized. The residue is dissolved in Known Excess Standard (KES) 0.5N sulphuric acid and the excess unreacted (EUR) sulphuric acid is titrated with 0.5N sodium hydroxide using methyl orange as an indicator. End point is the yellow colour. In this assay upon ignition of the potassium citrate, potassium carbonate is formed which when treated with sulphuric acid, the potassium carbonate (the base) goes into the solution in sulphuric acid and neutralization takes place, after this reaction the excess unreacted sulphuric acid is determined by titrating with sodium hydroxide. The indicator is orange colour in acidic medium and it changes to yellow colour upon neutralization which is the end point.

As the acid and alkali involved in this assay, it is called as acidimetry-alkalimetry method of titration and the neutralization takes place in this assay during titration hence this assay is also called as neutralization method. The chemical reactions of this assay are shown below.

$$\begin{array}{l} CH_2\text{-}COOK \\ \quad | \\ HO\text{-}C\text{-}COOK \; .H_2O \\ \quad | \\ CH_2\text{-}COOK \end{array} \xrightarrow{\Delta} K_2CO_3$$

$$K_2CO_3 + H_2SO_4 \longrightarrow K_2SO_4 + H_2O + CO_2$$

$$2\,NaOH + H_2SO_4 \longrightarrow Na_2SO_4 + 2\,H_2O$$

*Method 2:* It can also be assayed by nonaqueous titration. Potassium citrate is a very weak base, hence it is assayed by dissolving in acetic anhydride and glacial acetic acid and titrating against perchloric acid using 1-naphtholbenzein solution as indicator end point is the green colour.

***Procedure:*** Weigh accurately about 0.2 gm, dissolve in 20 ml of anhydrous glacial acetic acid, heat to about 50 °C, allow it to cool. Titrate with 0.1M perchloric acid, using 0.25 ml of 1-naphtholbenzein solution as indicator and titrating until a green colour is obtained. Carry out a blank titration.

***Uses:***

1. It is mainly used for its osmotic diuretic and diaphoretic action which is greater than other alkaline salts and ammonium compound.
2. It is also used as a systemic alkalinising agent and having slight laxative action.
3. It is used as an anticoagulant.

***Mechanism of action:*** The body tissues easily oxidize the potassium citrate and liberate carbon dioxide and water and equivalent amount of potassium bicarbonate which functions as an alkalinising agent.

***Dose:*** 4 to 10 gm.

***Storage:*** It should be stored in well closed containers, protected from moisture.

## Aluminium Hydroxide Gel I.P., B.P., U.S.P.

**(Synonym: Aluminium hydroxide suspension, Aluminium hydroxide mixture)**

It is an aqueous suspension of hydrated aluminium oxide together with various amounts of basic aluminium carbonate and bicarbonate. It may contain sweetening agents (sucrose, glucose, sorbitol etc.), flavouring agents (peppermint oil) and suitable antimicrobial agents (sodium benzoate).

It contains not less than 3.5% w/w and not more than 4.4% w/w of $Al_2O_3$.

***Preparation***

*From aluminium sulphate or potash alum:* A hot solution of potash alum is slowly added to a hot solution of sodium carbonate with constant stirring. During this reaction carbondioxide gas is evolved. After the complete evolution of carbondioxide, the precipitated aluminium hydroxide is separated by filtration. Wash thoroughly with hot water, until it is free from sulphate and the precipitate is suspended in distilled water for required strength.

$$3\,Na_2CO_3 + 2\,KAl(SO_4)_2 + 3\,H_2O \longrightarrow 2\,Al(OH)_3\downarrow + 3\,Na_2SO_4 + K_2SO_4 + 3\,CO_2\uparrow$$

***Precaution:*** The alum solution should be added to the sodium carbonate solution not vice versa since it would give a precipitate with alkali sulphate which is difficult to wash.

The aluminium hydroxide precipitate is washed with hot water only not by boiled water because the latter causes the decomposition of aluminium hydroxide.

***Physical properties:*** A white or colorless viscous suspension, translucent in nature, a small amount clear layer may be separated when it is kept on standing.

***Chemical properties***

*Reaction with hydrochloric acid:* Aluminium hydroxide gel reacts with gastric juice and gives aluminium chloride which is astringent in nature. So it leads to nausea, vomiting and constipation. So it should be administered along with magnesium salt which is a mild laxative.

$$Al(OH)_3 + 3\,HCl \longrightarrow AlCl_3 + 3\,H_2O$$

*Neutralization mechanism of aluminium hydroxide gel in Stomach:*

$$Al(OH)_3 + 3\,H_2O \rightleftharpoons [Al(H_2O)_3(OH)_3]$$

$$[Al(H_2O)_3(OH)_3] + H_3O^+ \longrightarrow [Al(H_2O)_4(OH)_2]^+ + H_2O$$

$$[Al(H_2O)_4(OH)_2]^+ + H_3O^+ \longrightarrow [Al(H_2O)_5(OH)]^{+2} + H_2O$$

$$[Al(H_2O)_5(OH)]^{+2} + H_3O^+ \longrightarrow [Al(H_2O)_6]^{+3} + H_2O$$

***Test for identification:*** An acidic solution of aluminium hydroxide gel gives the characteristic reactions of aluminium salts.

***Test for purity:*** It should be tested for arsenic, heavy metals, chlorides, sulphates and acid neutralizing capacity.

***Test for acid neutralizing capacity:*** Dissolve the required amount of sample in water, add 100 ml of 0.1M hydrochloric acid, stir it well, maintain the temperature at 37 °C and measure the pH of the solution with a time interval of 10, 15 and 20 minutes. The pH of the solution is not more than 1.8, 2.3 and 3 respectively. To this add 0.5 ml of 0.5M HCl, stir well at 37 °C and titrate with 0.1M sodium hydroxide solution to reach the pH 3.5. Not more than 50 ml of sodium hydroxide is needed to neutralize the solution.

**Assay**

***Principle:*** It is assayed by **Complexometry method of (Back) titration.**

In this assay the substance is dissolved in hydrochloric acid by warming, to this Known Excess Standard (KES) 0.05N disodium Ethylene Diamine Tetra Acetate (EDTA) added and the solution is neutralized with 1N sodium hydroxide using methyl red as an indicator (colour change from red to yellow). To this solution hexamine added as a buffer and xylenol orange as an indicator and titrated against 0.05M lead nitrate. End point is the appearance of violet colour due to the formation of lead-xylenol orange complex.

In this assay the aluminium ions of aluminium hydroxide reacts with EDTA, whereby the complexation takes place, after this reaction, the Excess Unreacted (EUR) disodium EDTA is determined by titrating with lead nitrate. The indicator is colourless before complexation and change into violet colour due to the formation of lead-xylenol orange complex. As the aluminium ions forms complex with disodium EDTA in this assay, it is called as complexometry method of titration. The chemical reactions of this assay are shown below.

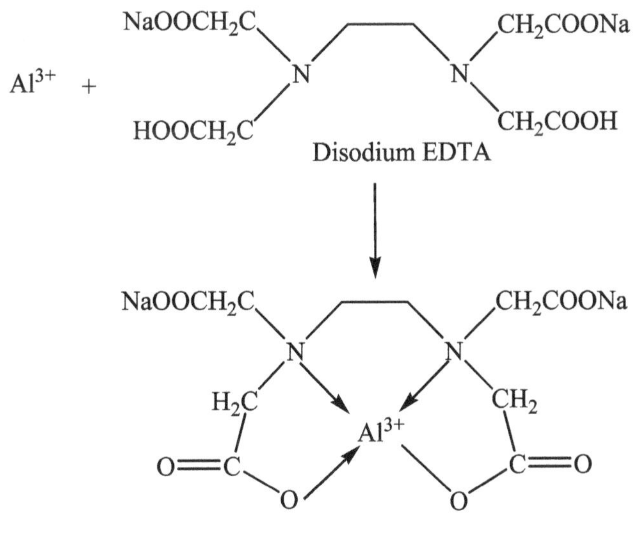

$Al^{3+}$ + $NaOOCH_2C$ / $HOOCH_2C$ >N–CH₂–CH₂–N< $CH_2COONa$ / $CH_2COOH$

Disodium EDTA

↓

$NaOOCH_2C$, $CH_2COONa$, N, N, $H_2C$, $CH_2$, $Al^{3+}$, O=C, C=O, O, O

Aluminium-EDTA Complex

***Procedure:*** Weigh accurately about 5 gm and dissolve in 3 ml of hydrochloric acid by warming on a water-bath; cool to below 20 °C and dilute to 100 ml with water. To 20 ml of this solution, add 40 ml of 0.05M disodium edetate, 80 ml of water, and 0.15 ml of methyl red solution and neutralize by the drop wise addition of 1M sodium hydroxide. Warm on a water-bath for 30 minutes, add 3 gm of hexamine and titrate with 0.05M lead nitrate using 0.5 ml of xylenol orange solution as indicator.

***Uses:***

1. Aluminium hydroxide gel is very effective slow acting antacid.
2. It has the advantage that it is not absorbed in the gastro intestinal tract (GIT) and doses not generate carbon dioxide and metallic carbonates.
3. It is used to absorb gastric toxins and gases.
4. It is widely used in the treatment of hyper chlorhydria and intestinal toxemia.

***Dose:*** 7.5 to 15 ml.

***Storage:*** It should be stored in well closed blue or amber colored container temperature of not exceeding to 30 °C. Do not freeze it.

## Dried Aluminium Hydroxide Gel I.P., B.P., U.S.P.

**(Synonym: Dried Aluminium hydroxide, Hydrated aluminium oxide, Aluminium hydroxide powder)**

It contains large amount of hydrated aluminium oxide with varying amounts of basic aluminium carbonate and bicarbonate.

It contains not less than 47% w/v and not more than 60% w/v of $Al_2O_3$.

***Physical properties:*** It is a white, highly amorphous powder with small aggregates, odourless, tasteless. It is soluble in dilute mineral acids and excess of caustic alkalis. It is insoluble in water and alcohol.

***Test for identification:*** A solution in hydrochloric acid gives the characteristic reactions of aluminium salts.

***Test for purity:*** It should be tested for pH, arsenic, heavy metals, chloride, sulphates, acid neutralizing capacity and microbial contamination.

***Test for pH of the solution:*** It should not be more than 10.

***Test for microbial contamination:*** The 1 gm of sample should be free from *Escherichia coli.*

**Assay**

***Principle:*** It is assayed by **Complexometry method of (Back) titration.**

In this assay the substance is dissolved in hydrochloric acid and water mixture by warming. Remaining procedure is similar to that of aluminium hydroxide gel.

***Procedure:*** Weigh accurately about 0.4 gm and dissolve in a mixture of 3 ml of hydrochloric acid and 3 ml of water by warming on a water-bath, cool to below 20 °C and dilute to 100.0 ml with water. To 20 ml of this solution, add 40.0 ml of 0.05M disodium edetate, 80 ml of water, and 0.15 ml of methyl red solution and neutralize by the drop wise addition of 1M sodium hydroxide. Warm on a water-bath for 30 minutes, add 3 gm of hexamine and titrate with 0.05M lead nitrate using 0.5 ml of xylenol orange solution as indicator.

***Uses:*** It is used as an antacid.

***Dose:*** 500 mg to 1 gm.

***Storage:*** It should be stored in tightly closed containers and protected from moisture.

## Aluminium Hydroxide Gel Tablet U.S.P.

It contains not less than 90% and not more than 110% of the aluminium hydroxide.

**Test for identification**

1. The tablet powder equivalent to 500 mg of dried aluminium hydroxide gel is placed in stoppered flask with glass tube and the tip of the tube is immersed in a test tube containing calcium hydroxide solution. To this add 5 ml of 3N hydrochloric acid, it gives precipitate in the test tube.
2. The solution obtained from the above method gives the characteristic reactions of aluminium.

***Test for acid neutralizing capacity:*** The powder equivalent to 250 mg of dried aluminium hydroxide gel is employed for the procedure as mentioned under dried aluminium hydroxide gel. Not less than 130 ml of 0.1N hydrochloric acid is consumed.

**Assay**

***Principle:*** It is assayed by **Complexometry method of (Back) titration**.

In this assay twenty tablets are weighed and the required quantity of the powder taken and the substance is dissolved in hydrochloric acid and water mixture by warming. Remaining procedure is similar to that of aluminium hydroxide gel.

***Uses:*** It is used as an antacid.

***Storage:*** It should be stored in well closed containers.

***Label:*** The content of aluminium hydroxide in each tablet is equivalent to 0.765 mg of aluminium hydroxide.

***Other formulations:*** Dried aluminium hydroxide gel capsules U.S.P.

## Aluminium Glycinate B.P.

**(Synonym: Dihydroxy Aluminium Amino Acetate)**

**Mol. Formula:** $C_2H_6AlNO_4 . xH_2O$ **Mol. Weight:** 135.05

or $NH_2CH_2COOAl(OH)_2 . XH_2O$

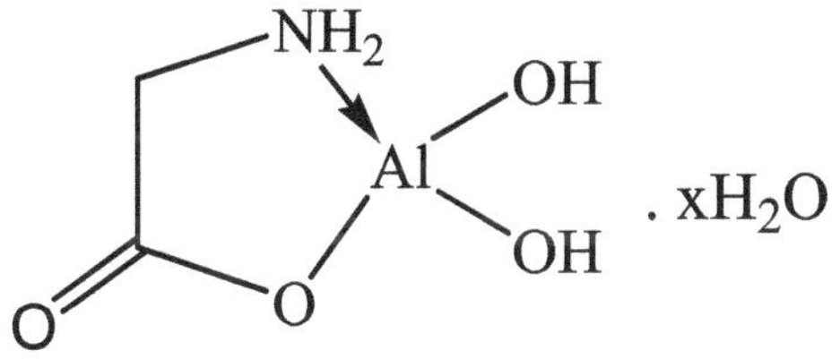

$NH_2$ OH Al OH O O . $xH_2O$

It is a basic aluminium monoglycinate, partly hydrated in nature.

It contains not less than 34.5% and not more than 38.5% of $Al_2O_3$ and not less than 9.9% and not more than 10.8% nitrogen which are calculated on dried basis.

***Preparation:*** It is prepared by the reaction between the aqueous solution of glycine and aluminium hydroxide.

$$NH_2CH_2COOH + Al(OH)_3 \longrightarrow NH_2CH_2COOAl(OH)_2 + H_2O$$

***Physical properties:*** It occurs as a white or almost white powder, insoluble in water and organic solvents. It is soluble in dilute mineral acids and aqueous alkali hydroxides.

***Test for identification:***

1. To the sample solution in citric acid, add 8 ml of 1M sodium hydroxide and diluted to 20 ml with water. To the above solution add 0.1% w/v of ninhydrin solution and warm it. A purple color is formed.
2. The sample solution in hydrochloric acid gives the characteristic reactions of aluminium.
3. To the sample solution add 0.15 ml of liquefied phenol, shake well and add 5 ml of dilute sodium hypochlorite solution. A blue color is produced.

***Test for purity:*** It should be tested for acidity or alkalinity, acid neutralizing capacity, arsenic, heavy metals, chloride, mercuric salts and loss on drying.

***Assay:*** It is assayed for aluminium trioxide content and for nitrogen content. Aluminium trioxide content is assayed by Complexometry method of (Back) titration as aluminium hydroxide (Refer aluminium hydroxide). The nitrogen content is assayed by Kjeldahl's method.

**For aluminium trioxide**

***Principle:*** It is assayed by **Complexometry method of (Back) titration**.

In this assay the substance is dissolved in hydrochloric acid by warming, to this Known Excess Standard (KES) 0.05N disodium Ethylene Diamine Tetra Acetate (EDTA) added and the solution is neutralised with 1N sodium hydroxide using methyl red as an indicator (colour change from red to yellow). To this solution hexamine added as a buffer and xylenol orange as an indicator and titrated against 0.05M lead nitrate.

In this assay aluminium ions of aluminium glycinate reacts with EDTA, whereby the complexation takes place, after this reaction, the Excess Unreacted (EUR) disodium EDTA is determined by titrating with lead nitrate. The indicator is colourless before complexation and change into violet colour due to the formation of lead-xylenol orange complex. As the aluminium ions forms complex with disodium EDTA in this assay, it is called as complexometry method of titration. The chemical reactions of this assay are shown below.

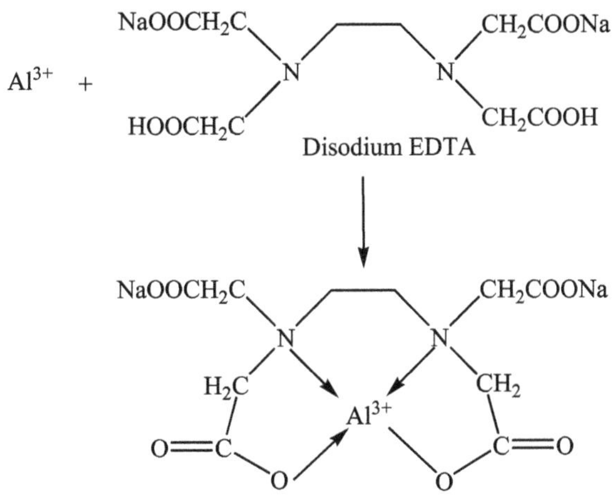

$Al^{3+}$ + $NaOOCH_2C$ / $HOOCH_2C$ > N — N < $CH_2COONa$ / $CH_2COOH$

Disodium EDTA

↓

$NaOOCH_2C$ — N — N — $CH_2COONa$; $H_2C$, $CH_2$, $O=C$, $C=O$, O, O, $Al^{3+}$

Aluminium-EDTA Complex

***Procedure:*** Dissolve 0.25 gm in a mixture of 3 ml of 1M hydrochloric acid and 50 ml of water, add 50 ml of 0.05M disodium edetate and neutralise with 1M sodium hydroxide using methyl red solution as indicator. Heat the solution to boiling; allow to stand for 10 minutes on a water bath, cool rapidly, add about 50 mg of xylenol orange triturate and 5 gm of hexamine and titrate the excess of disodium edetate with 0.05M lead nitrate until the solution becomes red.

***Uses:***

1. It acts as a slow acting antacid, but it acts more promptly than other antacids.
2. It is not affected by ageing like other antacid preparations of aluminium.

***Storage:*** It should be stored in well closed containers.

## Basic Aluminium Carbonate Gel U.S.P.

**Mol. Formula:** $Al(OH)CO_3$ **Mol. Weight:** 104

It is similar to aluminium hydroxide.

**Assay**

***Procedure:*** Transfer the sample equivalent to 1.2 gm of aluminium hydroxide, to a beaker containing hydrochloric acid to get a clear solution. After diluting it with water, add about 20 ml of standard EDTA solution, and acetic acid – ammonium acetate buffer. After heating the solution near the boiling point for 5 minutes and cool, and add 50 ml of alcohol and 2 ml of dithizone. Titrate with 0.05M zinc sulphate until get bright rose- pink color.

***Uses:*** It is mainly used in the management of phosphatic urinary calculi.

***Disadvantage:*** Mainly it causes phosphate deficiency by increasing the phosphate excretion in the feaces.

***Storage:*** It should be stored in well closed containers.

## Dried Aluminium Phosphate U.S.P.

**(Synonym: Dried aluminium phosphate gel )**

**Mol. Formula:** $AlPO_4.XH_2O$ - Dried Aluminium phosphate **Mol. Weight:** 122

$Al(OH)_x(PO_4)_y$ - Dried aluminium phosphate gel.

It consists of hydrated aluminium phosphate.

It contains not less than 19% and not more than 21% of aluminium phosphate.

***Preparation:*** It is mainly prepared by the reaction between aqueous solution of aluminum chloride and sodium phosphate. The soluble salts formed can be removed by washing with water and decantation or dialysis through suitable membrane. The product is then dried under suitable condition for controlling the particle size. The particle size depends upon the concentration of reactants, pH maintained during the process, temperature and the manner of addition etc.

$$AlCl_3 + Na_2PO_4 \longrightarrow AlPO_4.XH_2O$$

***Properties:*** It occurs as a white powder with some aggregates. It is practically insoluble in water and alcohol but soluble in dilute acids.

***Test for identification:*** The sample solution gives the characteristic reactions of aluminum and phosphate ions.

***Test for purity:*** It should be tested for chlorides, soluble phosphates, sulphate, soluble aluminium, arsenic, heavy metals, acid neutralizing capacity, residue on ignition and microbial contamination.

**Assay**

***Principle:*** It is assayed by **Complexometry method of (Back) titration**.

In this assay the substance is dissolved in 1N hydrochloric acid by warming, to this Known Excess Standard (KES) 0.05N disodium Ethylene Diamine Tetra Acetate (EDTA) added and the solution is treated with strong ammonium acetate and titrate it against 0.05M zinc sulphate. End point is determined potentiometrically.

In this assay aluminium ions of dried aluminium phosphate reacts with EDTA, whereby the complexation takes place, after this reaction, the excess unreacted disodium EDTA is determined by titrating with zinc chloride. As the Aluminium ions forms complex with disodium EDTA in this assay, it is called as complexometry method of titration. The chemical reactions of this assay are shown below.

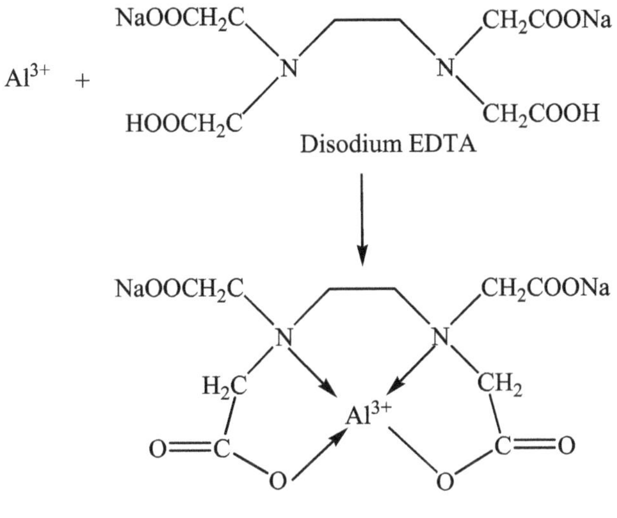

$$Al^{3+} + \text{Disodium EDTA} \longrightarrow \text{Aluminium-EDTA Complex}$$

Disodium EDTA: $NaOOCH_2C$ and $HOOCH_2C$ on one N, $CH_2COONa$ and $CH_2COOH$ on the other N; N–$CH_2$–$CH_2$–N bridge.

Aluminium-EDTA Complex

***Procedure:*** Dissolve with heating 0.300 gm in 5 ml of dilute hydrochloric acid. Add 45 ml of water, 10 ml of 0.1M sodium edetate and 30 ml of a mixture of equal volumes of ammonium acetate solution and dilute acetic acid. Heat to boiling and maintain boiling for 3 min. Cool, then add 25 ml of ethanol (96%). Titrate with 0.1M zinc sulphate, determining the endpoint potentiometrically.

***Uses:*** It is mainly used as an antacid and vaccine adjuvant.

***Mechanism of action of acid neutralizing capacity:*** The antacid action of aluminium phosphate is due to the release of strongly basis tertiary phosphate anion.

$$AlPO_4 \rightleftharpoons Al^{3+} + PO_4^{3-}$$

$$PO_4^{3-} + H_3O^+ \longrightarrow HPO_4^{2-} + H_2O$$

$$HPO_4^{2-} + H_3O^+ \longrightarrow H_2PO_4^- + H_2O$$

***Advantage:*** It contains 50% acid neutralizing capacity when compared with aluminium hydroxide gel.

***Storage:*** It should be stored in well closed containers.

## Magnesium Hydroxide I.P., B.P., U.S.P.

**Mol. Formula**: $Mg(OH)_2$ **Mol. Weight:** 58.3

It contains not less than 95% and not more than 100.5% of $Mg(OH)_2$.

***Preparation***

*Method 1:* It is prepared by evaporating the creamy magnesium hydroxide which is obtained from the preparation of milk of magnesia.

$$MgO + H_2O \longrightarrow \underset{\text{(Creamy consistancy)}}{Mg(OH)_2\downarrow} \xrightarrow{\text{Evaporation to dryness}} Mg(OH)_2$$

*Method 2:* It is also prepared by the treatment of brine solution or sea water with required amount of calcium hydroxide. The magnesium ion in the brine solution is converted into magnesium hydroxide as precipitate which is washed and dried.

***Physical properties:*** It is a bulky white powder, insoluble in water, which is alkaline in nature. It is soluble in dilute acids. It absorbs carbon dioxide from atmosphere slowly.

***Test for identification:*** The neutral solution of sample gives the characteristic reactions of magnesium ion.

***Test for purity:*** It should be tested for appearance of solution, arsenic, heavy metals, iron, chloride, sulphate, calcium, soluble substances, substances insoluble in acetic acid and loss on ignition.

**Assay**

***Principle:***

*Method 1:* It is assayed by **Acidimetry-alkalimetry method of (Back) titration** (also called **neutralization method**).

In this assay the substance is treated with Known Excess Standard (KES) 1N sulphuric acid and the excess unreacted sulphuric acid is titrated with 1N sodium hydroxide using methyl red as an indicator. End point is the yellow colour.

In this assay the Magnesium hydroxide (the base) reacts with sulphuric acid and neutralization takes place, after this reaction the excess unreacted sulphuric acid is determined by titrating with sodium hydroxide. The indicator is red colour in acid medium and it changes to yellow colour upon neutralization which is the end point.

As the acid and alkali involved in this assay, it is called as acidimetry-alkalimetry method of titration and the neutralization takes place in this assay during titration hence this assay is also called as neutralization method. The chemical reactions of this assay are shown below.

$$Mg(OH)_2 + H_2SO_4 \longrightarrow MgSO_4 + 2\,H_2O$$

$$H_2SO_4 + 2\,NaOH \longrightarrow Na_2SO_4 + 2\,H_2O$$

*Method 2:* It is assayed by **Complexometry method of (Direct) titration.**

In this assay the substance is dissolved in hydrochloric acid, to this strong ammonia-ammonium chloride solution added as buffer. The solution is then titrated against 0.05M disodium Ethylene Diamine Tetra Acetate (EDTA) using mordant black II mixture added as indicator. End point is the appearance of blue color.

In this assay magnesium ions of magnesium hydroxide reacts with disodium EDTA, whereby the complexation takes place. As the magnesium ions forms complex with disodium EDTA in this assay, it is called as complexometry method of titration. The chemical reactions of this assay are shown below.

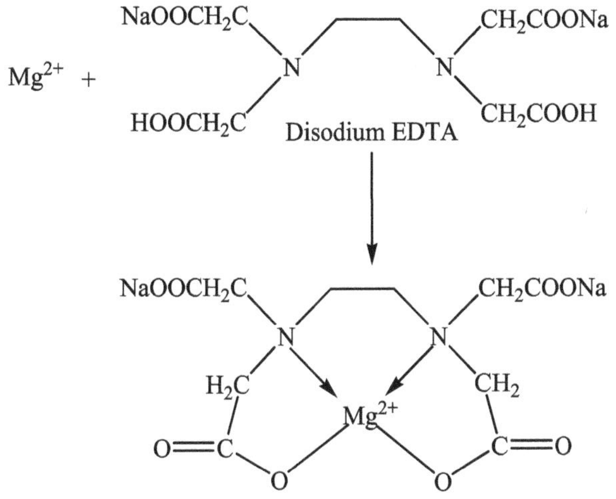

$Mg^{2+}$ + $(NaOOCH_2C)(HOOCH_2C)N-CH_2CH_2-N(CH_2COONa)(CH_2COOH)$

Disodium EDTA

↓

$NaOOCH_2C$, $CH_2COONa$, N, N, $H_2C$, $CH_2$, $Mg^{2+}$, O=C, C=O, O, O

Magnesium-EDTA Complex

***Procedure:*** Weigh accurately about 0.1 gm, dissolve in 20 ml of 2M hydrochloric acid and dilute to 100.0 ml with water. To 50.0 ml of this solution add 5 ml of strong ammonia-ammonium chloride solution and titrate with 0.05M disodium edetate, using about 50 mg of mordant black II mixture as indicator.

***Uses:*** It is used as an antacid and osmotic laxative.

***Dose:*** As antacid 500 to 750 mg

As laxative 2 to 4 gm.

***Storage:*** It should be stored in well closed containers and protected from moisture.

## Magnesium Hydroxide Mixture I.P., B.P.

**(Synonym: Milk of Magnesia, Cream of Magnesia, Magnesium hydroxide oral suspension)**

**Mol. Formula:** $Mg(OH)_2$ **Mol. Weight:** 58.3

It is an aqueous suspension of hydrated magnesium oxide, as well as hydrated oxide.

It contains not less than 7% w/w and not more than 8.5% w/w of hydrated magnesium oxide in purified water, calculated as magnesium hydroxide. Sometimes it may contain one more suitable preservative. It should be dispensed in blue colored bottles for better appearance.

***Preparation:***

1. *From magnesium oxide:* Light magnesium oxide is mixed with sodium hydroxide solution to get a cream. It is diluted with water; the suspension is poured in thin stream in to a solution of magnesium sulphate with constant stirring. The precipitate is allowed to settle, the clear liquid is decanted off. The residue is transferred into a calico filter washed thoroughly with water until it is free from sulphate ions and finally mixed with the required quantity of purified water.

$$MgO + H_2O \longrightarrow Mg(OH)_2$$

$$MgSO_4 + 2\,NaOH \longrightarrow Mg(OH)_2 + Na_2SO_4$$

In this reaction sodium hydroxide reacts with magnesium sulphate and gives magnesium hydroxide. In the absence of magnesium oxide, this magnesium hydroxide would form a translucent, gelatinous aqueous suspension. Whereas the addition of magnesium oxide leads to the formation of white and creamy consistency product.

In the above formulae, Pharmacopoeia permits the use of following pharmaceutical aids.

(i) 0.1% citric acid which is used to minimize the reaction between glass containers and milk of magnesia during storage (otherwise, it imparts a bitter taste).

(ii) 0.5 ml /1000 ml of volatile oil as a flavouring agent.

(iii) 0.2% of sodium benzoate or 0.125% of methyl paraben as preservative.

***Test for identification:*** The sample solution in hydrochloric acid gives the characteristic reactions of magnesium ions.

***Test for purity:*** It should be tested for arsenic, sulphate; soluble alkali, soluble salts, heavy metals, microbial contamination and it also should complies with test for oral liquids.

***Test for soluble salt:*** The small quantity of filtrate which is obtained from filtering the acidic solution of sample, add small volume of sulphuric acid evaporate to dryness, ignited to the constant weight and the weight of the residue should not more than 12 mg.

**Assay**

***Principle:***

*Method 1:* It is assayed by **acidimetry-alkalimetry method** of (Back) titration (also called **neutralization method**).

In this assay the substance is treated with Known Excess Standard (KES) 1N sulphuric acid and the Excess Unreacted (EUR) sulphuric acid is titrated with 1N sodium hydroxide using methyl orange as an indicator. End point is the yellow colour.

In this assay the magnesium hydroxide (the base) reacts with sulphuric acid and neutralization takes place, after this reaction the Excess Unreacted (EUR) sulphuric acid is determined by titrating with sodium hydroxide. The indicator is orange colour in acid medium and it changes to yellow colour upon neutralization which is the end point.

As the acid and alkali involved in this assay, it is called as acidimetry-alkalimetry method of titration and the neutralization takes place in this assay during titration hence this assay is also called as neutralization method. The chemical reactions of this assay are shown below.

$$Mg(OH)_2 + H_2SO_4 \longrightarrow MgSO_4 + 2\,H_2O$$

$$H_2SO_4 + 2\,NaOH \longrightarrow Na_2SO_4 + 2\,H_2O$$

***Procedure:*** Weigh accurately about 10.0 gm, mix with 50 ml of water, add 50.0 ml of 0.5M sulphuric acid and titrate the excess of acid with 1M sodium hydroxide using methyl orange solution as indicator.

*Method 2:* It is assayed by **Complexometry method of (Direct) titration.**

In this assay the substance is dissolved in hydrochloric acid, to this strong ammonia-ammonium chloride solution added as buffer. The solution is then titrated against 0.05M disodium Ethylene Diamine Tetra Acetate (EDTA) using mordant black II mixture added as indicator. End point is the appearance of blue color.

In this assay magnesium ions of magnesium hydroxide mixture reacts with disodium EDTA, whereby the complexation takes place. As the magnesium ions forms complex with disodium EDTA in this assay, it is called as complexometry method of titration. The chemical reactions of this assay are shown below.

$Mg^{2+}$ + $NaOOCH_2C$ N N $CH_2COONa$ $HOOCH_2C$ $CH_2COOH$

Disodium EDTA

↓

$NaOOCH_2C$ N N $CH_2COONa$ $H_2C$ $CH_2$ $Mg^{2+}$ O=C C=O O O

Magnesium-EDTA Complex

***Procedure:*** Weigh accurately about 0.1 gm, dissolve in 20 ml of 2M hydrochloric acid and dilute to 100.0 ml with water. To 50.0 ml of this solution add 5 ml of strong ammonia-ammonium chloride solution and titrate with 0.05M disodium edetate, using about 50 mg of mordant black II mixture as indicator.

***Uses:***

1. It is used as an antacid and laxative.
2. It is also used as an alkaline mouthwash (due to the alkaline property).
3. Due to the alkalinity, it is used to liberate alkaloids from their solutions.

***Dose:*** As antacid - 5 to 10 ml

As laxative - 15 to 30 ml

***Storage:*** It should be stored in tightly closed containers protected from moisture and do not refrigerate.

***Labelling:*** The label should contain "Shake well before use".

## Magnesium Trisilicate I.P., U.S.P.

**(Synonym: Epsom salt, Hydrated magnesium silicate)**

**Mol. Formula:** $2MgO.3SiO_2.xH_2O$ (or) $2MgO.3SiO_2.4H_2O$ **Mol. Weight:** 330

Magnesium trisilicate was introduced into medicine by Mutch. Pharmacopoeia describes that it is hydrated magnesium silicate of the approximate formula which is mentioned above. It contains not less than or equivalent of 29.0% of MgO and not less than or equivalent of 65.0% of $SiO_2$, which is calculated on ignited basis.

***Preparation:*** It is obtained from sodium silicate and magnesium sulphate. The solution of magnesium sulphate is slowly added to the solution of sodium silicate which is prepared by the reaction between sodium hydroxide and silicic acid, the magnesium trisilicate is precipitated out. The precipitate obtained is filtered, washed and dried.

***Preparation of sodium silicate ($Na_2O$: $SiO_2$):*** The 2:3 ratio of sodium silicate is prepared by adding sodium hydroxide to sodium silicate.

***Physical properties:*** It is fine, white or nearly white powder, free from grittiness, odourless, tasteless. It is insoluble in water and alcohol. It is slightly hygroscopic in nature.

***Chemical properties:***

1. *Decomposition reaction with acids:* The mineral acids decompose magnesium trisilicate and gives magnesium salt and silicic acid.

$$2\,MgO.\,3\,SiO_2 + 4\,HCl \longrightarrow 2\,MgCl_2 + \underset{\text{Trisilicic acid}}{H_4Si_3O_8}\downarrow$$

2. *Reaction with alkali decomposition:* Alkali carbonate decomposes it with the formation of magnesium carbonate and the corresponding soluble silicate.

$$2\,Na_2CO_3 + 2\,MgO.\,3\,SiO_2 \longrightarrow 2\,MgCO_3 + Na_4Si_3O_8$$

***Test for identification:*** The neutral solution of the sample gives the characteristic reactions of magnesium salts and silicates.

***Test for purity:*** It should be tested for alkalinity, arsenic, heavy metals, chlorides, sulphates, acid absorption capacity, water soluble salts and loss on ignition.

***Test for acid absorption capacity:*** A weighed quantity of sample and 0.1M hydrochloric acid allowed to stand in water bath at 37 °C for 2 hr. Allow to cool the solution and add bromophenol solution and titrated with 0.1M sodium hydroxide solution until a blue color is obtained. The titre volume should be within a limit.

**Assay**

***Principle:*** It is assayed for magnesium oxide and silicon dioxide.

1. *Magnesium oxide:* It is assayed by **Complexometry method of (Direct) titration**.

   In this assay the substance is dissolved in hydrochloric acid, to this 1N sodium hydroxide added until the pH reaches to 12. The solution is then titrated against 0.05M disodium Ethylene Diamine Tetra Acetate (EDTA) using mordant black II mixture as indicator. End point is the appearance of deep blue colour.

   In this assay magnesium ions of magnesium trisilicate reacts with disodium EDTA, whereby the complexation takes place. As the magnesium ions forms complex with disodium EDTA in this assay, it is called as complexometry method of titration. The chemical reactions of this assay are shown below.

$Mg^{2+}$ + $NaOOCH_2C$, $HOOCH_2C$–N–$CH_2CH_2$–N–$CH_2COONa$, $CH_2COOH$

Disodium EDTA

↓

$NaOOCH_2C$–N–$CH_2CH_2$–N–$CH_2COONa$; $H_2C$–C(=O)–O → $Mg^{2+}$ ← O–C(=O)–$CH_2$

Magnesium-EDTA Complex

2. *Silicon dioxide:* It is assayed by **Gravimetric method**.

   In this assay the substance is treated with sulphuric acid and heated, filtered, the filter paper and the contents are transferred into platinum crucible dried and incinerated. To it hydrofluoric acid and sulphuric acid are added and evaporated to dryness, ignited and weighed. From the difference in weight represent the weight of silicon dioxide.

*Uses:*

1. It is used as an antacid and absorbent.
2. It is also used for the treatment of hyper chlorhydria, gastric and duodenal ulcers.
3. In proper proportions it acts as emulsifying agent

In larger doses, it leads to diarrhoea (due to the formation of magnesium chloride).

**Advantage of magnesium trisilicate:** Magnesium trisilicate is insoluble in water so it neutralizes the excess acidity of the stomach (gastric acidity) without alkanisation of the system over other carbonate and alkaline earth hydroxide type antacids. Magnesium trisilicate forms a protective layer on the ulcers and prevents the further attack of acids on peptic ulcers.

***Dose:*** 500 mg to 2 gm repeated dose depends upon the needs of patients.

## Heavy Magnesium Carbonate I.P., U.S.P.

**Mol. Formula:** $3MgCO_3 . Mg(OH)_2 . 5H_2O$ **Mol. Weight:** 401.34

Heavy magnesium carbonate is a hydrated basic carbonate. It differs from light magnesium carbonate in density. 15 gm of heavy magnesium carbonate occupies a volume of 30 ml while 15 gm of light magnesium carbonate occupies a volume of 125 ml

It contains equivalent not less than 40% w/w and not more than 45% w/w MgO.

***Preparation:*** It is prepared by double decomposition of magnesium sulphate and sodium carbonate. The magnesium sulphate (125 parts) and crystalline sodium carbonate (150 parts) are dissolved in boiling water separately. The two solutions are mixed, evaporated and the resulting residue is digested with boiling water for half an hour. The insoluble carbonate is filtered through on a calico filter, washed until completely free from sulphate ions and dried in an oven.

$$MgSO_4 + Na_2CO_3 \longrightarrow MgCO_3\downarrow + Na_2SO_4$$

***Physical properties:*** Heavy magnesium carbonate is a white, granular powder, odourless, tasteless and insoluble in water.

When heated to redness it loses carbondioxide and water, leads to the formation of magnesium oxide.

$$3MgCO_3 . Mg(OH)_2 . 5H_2O \xrightarrow[\text{red hot}]{\text{Heated to}} 4\,MgO + 3CO_2 + 6H_2O$$

***Test for identification:*** The sample solution in acetic acid gives the characteristic reactions of magnesium ion and carbonate.

***Test for purity:*** It should be tested for color, clarity of solution, arsenic, heavy metals, iron, chlorine, sulphate, calcium, copper, soluble substances, substances insoluble in acetic acid and residue on ignition.

### Assay

***Principle:*** It is assayed by **Complexometry method of (Direct) titration**.

In this assay the substance is dissolved in hydrochloric acid, to this 1N sodium hydroxide added until the pH reaches to 12. The solution is then titrated against 0.05M disodium Ethylene Diamine Tetra Acetate (EDTA) using mordant black II as indicator. End point is the appearance of blue color.

In this assay magnesium ions of magnesium carbonate reacts with disodium EDTA, whereby the complexation takes place. As the magnesium ions forms complex with disodium EDTA in this assay, it is called as complexometry method of titration. The chemical reactions of this assay are shown below.

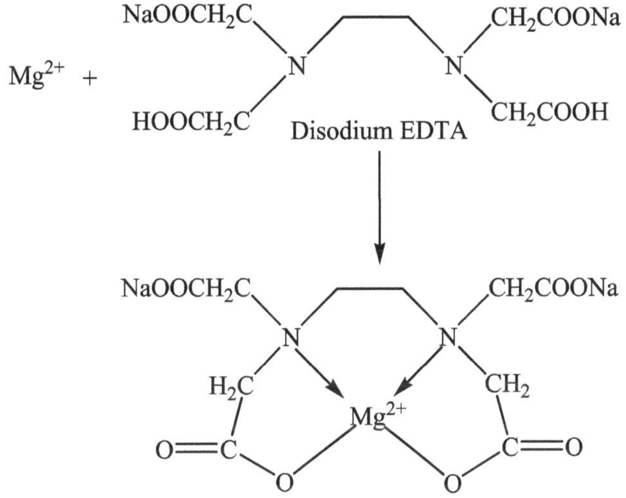

Disodium EDTA

Magnesium-EDTA Complex

***Procedure:*** Weigh accurately about 0.15 gm, dissolve in a mixture of 20 ml of water and 2 ml of 2M hydrochloric acid and add 50 ml of water, 10 ml of strong ammonia-ammonium chloride solution and titrate with 0.05M disodium edetate, using 0.1 gm of mordant black II mixture as indicator, until a blue colour is obtained.

***Uses:***

1. It is used as an antacid and osmotic laxative.
2. It is also used as a pharmaceutical aid (diluents for tablet powder).
3. It acts as a slow acting antacid. It is also used during pregnancy and lactation.
4. It is used as a catharatic; its pharmacological properties are equal to magnesium oxide.

***Dose:*** As antacid - 300 to 600 mg for four times a day.

As laxative - 2 to 4 gm.

***Storage:*** It should be stored in tightly closed container.

## Light Magnesium Carbonate I.P., U.S.P.

**Mol. Formula:** $3MgCO_3 . Mg(OH)_2 . 3H_2O$ **Mol. Weight:** 365.31

It is a hydrated basic carbonate which differs only slightly in composition from the heavy magnesium carbonate (bulk density). It contains not less than 40% and not more than 45% of MgO.

***Preparation:*** It is prepared by the similar method to that of heavy magnesium carbonate the only difference is concentration of reagents used and the reaction condition (temperature) and the subsequent treatment of the precipitate. When the solution of magnesium sulphate and sodium carbonate are heated it produce heavy magnesium carbonate, while under cold conditions light magnesium carbonate is produced.

The solution of magnesium sulphate (125 parts) mixed with the solution of sodium carbonate (150 parts which are dissolved in cold water), heated for 5 minutes then the precipitate is collected washed until it gives a slight reaction for sulphate and dried in an oven.

$$MgSO_4 + Na_2CO_3 \longrightarrow MgCO_3\downarrow + Na_2SO_4$$

***Physical properties:*** A very light white powder, odorless, tasteless, practically insoluble in water and alcohol but soluble in dilute acids with brisk effervescence.

**Assay**

***Principle & Procedure:*** Similar to that of heavy magnesium carbonate.

***Uses:***

1. It is used as an antacid and osmotic laxative.
2. It is also used as a pharmaceutical aid (diluents for tablet powder).
3. It acts as a slow acting antacid. It is also used during pregnancy and lactation.
4. It is also used as a cathartic; its pharmacological properties are equal to magnesium oxide.

***Storage:*** It should be stored in tightly closed container.

***Dose:*** Antacid = 300 to 600 mg.

Laxative = 2 to 4 gm.

## Heavy Magnesium Oxide I.P., U.S.P.

**(Synonym: Heavy magnesia)**

**Mol. Formula:** MgO **Mol. Weight:** 40.3

Heavy magnesium oxide is different from light magnesium oxide in density. 15 gm of light magnesium oxide occupies a volume of about 150 ml, but 15 gm of heavy magnesium oxide occupies only 30 ml. Heavy Magnesium oxide contains not less than 98% and not more than 100.5% of MgO which is calculated on ignited basis.

***Preparation:***

*From magnesium carbonate:* Heavy Magnesium carbonate when heated in a crucible or oven, it gives heavy magnesium oxide with expulsion of carbon dioxide and water.

$$3MgCO_3 \cdot Mg(OH)_2 \cdot 5H_2O \xrightarrow[\text{red hot}]{\text{Heated to}} 4\,MgO + 3CO_2 + 6H_2O$$

***Physical properties:*** It is a fine white powder, odorless, slight alkaline taste. It is soluble in dilute alkali, practically insoluble in water and alcohol. 15 gm occupies a volume of 30 ml. It absorbs carbon dioxide and moisture on exposure to air.

***Test for identification:*** The solution in dilute nitric acid and dilute sodium hydroxide gives the characteristic reactions of magnesium ions.

***Test for purity:*** It should be tested for arsenic, calcium, copper, ferrous, chlorides, sulphates, soluble substances, insoluble matter in acetic acid and loss on ignition.

***Test for loss on ignition:*** It should not be more than 8% which is determined by 0.5 gm of sample by ignition at 900 °C.

**Assay:**

***Principle:*** It is assayed by **Complexometry method of (Direct) titration**.

In this assay the substance is dissolved in hydrochloric acid, to this ammonia-ammonium chloride solution is added as buffer solution and it is then titrated against 0.05M disodium Ethylene Diamine Tetra Acetate (EDTA) using mordant black II mixture as an indicator. End point is the appearance of blue colour.

In this assay magnesium ions of heavy magnesium oxide reacts with disodium EDTA, whereby the complexation takes place. As the magnesium ions forms complex with disodium EDTA in this assay, it is called as complexometry method of titration. The chemical reactions of this assay are shown below.

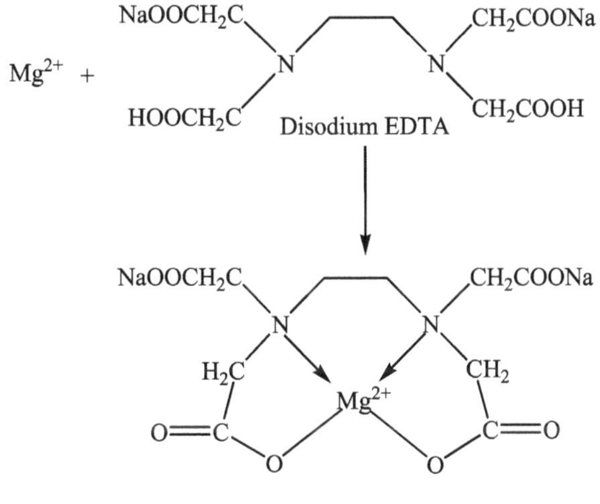

$Mg^{2+}$ + $NaOOCH_2C$, $CH_2COONa$, N, N, $HOOCH_2C$, $CH_2COOH$

Disodium EDTA

↓

$NaOOCH_2C$, $CH_2COONa$, N, N, $H_2C$, $CH_2$, $Mg^{2+}$, O=C, C=O, O, O

Magnesium-EDTA Complex

***Procedure:*** Weigh accurately about 0.35 gm, dissolve in 10 ml of 2M hydrochloric acid and dilute with water to 100 ml. To 10 ml add 5 ml of strong ammonia-ammonium chloride solution and titrate with 0.05M disodium edetate using about 50 mg of mordant black II mixture as indicator.

***Uses:***

1. It is used as an antacid and osmotic laxative. It is a quite effective and given as a non systemic antacid.
2. It is also used as a catharatic. It reacts with water, it is converted into hydroxide and it sets like cement.
3. When compared to heavy magnesium carbonate, it does not produce any carbon dioxide and it is fairly a long acting antacid.

***Dose:*** As antacid 300 to 600 mg

As laxative 2 to 4 gm.

***Storage:*** It should be stored in tightly closed container and protected from moisture.

## Light Magnesium Oxide I.P., U.S.P.

**(Synonym: Light magnesia)**

**Mol. Formula:** MgO **Mol. Weight:** 40.3

It contains not less than 98% and not more than 100.5% calculated on ignited basis.

***Preparation:*** It is prepared by heating light magnesium carbonate to a dull redness until carbondioxide evolution ceases.

$$3MgCO_3 \,.\, Mg(OH)_2 \,.\, 3H_2O \xrightarrow{\text{Heat}} 4MgO + 6H_2O + 3CO_2\uparrow$$

***Physical properties:*** It is a white very fine, light powder. It is slowly absorb water and carbon dioxide from the atmosphere forming basic carbonates. It is very slightly soluble in water but the particular amount of sample is dissolve in water and the resulting solution is distinctly alkaline to phenolphthalein and contains magnesium hydroxide. The difference between light magnesium oxide from heavy magnesium oxide is only its bulk density. 15 gm of sample occupies a volume of about 150 ml.

***Test for identification:*** The solution in dilute nitric acid and dilute sodium hydroxide gives the characteristic reactions of magnesium ions.

***Test for purity:*** It should be tested for arsenic, calcium, copper, ferrous, chlorides, sulphates, soluble substances, insoluble matter in acetic acid and loss on ignition.

***Test for loss on ignition:*** It should not be more than 8% which is determined by 0.5 gm of sample upon ignited at 900 °C.

**Assay**

***Principle & Procedure:*** Similar to heavy magnesium oxide.

*Uses:*

1. It is used as an antacid and laxative (it is quite effective and given as a non systemic antacid).
2. It is also used as a catharatic. It reacts with water, converted into hydroxide and it sets like cement.
3. Compared to heavy magnesium carbonate, it does not produce any carbon dioxide and it is fairly a long acting antacid.

***Dose:*** As antacid = 300 to 600 mg

As laxative = 2 to 4 gm.

***Storage:*** It should be stored in tightly closed containers and protected from moisture.

## Magnesium Phosphate U.S.P.

**Mol. Formula:** $Mg_3(PO)_4.5H_2O$ **Mol. Weight:** 350.88

The chemistry and other properties are similar to that of tribasic calcium phosphate.

***Physical properties:*** It is a white, odorless, tasteless powder. Insoluble in water and freely soluble in dilute mineral acids.

***Test for identification:*** The sample solution gives the characteristic reactions of magnesium and phosphate ions.

**Assay:** It is assayed by **Complexometry method of titration**.

***Use:*** It is used as an antacid with potent laxative action.

***Dose:*** 1 gm.

***Storage:*** It should be stored in well closed container.

## Calcium Carbonate I.P., B.P., U.S.P.

**(Synonym: Precipitated chalk)**

**Mol. Formula:** $CaCO_3$ **Mol. Weight:** 100.1

It contains not less than 98% and not more than 100.5% calcium carbonate, which is calculated on dried the sample at 105 °C. In nature it is widely distributed in chalk, lime stone, marble, aragonite and calcite. It is the one of the main constituents of corals, pearls and shells.

***Preparation:*** For commercial process, the boiling solution of calcium chloride and sodium carbonate are mixed and allowed the resulting precipitate to settle down. The precipitated calcium carbonate is filtered through a calico filter, washed and dried.

$$CaCl_2 + Na_2CO_3 \longrightarrow CaCO_3\downarrow + 2\,NaCl$$

***Physical properties:*** Calcium carbonate is a fine, white, micro crystalline powder, odorless and tasteless. It is insoluble in water but soluble in carbondioxide free water (boiling water) and ammonium salts due to the formation of calcium bicarbonate and free calcium ions respectively.

$$CaCO_3 + H_2CO_3 \longrightarrow Ca(HCO_3)_2$$

$$CaCO_3 + 2\,NH_4^+ \longrightarrow Ca^{2+} + 2\,NH_3 + H_2O + CO_2$$

***Chemical properties:*** It reacts with mineral acids produce effervescence due to elimination of carbondioxide (neutralization reaction).

$$CaCO_3 + 2\,HCl \longrightarrow CaCl_2 + CO_2\uparrow + H_2O$$

***Test for identification:*** The solution in acetic acid gives the characteristic reactions of calcium salts and carbonates.

***Test for purity:*** It should be tested for arsenic, heavy metals, aluminium, iron, phosphate and matter insoluble in acetic acid, barium, magnesium, alkali metals, chlorides, sulphates and loss on drying.

***Mechanism of acid neutralizing capacity of calcium carbonate:*** The antacid property of precipitated chalk is explained by as follows.

Calcium carbonate undergoes dissociation to forms free calcium ions.

$$CaCO_3 \rightleftharpoons Ca^{2+} + CO_3^{2-}$$

The carbonate ion reacts with hydronium ions and forms carbonic acid.

$$CO_3^{2-} + H_3O^+ \longrightarrow HCO_3^- + H_2O$$

$$HCO_3^- + H_3O^+ \longrightarrow H_2CO_3 + H_2O$$

Finally the carbonic acid is converted in to water and $CO_2$.

$$H_2CO_3 \longrightarrow H_2O + CO_2$$

**Assay**

***Principle:*** It is assayed by **Complexometry method of (Direct) titration.**

In this assay the substance is dissolved in hydrochloric acid, to this 1N sodium hydroxide added until the pH reaches to 12. The solution is then titrated against 0.05M disodium Ethylene Diamine Tetra Acetate (EDTA) using calcon mixture as indicator end point is the colour change from pink to a full blue colour.

In this assay calcium ions of calcium carbonate reacts with disodium EDTA, whereby the complexation takes place. As the calcium ions forms complex with disodium EDTA in this assay, it is called as complexometry method of titration. The chemical reactions of this assay are shown below.

***Procedure:*** Weigh accurately about 0.1 gm and dissolve in 3 ml of dilute hydrochloric acid and 10 ml of water. Boil for 10 minutes, cool, dilute to 50 ml with water. Titrate with 0.05M disodium edetate to within a few ml of the expected end-point, add 8 ml of sodium hydroxide solution and 0.1 gm of calcon mixture and continue the titration until the colour of the solution changes from pink to a full blue colour.

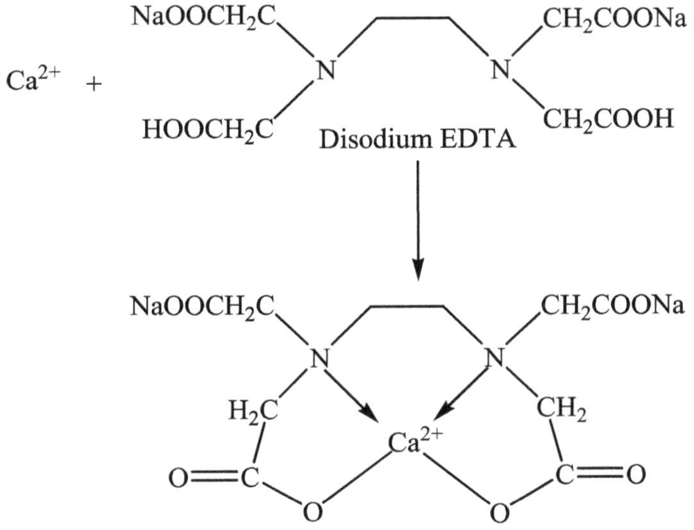

$Ca^{2+}$ + $NaOOCH_2C$, $CH_2COONa$, N, N, $HOOCH_2C$, $CH_2COOH$

Disodium EDTA

↓

$NaOOCH_2C$, $CH_2COONa$, N, N, $H_2C$, $CH_2$, $Ca^{2+}$, O=C, C=O, O, O

Calcium-EDTA Complex

***Uses:***

1. It is used as an antacid internally.
2. Due to the lack of water solubility it can produce alkalosis so the long term use is not advisable.
3. It is having a tendency to produce constipation so it is co-administered with magnesium antacids (combination antacid therapy).
4. It is externally used as a dentifrice due to its abrasiveness.

***Dose:*** 1 to 5 gm six times daily according to the patients need.

***Storage:*** It should be stored in tightly closed containers.

## Tribasic Calcium Phosphate I.P., U.S.P.

**(Synonym: Calcium hydroxide phosphate, Calcium phosphate)**

**Mol. Formula:** $Ca_3(PO_4)_2$ **Mol. Weight:** Variable

It is a mixture of tricalcium diortho phosphate ($Ca_3(PO_4)_2$) together with acidic or basic calcium phosphate. It contains not less than 90% w/w and not more than 100.5% w/w of calcium phosphate.

***Preparation (Laboratory preparation):***

*Method 1 (From calcium chloride):* The solution of calcium chloride mixed with secondary sodium phosphate, white precipitate of tribasic calcium phosphate is formed.

The precipitate obtained is washed with hot water until it becomes free from chloride and dried.

$$3\,CaCl_2 + 2\,Na_2HPO_4 + 2\,NH_3.\,2\,H_2O \longrightarrow Ca_3(PO_4)_2\downarrow + 4\,NaCl + 2\,NH_4Cl + 2H_2O$$

*Method 2 (From Bones):* Bones are collected calcined, powdered and digested with sulphuric acid. The insoluble phosphates are converted in to soluble phosphoric acid and insoluble calcium sulphate. The solution is filtered, to the filtrate add calcium hydroxide and the product is precipitated.

$$Ca_3(PO_4)_2 + 3\,H_2SO_4 \longrightarrow 2\,H_3PO_4 + 3\,CaSO_4$$

$$2\,H_3PO_4 + 3\,Ca(OH)_2 \longrightarrow Ca_3(PO_4)_2\downarrow + 6\,H_2O$$

***Physical properties:*** It is a white or colorless amorphous powder, odorless and tasteless, insoluble in water but soluble in dilute mineral acids.

***Mechanism of action:*** Neutralization of gastric juice by phosphate ion.

$$Ca_3(PO_4)_2 \longrightarrow 3\,Ca^{2+} + 2\,PO_4^{3-}$$

$$PO_4^{3-} + H_3O^+ \longrightarrow HPO_4^{2-} + H_2O$$

$$HPO_4^{2-} + H_3O^+ \longrightarrow H_2PO_4^- + H_2O$$

***Test for identification:*** The sample solution in nitric acid gives the characteristic reactions of calcium ions and phosphate ions.

***Test for purity:*** It should be tested for arsenic, heavy metals, iron, carbonates, chlorides, sulphates, water soluble substances, acid soluble substances, loss on ignition and protineous impurities.

***Test for protineous impurities:*** A small quantity of sample is heated in a dry test tube, no color change and no pleasant odour is emitted.

**Assay**

***Principle:*** *I.P. Method:* It is assayed for its content of calcium and calcium phosphate.

**Calcium** is assayed by adopting the method descried under dibasic calcium phosphate.

**Calcium phosphate** is assayed by dissolving the sample in a mixture of water and dilute nitric acid and filtered. Basify the filtrate using ammonia, a slight precipitation occurs, it is again dissolved in dilute nitric acid. By adding ammonium molybdate solution phosphomolybdate is precipitated. The precipitate is washed well until free from acidity and dissolves the precipitate in known excess standard sodium hydroxide and the excess unreacted sodium hydroxide is titrated with sulphuric acid using phenolphthalein as indicator. End point is the disappearance of pink colour.

$$2\,NaOH + H_2SO_4 \longrightarrow Na_2SO_4 + 2\,H_2O$$

*B.P. Method:* It is assayed by **Complexometry method of (Direct) titration.**

In this assay the substance is dissolved in a mixture of water and hydrochloric acid and strong ammonia solution, to this ammonia-ammonium chloride solution is added as buffer solution. Known Excess Standard (KES) 0.05N disodium Ethylene Diamine Tetra Acetate (EDTA) added to the above mixture and the excess unreacted EDTA is titrated against zinc chloride using mordant black II as an indicator.

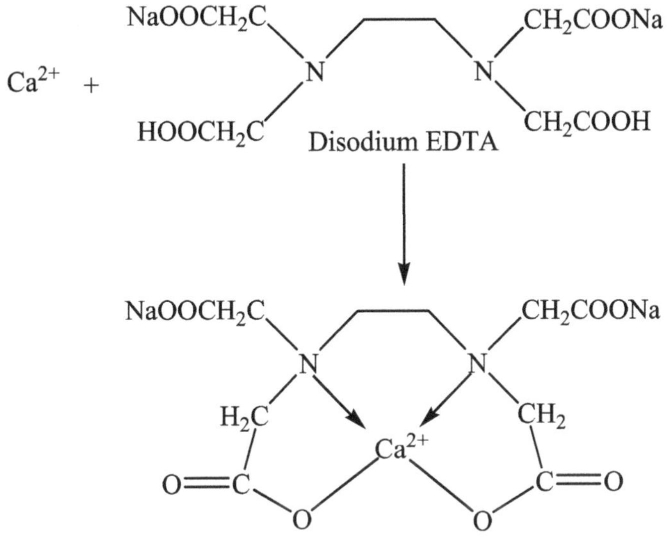

$Ca^{2+}$ + $(NaOOCH_2C)(HOOCH_2C)N\text{–}CH_2CH_2\text{–}N(CH_2COONa)(CH_2COOH)$

Disodium EDTA

↓

Calcium-EDTA Complex

**Procedure (I.P. Method):** Weigh accurately about 1.0 gm and dissolve in 10 ml of hydrochloric acid by heating on a water-bath, add 50 ml of water cool and dilute to 250.0 ml with water. To 25.0 ml of the resulting solution add 30.0 ml of 0.05M disodium edetate, 10.0 ml of ammonia buffer pH 10.9 and 100 ml of water and titrate the excess of disodium edetate with 0.05M zinc chloride using mordant black II solution as indicator.

***Uses:***

1. It is used as an antacid during pregnancy and lactation also.
2. Commonly used as a tablet excipient and non hygroscopic diluent.

***Storage:*** It should be stored in tightly closed containers.

## Sodium Citrate I.P., B.P.

**(Synonym: Trisodium citrate)**

**Mol. Formula:** $C_6H_5Na_3O_7.\ 2H_2O$ **Mol. Weight:** 294.1

$$\begin{array}{ccc} HO & & COONa \\ & C & \\ NaOOCH_2C & & CH_2COONa \end{array} \cdot 2H_2O$$

Sodium citrate is trisodium-2-hydroxy propane-1,2,3-tricarboxylate dihydrate. It contains not less than 99% and not more than 101% of citric acid calculated on dried basis.

***Preparation:*** Sodium citrate is prepared by a reaction between the hot solution of citric acid and sodium bicarbonate or sodium carbonate in the required proportions until the effervescence ceases. The product is obtained by crystallization.

$$HO-\underset{CH_2COOH}{\overset{CH_2COOH}{C}}-COOH + 3\,NaHCO_3 \longrightarrow HO-\underset{CH_2COONa}{\overset{CH_2COONa}{C}}-COONa + 3\,CO_2 + 3\,H_2O$$

***Physical properties:*** It is white granular crystals or a white crystalline powder odorless, the salt is neutral to phenolphthalein; it is soluble in water but insoluble in alcohol. The salt is slightly deliquescent in nature.

***Chemical properties:*** Sodium citrate when heated to 150 °C, it completely loses its water molecules and becomes anhydrous.

$$Na_3C_6H_5O_7\,.2\,H_2O \xrightarrow[\Delta]{150\,^{\circ}C} Na_3C_6H_5O_7 + 2\,H_2O$$

When it is further heated to charring it produces sodium carbonate.

$$2\,Na_3C_6H_5O_7\,.2\,H_2O + 9\,O_2 \longrightarrow 3\,Na_2CO_3 + 9\,CO_2\uparrow + 7\,H_2O$$

Sodium citrate solution is easily ionized in to sodium and citrate ions. The citrate ions are used for its buffering action.

***Test for identification:*** The solution of sodium citrate gives the characteristic reactions of sodium and citrate.

***Test for purity:*** It should be tested for clarity and color of the solution, acidity or alkalinity, arsenic, heavy metals, oxalate, tartarates, readily carbonisable substances and water.

**Assay**

***Principle:*** As the sodium citrate is very weak base, it cannot be assayed by the usual acid-base titration and hence it is assayed by **non-aqueous method of titration**.

In this assay the substance is dissolved in a mixture of glacial acetic acid and acetic anhydride and solution is titrated against perchloric acid. End point is determined potentiometrically or by using the indicator 1-naphtholbenzein solution. As the assay is carried out in a non-aqueous medium it is called nonaqueous assay.

***Procedure:*** Weigh accurately about 0.15 gm and dissolve in 20 ml of anhydrous glacial acetic acid, warming to about 50 °C. Allow to cool. Titrate with 0.1M perchloric acid, using 0.25 ml of 1-naphtholbenzein solution as indicator. Carry out a blank titration.

***Uses:***

1. It used to prepare buffer solution.
2. It is also used as a systemic antacid and acts as an anticoagulant.
3. It also finds use in the preparation of expectorant and acts as a systemic alkalizer.

***Dose:*** 1 to 10 gm.

***Storage:*** It should be stored in well closed container and protected from sun light.

***Official formulation:*** Sodium citrate tablets B.P, Anticoagulant sodium citrate solution B.P, Anticoagulant acid citrate dextrose solution B.P.

## Bismuth Subcarbonate I.P., B.P., U.S.P.

This compound is dicussed under the topic **adsorbents and protectives**.

## Magaldrate I.P., B.P., U.S.P.

**Mol. Formula:** $Al_5Mg_{10}(OH)_{31}(SO_4)_2.\ xH_2O$ **Mol. Weight:** 1097.4

It is a chemical composition of aluminium and magnesium hydroxides and sulphates corresponding to the above molecular formula.

It contains not less than 90% and not more than 105% of magaldrate.

***Preparation:*** It is prepared by the reaction between sodium potassium aluminate with magnesium sulphate. The product is obtained by controlling the concentration of reactants, temperature of the reaction. The precipitate is filtered, washed and dried.

***Physical properties:*** It is a white or almost white crystalline powder, odorless, insoluble in water and alcohol.

***Test for identification:*** The sample solutions are prepared by using water and dilute hydrochloric acid. To this add methyl red solution and heat to boil. Add dilute ammonia solution until the color changes to just yellow, continue boiling. Filter it. The filtrate gives the characteristic reactions of magnesium salts and the precipitate obtained from this test is treated with hydrochloric acid and ammonium chloride gives the characteristic reactions of aluminium.

***Test for purity:*** It should be tested for arsenic, heavy metals, soluble chloride, soluble sulphate, sodium, aluminium hydroxide, magnesium hydroxide, sulphates, microbial contamination and loss on drying.

***Assay:*** It is assayed by **alkalimetry method (back titration)**. It is similar to magnesium hydroxide.

***Procedure:*** Weigh accurately about 3 gm and transfer to a 250 ml conical flask. Add 100 ml of 1M hydrochloric acid and stir well until a clear solution is obtained. Titrate the excess acid with 1M sodium hydroxide to a pH of 3, determined potentiometrically. Repeat the procedure without the substance under examination. The difference between the titrations represents the amount of hydrochloric acid required.

***Test for sodium:*** It is determined by flame photometry.

***Test for microbial contamination:*** 1 gm of sample should be free from *E-coli.*

$Al(OH)_2$ = 32.1 to 45.9%

$Mg(OH)_2$ = 49.2 to 66.6%

***Uses:*** It is mainly used as an antacid.

***Storage:*** It should be stored in well closed container and protected from moisture.

***Official preparation:*** Magaldrate tablets (800 mg)

Magaldrate oral suspension (800 mg/5 ml).

## 6.1.5 Combination Antacid Preparations

None of the single antacid satisfies all the requirements of an ideal antacid, even though several products of mixed antacids are available in the market. Combination antacid therapy is given to get maximum therapeutic effect with less or least adverse effects. These are preferred for the following reasons.

1. To achieve quick and prolonged effect
2. Neutralizing the side effects
3. Additive effect
4. Gastric emptying
5. To compensate the constipative effect of calcium and aluminium with the laxative effect of magnesium.
6. To have long duration of action with rapid onset of action.

**Examples for combination antacid preparations**

***Aluminium Hydroxide Gel – Magnesium Trisilicate Combination (Gelusil):*** It is not official but used commonly as a combination antacid preparation. The constipative effect of aluminium is balanced by the laxative effect of magnesium and the trisilicate shows protective action in the stomach.

***Aluminium Hydroxide Gel – Magnesium Hydroxide Combination (Creamalin):*** It is official in U.S.P. It is also available in tablet and suspension forms.

**Magaltrate:** This compound is discussed under the topic **antacids**.

## 6.1.6 Adsorbents and Protectives

**Introduction:** These are class of anti-diarrheal agents. Diarrhoea is an abnormal increase in the frequency and liquidity of stools. The increased motility of GIT and the decreased ability of intestine to absorb water from the stool are the major factors for the cause of diarrhoea. The causes of diarrhoea may be virus (*Norovirus* and *Rotavirus*), bacteria (*Salmonella*, *Shigella* and *E. coli)* or protozoa (*Giardia*).

The adsorbent drugs used in diarrhea are kaolin, pectin and bismuth subsalicylate. Kaolin and Pectin adsorb bacteria, enterotoxins and fluid to increase the consistency of faecal matters. Bismuth subsalicylate reduces stool frequency and liquidity in acute diarrhea due to inhibition of prostaglandin synthesis and at secretion by its salicylate counterpart. As these adsorbents are not absorbed, they may cause constipation, even at therapeutic doses.

## Light Kaolin I.P., B.P., U.S.P.

**Mol. Formula:** Approx. chemical formula is $Al_2O_3.2SiO_2. 2H_2O$ **Mol. Weight:** 258

Light kaolin is a native hydrated aluminium silicate freed from most of its impurities and dried. It may contain a suitable dispersing agent. It is a finely divided form of kaolin specially intended for internal use.

***Preparation:*** It is prepared by electrical sedimentation process from natural sources.

***Physical properties:*** It is a light, white powder, free from gritty particles, almost tasteless, odorless and unctuous to the touch.

***Test for identification:***

1. Fuse small quantity of light kaolin with required amount of anhydrous sodium carbonate add water and warm it, filter, wash the filtrate with water and keep the residue separately. Combine the washings and filtrate, add hydrochloric acid. A gelatinous white precipitate is formed.

$$\text{Sample} + \text{anhydrous } Na_2CO_3 \xrightarrow[\text{add } H_2O\text{, warm Filter}]{\text{Fusion}} \text{Filterate} \longrightarrow \text{wash with water}$$

$$\downarrow$$

$$\text{Gelatinous White ppt is formed} \longleftarrow \text{add HCl} \longleftarrow \text{Combine washings and filterate}$$

2. To The residue obtained from the above test, add dilute hydrochloric acid which gives the characteristic reactions of aluminium.
3. A small quantity of sample upon triturated with water, the resulting mixture easily flows.

***Test for purity:*** It should be tested for coarser particles, fine particles, arsenic, heavy metals, chlorides, soluble matters, loss on drying and loss on ignition.

***Test for coarser particles:*** Transfer 5 gm of sample in a stoppered cylinder, add 60 ml of sodium pyro phosphate solution shake well, kept aside for 5 minutes. Then pipette out 50 ml of the supernatant liquid, then add 50 ml water, shake well, allow standing for 5 minutes, once again collecting the 50 ml supernatant liquid. This procedure is repeated until the collection of 400 ml of supernatant liquid. The remaining portions are evaporated to dryness; take the weight of the residue. It should not be more than 25 mg.

***Test for fine particles:*** The required amount of heavy kaolin is dispersed in prescribed amount of water, shake it well, transferred in to a measuring cylinder, from this, 20 ml of the solution is taken and evaporated to dryness. Take the weight of the residue. The remaining portion of the suspension is allowed to stand for 4 hours. Then once again collect the 20 ml of the supernatant, evaporate it, take the weight of the residue. The weight of second residue is not less than 70% that of the weight of the first residue.

When kaolin is prescribed it means light kaolin has to be supplied.

***Uses:***

1. It is used to adsorb toxins so it is mainly used of food and alkaloid poisoning.
2. Light kaolin mixture is used for the treatment of dysentery, diarrhoea, cholera and symptomatic treatment of colitis.

***Dose:*** 15 to 75 gm.

***Storage:*** It should be stored in tightly closed containers.

## Heavy Kaolin I.P., B.P., U.S.P.

**(Synonym: China clay)**

**Mol. Formula:** $Al_2O_3.2SiO_2.2H_2O$ **Mol. Weight:** 258

Heavy Kaolin is a purified, natural, hydrated aluminium silicate with variable composition with trace quantities of iron, calcium and magnesium. It is mainly derived from the decomposition of feldspar of granite rocks and occurs in various parts of the world.

***Preparation:*** For pharmaceutical grade of the substance, it is prepared by powdering the natural substance, freezing it and removing the gritty particles by elutriation.

***Properties:*** It is a white or greyish fine powder, odorless and tasteless.

***Test for identification:***

1. To the small amount of sample in a metal crucible, add required amount of potassium nitrate and small amount of anhydrous sodium carbonate. Heat the mixture until it was melt and allow it to cool. To the residue add water, filter, collect the residue and to the residue add small amount of dilute hydrochloric acid and water then filter. To the filtrate, add ammonium chloride solution. A white gelatinous precipitate is produced.

To the Sample + $KNO_3$ + $Na_2CO_3$ ⟶ Heat until melt and cool ⟶ Residue + $H_2O$

↓ Filter

Ammonium Chloride solution + Filterate ⟵(Filter) Residue + $H_2O$ + HCl

↓

White gelatinous precipitate

2. The sample solution gives the characteristic reactions of silicates.

***Test for purity:*** It should be tested for acidity and alkalinity, arsenic, heavy metals, chlorides, sulphates, substance soluble in mineral acids, organic impurities, adsorption power, swelling power and loss on ignition.

***Test for adsorption power:*** In a glass-ground stoppered test tube, take small amount of sample add required quantity of methylene blue and allowed to settle for 2 minutes.

Centrifuge and dilute to 100 ml with water. The solution is not more intense than that of standard methylene blue solution.

***Test for swelling power:*** Small quantity of sample is triturated with water, the mixture does not flow.

***Uses:***

1. It is used in the preparation of poultices. It must be thoroughly sterilized because it is liable to contaminate with spore bearing *Bacilli.*
2. Internally it is used as an adsorbent.

***Storage:*** It should be stored in well closed containers and protected from light.

## Activated Charcoal I.P., B.P.

**(Synonym: Decolorizing charcoal)**

***Preparation:*** It is obtained by carbonization of organic matter or a residue obtained during destructive distillation of organic matters. The coarse material obtained is crushed and powdered.

***Properties:*** It is a light, black color powder, free from grittiness, odorless, tasteless. It is insoluble in all solvents. The fine powder provides more surface area for adsorbent properties.

***Test for identification:*** It must comply with test for adsorbing power. When heated to red hot, burns slowly without flame.

***Test for purity:*** It should be tested for acidity or alkalinity, acid soluble substances, ethanol soluble substances, alkali soluble colored substances, chlorides, sulphates, copper, uncarbonisable substances, lead, zinc, sulphated ash, adsorbing power and loss on drying.

***Test for uncarbonisable substances:*** Boil the small amount of sample with required amount of sodium hydroxide solution for few seconds and filter. The filtrate is colorless.

***Uses:***

1. It is a common type of adsorbent in the treatment of diarrhoea.
2. It is used as an antidote for certain type of poisoning.
3. It is not only adsorbing heavy metals but also adsorb drugs like alkaloids, sedative and hypnotics etc.

***Dose:*** 50 gm. It is normally used in the ratio of 5:1 or 10:1 of charcoal to poison.

***Storage:*** It should be stored in tightly closed containers and protected from moisture.

## Bismuth Subcarbonate I.P.

**(Synonym: Bismuth carbonate)**

**Mol. Formula:** $Bi_2O_2\,CO_3$ **Mol. Weight:** 510

Bismuth subcarbonate contains not less than 80.0% and not more than 82.5% of $BiO_2$ calculated with reference to the dried substance. It is basic salt with various compositions.

***Preparation:*** Metallic bismuth or bismuth metal is dissolved in dilute nitric acid (50%) and the resulting solution is evaporated to small volume. To the above solution add cold sodium carbonate solution with constant stirring. The basic carbonate is precipitated out which is collected on the calico filter, washed with cold water and dried at a temperature not more than 60 °C.

$$4\,Bi(NO_3)_3 + 6\,Na_2CO_3 + H_2O \longrightarrow [(BiO)_2CO_3]_2\,H_2O + 12\,NaNO_3 + 4\,CO_2$$

***Caution:*** Repeated washing should be avoided, because it will leads to decomposition of basic carbonate into hydroxide.

***Physical properties:*** It is a white powder, odorless and tasteless. It is insoluble in water and alcohol but soluble in hydrochloric acid and nitric acid with effervescence and forming respective salts. The density of the compound is variable one depend upon its method of preparation. It is stable in pure air but on exposure to air, it slowly darkens.

***Chemical properties:*** When it is heated, it decomposes and yields bismuth trioxide (yellow color), water and carbon dioxide.

$$[(BiO)_2CO_3]_2.H_2O \xrightarrow{\Delta} \underset{\text{Yellow color}}{2\,Bi_2O_3} + 2\,CO_2\uparrow + H_2O$$

***Test for identification:*** It gives the characteristic reactions of bismuth and carbonate ions.

***Test for purity:*** It should be tested for clarity, color of the solution, alkalis and alkaline earth metals, arsenic, copper, lead, silver, chlorides and loss on drying.

**Assay**

$$4\,Bi(NO_3)_3 + 6\,Na_2CO_3 + H_2O \longrightarrow [(BiO)_2CO_3]_2\,H_2O + 12\,NaNO_3 + 4\,CO_2$$

It is assayed by two methods

1. ***Gravimetric method:***

   *Principle:* In this assay the substance is ignited in a tared crucible to a constant weight. Upon ignition bismuth sub carbonate is oxidised to bismuth trioxide, from the weight of bismuth trioxide obtained bismuth sub carbonate is calculated. As the test substance is converted to a precipitate, which is used for calculating the actual amount of bismuth subcarbonate present this is called Gravimetric assay.

2. ***Complexometry method:***

   *Principle:* It is assayed by **Complexometry method of (Back) titration**

   In this assay the substance is dissolved in nitric acid to this add ammonia-ammonium chloride as buffer. Add xylenol orange mixture and titrate with 0.1M disodium edetate until the colour changes from pinkish-violet to lemon yellow.

In this assay Bismuth ions reacts with EDTA, whereby the complexation takes place, As the Bismuth ions forms complex with disodium EDTA in this assay, it is called as complexometry method of titration. The chemical reactions of this assay are shown below.

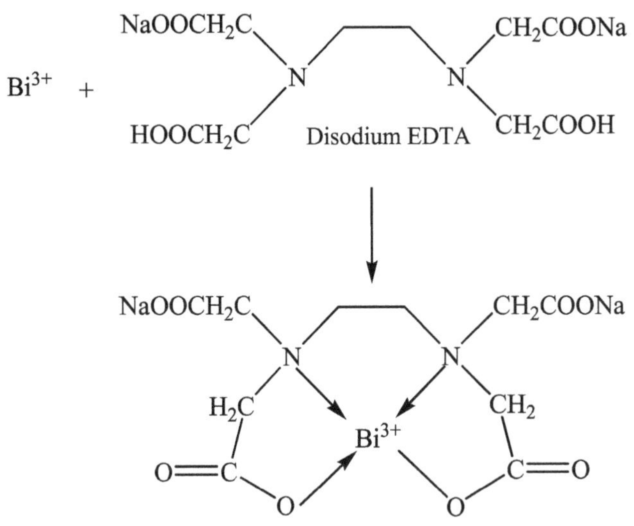

$$Bi^{3+} + \text{Disodium EDTA } (NaOOCH_2C, HOOCH_2C)N-CH_2CH_2-N(CH_2COONa, CH_2COOH) \longrightarrow \text{Bismuth-EDTA Complex}$$

Bismuth-EDTA Complex

***Procedure:*** Weigh accurately about 0.5 gm, dissolve in 3 ml of nitric acid and dilute to 250 ml with water. Add strong ammonia solution until cloudiness is first observed, add 0.5 ml of nitric acid and heat to 70 °C, maintaining the solution at this temperature until the solution becomes completely clear. Add about 50 mg of xylenol orange mixture and titrate with 0.1M disodium edetate until the colour changes from pinkish-violet to lemon yellow.

***Uses:***

1. It is mainly used as mild antacid.
2. Sub carbonate ointments and lotions are used as protectives.
3. It is also used as an absorbent and astringent, antiseptic and treating ulcerative colitis and diarrhoea etc.

***Official preparations:*** Emetine and Bismuth iodide.

***Dose:*** 1 to 4 gm in divided doses.

***Storage:*** It should be stored in well tightly closed containers and protected from light.

## Bismuth Subgallate B.P., U.S.P.

**(Synonym: Basic bismuth gallate, Bismuth oxygallate)**

**Mol. Formula:** $Bi(OH)_2.C_7H_5O_5$ **Mol. Weight:** 394.1

It contains not less than 48% and not more than 51% of bismuth which is calculated with reference to the dried basis.

***Preparation:*** It is prepared by the reaction between bismuth sub nitrate and dilute acetic acid and precipitated by the addition of gallic acid.

$$[Bi(OH)_4NO_3] \,.\, BiO[OH] + CH_3COOH + \text{Gallic acid} \longrightarrow \underset{\text{Bismuth sub gallate}}{Bi(OH)_2 \,.\, C_7H_5O_5}$$

***Physical properties:*** It is a bright yellow, amorphous powder, odorless and tasteless. It is insoluble in water, alcohol and ether. It is affected by light. But when it dissolves in mineral acids and alkali hydroxide, yields yellow color solution which change to deep red on standing.

***Test for identification:*** To the small amount of sample add hydrogen sulphide gas and filter. Then the filtrate is boiled to expel hydrogen sulphide gas, cool it and add one drop of ferric chloride solution, a bluish black color is formed. The sample solution gives the characteristic reactions of bismuth.

***Test for purity:*** It should be tested for arsenic, copper, lead, silver nitrate, alkali and alkaline earths, gallic acid and loss on drying.

***Test for nitrate:*** To the small amount of sample in water add required amount of nitrogen free sulphuric acid and superimposed with required quantity of ferrous sulphate solution. No brown or red color is produced at the interface between the two solutions.

**Assay**

***Principle:*** It is assayed by **Gravimetric method.**

In this assay the substance is dried and dissolved in concentrated nitric acid. After evaporation the solid ignited in a tared crucible to a constant weight. Upon ignition bismuth subgallate is oxidised to bismuth trioxide, from the weight of bismuth trioxide obtained bismuth subgallate is calculated. As the test substance is converted to a precipitate, which is used for calculating the actual amount of bismuth subgallate present this is called Gravimetric assay.

***Procedure:*** Dry about 1 gm of Bismuth Subgallate at 105 °C for 3 hours, then weigh accurately and ignite in a porcelain crucible. Allow it to cool and add nitric acid to the residue, drop wise, warming until complete solution has been effected. Evaporate the solution to dryness and carefully ignite the residue to constant weight. From the weight of the residue so obtained, determine the percentage of $Bi_2O_3$ in the portion of Bismuth subgallate taken.

***Uses:*** It is used as an astringent and antacid.

***Dose:*** 1 gm.

***Storage:*** It should be stored in well closed containers and protected from light.

## Bismuth Subnitrate I.P., B.P., U.S.P.

**Mol. Formula:** $[Bi(OH)_2NO_3]_4.BiO(OH)$. **Mol. Weight:** 1462

It contains not less than 79% of $Bi_2O_3$. It is a basic subnitrate.

***Preparation:*** It is obtained by adding a solution of bismuth nitrate to sodium hydroxide solution at 15 °C with stirring until the pH reached 5. The sodium subnitrate is precipitated out until the stirring is continued. Filter it, wash with cold water and dried at about 50 °C.

***Properties:*** It is a colorless or white powder with slightly hygroscopic in nature. It is insoluble in water and alcohol, but soluble in excess of hydrochloric and nitric acid. It undergoes hydrolysis with water and liberates nitric acid.

***Test for identification:*** To the small amount of sample add $H_2S$ and filter. Then the filtrate is boiled to expel $H_2S$ gas, then cool and add one drop of ferric chloride solution, a bluish black color is formed. The sample solution gives the characteristic reactions of bismuth.

***Test for purity:*** It should be tested for arsenic, copper, lead, silver nitrate, alkali and alkaline earths, gallic acid and loss on drying.

**Assay**

***Principle:***

*Method 1:* It is assayed by **Gravimetric method**. In this assay the substance is ignited in a tared crucible to a constant weight. Upon ignition bismuth subnitrate is oxidized to bismuth trioxide, from the weight of bismuth trioxide obtained bismuth subnitrate is calculated. The chemical reactions of this assay are shown below. As the test substance is converted to a precipitate, which is used for calculating the actual amount of bismuth subnitrate present this is called Gravimetric assay.

*Method 2:* It is assayed by **Complexometry method of (Back) titration**.

In this assay the substance is dissolved in perchloric acid. Add xylenol orange mixture and titrate with 0.1M disodium edetate until the colour changes from pinkish-violet to lemon yellow.

In this assay Bismuth ions reacts with EDTA, whereby the complexation takes place, As the Bismuth ions forms complex with disodium EDTA in this assay, it is called as complexometry method of titration. The chemical reactions of this assay are shown below.

$Bi^{3+}$ + $NaOOCH_2C$ / $HOOCH_2C$ N–$CH_2CH_2$–N $CH_2COONa$ / $CH_2COOH$

Disodium EDTA

↓

$NaOOCH_2C$ N–$CH_2CH_2$–N $CH_2COONa$; $H_2C$, $CH_2$; $Bi^{3+}$; O=C–O, O–C=O

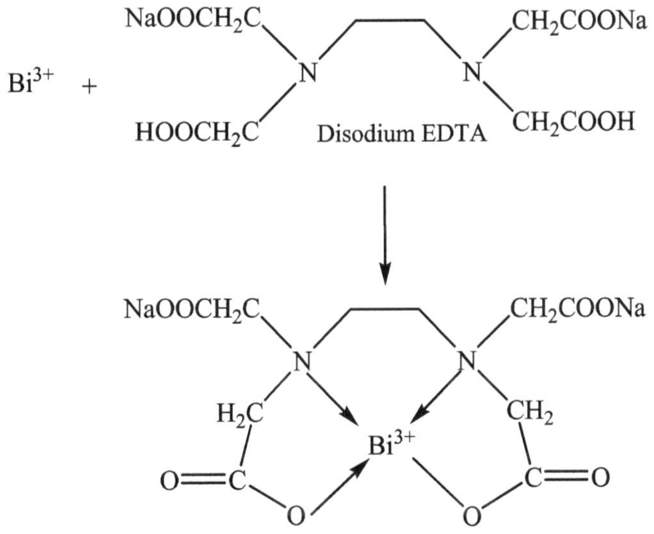

Bismuth-EDTA Complex

***Procedure:*** Dissolve with heating 0.250 gm in 10 ml of a mixture of 2 volumes of perchloric acid and 5 volumes of water. To the hot solution, add 200 ml of water and 50 mg of xylenol orange triturate. Titrate with 0.1M sodium edetate until a yellow colour is obtained.

***Uses:***

1. It is mainly used as an astringent, adsorbent and protective.
2. It is commonly used for the treatment of intestinal inflammation and diarrhoea. It is a main constituent of milk of bismuth.

***Storage:*** It should be stored in tightly closed containers and protected from sunlight.

---

### Milk of Bismuth U.S.P.

**(Synonym: Bismuth cream, Bismuth magma)**

It contains not less than 5.2% and not more than 5.8% $Bi_2O_3$.

***Preparation:*** It is prepared by dissolving bismuth sub carbonate and bismuth hydroxide in water.

***Uses:*** It is mainly used as an antacid and astringent.

***Dose:*** 4 to 5 ml.

---

## 6.1.7 Saline Catharatics

**Introduction:** Catharatics are drugs that relieve constipation and promote defecation. These are otherwise called as laxatives or purgatives. Constipation is a delayed passage of faeces through the intestine along with defecation and evacuation of bowel.

Dyschezia is a derangement of defecation which is due to

1. Presence of hard dehydrated fecal matter in the rectum.
2. Habitual use of purgatives.
3. Presence of haemorrhoids and fissures.

In majority of the cases, constipation is relieved by non therapeutic measures, like increasing the fiber content of daily diet intake or increase daily fluid intake etc. If all the above non therapeutic measures are failed laxatives or purgative are used. The order of effectiveness is described as follows. Aperients (to smooth and soft) < Evacuant (to empty) < Purgative (to clean) < Catharatic (to completely clean).

The intensity of their action depends of dose. A purgative in smaller dose acts as a laxative and vice versa. Generally laxatives eliminates soft semisolid stool and the purgatives leads to watery evacuation.

**Types of laxatives:** Laxatives are classified in to four types

1. Bulk forming laxatives
2. Osmotic laxatives
3. Lubricants laxatives
4. Surfactant laxatives

1. ***Bulk forming laxatives:*** These are acting on intestinal luminal. Normally these are hydrophilic, indigestible vegetable fibres which stimulate peristalsis and defecation reflexes by increasing fecal bulk due to their water absorbing and retaining capacity.

   *For example:* Wheat bran, isphagula, semisynthetic cellulose such as carboxy methyl cellulose and poly carbophils. Bulk forming laxatives must be administered along with plenty or adequate amount of water.

   *Side effects:* Bacterial digestion of vegetable fibres within the colon may leads to abdominal discomfort.

2. ***Osmotic laxatives:*** These are non absorbable, indigestible disaccharides. Due to their osmotic action and hydrophilic action they increases the faecal bulk.

   *Example:* Sorbitol and lactulose.

   *Dose:* 10 gm two times per day with plenty of water.

   *Side effects:* It may leads to flatulence, nausea and cramps.

3. ***Lubricant laxatives:*** These are pharmacologically inert mineral oils. These are acting on intestinal lumen. These are generally fecal lubricants and stool softeners by decreasing the water absorption from the stool (lubricating effect).

   *Example:* Liquid paraffin.

   *Dose:* 15- 30 ml/day at bed time.

   *Side effect:* Long term use of liquid paraffin leads to deficiency of fat soluble vitamins.

4. ***Surfactant laxatives:*** It is again a luminally active laxative agent. It is generally an anionic surfactant which softens the stool by decreasing the surface tension of fluids in the bowel.

Sometimes it also acts as a wetting agent for the bowel by emulsifying the colonic contents which facilitates the mixing of water in to fatty substances of faces.

*Example:* Docusate sodium (Dioctyl sodium sulfosuccinate).

***Dose:*** 100 - 400mg/day by oral route.

---

### 6.1.8 Purgatives

Purgatives provide either semi fluid stool or leads to watery evacuation. These are used for complete cleaning of bowel prior to gastrointestinal endoscopic procedures or to flush out the worms of post bed ridden or post operative patients after the use of anthelmintic drugs or cleaning the bowel before surgery or taking abdominal x-ray. In low doses these are acting as laxatives also.

Purgatives are majorly classified in to two types

1. Osmotic purgatives
2. Irritant purgatives

***Osmotic purgatives:*** It is of two types

1. *Electrolyte osmotic purgative :* Poly ethylene glycol
2. *Saline purgatives:* Magnesium sulphate, magnesium hydroxide mixture.

***Mechanism of action of electrolyte osmotic purgative:*** It contains non absorbable PEG. It retains water due to its high osmotic nature. It is given along with a balanced isotonic solution which contains sodium chloride, sodium bicarbonate, sodium sulphate and potassium chloride. So this is safer for all patients.

***Mechanism of action of saline purgatives:*** These are soluble inorganic salts which acts by increasing the fecal bulk by retaining water due to its osmotic effect thus increases the peristalsis indirectly. Magnesium salts also releases "cholecytokinin" which is used to increases the intestinal secretions and peristalsis.

***Common side effects:***

1. It is given along with plenty of water because being irritant it may induce vomiting.
2. Due to their high osmolar property leads to intra vascular fluid depletion and electrolyte disturbances.
3. Long term usage should be avoided for hypertensive and congestive cardiac failure patients.
4. Long term use of magnesium salts for renal failure patients leads to a risk of hyper magnesemia.

***Irritant purgatives:*** These are providing semisolid stools.

These are further classified into three types

1. Anthraquinone derivatives- Senna, cascara and aloe.
2. Oils- Castro oil.
3. Organic irritants - Phenolphthalein, bisacodyl etc.

All of the above irritant purgatives stimulate the intestinal peristalsis due to their irritant action. They also stimulate colonic electrolyte and fluid secretion by alters the secretary and absorptive activity of the intestinal mucosal cells.

***Common side effects:***

1. Senna glycosides leads to melanosis coli when long term use.
2. Long term uses of castor oil leads to damaging the intestinal mucosa.
3. Bisacodyl leads to hypokalemia.

## Magnesium Hydroxide I.P., B.P., U.S.P.

This compound is discussed under the topic **antacids**.

## Magnesium Sulphate I.P., B.P., U.S.P.

**(Synonym: Epsom salt)**

**Mol. Formula:** $MgSO_4.7H_2O$ **Mol. Weight:** 246.5

It contains not less than 99% and not more than 100.5% of $MgSO_4$ with reference to the dried substance.

***Preparation:***

1. *Laboratory preparation:* Epsom salt can be prepared in the laboratory scale by neutralization of magnesium carbonate with hot sulphuric acid. Filter the solution and collect the filtrate. The filtrate is evaporated to crystallization and dried.

$$MgCO_3 + H_2SO_4 \longrightarrow MgSO_4 + H_2O + CO_2\uparrow$$

2. *From Magnesite or Calcined Dolomite:* It is manufactured by the reaction of sulphuric acid with magnesite (native carbonate of magnesium) or previously powdered and calcined dolomite.

   When dolomite is used means, magnesium sulphate goes in to solution and sparingly soluble calcium sulphate is deposited.

$$MgCO_3.CaCO_3 + 2\,H_2SO_4 \longrightarrow MgSO_4 + CaSO_4 + 2CO_2 + 2H_2O$$

3. *From native sulphate, kieserite:* These are dissolved in hot water; the solution deposits, the rhombic crystals of magnesium sulphate hepta hydrate is formed on cooling.

4. *From Brine solution:* More quantities of magnesium salts are present in brine solution after extraction of bromine from the brine solution, the brine is treated with milk of lime the magnesium salts are precipitated as magnesium hydroxide suspension. The sulphur dioxide and air is passed through this suspension so that magnesium sulphate precipitate is formed upon crystallization.

$$2\,Mg(OH)_2 + 2\,SO_2 + O_2 \longrightarrow 2\,MgSO_4 + 2\,H_2O$$

***Physical properties:*** Magnesium sulphate is colorless crystals or a white crystalline powder having cool saline taste. It is soluble in water and insoluble in alcohol. The crystals effloresce slightly in warm air.

***Chemical properties:*** When heated gently it losses some of the water molecules and produce monohydrate.

$$MgSO_4.7\,H_2O \xrightarrow{\Delta} MgSO_4.H_2O + 6\,H_2O$$

But when heated up to 200 °C it produces anhydrous magnesium sulphate by total loss of water molecules.

$$MgSO_4.7\,H_2O \xrightarrow[200\,^{\circ}C]{} MgSO_4 + 7\,H_2O$$

***Test for identification:*** The solution of magnesium sulphate in water gives the characteristic reactions of magnesium and sulphate ions.

***Test for purity:*** It should be tested for color and clarity of the solution, acidity or alkalinity, arsenic, heavy metals, iron, lead, chloride, zinc and loss on drying.

***Test for loss on drying:*** It should be 48 to 52% which is determined by drying the substance at 110 °C -120 °C for 1 hr in oven.

***Mechanism of Action:*** It does not get absorbed from intestine, so it retains sufficient water within the lumen which leads to increase in the hydrostatic pressure of the lumen to promote the peristalsis of bowel.

**Assay**

***Principle:*** It is assayed by **Complexometry method of (Direct) titr**ation.

In this assay the substance is dissolved in hydrochloric acid, to this ammonia-ammonium chloride solution is added as buffer solution and it is then titrated against 0.05M disodium Ethylene Diamine Tetra Acetate (EDTA) using mordant black II mixture as an indicator. End point is the blue colour.

In this assay magnesium ions of magnesium sulphate reacts with disodium EDTA, whereby the complexation takes place. As the magnesium ions forms complex with disodium EDTA in this assay, it is called as complexometry method of titration. The chemical reactions of this assay are shown below.

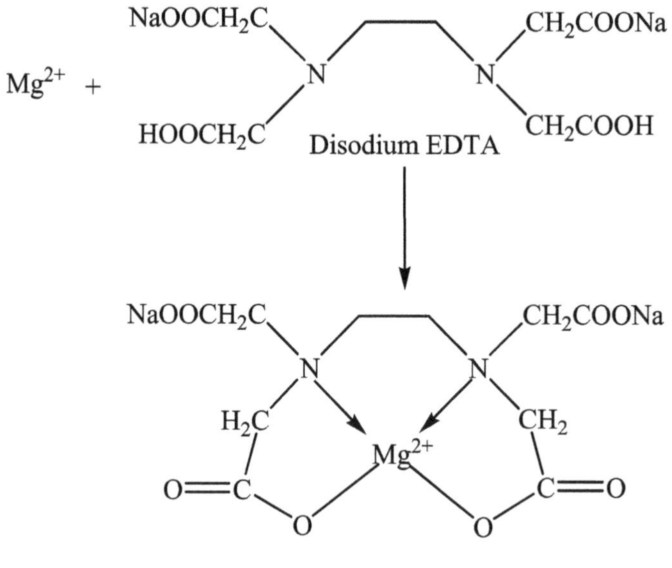

$Mg^{2+}$ + $(NaOOCH_2C)(HOOCH_2C)N-CH_2CH_2-N(CH_2COONa)(CH_2COOH)$

Disodium EDTA

↓

$NaOOCH_2C$, $CH_2COONa$, N, N, $H_2C$, $CH_2$, $Mg^{2+}$, O=C, C=O, O, O

Magnesium-EDTA Complex

***Procedure:*** Weigh accurately about 0.3 gm, dissolve in 50 ml of water, add 10 ml of strong ammonia-ammonium chloride solution and titrate with 0.05M disodium edetate, using 0.1 gm of mordant black II mixture as indicator, until a blue colour is obtained.

***Uses:***

1. The solution of magnesium sulphate is given by oral route which is used as an osmotic laxative and electrolyte replenishers.
2. It is given along with fruit juices due to its bitter taste and unpleasant odour.
3. It also used in renal function impaired patients as laxative.

***Dose:*** 2 to 16 gm usual dose.

5 gm as laxative.

**Storage:** It should be stored in tightly closed container and protected from moisture.

## Magnesium Citrate Solution N.F.

**(Synonym: Purgative lemonade, Citrate of magnesia)**

**Mol. Formula:** $MgHC_6H_5O_7$ **Mol. Weight**: 215

***Preparation:*** It is prepared by treating magnesium carbonate with citric acid which gives soluble magnesium citrate. Sodium or potassium carbonate is added to react with excess unreacted citric acid to yield carbonated, palatable and lemon flavored solution. The resulting solution must be sterilized or pasteurized.

$$3\,MgCO_3 + 2\,HO{-}C(CH_2COOH)_2{-}COOH \xrightarrow[-3\,H_2O,\ -3\,CO_2]{} \left[HO{-}C(CH_2COO^-)_2{-}COO^-\right]_2\ 3Mg^{2+}$$

***Test for identification:*** The sample solution gives the characteristic reactions of magnesium and citrate ions.

***Assay:*** Similar to that of sodium citrate.

***Uses:*** It is used as a saline catharatic.

***Dose:*** 200 ml.

## Magnesium Carbonate

This compound is discussed under the topic **antacids**.

## Sodium Phosphate

This compound is discussed under the topic **acidifiers and alkalinising agents**.

## Disodium Hydrogen Phosphate (Sodium phosphate)

This compound is discussed under **acidifiers and alkalising agents**.

## Potassium Bitartarate U.S.P.

**(Synonym: Potassium hydrogen tartarate, Cream of tartar)**

**Mol. Formula:** $C_4H_5O_6K$ **Mol. Weight:** 188.2

It contains not less than 99.5% of calculated with reference to the substance dried to a constant weight at 105 °C.

$$\begin{array}{c} \text{H} \\ | \\ \text{OH}-\text{C}-\text{COOK} \\ | \\ \text{OH}-\text{C}-\text{COOH} \\ | \\ \text{H} \end{array}$$

### *Preparation*

*From Grape Juice:* After fermentation of grape juice the crude tartar obtained is called as argol (mixture of calcium tartarate and potassium acid tartarate).

Argol is dissolved in hot water, neutralized with the addition of sodium carbonate and the resulting solution is allowed to pass through the soda ash beds and then filtered through charcoal to remove colored impurities.

The filtered solution is treated with acetic acid (decomposition reaction), the pure potassium bitartarate settled down as a very fine precipitate. Then purify the substance by recrystallisation.

$$\underset{\text{Sodium potassium tartarate}}{\begin{array}{c} \text{H} \\ | \\ \text{OH}-\text{C}-\text{COONa} \\ | \\ \text{OH}-\text{C}-\text{COOK} \\ | \\ \text{H} \end{array}} + \underset{\text{Acetic acid}}{CH_3COOH} \longrightarrow \underset{\text{Potassium bitartarate}}{\begin{array}{c} \text{H} \\ | \\ \text{OH}-\text{C}-\text{COOH} \\ | \\ \text{OH}-\text{C}-\text{COOK} \\ | \\ \text{H} \end{array}} + \underset{\text{Sodium acetate}}{CH_3COONa}$$

***Properties:*** It is a white or colorless, slightly opaque, gritty, white crystalline powder. It is soluble in water and insoluble in alcohol.

***Test for identification:*** The sample solution in water gives the characteristic reactions of potassium and tartarate ions.

***Test for purity:*** It should be tested for color and clarity of the solution, acidity or alkalinity, arsenic, heavy metals, iron, lead, chloride, zinc and loss on drying.

***Assay: Principle:*** It is assayed by **acidimetry-alkalimetry method of titration** (also called **neutralization method**).

In this assay the substance is dissolve in boiling water and titrated against sodium hydroxide, using phenolphthalein as an indicator. End point is the appearance of permanent pale pink colour. In this assay the sodium hydroxide (the base) reacts with potassium bitartarate and neutralization takes place during the titration. The indicator is colorless in acid medium and it changes to pink colour in alkali medium which is the end point.

As the acid and alkali involved in this assay, it is called as acidimetry-alkalimetry method of titration and the neutralization takes place in this assay during titration hence this assay is also called as Neutralization method.

$$\begin{array}{l} \text{CHOH-COOK} \\ | \\ \text{CHOH-COOH} \end{array} + \text{NaOH} \longrightarrow 2 \begin{array}{l} \text{CHOH-COOK} \\ | \\ \text{CHOH-COONa} \end{array} + H_2O$$

***Uses:***

1. It is used as saline purgative.
2. It also used as a dusting powder (bacteriostatic) in surgery.
3. It finds as the one of constituent of baking powder to increase the dough.

***Dose:*** As a saline purgative 2 gm (large doses cause renal impairment).

***Storage:*** It should be stored in tightly close containers.

## Calomel U.S.P.

**(Synonym: Mercurous chloride)**

**Mol. Formula:** HgCl **Mol. Weight:** 236.1

It contains not less than 99.6% of mercurous chloride.

***Preparation:***

*From mercuric chloride:* It is obtained by heating mercuric chloride with mercury and sublimating the product. The resulting sublimate is washed with water until it becomes free from $HgCl_2$.

$$Hg + HgCl_2 \rightleftharpoons Hg_2Cl_2 \text{ or } 2\,HgCl$$

*From soluble mercurous salt:* It is prepared by adding sodium chloride solution to soluble mercurous salts.

$$Hg_2(NO_3)_2 + 2\,NaCl \longrightarrow Hg_2Cl_2 + 2\,NaNO_3$$

*From mercurous sulphate:* It is obtained by heating mercurous sulphate with sodium chloride and the resulting mercurous chloride vapours are condensed. It is thoroughly washed with water to eliminate mercuric chloride, washed with dilute nitric acid to remove the metallic mercury, and then washed with water until all the nitric acid is removed. After heating and sublimating the product is collected.

$$Hg_2SO_4 + 2\,NaCl \longrightarrow 2\,HgCl + Na_2SO_4$$

The mercurous sulphate needed for the above preparation is obtained by heating mercury with sulphuric acid until dry mercuric sulphate is formed. Then sufficient quantity of mercury is added and triturated, all the mercuric sulphate is converted in to mercurous sulphate.

$$Hg + 2\,H_2SO_4 \longrightarrow HgSO_4 + SO_2\uparrow + 2\,H_2O$$

$$HgSO_4 + Hg \longrightarrow Hg_2SO_4$$

***Physical properties:*** It is a white or colorless, heavy powder, odorless, tasteless. It is insoluble in water, alcohol and in cold sulphuric acid also, when compressed it becomes yellowish white and when strongly heated it volatilizes. It is stable in air but gradually darkens, when exposed to light turns slightly grey.

***Chemical properties:***

1. *Decomposition reaction:* It undergoes decomposition give mercury and mercuric chloride.

$$Hg_2Cl_2 \longrightarrow Hg + HgCl_2$$

Upon heated under required conditions it forms metallic mercury and poisonous mercuric chloride when it is cooled it forms calomel.

$$Hg_2Cl_2 \overset{\Delta}{\rightleftharpoons} \underset{\text{Poisonous mercuric chloride}}{HgCl_2} + Hg$$

2. *Reaction with alkali hydroxides:* Calomel reacts with calcium hydroxide, ammonium hydroxide etc. and forms the respective hydroxide precipitate which is black in color.

$$2\,Hg_2Cl_2 + 4\,NH_4OH \longrightarrow HgNH_2Cl + Hg + 3\,NH_4Cl + Hg_2O + 3\,H_2O$$

$$Hg_2Cl_2 + Ca(OH)_2 \longrightarrow Hg_2(OH)_2\downarrow + CaCl_2$$

$$Hg_2(OH)_2 \longrightarrow Hg_2O + H_2O$$

3. *Reaction with reducing agents:* Reaction with hypo phosphorous acid: Calomel reduces hypo phosphorous acid in to phosphoric acid.

$$2\,Hg_2Cl_2 + H_3PO_2 + 2\,H_2O \longrightarrow H_3PO_4 + 4\,Hg + 4\,HCl$$

***Reaction with stannous chloride:*** Calomel reacts with stannous chloride to gives metallic mercury.

$$Hg_2Cl_2 + SnCl_2 \longrightarrow 2\,Hg + SnCl_4$$

***Test for identification:***

1. It reacts with dilute ammonia or alkali hydroxides and it blackens.
2. The solution in sodium carbonate and dilute nitric acid (heating and sublimation with sodium carbonate metallic Hg formed) gives the characteristic reactions of chlorides.

***Test for purity:*** It should be tested for ammoniated mercury, non volatile matter and mercuric chloride.

**Assay**

***Principle:*** It is assayed by **Iodimetry method** of titration (also called **Redox titration**).

In this assay the substance is dissolved in water and to this a known Excess Standard (KES) iodine solution and potassium iodide solution added in an iodine flask. The solution is kept aside, whereby the mercurous chloride is oxidized by iodine and potassium iodide and form $K_2(HgI_4)$ complex. After the completion of this reaction, the excess unreacted iodine is determined by titrating with N/10 sodium thiosulphate using starch mucilage as an indicator. End point is the disappearance of blue colour. During this titration iodine is reduced to sodium iodide and sodium thiosulphate is oxidised to sodium tetrathionate. As the oxidation and reduction takes place simultaneously this is called Redox titration. The chemical reactions of this assay are shown below.

$$2\,HgCl + I_2 \longrightarrow HgI_2 + HgCl_2$$

$$2\,HgCl + 6\,KI + I_2 \longrightarrow 2\,K_2HgI_4 + 2\,KCl$$

$$I_2 + 2\,Na_2S_2O_3 \longrightarrow 2NaI + Na_2S_4O_6$$

***Uses:***

1. Calomel has been used as cathartic.
2. It is also used in dusting powders in pruritis, ecezema and psoriasis.
3. Calomel containing ointments are used as a prophylactic in syphilis.
4. In recent years it should be replaced by some other drugs due to its toxicity. It is insoluble in gastric acid and not absorbed from the stomach. But it is absorbed by the intestine, it gets slowly dissociated in to mercury and the irritant mercuric compounds exerts cathartic action.

***Storage:*** It should be stored in well closed containers and protected from moisture.

## PROBABLE QUESTIONS

1. Define acidifiers. Write the official inorganic acidifiers.
2. Explain about the different type of acidifiers with one example and mention their uses.
3. Write about the mechanism of action of acidifiers.
4. Define the terms (a) Achlorhydria (b) Hypochlorhydria (c) Systemic acidosis (d) Systemic alkalosis.
5. Write the preparation, properties, test for identification and assay of dilute hydro chloric acid.

6. Write the preparation, properties, assay and uses of sodium phosphate.
7. Write the assay of dried sodium phosphate.
8. Write the preparation, assay and uses of any one sodium compound which is used as a urinary acidifier.
9. Write in detail about dilute ammonia solution.
10. Explain about the preparation of ammonium chloride by Sal ammoniac process.
11. Write in brief about the assay methods of ammonium chloride.
12. Why previously neutralized formaldehyde solution is added in the assay of ammonium chloride.
13. Explain about the preparation, properties and uses of aromatic spirit of ammonia.
14. Describe the assay of aromatic spirit of ammonia.
15. Write in detail about hypo phosphorous acid.
16. Explain about the old Leblanc process for the preparation of concentrated hydrochloric acid.
17. Write about the chemical properties of concentrated hydrochloric acid with chemical equations.
18. Why hydrochloric acid is called as spirit of salt?
19. What is the composition and uses of aqua regia?
20. Write the assay and uses of hydrochloric acid.
21. Write in detail about the uses and adverse effects of concentrated hydrochloric acid.
22. Write about the manufacturing process of sulphuric acid.
23. Write a brief note on acid-base regulators.
24. Explain about the preparation, properties and uses of the following compounds.
    (a) Phosphoric acid (b) Strong ammonia solution
25. Write about the Haber's process for the preparation of strong ammonia solution.
26. Define the term alkalizing agent and explain preparation and assay of any one of them.
27. Explain the preparation, chemical properties, test for identification, test for purity, assay and uses of caustic soda.
28. Write in detail about potassium hydroxide and its official formulations.
29. Describe Modified Winkder method of titration with one example.
30. Write in detail about hypo phosphorous acid.
31. What is mean by slaking?
32. Write the assay of calcium hydroxide.

33. What is meant by antacids? Enumerate the official inorganic antacids.
34. Explain about the mechanism of antacid with one example.
35. What are the ideal characteristics of antacids?
36. How will you measure the acid neutralizing capacity of antacids (Both *in- vivo* and *in-vitro*)?
37. Briefly explain about the aluminium compounds as antacids.
38. Write the preparation, properties, assay and uses of sodium bicarbonate and its official formulations.
39. Explain the principle involved in the assay of calcium carbonate.
40. Write the preparation, properties and test for purity of sodium carbonate.
41. What types of combination of antacid preparations are commercially available? Why is simethicone added in antacid preparation?
42. List out the antacid preparations contain both aluminium and magnesium compounds. What is the reason of this combination?
43. Define saline laxatives. Highlight their advantages and disadvantages.
44. Explain the properties, test for purity and uses of light and heavy kaolin.
45. Enumerate the bismuth compounds used as protectives. Write the method of preparation, action, properties and uses of bismuth subnitrate.
46. Describe the preparation, properties, assay and uses of following.
    (a) Kaolin (b) Activated charcoal
    (c) Bismuth compounds
47. Briefly explain about the followings.
    (a) Aluminium containing antacids
    (b) Magnesium containing antacids
    (c) Any three combination antacid preparations
    (d) Saline cathartics
48. Explain about saline cathartics with two examples.
49. Explain in detail about combination antacid therapy.
50. Write a detail account on antacids which are official in I.P.
51. Explain about the mechanism of action and assay of aluminium hydroxide gel.
52. Enumerate the preparation, properties and uses of the official compounds of aluminium hydroxide gel.
53. Write the preparation, properties and test for identification, assay and uses of aluminium glycinate.

54. Explain the acid neutralizing capacity of dried aluminium phosphate.
55. Write the preparation, properties, assay and uses of the following.
    (a) Magnesium hydroxide (b) Milk of magnesia
    (c) Magnesium trisilicate
56. Enumerate the advantages and disadvantages of magnesium antacids.
57. Write the common assay method for magnesium compounds.
58. Write about the preparation, properties, test for purity, uses and assay of the following.
    (a) Light and heavy magnesium carbonate.
    (b) Heavy magnesium oxide
    (c) Magnesium phosphate
59. Explain the preparation, properties, uses and mechanism of action of tribasic calcium phosphate.
60. Write the B.P method of assay of tribasic calcium phosphate.
61. Explain about the neutralization of gastric acid by phosphate ions.
62. How can you distinguish dibasic calcium phosphate from tribasic calcium phosphate?
63. Explain about mixed antacid preparations.
64. Write a note on activated charcoal.
65. How does the bismuth compounds assayed. Explain it with any one example.
66. Briefly explain about the following.
    (a) Test for purity of coarse particles
    (b) Fine particles
    (c) Adsorption and swelling power of heavy kaolin
67. Define saline cathartics and write one example.
68. Define the term purgatives and laxatives and mention a compound possessing this property.
69. Describe the type of cathartics.
70. Explain about the preparation, properties, assay and mechanism of action of magnesium sulphate.
71. List out the sodium compounds which are used as a saline cathartics. Explain any one compound.
72. Write a note on magnesium citrate solution.
73. Explain in detail about the following.
    (a) Potassium bitartarate
    (b) Mercurous chloride (calomel)

## 6.2 TOPICAL AGENTS

### 6.2.1 Protectives

**Introduction:** Adsorbents are finely powdered, inert and insoluble solids capable of binding to the surface of (adsorbing) noxious and irritant substances. They are also called 'protectives' because they offer physical protection to the skin or mucosa. Demulcents and emollients also serve as protectives. In general, the protectives form a continuous, adherent and flexible coating on the skin and there by protects it. Example: Talc, calamine, starch, aloe vera gel.

**Classification of topical agents:** According to their mechanism of action topical agents are classified as follows.

1. Protectives.
2. Demulcents and adsorbents.
3. Emollients.
4. Astringents.
5. Caustics.

***Protectives:*** These are compounds which protect the exposed skin or mucous membrane by forming a thin coat from external stimuli like heat etc. or annoying stimuli. This protection is produced by either physical or mechanical way. These compounds does not show any biological activity. Examples for protectives: Zinc oxide, dimethicone etc.

***Demulcents & Adsorbents:*** These are similar to that of protectives. These are acts by adsorbing moisture from the skin surfaces, by this way it decreases the irritation and friction. These exert their surface action which depends upon the particle size. These are used internally to adsorb dissolved gases or toxins. It should not be applied to the abraded skin, because it would be absorbed by the systemic circulation.

***Emollients:*** These are substances, which make the external layers of the skin (epidermis) softer and more pliable. They increase the skin's hydration (water content) by reducing evaporation. Naturally occurring skin lipids and sterols, as well as artificial or natural oils, humectants, emollients, lubricants etc., may be part of the composition of commercial skin moisturizers. They prevent and treat dry skin, protect sensitive skin, improve skin tone and texture, and mask imperfections.

***Astringents:*** Astringents are the substances which precipitate the proteins, but do not penetrate into cells, thus affecting superficial layer only. They toughen the surface making it mechanically stronger and decrease exudation. These are generally described as a firming or shrinkage of the tissue. A very dilute solution of metal cation is applied to tissues primarily produces local or surface protein precipitation action. These are causes the constriction of small capillaries and small blood vessels, hence they are used to styptics (stop bleeding from small cuts). Example: Tannic acid and tannins, alcohol, mineral astringents (Heavy metal ions).

***Caustics:*** By using higher concentrated solution of astringents leads to irritation but further increases in concentration that solution have a corrosive effect on contact with tissues. This property is used for the removal of undesirable tissues like warts, moles and hyper plastic tissues.

**Properties of protectives and adsorbents:**

1. Protectives acts physically by blocking the pores present in the surface of the skin and leads to the formation of protective layers.
2. These are available in the form of ointments, suspensions and dusting powders.
3. They are also used to reduce the irritation caused by the allergic inflammation.
4. These agents also act mechanically by forming a flexible coat or protective coat on the surface of the skin.
5. Many of the inorganic topical agents are shows both protective and adsorbent properties.
6. They should be insoluble in water and does not absorb moisture.

## Talc I.P., B.P.

**(Synonym: Purified talc, Topalcum)**

**Mol. Formula:** Approximate formula $[Mg_6(Si_2O_5)_4(OH)_4]$

It is a native powdered hydrated magnesium silicate with small proportions of aluminium silicate and iron. It is having free flow property than that of kaolin.

***Preparation:*** Pharmaceutical grade talc is prepared by boiling purified talc with hydrochloric acid, then washed with water until becomes free from acid. Then hydrochloric acid is added to remove impurities like calcium oxide, iron, aluminium tri oxide and $Fe_2O_3$.

***Properties:*** It is a white or almost white powder, free from grittiness, odorless, tasteless and readily adheres to skin, unctuous to touch. It is insoluble in water, dilute solutions of acids and alkalis. When heated at 850 to 950 °C it loses water molecule and converted into $Mg_4SiO_{12}$.

$$Mg_6(Si_2O_5)_4(OH)_4 \xrightarrow[\Delta]{850\text{-}960\ ^{\circ}C} Mg_4SiO_{12} + H_2O$$

***Test for identification:***

1. It is identified by IR spectrophotometry.
2. Small amount of anhydrous sodium carbonate and potassium carbonate are melted in a platinum crucible. To the melted mass add small quantity of substance to be analyzed and heat it to melt. Cool it and transfer the mixture into china dish and add required amount of water. Then add hydrochloric acid until the effervescence ceases. Add excess hydrochloric acid and evaporate to dryness. Cool it, add water, boil the solution and filter it. To the small quantity of filtrate, add ammonia and ammonium chloride and again filter the solution.

   To the above filtrate add disodium hydrogen phosphate solution, a white crystalline precipitate is formed
3. The residue obtained from the above test gives the characteristic reactions of silicates.

***Test for purity:*** It should be tested for acidity or alkalinity, acid soluble substances, water soluble substances, carbonates, chlorides, organic compounds, loss on drying, loss on ignition and microbial contamination.

***Test for loss on drying:*** It should not be more than 1% which is determined on 1 gm of the sample is drying in an oven at 180 °C for 1 hr.

***Test for microbial contamination:*** If topical use viable aerobic count is not more than $10^2$ bacteria and fungi/gm. If it is in oral administration, the total viable count is not more than $10^3$ bacteria and $10^2$ fungi/gm.

***Uses:***

1. It is mainly used as a pharmaceutical aid, dusting powder in cosmetic preparations.
2. It is commonly used with zinc oxide, starch and very less quantity of boric acid.
3. Sometimes it may be medicated or perfumed.
4. It is also used as lubricating agent for tablet granules.
5. It is also used as a filtering media for liquids and distributing media for water and elixirs, since it does not adsorb active ingredients.

***Storage:*** It should be stored in a well closed container and protected from moisture.

## Zinc Oxide I.P., U.S.P.

**Mol. Formula:** ZnO **Mol. Weight:** 81.4

It contains not less than 99% and not more than 100.5% of ZnO which is calculated on the dried basis of the substance.

***Preparation***

*From zinc sulphate:* The medicinally pure zinc oxide is obtained by this process. A solution of zinc sulphate is mixed to a boiling sodium carbonate solution. The basic zinc carbonates gets precipitated out. Wash it until free from sulphate and dried. The dried zinc carbonate is ignited gently, it loses carbon dioxide and forms zinc oxide.

$$ZnSO_4 + Na_2CO_3 \longrightarrow ZnCO_3 + Na_2SO_4$$

$$ZnCO_3 \xrightarrow{\Delta} ZnO + CO_2\uparrow$$

*Large scale preparation:* By this method, zinc oxide is prepared by heating zinc metal to bright redness in a current of air. The vapours off the metal burns to form the oxide, which is collected as a fine white powder.

$$2\,Zn + O_2 \xrightarrow{\Delta} 2\,ZnO$$

***Properties:*** Zinc oxide is a soft white or faintly yellowish white amorphous powder, free from grittiness. It slowly absorbs small amount of water and carbon dioxide when it is exposed to moist air. It is insoluble in water and alcohol but soluble in dilute acids and alkali hydroxides. It is amphoteric in nature.

$$ZnO + H_2SO_4 \longrightarrow ZnSO_4 + H_2O$$

$$ZnO + 2\,NaOH \longrightarrow Na_2ZnO_2 + H_2O$$

***Test for identification:***

1. When zinc oxide is heated strongly, it produces yellow color, which disappears on cooling.
2. The solution of zinc oxide gives the characteristic reactions of zinc salts.

***Test for purity:*** It should be tested for alkalinity, carbonates and substances insoluble in acids, arsenic, iron, lead, metallic zinc and loss on ignition.

**Assay**

***Principle:***

*Method 1:* It is assayed by **acidimetry-alkalimetry method of (Back) titration** (also called **neutralization method**).

In this assay the substance is dissolved in Known Excess Standard (KES) 1N sulphuric acid and the Excess Unreacted (EUR) sulphuric acid is titrated with 1N sodium hydroxide using methyl orange as an indicator. End point is the yellow colour. As the zinc hydroxide interferes in detection of end point results in poor end point. Hence ammonium chloride is used to prevent the precipitation of zinc hydroxide.

In this assay the zinc oxide (the base) reacts with sulphuric acid and neutralization takes place, after this reaction the excess unreacted sulphuric acid is determined by titrating with sodium hydroxide. The indicator is orange colour in acid medium and it changes to yellow colour upon neutralization which is the end point.

As the acid and alkali involved in this assay, it is called as acidimetry-alkalimetry method of titration and the neutralization takes place in this assay during titration hence this assay is also called as Neutralization method. The chemical reactions of this assay are shown below.

$$ZnO + H_2SO_4 \longrightarrow ZnSO_4 + H_2O$$

$$H_2SO_4 + 2\,NaOH \longrightarrow Na_2SO_4 + 2\,H_2O$$

*Method 2:* It is assayed by **Complexometry method of titration**.

In this assay the substance is dissolved 2M acetic acid and dilute to 50 ml with water. To this solution hexamine added as a buffer and xylenol orange as an indicator and titrated against disodium EDTA. End point is the appearance of yellow colour.

In this assay zinc ions of zinc oxide reacts with EDTA, whereby the complexation takes place. As the zinc ions forms complex with disodium EDTA in this assay, it is called as complexometry method of titration. The chemical reactions of this assay are shown below.

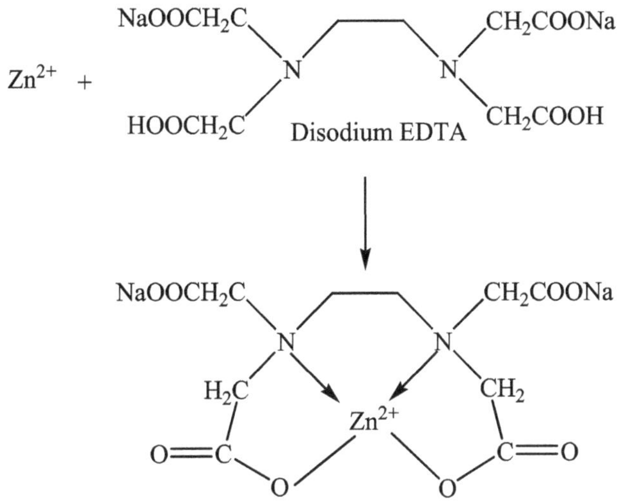

$Zn^{2+}$ + $NaOOCH_2C$, $HOOCH_2C$, N, N, $CH_2COONa$, $CH_2COOH$

Disodium EDTA

↓

$NaOOCH_2C$, N, N, $CH_2COONa$, $H_2C$, $CH_2$, $Zn^{2+}$, O=C, C=O, O, O

Zinc-EDTA Complex

***Procedure:*** Dissolve 0.15 gm in 10 ml of 2M acetic acid and dilute to 50 ml with water. To the resulting solution add about 50 mg of xylenol orange, triturate and add sufficient hexamine to produce violet-pink colour. Add a further 2 gm of hexamine and titrate with 0.1M disodium edetate until the solution becomes yellow.

***Uses:***

1. It is mainly act as mild astringent and topical protectants.
2. It is also used for the treatment of eczema, varicose, ulcers, psoriasis and various types of skin diseases.
3. In dentistry it is used as dental cement for temporary filling of teeth.
4. It is also used in the manufacturing of bandages and adhesive tapes.

***Storage:*** It should be stored in tightly closed containers and protected from moisture.

## Zinc Oxide Compound Paste

**(Synonym: Zinc paste)**

It contains not less than 24% and not more than 26% of ZnO.

***Preparation:***

***Ingredients:***

Zinc oxide = 250 gm

Starch = 250 gm

White petrolatum or White soft paraffin = 500 gm

***Procedure:*** The finely sifted zinc oxide, starch are added to the melted white petrolatum base with constant stirring. The stirring is continued until cold.

***Test for identification:*** The residue obtained after igniting the paste is yellow when hot and white upon cooling.

***Test for purity:*** Similar to zinc oxide.

**Assay**

It is assayed by **Gravimetric method**.

In this assay the substance is taken in a crucible, melted gently and heated to charring. The charred mass ignited until the residue becomes uniformly yellow. The residue represents zinc oxide and ignited to a constant weight. As the test substance is converted to a precipitate, which is used for calculating the actual amount of zinc oxide present this is called gravimetric assay.

***Storage:*** It should be preserved in well closed containers and avoid the temperatures exceeding 30 °C.

***Official formulation:*** Zinc oxide and Salicylic acid paste U.S.P.

Hydrous zinc oxide paste.

---

## Zinc Gelatin Paste I.P.

**(Synonym: Unna's paste)**

It contains 15% w/w of Zinc oxide.

***Preparation:***

***Ingredients:***

| | | |
|---|---|---|
| Zinc oxide | = | 150 gm |
| Gelatin | = | 150 gm |
| Glycerin | = | 350 gm |
| Purified water | = | 350 gm or quantity sufficient |

***Procedure:*** Gelatin is softened by treating with water, and then mixed with glycerin. This mixture is heated in a water bath until the clear solution is obtained. The required volume is adjusted by using purified water. Zinc oxide is then added, stirred well, allowed to settle in the form of paste.

**Assay**

***Principle:*** It is assayed by **acidimetry-alkalimetry method of (Back) titration** (also called **neutralization method**).

In this assay the substance is dissolved in water by warming, to this Known Excess Standard (KES) 1N sulphuric acid added and the Excess Unreacted (EUR) sulphuric acid is titrated with 1N sodium hydroxide using methyl orange as an indicator. End point is the yellow colour. As the zinc hydroxide interferes in detection of end point results in poor end point. Hence ammonium chloride is used to prevent the precipitation of zinc hydroxide.

In this assay zinc gelatin reacts with sulphuric acid, whereby the neutralization takes place, after this reaction, the excess unreacted sulphuric acid is determined by titrating with sodium hydroxide. The indicator is orange colour in acid medium and it changes to yellow colour upon neutralization which is the end point.

As the acid and alkali involved in this assay, it is called as acidimetry-alkalimetry method of titration and the neutralization takes place in this assay during titration hence this assay is also called as Neutralization method. The chemical reactions of this assay are shown below.

$$Zn^{2+} + H_2SO_4 \longrightarrow ZnSO_4 + 2H^+$$

$$H_2SO_4 + 2\,NaOH \longrightarrow Na_2SO_4 + 2\,H_2O$$

***Uses:***

1. It is used as a protective.
2. It is applied in the molten state between two layers of bandage for protective purpose and for supporting varicosities and lesion of the legs. The dressing is usually removed after fortnight.

***Storage:*** It should be stored in a well closed container.

## Zinc Undecylenate I.P.

**(Synonym: Zinc Undecenoate)**

**Mol. Formula:** $C_{22}H_{38}O_4Zn$ **Mol. Weight:** 431.9

**Structure:**

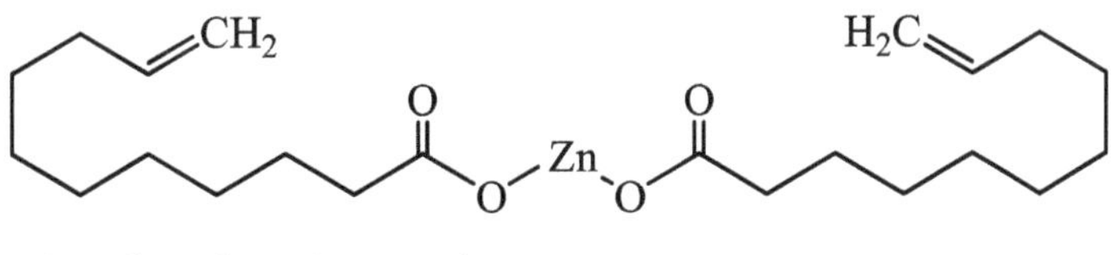

$CH_2$ $H_2C$ O O Zn O O

Chemically, it is zinc di(undec-10-enoate).

It contains not less than 98% and not more than 102% of zinc undecylenate, calculated on the dried basis.

***Preparation:*** It is prepared by the precipitation reaction from its sodium salt. It involves two step processes.

*Step1: Preparation of sodium undecenoate*

The required quantity of undecenoic acid is treated with required quantity of sodium hydroxide to give sodium undecenoate.

$$CH_2{=}CH\text{-}(CH_2)_8\text{-}COOH + NaOH \xrightarrow[-H_2O]{} CH_2{=}CH\text{-}(CH_2)_8\text{-}COONa + H_2O$$

*Step 2: Preparation of zinc undecenoate*

The sodium undecenoate obtained from the above method is treated with zinc salt (zinc sulphate) to yield zinc undecenoate.

$$2\,[CH_2{=}CH\text{-}(CH_2)_8\text{-}COONa] + ZnSO_4 \longrightarrow [CH_2{=}CH\text{-}(CH_2)_8\text{-}COO]_2Zn + Na_2SO_4$$

The unsaturated undecenoic acid needed for the above process is obtained from castor oil, which upon distillation gives undecenoic acid and an aldehyde.

***Properties:*** It occurs as a white or almost white, fine powder, soft to touch, practically insoluble in water and alcohol.

***Test for identification:***

1. A small amount of sample is ignited, cooled and dissolved in dilute hydrochloric acid to give the characteristic reaction of zinc salts.
2. Dissolve 0.1 gm of a substance in a mixture of sulphuric acid and glacial acetic acid and add drop wise, potassium permanganate solution, the pink color of the potassium permanganate is disappeared.

***Test for purity:*** It should be tested for alkalinity, alkalis and alkaline earths, sulphates, degree of unsaturation and loss on drying.

**Assay**

***Principle:***

*Method 1:* It is assayed by **acidimetry-alkalimetry method of (Back) titration** (also called **neutralization method**).

In this assay the substance is boiled with Known Excess Standard (KES) 0.1N sulphuric acid and the excess unreacted sulphuric acid is titrated with 0.1N sodium hydroxide using methyl orange as an indicator. End point is the yellow colour.

In this assay the zinc undecylenate (the base) reacts with sulphuric acid and neutralization takes place, after this reaction the excess unreacted sulphuric acid is determined by titrating with sodium hydroxide. The indicator is orange colour in acid medium and it changes to yellow colour upon neutralization which is the end point.

As the acid and alkali involved in this assay, it is called as acidimetry-alkalimetry method of titration and the neutralization takes place in this assay during titration hence this assay is also called as neutralization method. The chemical reactions of this assay are shown below.

$$\underset{\text{Zinc undecylenate}}{[CH_2{=}CH\text{-}(CH_2)_8COO]_2Zn} + H_2SO_4 \longrightarrow \underset{\text{Undeconoic acid}}{2\,CH_2{=}CH\text{-}(CH_2)_8COOH} + ZnSO_4$$

$$H_2SO_4 + 2\,NaOH \longrightarrow Na_2SO_4 + 2\,H_2O$$

*Method 2:* It is assayed by **Complexometry method of titration.**

In this assay the substance is dissolved 2M acetic acid and dilute to 50 ml with water. To this solution hexamine added as a buffer and xylenol orange as an indicator and titrated against 0.05M disodium EDTA. End point is the appearance of yellow colour.

In this assay zinc ions of zinc undecylenate reacts with EDTA, whereby the complexation takes place. As the zinc ions forms complex with disodium EDTA in this assay, it is called as complexometry method of titration. The chemical reactions of this assay are shown below.

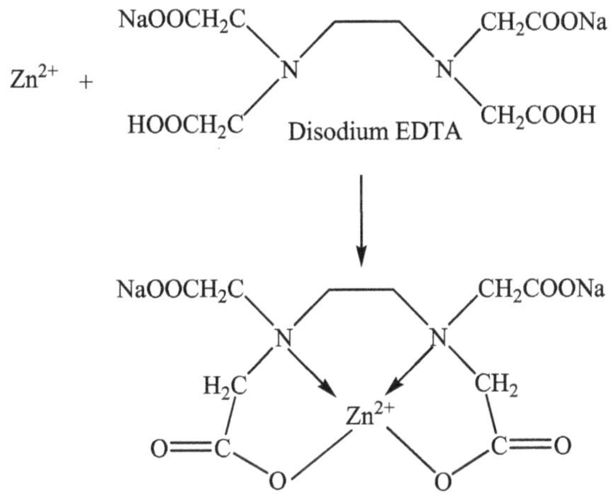

$Zn^{2+}$ + $NaOOCH_2C$, $HOOCH_2C$ – N – $CH_2CH_2$ – N – $CH_2COONa$, $CH_2COOH$

Disodium EDTA

↓

Zinc-EDTA Complex

***Procedure:*** Dissolve 0.15 gm in 10 ml of 2M acetic acid and dilute to 50 ml with water. To the resulting solution add about 50 mg of xylenol orange triturate and sufficient hexamine to produce violet-pink colour. Add a further 2 gm of hexamine and titrate with 0.1M disodium edetate until the solution becomes yellow.

***Uses:***

1. It is mainly used as a topical antifungal agent.
2. The antifungal activity is due to zinc ion and the undecenoic acid is helpful in wound healing.

***Storage:*** It should be preserved in well closed containers and protected from light and moisture.

## Zinc Undecylenate Ointment

**(Synonym: Zinc undecenoate ointment)**

**Mol. Formula:** $(CH_2{=}CH(CH_2)_8COO)_2Zn$ **Mol. Weight:** 431.9

It contains not less than 18% and not more than 22% of zinc undecenoate and not less than 4.5% and not more than 5.5% of free undecenoic acid.

***Composition:***

| | | |
|---|---|---|
| Zinc undecylenate | = | 200 gm |
| Undecenoic acid | = | 50 gm |
| Emulsifying ointment | = | 750 gm |

***Preparation:*** It is prepared by melting the emulsifying ointment to which two ingredients are added in the required amounts. The ointment is stirred and allowed to cool until reach the room temperature.

**Assay**

***Principle:*** It is assayed by **acidimetry-alkalimetry method of (Back) titration** (also called **neutralization method**).

In this assay the substance is warmed with chloroform until the ointment base is dissolved. To this Known Excess Standard (KES) 0.1N sulphuric acid and ammonium chloride added the excess unreacted sulphuric acid is titrated with 0.1N sodium hydroxide using methyl orange as an indicator. End point is the yellow colour.

In this assay the zinc undecylenate (the base) reacts with sulphuric acid and neutralization takes place, after this reaction the excess unreacted sulphuric acid is determined by titrating with sodium hydroxide. The indicator is orange colour in acid medium and it changes to yellow colour upon neutralization which is the end point.

As the acid and alkali involved in this assay, it is called as acidimetry-alkalimetry method of titration and the neutralization takes place in this assay during titration hence this assay is also called as neutralization method. The chemical reactions of this assay are shown below.

$$\underset{\text{Zinc undecylenate}}{[CH_2{=}CH\text{-}(CH_2)_8COO]_2Zn} + H_2SO_4 \longrightarrow \underset{\text{Undeconoic acid}}{2\,CH_2{=}CH\text{-}(CH_2)_8COOH} + ZnSO_4$$

$$H_2SO_4 + 2\,NaOH \longrightarrow Na_2SO_4 + 2\,H_2O$$

***Uses:***

1. It is used as a topical antifungal agent.
2. It is also used for treating tinea capitis and dermatophytosis.

***Storage:*** It should be stored in well closed container and stored in cool place.

## Calamine I.P., B.P., U.S.P.

**(Synonym: Prepared calamine)**

Calamine is zinc oxide colored with a small quantity ferric oxide, it is faint pink color. It contains not less than 98% and not more than 100.5% of ZnO with reference to ignition of the substance.

**Commercial preparation:** Calamine is commercially prepared by heating zinc carbonate. The zinc oxide obtained is mixed with 1% of ferric oxide.

$$ZnCO_3 \xrightarrow{\Delta} ZnO + CO_2\uparrow$$

***Properties:*** It is a fine amorphous impalpable pink or reddish brown powder (due to the presence of ferric oxide). It is almost odorless and tasteless. It is insoluble in water but completely soluble in mineral acids, the coloring matter is insoluble and harmless.

***Test for identification:*** To the small quantity of sample add dilute hydrochloric acid, heat it and filter. To the filtrate add one or two drops of ammonium thiocyanate solution. A reddish color is produced.

The solution of calamine in dilute hydrochloric acid gives the characteristic reactions of zinc ions.

***Test for purity:*** It should be tested for acid insoluble substances, arsenic, lead, calcium, chlorides, sulphate, alkaline substances, water and ethanol soluble dyes and loss on ignition.

***Test for water soluble substances:*** Small amount of sample is dissolved in water and filter it. The filtrate should be colorless.

***Test for ethanol soluble substances:*** Small amount of sample is dissolved in ethanol and filter it. The filtrate should be colorless.

**Assay**

***Principle:*** It is assayed by **acidimetry-alkalimetry method of (Back) titration** (also called **neutralization method**).

In this assay the substance is ignited and dissolved in Known Excess Standard (KES) 1N sulphuric acid and the Excess Unreacted (EUR) sulphuric acid is titrated with 1N sodium hydroxide using methyl orange as an indicator. End point is the yellow colour. As the zinc hydroxide intereferes in detection of end point results in poor end point. Hence ammonium chloride is used to prevent the precipitation of zinc hydroxide.

In this assay upon ignition of the calamine followed by treatment with sulphuric acid, the zinc oxide (the base) goes into the solution in sulphuric acid and neutralization takes place, after this reaction, the excess unreacted sulphuric acid is determined by titrating with sodium hydroxide. The indicator is orange colour in acid medium and it changes to yellow colour upon neutralization which is the end point.

As the acid and alkali involved in this assay, it is called as acidimetry-alkalimetry method of titration and the neutralization takes place in this assay during titration hence this assay is also called as neutralization method. The chemical reactions of this assay are shown below.

$$ZnO + H_2SO_4 \longrightarrow ZnSO_4 + H_2O$$

$$H_2SO_4 + 2\,NaOH \longrightarrow Na_2SO_4 + 2\,H_2O$$

***Procedure:*** Weigh accurately about 1.5 gm and digest with 50.0 ml of 0.5M sulphuric acid, applying gentle heat until no further solution occurs. Filter and wash the residue with hot water until the last washing is neutral to litmus paper. To the combined filtrate and washings, add 2.5 gm of ammonium chloride cool and titrate with 1 M sodium hydroxide using methyl orange solution as indicator.

*Uses:*

1. It is mainly used as an antiseptic, mild astringent and topical protectant for skin.
2. Due to its soothing effect, it is used in ointments and lotions.

***Dose:*** It varies according to the formulations.

***Storage:*** It should be stored in tightly closed containers and protected from sunlight.

***Official preparations of Calamine:*** The following preparations are the official formulations for calamine and are included in various pharmacopoeias.

1. Aqueous calamine cream I.P.
2. Calamine lotion I.P.
3. Calamine ointment I.P.

## Calamine Lotion I.P.

***Ingredients:***

| | | |
|---|---|---|
| Calamine | = | 150 gm |
| Zinc oxide | = | 50 gm |
| Bentonite | = | 30 gm |
| Sodium citrate | = | 5 gm |
| Liquefied phenol | = | 5 ml |
| Glycerin | = | 50 ml |

Purified water freshly boiled and cooled, sufficient to produce - 1000 ml.

***Procedure:*** Triturate the calamine, zinc oxide and bentonite with the solution of sodium citrate in 700 ml of purified water and add liquefied phenol, glycerin and sufficient quantity of purified water to make 1000 ml.

***Test for identification***

1. To the small amount of sample solution, add 2 ml of periodic acid solution shake and centrifuge. To the supernatant liquid, add 2 ml of ammonical silver nitrate solution. A silver mirror is produced on the walls of the test tube.
2. The neutral solution of sample gives the characteristic reactions of zinc salts.

***Test for purity:*** It should be tested for microbial contamination.

*Uses:*

1. It is used as a skin protective in sunburn preparation due to its soothing effect.
2. It is also acts as an anti-itching agent.

***Storage:*** Similar to calamine.

## Aqueous Calamine Cream I.P.

It contains not less than 6.3% and not more than 7.67% w/w of ZnO.

**Composition:**

| | | |
|---|---|---|
| Calamine | = | 40 gm |
| Zinc oxide | = | 30 gm |
| Liquid paraffin | = | 200 gm |
| Cetosteryl alcohol | = | 40 gm |
| Cetomacrogol 1000 | = | 10 gm |
| Phenoxy ethanol | = | 5 gm |
| Self emulsifying glyceryl monostearate | = | 50 gm |
| Purified water, freshly boiled and cooled | = | 625 gm |

Melt together the cetosteryl alcohol and cetomacrogol 1000, stir until cold and dissolve this mixture. Dissolve self emulsifying glyceryl mono stearate in the liquid paraffin at 60 °C. Add with rapid stirring to a phenoxy ethanol solution in purified water at the same temperature and stir until cold. Triturate the calamine and zinc oxide with the remaining of the purified water and incorporate or mix with the cream by stirring.

***Test for identification:*** The residue obtained after ignition is yellow when hot and white upon cooling.

***Test for purity:*** It should be complies with tests for creams.

**Assay**

Similar to calamine.

***Storage:*** It should be stored in well closed container at the temperature of not exceeding 30 °C. Do not freeze.

***Uses:*** It is used as a skin protective in sunburn preparation.

## Calamine Ointment I.P.

It contains not less than 7.8% and not more than 9.4% of ZnO.

***Ingredients:***

| | | |
|---|---|---|
| Calamine | = | 150 gm |
| White soft paraffin | = | 850 gm |

Triturate the required quantity of calamine with small amount of white soft paraffin until smooth and gradually add the remaining portion of white soft paraffin.

***Test for identification:*** Similar to calamine.

***Test for purity:*** It should be complies with the tests for ointments.

**Assay**

***Procedure:*** Weigh accurately about 1.0 gm. Heat gently until the base is completely volatilized or charred. Increase the heat until all the carbon is removed and ignite the residue until, after further ignition, two successive weighing do not differ by more than 0.2% of the weight of the residue.

***Storage:*** It should be stored in well closed containers, the temperature of not exceeding 30 °C

***Labelling:*** The label of this preparation should states that

(i) The concentration of calamine

(ii) The preparation is intended for external use only and

(iii) The storage conditions

## Zinc Stearate I.P., B.P., U.S.P.

**Mol. Formula:** $[C_{17}H_{35}COO]_2Zn$ **Mol. Weight:** 632.3

It mainly consists of zinc stearate but many of them contain various proportions of zinc palmitate and zinc oleate. It contains not less than 10% and not more than 12% of zinc.

***Preparation:*** Zinc stearate is prepared by the reaction between zinc sulphate or various zinc salts and commercial stearic acid or its salts (sodium stearate) and washing the precipitate until completely free from sulphate and dry it. Preparation of zinc stearate involves the following steps:

*Step 1:* Sodium stearate is prepared by gradually adding the calculated amount of stearic acid to a hot solution of sodium hydroxide or sodium carbonate with constant stirring. The commercial stearic is used for the preparation of sodium stearate.

$$NaOH + C_{17}H_{35}COOH \longrightarrow C_{17}H_{35}COONa + H_2O$$

$$Na_2CO_3 + 2\,C_{17}H_{35}COOH \longrightarrow 2\,C_{17}H_{35}COONa + CO_2\uparrow + H_2O$$

*Step 2: Preparation of zinc stearate:* The sodium stearate produced by the above method is cooled and the zinc sulphate solution is added to it. Zinc stearate is precipitated out and then washed with water, filtered and dried.

$$2\,C_{17}H_{35}COONa + ZnSO_4 \longrightarrow [C_{17}H_{35}COO]_2Zn + Na_2SO_4$$

***Physical properties:*** It is a white, fine amorphous powder, free from grittiness. It has faint and characteristic odour, tasteless, unctuous to touch and readily adheres to the skin. It is insoluble in water and alcohol. Its suspension has neutral pH.

***Test for identification***

1. The neutral solution of the sample gives the characteristic reactions of zinc salts.
2. To a small amount of sample in ether solution, add little dilute nitric acid and distilled water. Allow to cool, separate the aqueous layer, washed with water and heat it until the complete evolution of ether. Allow to cool, dilute with required volume of water, evaporate to dryness and dry the residue at 105 °C. The freezing point of the residue is not less than 53 °C.

***Test for purity:*** It should be tested for clarity and color of the solution, acidity and alkalinity, alkalis and alkaline earths, arsenic, heavy metals, chlorides, sulphates and free fatty acids.

## Assay

### *Principle:*

*Method 1:* It is assayed by **acidimetry-alkalimetry method of (Back) titration** (also called **neutralization method**).

In this assay the substance is boiled with Known Excess Standard (KES) 0.1N sulphuric acid and the excess unreacted sulphuric acid is determined by titrating with 0.1N sodium hydroxide using methyl orange as an indicator. End point is the yellow colour.

In this assay the zinc stearate (the base) reacts with sulphuric acid and neutralization takes place, after this reaction the excess unreacted sulphuric acid is determined by titrating with sodium hydroxide. The indicator is orange colour in acid medium and it changes to yellow colour upon neutralization which is the end point.

As the acid and alkali involved in this assay, it is called as acidimetry-alkalimetry method of titration and the neutralization takes place in this assay during titration hence this assay is also called as neutralization method.

$$(C_{17}H_{35}COO)_2Zn + H_2SO_4 \longrightarrow 2\,C_{17}H_{35}COOH + ZnSO_4$$

$$H_2SO_4 + 2\,NaOH \longrightarrow Na_2SO_4 + 2\,H_2O$$

*Method 2:* It is assayed by **Complexometry method of (Back) titration.**

In this assay the substance is dissolved 2M acetic acid and dilute to 50 ml with water. To this solution hexamine added as a buffer and xylenol orange as an indicator and titrated against disodium edetate. End point is the appearance of yellow colour.

In this assay zinc ions of zinc sterate reacts with EDTA, whereby the complexation takes place. As the zinc ions forms complex with disodium EDTA in this assay, it is called as complexometry method of titration. The chemical reactions of this assay are shown below.

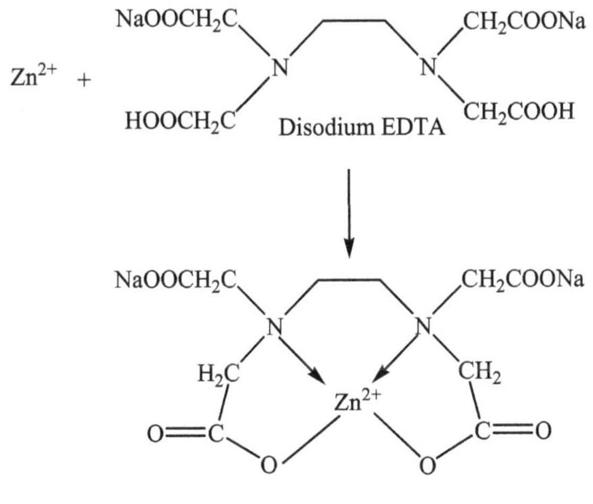

$Zn^{2+}$ + $(NaOOCH_2C)(HOOCH_2C)N{-}CH_2CH_2{-}N(CH_2COONa)(CH_2COOH)$

Disodium EDTA

↓

Zinc-EDTA Complex

***Procedure:*** Weigh accurately about 1.0 gm and boil with 50 ml of 2M acetic acid until the fatty acid layer which separates is clear, adding more water if necessary to maintain the original volume. Cool, filter and wash the filter and the flask thoroughly with water until the last washing is not acidic to blue litmus paper. To the combined filtrate and washings add about 50 mg of xylenol orange triturate and sufficient hexamine to produce violet-pink colour. Add a further 2 gm of hexamine and titrate with 0.1M disodium edetate until the colour changes to yellow.

***Uses:***

1. It is mainly used as mild astringent and it contains antimicrobial properties
2. Due to its protective property, it is used in dermatology.
3. It is also used in water repellant ointments and dusting powders.
4. In children its use should be discouraged because its inhalation causes pulmonary inflammation.
5. It acts as a lubricant in tablet preparation.

***Storage:*** It should be stored in non metallic containers and protected from sunlight.

## Titanium Dioxide I.P., U.S.P.

**Mol. Formula:** $TiO_2$ **Mol. Weight:** 79.9

Titanium is having valences of three and four. Titanium is mainly present in the minerals as dioxide form. The minerals of titanium are Rutile, brookite, anatase and the very important mineral is ilmenite (Ferrous titanate).

It contains not less than 98% and not more than 100.5% of $TiO_2$.

***Preparation:***

1. *From ilmenite:* Titanium dioxide is prepared by treating ilmenite with hydrochloric acid and chlorine.

$$2\,FeTiO_3 + 4\,HCl + Cl_2 \rightleftharpoons 2\,TiO_2 + 2\,FeCl_3 + 2\,H_2O$$

The resulting precipitate of titanium dioxide is filtered off, washed and calcined to give the anhydrous titanium dioxide.

2. *From Rutile:* The rutile ore is heated with concentrated sulphuric acid when iron sulphate and titanium sulphate is dissolved in water, the titanium dioxide obtained is separated by hydrolysis.

***Physical properties:*** It is a white or white fluffy powder or infusible powder, odorless and tasteless. It is practically insoluble in water and dilute mineral acids. It is slowly soluble in hot sulphuric acid, hydrofluoric acid; the solubility in water is increased by fusion with potassium bisulphate or with alkali hydroxides or carbonates to form alkali titanates. It is a high opaque compound.

***Chemical properties:*** *Reaction with hydrogen peroxide:* Titanium dioxide reacts with hydrogen peroxide in the presence of dilute sulphuric acid and gives orange red color solution (due to the formation of titanium trioxide).

$$TiO_2 + H_2O_2 \xrightarrow{Dil.H_2SO_4} TiO_3 + H_2O$$

***Test for identification***

1. When strongly heated it becomes pale yellow, the color is discharged when cooling.
2. To the required quantity of the sample add very less amount of zinc (0.5 gm) granules, keep it stand for 45 minutes. Violet blue color is formed.
3. To a small quantity of sample add anhydrous sodium sulphate, water and sulphuric acid. Heat on water bath, cool slowly, add 25% v/v solution of sulphuric acid and make up to 100 ml. To the 10 ml of above solution, add strong hydrogen peroxide solution, an orange red color is produced.

***Test for purity:*** It should be tested for clarity and color of the solution, acidity or alkalinity, water soluble substances, arsenic, barium, heavy metals and iron.

**Assay**

***Principle:*** It is assayed by **Complexometry method of (Back) titration**.

In this assay the substance is dissolved in a mixture of sulphuric acid and ammonium sulphate by heating. To the solution was added strong ammonia solution, hydrogen peroxide and Known Excess Standard (KES) 0.05N disodium Ethylene Diamine Tetra Acetate (EDTA) and allow it to stand. Adjust the pH to 5.0 by adding sodium hydroxide solution and add hexamine as a buffer and xylenol orange as an indicator and titrate against 0.05M zinc chloride. End point is the appearance of violet colour due to the formation of zinc-xylenol orange complex.

In this assay titanium ions of titanium dioxide reacts EDTA, whereby the complexation takes place, after this reaction, the Excess Unreacted (EUR) disodium EDTA is determined by titrating with zinc chloride. The indicator is colourless before complexation and change into violet colour due to the formation of zinc-xylenol orange complex. As the titanium ions forms complex with disodium EDTA in this assay, it is called as complexometry method of titration. The chemical reactions of this assay are shown below.

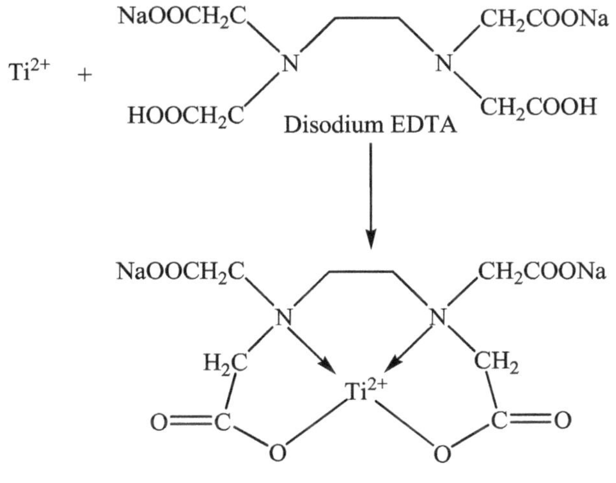

$Ti^{2+}$ + ($NaOOCH_2C$, $HOOCH_2C$)N–CH₂CH₂–N($CH_2COONa$, $CH_2COOH$)

Disodium EDTA

↓

($NaOOCH_2C$)N(–$H_2C$–C(=O)–O–)→$Ti^{2+}$←N(–$CH_2$–C(=O)–O–)($CH_2COONa$)

Titanium-EDTA Complex

***Uses:***

1. It is mainly used as a good topical protective in eczema.
2. It is used for the relief of pruritus and in certain case of exudative dermatoses.
3. It is used to prevent sun burns.
4. Due to its high refractive index, it is useful for preparation of various sun creams and also acts as delustering agent for regenerated cellulose.
5. Purified grade is used for food colors.
6. Due to its solar ray protective property it is useful in a concentration of 5 to 25% in ointments and lotions.
7. It is also used as a white pigment in cosmetics and paints.
8. It is also used as an opacifying agent for the preparation of hard gelatin capsules and tablet coatings.

***Storage:*** It should be stored in tightly closed containers and protected from light. Avoid contact with aluminium.

---

## Light Kaolin

This compound is discussed under **adsorbents and protectives**.

---

## Heavy Kaolin

This compound is discussed under **adsorbents and protectives**.

---

## Silicone Polymers
## Silicone

**Atomic symbol:** Si **Atomic Weight:** 28.09

It is the most abundant of all the elements apart from oxygen and makes up more than a quarter of the material of solid crust of the earth (28%). It belongs to the Group IV element in the periodic table. It is distributed as its oxide ($SiO_2$) and silicates. Silicon forms covalent compound, which leads to chains and polymers. It also undergo substitution with carbon containing radicals like methyl, ethyl etc. These are called as organo-silicon compounds.

***Preparation:*** Silicon dioxide is an anhydride of silicic acid ($H_4SiO_4$ or thiosilicic acid). Two molecules of silicic acid lose one water molecule between themselves giving rise to disilicic acid. Similarly a chain compound polysilicic acid can be obtained by condensation of several silicic acid molecules. Polysilicic acid has high affinity with water. These are called as silica gels and have many applications.

Silicone polymers are obtained by substitution of silicic acid by organic alkyl or aryl radicals.

The inter relationship of these compounds are mentioned as follows.

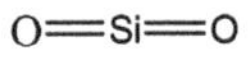

Silicon dioxide

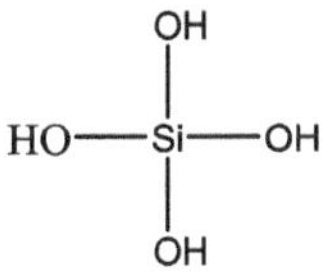

Orthosilicic acid

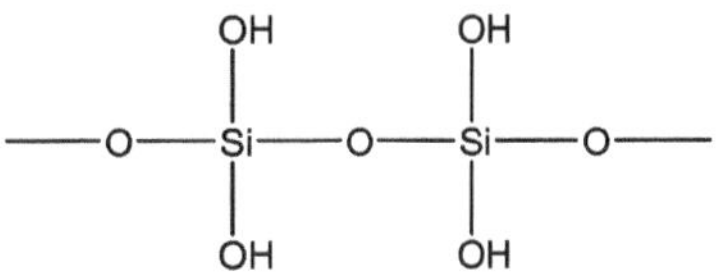

Part of poly silicic acid chain

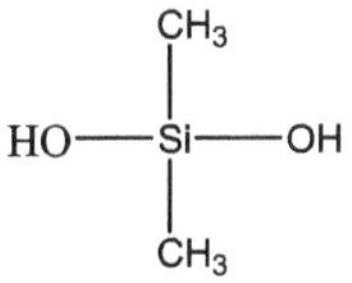

Dimethyl silanediol

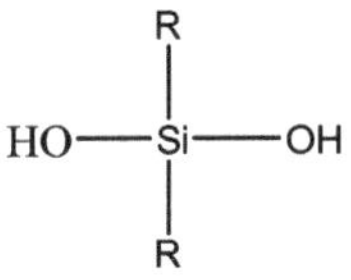

Organo silanediol

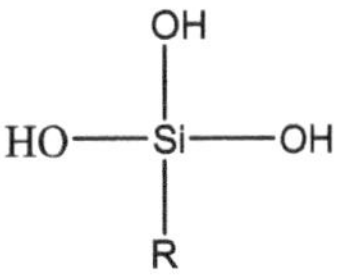

Organo silanetriol

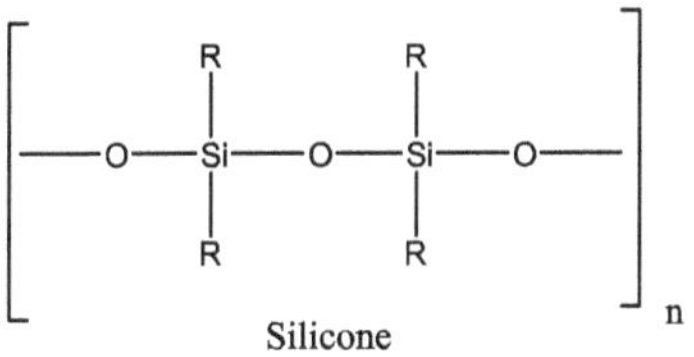

Silicone
(Poly-organo-siloxane)
Linear polymer

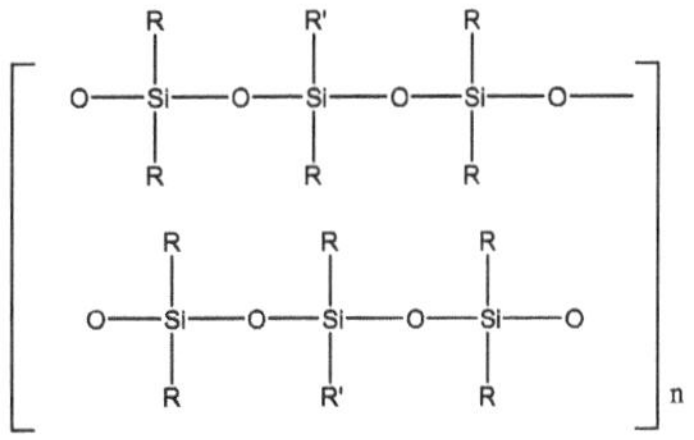

Silicone (poly-organo-siloxane) cross linked polymer. The above silicone polymers are otherwise called as silicone oils. The "n" indicates the changes in viscosity. These are prepared synthetically by the following methods.

$$\underset{\text{Silicone tetrachloride}}{SiCl_4} \xrightarrow{RMgX} \underset{\text{Dichlorosilane}}{R_2SiCl_2} \xrightarrow{H_2O} \underset{\text{Dialkyl silanediol}}{R_2Si(OH)_2}$$

$$R_2Si(OH)_2 \xrightarrow{\text{Polymerisation}} \text{Silicone linear polymer}$$

$$R_2Si(OH)_2 + RSi(OH)_3 \xrightarrow{\text{Polymerisation}} \text{Silicone Cross linked Polymer}$$

The molecular weight, cross linking of the polymers is controlled by limiting the amounts of polymerizing molecules and conditions of polymerization.

***Properties:*** These are colorless, odorless, oily liquids which repels water. They are miscible with organic low polar and non-polar solvents like benzene, ether, chloroform, xylene, cyclohexane, kerosene, ethyl acetate etc. Silicon fluids with almost every viscosity are available. The marketed products are actually graded on this property and numbered accordingly. For example, dimethicone 200, the viscosity between 190 and 200 centistokes. These are highly stable, chemically and biologically inactive fluids, which withstand high temperatures. These find a variety of application in pharmacy and industry.

## Dimethicone U.S.P.

It is a poly dimethyl siloxane of grade 200 obtained by hydrolysis and poly condensation of dichloro dimethyl silane and chloro trimethyl silane. Other grades up to 500 may also be available.

$$(H_3C)_3Si-O-[Si(CH_3)_2-O]_n-Si(CH_3)_3$$

It contains not less than 97% and not more than 103% of poly dimethyl siloxane.

***Properties:*** It is a clear, colorless liquid with various viscosities, practically insoluble in water.

***Test for identification***

1. It is identified by its kinematic viscosity at 25 °C and examined by IR spectrophotome try.
2. The residue obtained after ignition of the sample gives the characteristic reactions of silicates.

***Test for purity:*** It should be tested for acidity, viscosity, heavy metals, phenylated compounds, mineral oils and volatile matters.

***Uses:***

1. It is mainly used as an anti foaming agent and water repellant.
2. It has skin adherent properties. The adherent layer remains for several hours and it will not be washed away by water or soap solution. Organic solvents are used to remove the film.
3. These are also used in barrier creams, lotions, ointments etc. to help in protecting skin.
4. It is also used in pulmonary edema and in flatulence.
5. It is used as pharmaceutical aid and in cosmetics.
6. It is also used as bacterial endo toxins.

## Activated Dimethicone or Simethicone I.P., B.P., U.S.P.

**(Synonym: Activated polydimethyl siloxane)**

**Mol. Formula:** $(CH_3)_3Si[OSi(CH_3)_2]_nCH_3 \cdot SiO_2$

It is a mixture of fully methylated linear siloxane polymer containing repeating units of $(CH_3)_2SiO$ stabilized with tri methylsiloxy, $(CH_3)_3Si$ end blocking units and finely divided silicon dioxide. It contains not less than 90% and not more than 99% of poly dimethyl siloxane $[-(CH_3)_2\ SiO-]_n$ and not less than 4% and not more than 7% of silicon dioxide $(SiO_2)$.

$$H_3C-\left[Si(CH_3)_2-O\right]_n-Si(CH_3)_2-CH_3 \cdot SiO_2$$

***Properties:*** It occurs as a translucent, odorless, grey color and viscous liquid.

***Test for identification:*** Similar to dimethicone.

***Test for purity:*** It should be tested for acidity, heavy metals and defoaming activity.

**Assay**

***Procedure***

*For Silica:* Heat not less than 20.0 mg to 800 °C increasing the temperature by 20 °C/min under a current of nitrogen at a flow rate of 200 ml/min and weigh the residue (silica).

*Poly (dimethylsiloxane):* Infrared absorption spectrophotometry.

***Uses:***

1. It is used as a defoaming agent.
2. It is often used along with antacid preparation to facilitate defoaming and decrease distension caused by gas and gastric acid. It does not reduce the dose of antacid.
3. It also used as an antiflatulent, antacid, antispasmodic, sedative and digestant.

***Dose:*** 40 – 100 mg, four times daily.

***Storage:*** It should be stored in well closed container and protected from moisture.

## Aluminium as Protecting Agent - Aluminium

**Atomic symbol:** Al **Atomic weight:** 26.98

Aluminium is official in U.S.P XVII. It is a silver white metal with density of 2.7. It is a fine, free flowing, and silver colored powder free from grittiness. It possesses high affinity with oxygen atom. It is insoluble in water and alcohol. It reacts with concentrated HCl and sulphuric acid to give hydrogen and aluminium chloride.

**Assay**

***Procedure:*** Transfer 0.2 gm, previously freed from lubricant by successive washing with acetone and drying, to a three-necked 500 ml flask fitted with a 150 ml dropping funnel, an inlet tube connected to a cylinder of carbon dioxide and an outlet tube dipping into a water trap. Add 60 ml of water and disperse the substance being examined; replace the air by carbon dioxide and add 100 ml of a solution containing 56 gm of ammonium iron (III) sulphate and 7.5 ml of sulphuric acid in water. While maintaining an atmosphere of carbon dioxide in the flask, heat to boiling, boil for 5 minutes after the sample has dissolved, cool rapidly to 20 °C and dilute to 250 ml with water. To 50 ml add 15 ml of orthophosphoric acid and titrate with 0.02M potassium permanganate.

***Uses***:

1. 10% of aluminium is present in aluminium paste, which is used as a protective to prevent the irritation around the intestinal fistulae.
2. The pure aluminium foil is used for the dressings of burns.
3. It is also used in application around the colostomy opening after surgery for intestinal cancer.
4. Aluminium acetate solution or Burow's solution is used as an antiseptic and astringent.
5. Aluminium hydroxy chloride solution is used as an antiperspirant.

### 6.2.2 Minor Topical Agents

Other than all of the above individual compounds some of the compounds are used as minor topical agents. Sometimes zirconium compounds are used as minor topical agents.

***For example***:

1. Zirconium carbonate is used as a medicament for athlete's foot, antiperspirant.
2. Zirconium silicate is showing the property similar to that of titanium dioxide like shipping and clinging powder on the skin, so it is used in cosmetics. Now a days the usage of zirconium compounds are stopped due to their skin irritating properties.
3. White lotion is used for the treatment of seborrhea dermatitis.

### 6.2.3 Astringents

***Introduction***: Astringents are the substances which precipitate the proteins, but do not penetrate into cells, thus affecting superficial layer only. They toughen the surface making it mechanically stronger and decrease exudation. These are generally describes as a firming or shrinkage of the tissue. A very dilute solution of metal cation is applied to tissues primarily produces local or surface protein precipitation action. These agents causes the constriction of small capillaries and small blood vessels, hence they are used to styptics (stop bleeding from small cuts). Example: Tannic acid and tannins, alcohol, mineral astringents (Heavy metal ions). By this way they protect the mucosa by firming up the mucosal surface. They are also used to decrease the exudates from wounds and skin eruption. These are present as antiperspirants in deodorants due to their ability to constrict pores and destroy microbes that induce or produce body odors but the concentration needed is more than that of antimicrobial activity.

During the application of astringents to the wounds topically they stimulate the growth of new tissue. By using higher concentrated solution leads to irritation but further increases in concentration that solution have a corrosive effect on contact with tissues. This property is used for the removal of undesirable tissue for e.g.: warts. Astringents are used to check discharge of blood serum or mucus secretions in conditions like sore throat, diarrhea and peptic ulcers. Topically, these are used in cuts, insect bites, acne and athlete's foot.

***Control of antiseptic/astringent action***: The inorganic antimicrobials are non specific in their action on pathogenic organism. The action against microbes versus host cells, the action depends upon their concentration according to this factor only their microbial effect and for minimizing unwanted action on host cells.

1. For water soluble compounds the antimicrobial activity depends upon the concentration of solution for the desired use. It varies according to their area of use. For example: Higher concentrations are used on the skin than in the eye.
2. Slow release preparations of the soluble substance are also used for controls their activity. For example: Controlled release antimicrobial action of hydrogen peroxide in glycerin or poly ethylene glycol (Glycerite of hydrogen peroxide).
3. For minimizing the toxicity and activity against the host cells is accomplished by complexation. For example: Povidone iodine.

The other insoluble synthetic compounds are used in the form of creams, ointments and suspensions to obtain better antimicrobial activity.

## Alum U.S.P.

**(Synonym: Potash alum, Ammonia alum)**

**Mol. Formula:** $KAl(SO_4)_2.\ 12H_2O$ **Mol. Weight:** 474.4

Alum is potassium aluminium sulphate. It is a double salt contains an amount of aluminium equivalent to not less than 99.5% and not more than the equivalent of 100.5% of $KAl(SO_4)_2.\ 12H_2O$.

In pharmacopoeia two types of alums are there. They may be either potassium or ammonium.

***Preparation*:** Alum is prepared by a adding a hot concentrated solution of potassium sulphate to the equimolar proportion of aluminium sulphate. Then the solution is concentrated and cooled, the octahedral crystals of alum is separated out. By slow crystallization large characteristic regular octahedral crystals are obtained.

$$K_2SO_4 + Al_2(SO_4)_3 + 24\ H_2O \longrightarrow 2\ KAl(SO_4)_2 \cdot 12\ H_2O$$

***Physical properties*:** It is a colorless, crystalline powder, deliquescent in nature. It has a sweet astringent taste. It is soluble in water but insoluble in alcohol.

***Chemical properties*:** When it is slowly heated on water bath it melts in water. At 200 °C it completely loses its water and becomes anhydrous.

$$2\ KAl(SO_4)_2 .12\ H_2O \xrightarrow{200\ ^\circ C} 2\ KAl(SO_4)_2 + 12\ H_2O$$

***Test for identification*:** The solution of alum gives the characteristic reactions of aluminium, potassium and sulphate ions.

***Test for purity*:** It should be tested for arsenic, iron, ammonium salts and heavy metals.

**Assay**

***Principle:***

*Method 1:* It is assayed by **gravimetric method**.

In this assay the substance is dissolved in water, to it ammonium chloride, methyl red and sufficient ammonia added to get distinct yellow colour. Heat the solution, filter and wash the filtrate with ammonium nitrate until it become free from chloride. The precipitate of aluminium trioxide is dried to a constant weight at 120 °C. As the test substance is converted to a precipitate, which is used for calculating the actual amount of alum present this is called Gravimetric assay.

*Method 2:* It is assayed by **Complexometry method of (Back) titration.**

In this assay the substance is dissolved in a mixture of water and acetic acid, add acetic acid-ammonium acetate buffer, Known Excess Standard 0.1M disodium edetate and dithizone as indicator and titrate the excess of disodium edetate with 0.1M zinc sulphate. End point is the appearance of bright rose pink color.

In this assay, aluminium ions of alum react with disodium EDTA, whereby the complexation takes place. As the aluminium ions forms complex with disodium EDTA in this assay, it is called as complexometry method of titration. The chemical reactions of this assay are shown below.

$Al^{3+}$ + $NaOOCH_2C$, $HOOCH_2C$ –N–$CH_2CH_2$–N– $CH_2COONa$, $CH_2COOH$

Disodium EDTA

↓

$NaOOCH_2C$ –N–$CH_2CH_2$–N– $CH_2COONa$; $H_2C$–C(=O)–O → $Al^{3+}$ ← O–C(=O)–$CH_2$; N → $Al^{3+}$ ← N

Aluminium-EDTA Complex

***Procedure*:** Accurately weigh 800 mg of sample, transfer in to a 400 ml beaker, moisten with 1 ml of glacial acetic acid, and add 50 ml of disodium edetate and 20 ml of acetic acid-ammonium acetate buffer. Warm on a steam bath until get a clear solution, and boil gently for 5 minutes. Cool, add 50 ml of alcohol and 2 ml of dithizone and titrate against 0.05M zinc sulphate. End point is the appearance of bright rose pink color. Perform blank determination also.

*Uses*:

1. It is mainly used as a pharmaceutical aid.
2. It is also used for the preparation of oxides.
3. Alum precipitates proteins and it is a powerful topical astringent.
4. It is also used as a haemostatic agent and for hyperhydrosis and local styptic

***Caution***: Large doses of alum may be corrosive and irritant. It causes gum necrosis and GIT hemorrhage. Adverse effects on muscles and kidneys have been reported.

***Storage:*** It should be stored in well closed containers.

---

## Aluminium Chloride U.S.P.

**Mol. Formula:** $AlCl_3.\ 6H_2O$ **Mol. Weight:** 241.43

It contains not less than 95% of aluminium chloride hexahydrate which is calculated on dried basis.

***Preparation:***

*Method 1:* Aluminium hydroxide is treated with hydrochloric acid, concentrate the liquid, allow it to cool. The crystals of aluminium chloride separates out.

$$Al(OH)_3 + 3\ HCl + 3H_2O \longrightarrow AlCl_3.\ 6H_2O$$

*Method 2:* Aluminium metal is heated with a current of chlorine and the product obtained is dissolved in water and crystallized.

$$2\ Al + 3\ Cl_2 \longrightarrow 2\ AlCl_3$$

***Physical properties***: It is a colorless, crystalline powder. It is deliquescent in nature. It has sweet astringent taste, mild odor. It is freely soluble in water and alcohol. The solution of the sample is acidic to litmus due the liberation of hydrochloric acid by hydrolysis. The hydrochloric acid formed irritates body tissues hence buffering of the solution is necessary one.

***Test for identification***: The solution of aluminium chloride gives the characteristic reactions of aluminium, and chloride ions.

***Test for purity***: It should be tested for arsenic iron, sulphate and heavy metals.

**Assay**

***Principle***: It is assayed by **Complexometry method of (Back) titration**.

In this assay the substance is dissolved in 1N hydrochloric acid by warming, to this Known Excess Standard (KES) 0.05N disodium Ethylene Diamine Tetra Acetate (EDTA) added and the solution is neutralised with 1N sodium hydroxide using methyl red as an indicator (colour change from red to yellow). To this solution hexamine added as a buffer and xylenol orange as an indicator and titrated against 0.05M lead nitrate. End point is the appearance of violet colour due to the formation of lead-xylenol orange complex.

In this assay aluminium ions of aluminium chloride reacts with EDTA, whereby the complexation takes place, after this reaction, the excess unreacted disodium EDTA is determined by titrating with lead nitrate. The indicator is colourless before complexation and change into violet colour due to the formation of lead-xylenol orange complex. As the aluminium ions forms complex with disodium EDTA in this assay, it is called as complexometry method of titration. The chemical reactions of this assay are shown below.

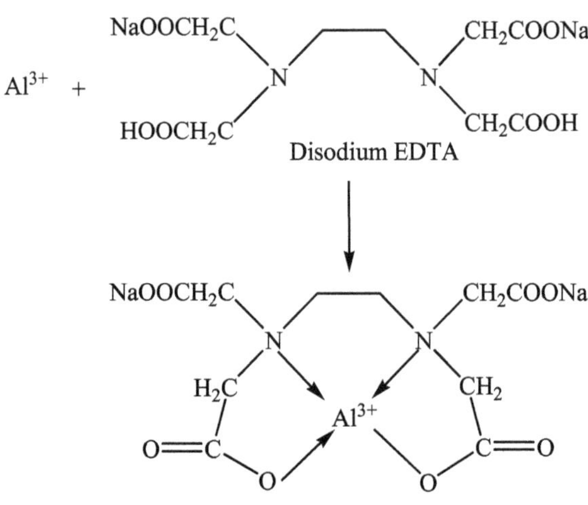


Aluminium-EDTA Complex

***Uses:***

1. It is used as local, external mild antiseptic and astringent.
2. It is used in aqueous solution in the concentration ranges between 10 to 25%. The solutions are too irritating to the sensitive tissues, so it cannot be used currently.

***Storage*:** It should be stored in well closed containers.

## Aluminium Sulphate B.P., U.S.P.

**Mol. Formula:** $Al_2 (SO_4)_3 . X H_2O$ **Mol. Weight:** 342.12

It contains not less than 51% and not more than 59% of aluminium sulphate with varying amount of water for crystallization.

***Preparation*:** It is prepared by dissolving aluminium hydroxide in sulphuric acid.

The solution is concentrated and allowed to crystallize, when the octadecahydrate is obtained.

$$2\,Al(OH)_3 + 3\,H_2SO_4 \longrightarrow Al_2(SO_4)_3 + 6\,H_2O$$

***Properties*:** It occurs as a white, crystalline powder or crystalline fragment or shining plates with sweet taste, very soluble in water to gives acidic solution due to hydrolysis.

$$Al_2(SO_4)_3.6\,H_2O \longrightarrow 2\,Al(OH)_3 + 3\,H_2SO_4$$

***Test for identification***: It gives the characteristic reactions of aluminium and sulphate ions.

***Test for purity***: It should be tested for pH, alkalis, alkaline earths, ammonium salts, arsenic, heavy metals and iron.

**Assay**

***Principle***: It is assayed by **Complexometry method of (Back) titration.**

In this assay the substance is dissolved in 1N hydrochloric acid by warming, to this Known Excess Standard (KES) 0.05N disodium Ethylene Diamine Tetra Acetate (EDTA) added and the solution is neutralised with 1N sodium hydroxide using methyl red as an indicator (colour change from red to yellow). To this solution hexamine added as a buffer and xylenol orange as an indicator and titrated against 0.05M lead nitrate. End point is the appearance of violet colour due to the formation of lead-xylenol orange complex.

In this assay aluminium ions of aluminium sulphate reacts with EDTA, whereby the complexation takes place, after this reaction, the excess unreacted disodium EDTA is determined by titrating with lead nitrate. The indicator is colourless before complexation and change into violet colour due to the formation of lead-xylenol orange complex. As the Aluminium ions forms complex with disodium EDTA in this assay, it is called as complexometry method of titration. The chemical reactions of this assay are shown below.

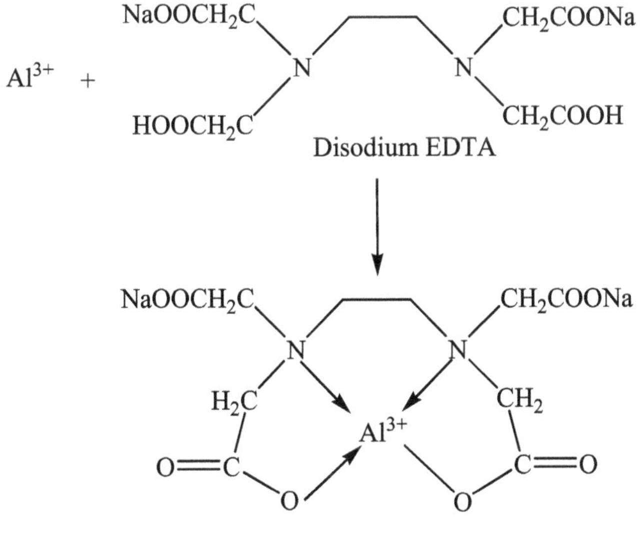

$Al^{3+}$ + $NaOOCH_2C$, $CH_2COONa$, N, N, $HOOCH_2C$, $CH_2COOH$

Disodium EDTA

↓

$NaOOCH_2C$, $CH_2COONa$, N, N, $H_2C$, $CH_2$, $Al^{3+}$, O=C, C=O, O, O

Aluminium-EDTA Complex

***Procedure***: Weigh accurately about 0.6 gm and dissolve in 2 ml of 1M hydrochloric acid and 50 ml of water. Add 50.0 ml of 0.05M disodium edetate and neutralise to methyl red solution with 1M sodium hydroxide. Heat the solution to boiling, leave on a water-bath for 10 minutes, cool rapidly and add about 50 mg of xylenol orange mixture and 5 gm of hexamine. Titrate with 0.05M lead nitrate. Carry out a blank titration.

***Uses:***

1. A 10% solution is used for disinfection of dental cavities (disinfectant)
2. A 5.25% solution is used for topical application.
3. A 10-15% is solution used as an anti perspirant in creams.
4. In solutions, the liquid form is used as deodorants.

***Storage*:** It should be stored in well closed containers.

---

## Aluminium Subacetate Solution U.S.P.

A 100 ml of aluminium subacetate solution is having not less than 2.3 gm and not more than 2.6 gm aluminium oxide, and not less than 5.4 gm and not more than 6.1 gm of acetic acid.

***Preparation*:** To prepare this, the dried precipitated calcium carbonate is added to a solution of aluminium sulphate.

$$3\ CaCO_3 + Al_2(SO_4)_3 + 3\ H_2O \longrightarrow 2\ Al(OH)_3 + 3\ CaSO_4 + 3\ CO_2\uparrow$$

To the above solution, acetic acid is added, and the mixture is filtered from the calcium sulphate, washed with water and volume is made. Sometimes boric acid is used as a stabilizer.

$$Al(OH)_3 + 2\ CH_3COOH \longrightarrow (CH_3COO)_2AlOH + 2\ H_2O$$

***Properties*:** It is a colorless or faint yellow liquid with acetous odor, on standing becomes turbid due to precipitation of a more basic salt.

***Uses*:**

1. It is used as a mouth wash or gargle for deodorant purpose.
2. It is diluted up to 20 to 40 times with water, the solution is used as an astringent wash or it is applied in wet dressings.

***Storage*:** It should be stored in well closed containers.

---

## Zinc Sulphate I.P., U.S.P.
### (Synonym: Hydrated zinc sulphate)

**Mol. Formula:** $ZnSO_4.\ 7H_2O$ **Mol. Weight:** 287.5

It contains not less than 99% and not more than 104% of $ZnSO_4.7H_2O$

***Preparation*:** For Pharmaceutical needs the zinc sulphate is prepared by treating or boiling zinc metal with dilute sulphuric acid. A slight excess of zinc metal is used and the reaction should be allowed to continue until evolution of $H_2$ gas ceases. Then the liquid is filtered off to remove the undissolved zinc metal and the resulting filtrate is treated with chlorine to remove the ferrous impurity. Then the filtrate is evaporated to crystallization and collect the crystals formed.

$$Zn + H_2SO_4 \longrightarrow ZnSO_4 + H_2\uparrow$$

***Common method***: Zinc sulphate is prepared by heating zinc blend (zinc sulphide) in the presence of air under specified conditions. The heated mass is dissolved in boiling water, filtered off; the resulting filtrate is collected and evaporated to crystallization.

$$ZnS + 2O_2 \longrightarrow ZnSO_4$$

***Properties***: It is a colorless, transparent crystals or a white crystalline powder, odorless, astringent and metallic taste, efflorescent in dry air. It is very soluble in water, freely soluble in glycerin and insoluble in alcohol. Aqueous solutions are acidic to litmus due to hydrolysis and the pH of the solution is 5.

***Test for identification***: The aqueous of solution sample in carbon dioxide free water gives the characteristic reactions of zinc and sulphate ions.

***Test for purity***: It should be tested for clarity and color of the solution, pH, arsenic, iron, aluminium, copper, magnesium, manganese and nickel, arsenic, chloride, alkalis and alkaline earths.

***Chemical properties:***

*Reaction with sodium hydroxide*: Zinc sulphate reacts with sodium hydroxide and forms zinc hydroxide as a white precipitate which is soluble in excess sodium hydroxide.

$$ZnSO_4 + 2\,NaOH \longrightarrow Zn(OH)_2 + Na_2SO_4$$

$$\underset{}{Zn(OH)_2} + \underset{\text{(Excess)}}{2\,NaOH} \longrightarrow \underset{\text{Sodium Zincate}}{Na_2ZnO_2} + 2\,H_2O$$

*Reaction with hydrogen sulphide*: Zinc sulphate reacts with hydrogen sulphide and forms white color zinc sulphide precipitate which is soluble in hydrochloric acid but remains insoluble in acetic acid.

$$ZnSO_4 + H_2S \longrightarrow \underset{\text{(White)}}{ZnS\downarrow} + H_2SO_4$$

*Reactions with potassium and ammonium salts*: It reacts with potassium and ammonium salts and forms double salts.

$$ZnSO_4 + K_2SO_4 \longrightarrow ZnSO_4.\,K_2SO_4$$

$$ZnSO_4 + (NH_4)_2SO_4 + 6\,H_2O \longrightarrow ZnSO_4.(NH_4)_2SO_4.6H_2O$$

*Decomposition reaction or reaction on heat or dehydration reaction:* Zinc sulphate when heated to 50 °C it losses the five water molecules and produce dihydrate, further it is heated up to 100 °C and 450 °C and it forms monohydrate and anhydrous salt respectively. When heated to higher temperature it forms zinc oxide and sulphur dioxide.

$$ZnSO_4.7H_2O \xrightarrow[-5H_2O]{50\ ^\circ C} ZnSO_4.2H_2O \xrightarrow[-H_2O]{100\ ^\circ C} ZnSO_4.H_2O$$

$$ZnSO_4.H_2O \xrightarrow[-H_2O]{450\ ^\circ C} ZnSO_4$$

$$SO2\uparrow + ZnO \xleftarrow{740\ ^\circ C} ZnSO_4$$

*Reaction with potassium ferro cyanide*: Zinc sulphate reacts with potassium ferro cyanide and forms zinc ferrous cyanide (white color precipitate).

$$2\ ZnSO_4 + K_4Fe(CN)_6 \longrightarrow Zn_2[Fe(CN)_6] + 2\ K_2SO_4$$

**Assay**

***Principle:*** *1st method:* It is assayed by **gravimetric method** of titration.

In this assay the substance is dissolved in water, heated. To the hot solution was added sodium carbonate solution until complete precipitation of zinc carbonate. The precipitate is washed, dried and ignited in Gooch crucible. During this assay, zinc sulphate reacts with sodium carbonate, whereby zinc carbonate is formed. Thus the formed zinc carbonate upon ignition yields zinc oxide, which is weighed, from the amount of zinc oxide the amount of zinc sulphate is calculated. As the test substance is converted to a precipitate, which is used for calculating the actual amount of zinc sulphate present this is called Gravimetric assay.

$$ZnSO_4 + Na_2CO_3 \longrightarrow ZnCO_3\downarrow + Na_2SO_4$$

$$ZnCO_3 \xrightarrow{\Delta} ZnO + CO_2\uparrow$$

*2nd method:* It is assayed by **complexometry method of (Direct) titration.**

In this assay the substance is dissolved in acetic acid, dilute and add hexamine and titrate against 0.05M disodium Ethylene Diamine Tetra Acetate (EDTA) using xylenol orange as an indicator. End point is the colour change to yellow.

In this assay zinc ions of zinc sulphate reacts with disodium EDTA, whereby the complexation takes place. As the zinc ions forms complex with disodium EDTA in this assay, it is called as complexometry method of titration. The chemical reactions of this assay are shown below.

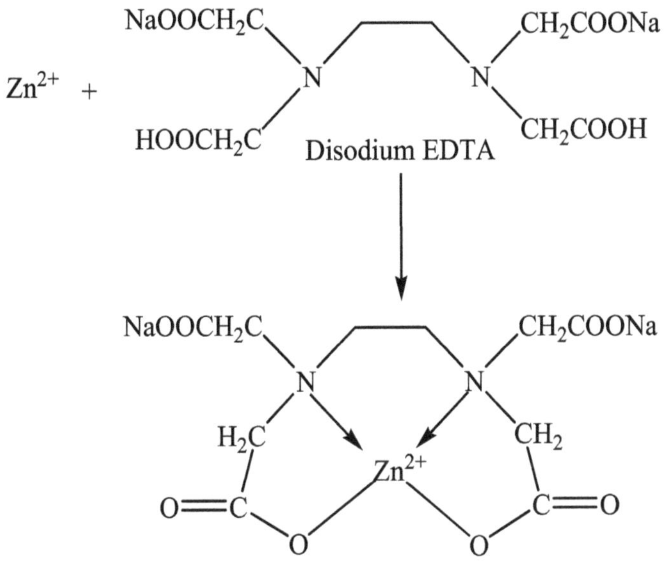

$$Zn^{2+} + \text{Disodium EDTA} \ (NaOOCH_2C, HOOCH_2C)N-CH_2CH_2-N(CH_2COONa, CH_2COOH) \longrightarrow \text{Zinc-EDTA Complex}$$

Disodium EDTA

Zinc-EDTA Complex

***Procedure*:** Weigh accurately about 0.5 gm and dissolve in 5 ml of 2M acetic acid and dilute to 50 ml with water. To the resulting solution add about 50 mg of xylenol orange triturate and sufficient hexamine to produce violet-pink colour. Add a further 2 gm of hexamine and titrate with 0.1M disodium edetate until the colour changes to yellow.

***Uses:***

1. It is mainly used as an astringent in lotions and eye drops.
2. It is used to treat zinc deficiency conditions like acrodermatitis, enteropathica.
3. It is also used as an emetic internally.
4. It is the one of the main ingredient of zinc sulphate eye drops.
5. A 0.2% solution is used for ophthalmic purpose:

***Dose*:** 0.6 to 2 gm.

***Storage*:** It should be stored in tightly closed, non metallic containers and protected from moisture.

**Other official formulations:** Zinc sulphate eye drops I.P.

## Zinc Chloride I.P., U.S.P.

**Mol. Formula:** $ZnCl_2$ **Mol. Weight:** 136.3

It contains not less than 95% and not more than 100.5% of $ZnCl_2$.

***Preparation*:**

1. *From metallic zinc*: Zinc chloride is prepared by treating metallic zinc with hydrochloric acid. The solution is evaporated to dryness.

$$Zn + 2\,HCl \longrightarrow ZnCl_2 + H_2\uparrow$$

2. *From zinc oxide or zinc carbonate*: Zinc oxide or zinc carbonate is reacted with hydrochloric acid to gives zinc chloride.

$$ZnO + 2\,HCl \longrightarrow ZnCl_2 + H_2O$$

$$ZnCO_3 + 2\,HCl \longrightarrow ZnCl_2 + H_2O + CO_2\uparrow$$

***Properties*:** A white crystalline powder or granules, odorless and very deliquescent in nature. It is very soluble in water, freely soluble in alcohol and glycerin. It is soluble in polar organic solvents. The aqueous solution is acidic to litmus.

It easily undergoes hydrolysis to gives hydrochloric acid and basic zinc chloride.

$$ZnCl_2 + H_2O \rightleftharpoons Zn(OH)Cl + HCl$$

***Test for identification*:** The aqueous solution of sample gives the characteristic reactions of zinc ion. A 5% w/v solution of sample in nitric acid gives the reactions of chloride ion.

***Test for purity*:** It should be tested for the pH of the solution, aluminium, calcium, heavy metals, iron and magnesium, ammonium salts, sulphate and oxychlorides.

***Test for oxychlorides*:** The aqueous solution of sample in boiling water is not more opalescence than that of standard opalescence which is prepared as per the monograph. Then add small volume of ethanol, the solution becomes cloudy within 10 minutes but becomes clear on the addition of one drop of hydrochloric acid.

**Assay**

***Principle*:** It is assayed by **Complexometry method of (Direct) titration.**

In this assay the substance is dissolved in water, to this ammonia-ammonium chloride solution is added as buffer solution and it is then titrated against 0.05M disodium Ethylene Diamine Tetra Acetate (EDTA) using eriochrome black T as an indicator. End point is the appearance of deep blue colour.

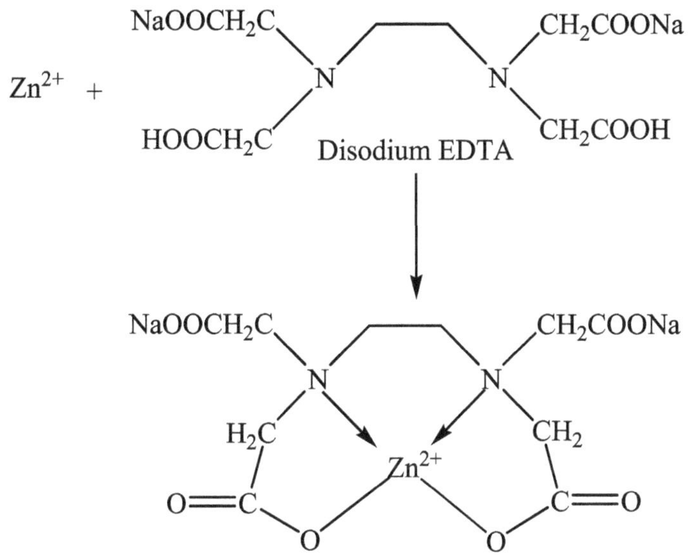

$Zn^{2+}$ + $NaOOCH_2C(HOOCH_2C)N{-}CH_2{-}CH_2{-}N(CH_2COONa)CH_2COOH$

Disodium EDTA

↓

Zinc-EDTA Complex

In this assay zinc ions of zinc chloride reacts with disodium EDTA, whereby the complexation takes place. As the zinc ions forms complex with disodium EDTA in this assay, it is called as complexometry method of titration. The chemical reactions of this assay are shown above.

***Procedure***: Weigh accurately about 3.0 gm, dissolve in 125 ml of water, add 3 gm of ammonium chloride and add sufficient water to produce 250 ml. To 25 ml of the resulting solution add 100 ml of water and 10 ml of strong ammonia-ammonium chloride solution. Titrate with 0.1M disodium edetate, using eriochrome black T solution as indicator until a deep blue colour is obtained.

***Uses:***

1. Zinc chloride is mainly used as a strong astringent and mild antiseptic.
2. Anhydrous zinc chloride is used as a condensing agent for the preparation of brilliant green.
3. The antiseptic and the protein precipitation properties are due to its interaction with some microbial enzymes.
4. It is also used as an astringent in various insulin preparations.
5. In dentistry, it is used as a desensitizer of dentin (Mouth washes).
6. It is also used in ulcers, pododermatitis and fistulas.

***Storage***: Due to its deliquescent property, it should be stored in tightly closed non metallic containers and protected from moisture.

## Zinc Peroxide U.S.P.

**(Synonym: Medicinal Zinc peroxide)**

**Mol. Formula:** $ZnO_2$ **Mol. Weight:** 97.39

***Preparation*:** It is prepared by treating concentrated hydrogen peroxide with very pure zinc oxide.

$$Zn(OH)_2 + H_2O_2 \longrightarrow ZnO_2 + 2\,H_2O$$

The final product contains zinc hydroxide ($Zn(OH)_2$) and zinc carbonate ($ZnCO_3$) due to unchanged zinc oxide and carbon dioxide. The composition of the particular compound is varying according to the conditions of the preparation.

***Physical properties:*** It is a white or slightly white powder.

***Test for identification:*** Similar to that of hydrogen peroxide.

***Test for purity:*** It should be tested for chloride, sulphate, alkali and alkaline earth metals.

***Test for alkali and alkaline earth metals:*** A small amount of sample solution is prepared by using dilute hydrochloric acid (zinc is converted into $ZnCl_2$). To this add ammoniacal ammonium sulphide solution. The zinc sulphide is filtered, acidified with dilute sulphuric acid, evaporated, ignited and the residue is weighed.

**Assay**

***Principle:*** It is assayed by **permanganometry method of titration** (also called **redox titration**).

In this assay the substance is dissolved in a mixture of water and dilute hydrochloric acid and solution is titrated against 0.1N potassium permanganate. Potassium permanganate is acting as a self indicator. End point is the appearance of permanent pale pink colour.

During this assay, hydro chloric acid first reacts with potassium permanganate and liberate nascent oxygen. Thus the liberated nascent oxygen oxidizes zinc peroxide. After the completion of this reaction, addition of potassium permanganate remains in the flask and its colour is retained i.e., permanent pale pink colour. As the oxidation and reduction takes place simultaneously this is called Redox titration. The chemical reactions of this assay are shown below.

$$2\,KMnO_4 + 6HCl \longrightarrow 2\,KCl + 2MnCl_2 + 3H_2O + 5(O)$$

$$3\,ZnO_2 + 3(O) \longrightarrow 3ZnO + 3\,O_2$$

*These equations can also be written as*

$$2\,KMnO_4 + 6HCl + 5ZnO_2 \longrightarrow 2KCl + 2\,MnCl_2 + 3\,H_2O + 5\,O_2 + 5ZnO$$

***Uses***

1. It is used as astringent, antiseptic and protective.
2. Due to its oxidative properties it is used in the treatment of infected wounds and dressings in post operative treatment.

### Calcium Hydroxide

This compound is discussed under the topic of **acidifiers and alkalinising agents**.

## 6.2.4 Oxidative Antimicrobials

***Introduction:*** Antimicrobials are drugs which are used for the treatment of systemic infections. There are different types of terms are applied or used for describing the antimicrobial activity.

**Terms used for describing antimicrobial activity**

***Germicides:*** The chemical substances or other agents which destroy microorganisms. These are having low margin of safety and for non systemic use.

Other terms used are as follows.

1. Disinfectants
2. Antiseptics
3. Sterilizing agents
4. Pasteurization
5. Decontamination agents
6. Sanitising agents
7. Preservatives

***Disinfectants:*** These are chemical substances or agents that are used to inhibit or destroy the growth of pathogenic vegetative bacteria on non- living surfaces like surgical instruments and glass wares. E.g.: Soaps, Ethanol, Phenols and Formaldehyde.

***Antiseptics:*** These are chemical substances or agents that are used to destroy pathogenic bacteria on living surfaces like skin and mucosal membranes. Some times at lower concentration disinfectants acts as antiseptic while at higher concentration same antiseptics acts as disinfectants. Both disinfectants and antiseptics are used to destroy the pathogenic organisms not their spores.

***Sterilizing agents:*** Chemical substances, which are used to destroy all living microorganism and their spores includes viruses and fungi are called as sterilizing agents.

***Pasteurization:*** Pasteurization means heating milk or semisolids or other liquids at 60 °C - 80 °C for half an hr that kills the non sporulating pathogens and prevents the food borne pathogens for a particular period of time.

***Decontamination:*** It means the destruction of viable microbes to a level that will allow a healthy person natural defenses to prevent any infection. Chemical substances, which are used for this purpose is called as decontamination agents. Example: Decontamination of water.

***Sanitization:*** It is a process of reduction in microbial load (surface up to levels to be considered acceptable for the health of population). Chemical substances, which are used for this purpose is called as Sanitizing agents.

***Preservation:*** It means to prevent the deterioration and to preserve the efficacy of drug or its formulations up to their expiry period. E.g.: Antioxidants, which are used to protect the drug from oxidation or may kill or inhibit the microbes inadvertently introduced during manufacturing or uses (antimicrobial/antifungal preservatives). These are mainly used in sterile preparations such as eye drops and parenteral preparations. These are also used in cosmetics and other non sterile formulations like oral liquids, creams and ointment to prevent deteriorations. Chemical substances, which are used for this purpose is called as preservatives.

Commonly used preservatives are benzoic acid and its salts, parabens etc. The most commonly used antimicrobial antioxidants are BHA (Butylated Hydroxy anisole) and BHT (Butylated Hydroxy Toluene). Some time the usage of citric acid and edetic acid along with antioxidant preservatives increases their efficacy.

Ideal characteristics of antiseptics:

1. It should be better effective even at shorter exposure.
2. It should have ability to kill the all vegetative forms of pathogens.
3. It should show the effectiveness at room temperature.
4. It should have the selective toxicity.

According to their site of action germicides are classified in to two types.

1. Internally used germicides.
2. Topically used germicides.

Internally used germicides are once again subdivided into systemic (absorbed) and non systemic (non absorbed).

***Systemic germicides:*** These compounds or substances are distributed through the blood stream and used to treat the infections of various organs and tissues.

***Non systemic germicide:*** They are producing the effects in the particular area where they applied for it.

**Mechanism of action:** According to their primary chemical interaction or reactions that occurs between antimicrobial agent and the microbial protein leads to the death of microbes or inhibition of their growth. The mechanism of action of inorganic antimicrobial agents are classified in to three types as mentioned here.

1. Oxidation
2. Halogenation and
3. Protein precipitation (or) coagulation

***Oxidation:*** Non metals and certain types of anions are acts by this mechanism. The main action of these types of agents involves the reducing groups present in the microbes. For example: The sulfhydryl group in cysteine. Compounds acts by this mechanism include iodophores (Iodine and all iodine solutions) chlorine and chlorophores (chlorinated lime, Dakin's solution and sodium hypochlorite solution) and other oxidizing agents such as potassium permanganate solution and hydrogen peroxide. The oxidizing antiseptic reacts

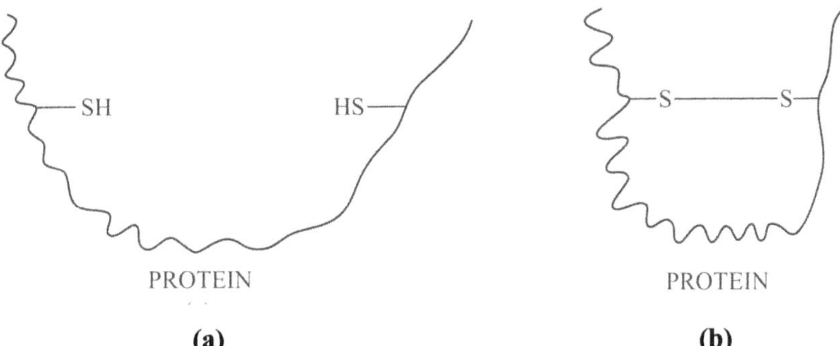


Fig. 6.2 An illustration of the action of oxidizing agents on protein-containing sulfhydryl groups. (a) The protein before oxidation showing the presence of free sulfhydryl groups. (b) The protein after oxidation showing the formation of a disulfide bridge between the two-SH groups

with the sulfhydryl group of bacterial enzyme (protein) which is having a specific function in the pathogens leads to the formation of disulfide bridge (Fig. 6.2). This chemical reaction leads conformation changes of the protein (shape) which alter its normal function. The total destruction or change the function in specific proteins is responsible for the ultimate death or destruction of microbes. During this reaction the oxidizing antiseptic agent gets reduced.

*Example*: hydrogen peroxide solution. It acts as a broad spectrum germicidal agent against bacteria, Tubercle bacilli, spores, virus and fungi when used particular concentrations. It liberates nascent oxygen which oxidizes the necrotic matter and kills bacteria or pathogenic organisms.

***Halogenation***: Compounds containing hypochlorite or hypohalite (OCl) group type antiseptics acts by this mechanism because these types of compounds are used as the reagents in the chlorination of primary and secondary amides. All of the pathogens are containing protein molecules which are made up of amino acid sequences. These amino acid sequences are connected through peptide linkages.

The compounds act by this mechanism includes sodium hypochlorite, chlorinated lime etc. These antiseptics provide the chlorine atom to the peptide linkage of microbial enzyme leads to the destruction of the function of specific proteins. The substitution of the chlorine atom for the hydrogen changes or weakens in the hydrogen bond forces which are responsible for the proper conformation of protein molecule.

$$\text{Protein}-\overset{\overset{\displaystyle O}{\|}}{C}-\underset{\underset{\displaystyle H}{|}}{N}-\text{Protein} \xrightarrow{OCl^-} \text{Protein}-\overset{\overset{\displaystyle O}{\|}}{C}-\underset{\underset{\displaystyle Cl}{|}}{N}-\text{Protein}$$

The changes in the proper confirmation lead to destruction of microbes.

***Protein precipitation or coagulation***: It involves the interaction between microbial enzymes with metallic ions having large or strong electrostatic forces. The metal ion in periodic table belongs to group IB and IIB exert this property. This reaction is takes place by formation of complexes with various polar groups on the protein molecule of microbe's acts as ligands (Fig. 6.3).

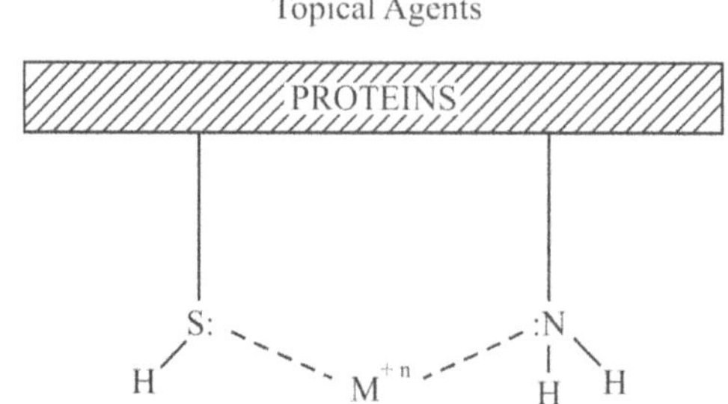


**Fig. 6.3** A model illustration of the interaction between a metal ion and a protein, resulting in protein precipitation

The complexation between metal ion and protein leads to changes in radical properties of the protein or precipitating the protein. The above said reaction is no specific one at sufficient concentration they reacts with host as well as microbial protein. Some of the metals are having the property to forms strong covalent bonds with microbial enzyme due to this "ties up" property with important functional group of the active site of the enzyme; they exert their protein precipitant properties.

Some of the metal cations except alkali and alkaline earth metals also show antiseptic (protein precipitant) properties. This is mainly depends upon the concentration of antiseptic at site of action.

## Hydrogen Peroxide I.P., B.P.

**(Synonym: Hydrogen peroxide solution (20 vol), dilute hydrogen peroxide solution, Hydrogen peroxide solution (6%))**

**Mol. Formula:** $H_2O_2$ **Mol. Weight:** 34

It is an aqueous solution of hydrogen peroxide with suitable stabilizing agent.

It contains not less than 5% w/v and not more than 7% w/v of hydrogen peroxide, corresponding to about 20 times of its volume of available oxygen.

***Preparation:***

1. *Industrial method of preparation:* It is prepared by mixing of hydrated barium peroxide ($BaO_2$. $8H_2O$) with sulphuric acid. But this process is not an absolute one since the yield is 10-20% only.

$$BaO_2 . 8\,H_2O + H_2SO_4 \longrightarrow H_2O_2 + BaSO_4\downarrow + 8\,H_2O$$

2. *Laboratory preparation:* A thin cream of barium peroxide with water is gradually added to dilute sulphuric acid with constant stirring, it should be kept in ice, adjust the pH of the mixture to acidic by using sulphuric acid and then cool it in ice for 1 hour, remove the precipitated barium sulphate.

$$BaO_2 + H_2SO_4 \longrightarrow H_2O_2 + BaSO_4 \downarrow$$

3. *From decomposition of barium peroxide:* Hydrogen peroxide can also be prepared by decomposition of barium peroxide with phosphoric acid or by passing carbon dioxide into barium peroxide in water.

$$3\,BaO_2 + 2\,H_3PO_4 \longrightarrow 3\,H_2O_2 + Ba_3(PO_4)_2$$

$$BaO_2 + H_2O + CO_2 \longrightarrow H_2O_2 + BaCO_3$$

4. *From decomposition of sodium peroxide:* Decomposition of sodium peroxide with sulphuric acid at low temperature gives hydrogen peroxide and most of the sodium sulphate formed is crystallized as its decahydrate and the hydrogen peroxide is subsequently distilled at 10 mm Hg pressure.

$$Na_2O_2 + H_2SO_4 \xrightarrow[\text{Pressure}]{\text{10 mmHg}} H_2O_2 + Na_2SO_4$$

5. *By electrolytic process:* The yield of hydrogen peroxide formed by this method is 30-40%. By using this method, 50% of ice cold sulphuric acid can be electrolyzed to give persulphuric acid by vacuum distillation; this is further hydrolyzed leads to the formation of hydrogen peroxide which is removed as vapour.

$$2\,H_2SO_4 \xrightarrow{\text{Electrolysis}} H_2S_2O_8 + H_2$$

$$H_2S_2O_8 + 2\,H_2O \xrightarrow[\text{reduced pressure}]{\text{Distilled under}} H_2O_2 + 2\,H_2SO_4$$

By the modification of this method ammonium sulphate is reacted with sulphuric acid to form ammonium peroxydisulphate. Thus the formed ammonium peroxydisulphate solution is electrolyzed to give hydrogen peroxide along with ammonium bisulphate as by product.

$$(NH_4)_2SO_4 + H_2SO_4 \longrightarrow \underset{\text{Ammonium peroxydisulphate}}{(NH_4)_2S_2O_8} + H_2$$

$$(NH_4)_2S_2O_8 + 2H_2O \longrightarrow 2\,NH_4\,HSO_4 + H_2O_2$$

***Physical properties:*** Hydrogen peroxide solution is acidic in taste. It is a clear, colorless and odorless solution. It is usually unstable one, easily decomposes in alkaline solution or contact with oxidisable substances. It is miscible with water.

$$2\,H_2O_2 \longrightarrow 2\,H_2O + O_2$$

The decomposition of hydrogen peroxide is also enhanced by catalysts like copper, iron or manganese ions. The pure hydrogen peroxide which is stored in the containers slowly decomposes. The stability of hydrogen peroxide solution is increased by adding sulphuric acid or phosphoric acid and also by the addition of very small amount of organic or inorganic stabilizers such as urea, acetanilide, hexamine and boric acid.

The pH of the commercial hydrogen peroxide solution is usually adjusted to 2-3 but even at pH 5-6 solutions as concentrated as 35%.

For industrial purposes, 90% concentrated solutions are prepared.

**Chemical properties:**

***Oxidation reactions:*** Hydrogen peroxide is a strong oxidizing agent and it oxidizes many organic materials. Some of the examples are as follows.

1. *Oxidation of lead sulphide:* Hydrogen peroxide oxidizes lead sulphide to lead sulphate.

$$PbS + 2\,H_2O_2 \longrightarrow PbSO_4 + 2\,H_2$$

2. *Oxidation of sodium sulphite:* Hydrogen peroxide oxidizes sodium sulphite to sodium sulphate.

$$Na_2SO_3 + H_2O_2 \longrightarrow Na_2SO_4 + H_2O$$

3. *Oxidation of ferrous sulphate:* Hydrogen peroxide oxidizes ferrous sulphate to ferric sulphate.

$$2\,FeSO_4 + H_2O_2 + H_2SO_4 \longrightarrow Fe_2(SO_4)_3 + 2\,H_2O$$

4. *Oxidation of potassium iodide:* Hydrogen peroxide oxidizes potassium iodide to iodine.

$$2\,KI + H_2O_2 \longrightarrow 2\,KOH + I_2$$

**Reducing properties:** Hydrogen peroxide also acts a reducing agent against other oxidizing agents. Example: It reduces silver oxide to silver, potassium permanganate to potassium sulphate, ozone to oxygen etc.

$$Ag_2O + H_2O_2 \longrightarrow 2\,Ag + H_2O + O_2$$

$$2\,KMnO_4 + 3\,H_2SO_4 + 5\,H_2O_2 \longrightarrow K_2SO_4 + 2\,MnSO_4 + 8\,H_2O + 5\,O_2\uparrow$$

$$3O_3 + H_2O_2 \longrightarrow 5O_2 + H_2O$$

**Acidic properties:** The dilute solution of hydrogen peroxide is acidic in nature and it is neutral to litmus. It reacts with alkalis and carbonates to form their respective peroxides.

$$H_2O_2 + 2\,NaOH \longrightarrow \underset{\text{Sodium Peroxide}}{Na_2O_2} + 2\,H_2O$$

$$H_2O_2 + Ba(OH)_2 \longrightarrow \underset{\text{Barium Peroxide}}{BaO_2} + 2\,H_2O$$

$$H_2O_2 + Na_2CO_3 \longrightarrow \underset{\text{Sodium Peroxide}}{Na_2O_2} + CO_2 + H_2O$$

***Test for identification:***

1. To the small amount of sample solution add one to two drops of sulphuric acid and one drop of potassium permanganate solution. The pink color of the solution disappears with the evolution of oxygen.

$$2\,KMnO_4 + 3\,H_2SO_4 + 5\,H_2O_2 \longrightarrow K_2SO_4 + 2\,MnSO_4 + 8\,H_2O + 5\,O_2\uparrow$$

2. To the sample solution add 2 ml of sulphuric acid, 2 ml of ether and one drop of potassium dichromate solution and shake well. A deep blue layer is formed between the ether and aqueous layer.

***Test for purity:*** It should be tested for acidity, organic stabilizers, non volatile matter and loss on evaporation.

***Test for organic stabilizers:*** Extract the required quantity of sample with required quantity of chloroform, evaporate the extract and weigh the residue. The residue weighs not more than 10 mg (50 ppm).

**Assay**

***Principle:*** It is assayed by **permanganometry method of titration (also called redox titration)** to find out the "available oxygen".

In this assay the substance is diluted with 1M sulphuric acid and the solution is titrated against potassium permanganate. Potassium permanganate is acting as a self indicator. End point is the appearance of permanent pale pink colour.

During this assay, sulphuric acid first reacts with potassium permanganate and liberate nascent oxygen. Thus the liberated nascent oxygen oxidises the hydrogen peroxide to water and oxygen. After the completion of this reaction, addition of potassium permanganate remains in the flask and its colour is retained i.e., permanent pale pink colour. As the oxidation and reduction takes place simultaneously this is called Redox titration. The chemical reactions of this assay are shown below.

$$2\,KMnO_4 + 3\,H_2SO_4 \longrightarrow K_2SO_4 + 2\,MnSO_4 + 3\,H_2O + 5(O)$$

$$5\,H_2O_2 + 5(O) \longrightarrow 5\,H_2O + 5\,O_2\uparrow$$

It can also be written as

$$2\,KMnO_4 + 3\,H_2SO_4 + 5\,H_2O_2 \longrightarrow K_2SO_4 + 2\,MnSO_4 + 8\,H_2O + 5\,O_2\uparrow$$

***Procedure*:** To 1 ml of the substance add 20 ml of 1M sulphuric acid and titrate with 0.02M potassium permanganate.

*Uses*

1. It is a powerful oxidizing agent and gives nascent oxygen, so it acts as bleaching agent, bleaching for hair also.
2. It is also used as a mild oxidizing antiseptic to cleanse wounds and cuts up to the concentration of 6% solution.
3. It kills the most of the pathogenic bacteria like *E. coli*, *S. aureus* and *typhoid bacilli.*
4. 1.5% solution of hydrogen peroxide is used as mouth wash in the treatment of acute stomatitis and deodorant gargle.
5. It used to clean septic sockets and root canals in dentistry.
6. Hydrogen peroxide ear drops are used to remove wax, dirt, debris from the ear.
7. Strong solution of hydrogen peroxide or high concentrated solutions produce irritation and burns on the skin and mucous membrane with eschar.
8. It may cause reversible hypertrophy of the papillae of tongue, so continuous use of hydrogen peroxide solution should be avoided.
9. 3% solution of hydrogen peroxide is used as a mouth wash.
10. The nascent oxygen liberated during the decomposition of hydrogen peroxide, kills bacteria, hence it can be used as an antiseptic.
11. The fine foam of evolving oxygen is able to mechanical cleaning between the teeth, cervices and cavities.

***Storage:*** It should be stored in a tightly closed, light resistant container with stopper which is made up of glass or plastic not affected by temperature more than 30 °C. If the solution does not contain a preservative it should be stored in a refrigerator (2 to 8 °C). It should not be stored for longer periods.

***Labelling:*** The label states that either it contains stabilizers or not.

***Other official preparations:*** Strong hydrogen peroxide solution (100 vol) I.P, B.P.

## Potassium Permanganate I.P., B.P., U.S.P.

**Mol. Formula:** $KMnO_4$ **Mol. Weight:** 158

Potassium permanganate contains not less than 99% and not more than 100.5% of potassium permanganate.

***Preparation:***

1. *From manganese dioxide:* In this method, manganese dioxide is fused with excess of potassium hydroxide either in the presence of free air or with addition of oxidizing agent like potassium nitrate or potassium chlorate so that a green mass of potassium manganate is formed.

$$2\,KOH + MnO_2 + (O) \longrightarrow K_2MnO_4 + H_2O$$

The resulting potassium manganate is extracted with water and treated with $CO_2$. During this reaction 1/3 of manganate is converted to its dioxide and remaining manganate is converted into permanganate which is in solution.

$$3\,K_2MnO_4 + 2\,CO_2 \longrightarrow 2\,KMnO_4 + MnO_2 + 2\,K_2CO_3$$

Instead of $CO_2$ if chlorine is passed to the potassium manganate solution, all the manganate in the manganate solution is converted into permanganate.

$$6\,K_2MnO_4 + 3\,Cl_2 \longrightarrow 6\,KMnO_4 + 6\,KCl$$

2. *By electrolytic hydrolysis of potassium manganate (Large scale process):* This method consists of the conversion of potassium manganate to potassium permanganate by electrolytic hydrolysis of the warm manganate solution with the liberation of hydrogen gas.

$$2\,K_2MnO_4 + 2\,H_2O \longrightarrow 2\,KMnO_4 + 2\,KOH + H_2\uparrow$$

The solution obtained from any of the above methods is filtered, evaporated and cooled to get potassium permanganate crystals.

**Physical properties:** It is a dark purple or brownish black, granular powder or dark purple or almost black slender, prismatic crystals with a metallic luster, odorless. It is completely soluble in water and slightly soluble in alcohol.

The solution of potassium permanganate is sweetish astringent taste. It gets decomposed when contact with some organic matters.

***Chemical properties:***

1. *Action of heat:* When it is heated, it deprecipitates at higher temperatures. It decomposes into potassium manganate with the evolution of oxygen.

$$2\,KMnO_4 \xrightarrow[\Delta]{240\,^{\circ}C} K_2MnO_4 + MnO_2 + O_2\uparrow$$

2. It is a powerful oxidizing agent so it oxidizes many compounds.

(a) *Reaction with hydrogen peroxide:* When a solution of acidified potassium permanganate is added to the hydrogen peroxide solution, the pink color gets disappeared.

$$2\,KMnO_4 + 3\,H_2SO_4 \longrightarrow K_2SO_4 + 2\,MnSO_4 + 3H_2O + 5\,(O)$$

$$5\,H_2O_2 + 5\,(O) \longrightarrow 5\,H_2O + 5\,O_2$$

(b) *Reaction with hydrogen sulphide:* When $H_2S$ gas is passed through the acidified solution of potassium permanganate, the violet color disappears and sulphur gets precipitated.

$$2\,KMnO_4 + 6\,HCl + 5\,H_2S \longrightarrow 2\,MnCl_2 + 2\,KCl + 5\,S\downarrow + 8\,H_2O$$

(c) *Reaction with hydrochloric acid:* When hydrochloric acid is added to potassium permanganate solution, chlorine gas is evolved.

$$2\ KMnO_4 + 16\ HCl \longrightarrow 2\ MnCl_2 + 2\ KCl + 8\ H_2O + 5\ Cl_2\uparrow$$

The alkaline or neutral solution of potassium permanganate oxidizes potassium iodide to potassium iodate.

$$2\ KMnO_4 + KI + H_2O \longrightarrow KIO_3 + 2\ MnO_2 + 2\ KOH$$

In acidic solution potassium permanganate reacts with potassium iodide and liberates iodine.

$$2\ KMnO_4 + 8\ H_2SO_4 + 10\ KI \longrightarrow 6\ K_2SO_4 + 2\ MnSO_4 + 5\ I_2 + 8\ H_2O$$

The acidic potassium permanganate solution reacts with ferrous sulphate and forms ferric sulphate.

$$2\ KMnO_4 + 10\ FeSO_4 + 8\ H_2SO_4 \longrightarrow 5\ Fe_2(SO_4)_3 + K_2SO_4 + 2\ MnSO_4 + 8\ H_2O$$

***Test for identification:***

1. A solution in water acidified with sulphuric acid and heated to 70 °C; add hydrogen peroxide solution. The color of the solution gets decolorized.
2. When heated to redness it deprecipitate with the evolution of oxygen and leaves black residue. When water is added to this residue, potassium hydroxide is formed. The resulting solution gives the characteristic reactions of potassium ion.

***Test for purity:*** It should be tested for appearance of solution, chlorides, sulphates and water insoluble matter. Before performing the above tests the color of the solution should be decolorized, this will not interfere with the limit tests. The decolorisation of the solution is done by boiling the aqueous solution with 95% alcohol and removes the precipitated manganese dioxide through filtration.

$$2\ KMnO_4 + 3\ C_2H_5OH \longrightarrow 2\ KOH + 2\ MnO_2 + 3\ CH_3CHO + 2\ H_2O$$

**Assay**

***Principle*:**

*Method 1*: It is assayed by **permanganometry method of titration (also called redox titration)**.

In this assay oxalic acid is dissolved in water and acidified with dilute sulphuric acid and the solution is titrated by warmed at 70 °C and titrated against 0.1N potassium permanganate. Potassium permanganate is acting as a self indicator. End point is the appearance of permanent pale pink colour.

During this assay, sulphuric acid first reacts with potassium permanganate and liberate nascent oxygen. Thus the liberated nascent oxygen oxidises the oxalic acid to carbon dioxide and water. After the completion of this reaction, addition of potassium permanganate remains in the flask and its colour is retained i.e., permanent pale pink colour. As the oxidation and reduction takes place simultaneously this is called Redox titration. The chemical reactions of this assay are shown below.

$$2\,KMnO_4 + 3\,H_2SO_4 \longrightarrow K_2SO_4 + 2\,MnSO_4 + 3\,H_2O + 5(O)$$

$$5\begin{array}{c}COOH\\ |\\ COOH\end{array} + 5(O) \longrightarrow 10\,CO_2 + 5\,H_2O$$

It can also be written as

$$2\,KMnO_4 + 3\,H_2SO_4 + 5\begin{array}{c}COOH\\ |\\ COOH\end{array} \longrightarrow K_2SO_4 + 2\,MnSO_4 + 8\,H_2O + 10\,CO_2\uparrow$$

*Method 2:* It is assayed by **iodometry method of titration (also called redox titration).**

In this assay the substance is treated with potassium iodide and hydrochloric acid and titrate the liberated iodine with 0.1M sodium thiosulphate using starch solution, added towards the end of the titration, as indicator.

In this assay when the substance is reacted with hydrochloric acid in presence of excess of potassium iodide, iodine is liberated from potassium iodide. The liberated iodine is determined by titrating with N/10 sodium thiosulphate using starch mucilage as an indicator. End point is the disappearance of blue colour.

During this titration iodine is reduced to sodium iodide and sodium thiosulphate is oxidised to sodium tetrathionate. As the oxidation and reduction takes place simultaneously this is called Redox titration. The chemical reactions of this assay are shown below.

$$HCl + 2KI \xrightarrow{KMnO_4} I_2 + 2\,KCl$$

$$\underset{\text{Sodium thiosulphate}}{I_2 + 2\,Na_2S_2O_3} \longrightarrow 2\,NaI + \underset{\text{Sodium tetrathionate}}{Na_2S_4O_6}$$

***Procedure:*** Weigh accurately about 0.3 gm, dissolve in sufficient water to produce 100 ml. To 20 ml add 20 ml of water, 1 gm of potassium iodide and 10 ml of 2M hydrochloric acid and titrate the liberated iodine with 0.1M sodium thiosulphate using starch solution, added towards the end of the titration, as indicator.

***Uses***

1. It is used as an antiseptic in mouth wash.
2. It is also used as an astringent, anti-infective, disinfectant and deodorant.
3. It is mainly used for treatment of snake venom poison due to its oxidizing property.
4. It is also used as an antidote for opium, morphine and strychnine poisoning.

5. The solution of potassium permanganate is used to clean ulcers, abscesses in eczematous conditions and acute dermatoses. It is also used in bromhidrosis.
6. The concentrated solution of potassium permanganate is caustic and irritant to tissues.
7. Repeated use of dilute solutions may cause corrosive burns.

***Storage:*** It should be stored in well closed container and protected from moisture.

***Caution:*** Care should be taken for handling potassium permanganate as dangerous explosion occurs when come into contact with organic or readily oxidisable substances either in solution or in dry condition.

***Official formulations:*** Potassium permanganate tablets U.S.P.

## Sodium Perborate B.P.

**Mol. Formula:** $NaBO_3 . 4H_2O$ **Mol. Weight:** 153.9

It is a complex of sodium metaborate and hydrogen peroxide occurring as tri or monohydrates. It contains not less than 96% and not more than 103% sodium perborate.

***Preparation:***

*Method 1:* It is prepared by treating sodium hydroxide with double quantity of hydrogen peroxide to a saturated solution of borax.

$$Na_2B_4O_7 + 2NaOH + 4H_2O_2 \longrightarrow 4NaBO_3 + 5H_2O$$

*Method 2:* The solution of sodium peroxide is mixed with boric acid solution. Then carbon dioxide gas is passed through the above mixture. Finally the mother liquor is saturated with sodium chloride to yield sodium perborate crystals. The reaction is kept in ice cold condition.

$$2H_3BO_3 + 2Na_2O_2 + CO_2 \longrightarrow 2NaBO_3 + Na_2CO_3 + 3H_2O$$

***Physical properties:*** It occurs as a colorless, odorless prismatic crystals or white powder. Crystalline form is more stable. The monohydrate is less soluble than tri hydrate. Sparingly soluble in water with slow decomposition and soluble in dilute mineral acids.

***Test for identification:***

1. To the saturated solution of sample add one drop of dilute sulphuric acid and 0.2 ml of potassium dichromate solution and small amount of ether shake well; allow it to stand for five minutes. Ether layer shows blue color.
2. The sample solution gives the characteristic reactions of sodium ions.
3. The sample is treated with 0.1 ml of dilute sulphuric acid and methanol, resulting mixture is introduced into a flame, and a greenish flame is produced.

***Test for purity:*** It should be tested for chlorides, sulphate, iron and heavy metals.

**Assay**

***Principle***: It is assayed by **permanganometry method of titration (also called redox titration)**.

In this assay the substance is dissolved in water and it is acidified with dilute sulphuric acid and the solution is titrated against 0.1N potassium permanganate. Potassium permanganate is acting as a self indicator. End point is the appearance of permanent pale pink colour.

During this assay, sulphuric acid first reacts with potassium permanganate and liberate nascent oxygen. Thus the liberated nascent oxygen oxidizes the sodium perborate. After the completion of this reaction, addition of potassium permanganate remains in the flask and its colour is retained i.e., permanent pale pink colour. As the oxidation and reduction takes place simultaneously this is called redox titration. The chemical reactions of this assay are shown below.

$$2\ KMnO_4 + 3\ H_2SO_4 \longrightarrow K_2SO_4 + 2\ MnSO_4 + 3\ H_2O + 5(O)$$

$$NaBO_3.4\ H_2O \xrightleftharpoons{(O)} H_2O_2 + NaBO_2 + 3\ H_2O$$

***Procedure***: Dissolve 0.300 gm in 50.0 ml of water. Dilute 10.0 ml of the solution to 50 ml with water and add 10 ml of dilute sulphuric acid. Titrate with 0.02M potassium permanganate.

***Uses***

1. It is used as an antiseptic, disinfectant and deodorant.
2. The dilute solution (2%) is used in mouth washes and tooth powder.

***Storage:*** It should be stored in air tight containers.

---

## Chlorinated Lime I.P., B.P.

**(Synonym: Bleaching powder, Chloride of lime, Calcium chloro hypochlorite)**

**Mol. Formula:** $Ca(OCl)Cl.H_2O$ **Mol. Weight:** 144

It consists of calcium chloro hypochlorite $Ca(OCl)Cl$ with varying quantities of calcium hydroxide and moisture. It contains not less than 30% w/w of available chlorine.

***Preparation:*** It is mainly prepared by the action of chlorine on calcium hydroxide (slaked lime). The pure and fairly dried slaked lime is spread in layers, in lead chambers. The chlorine is passed into the chambers until the lime is saturated. The process takes place for 12 to 24 hr. When absorption of chlorine is completed, lime powder is blown in to the chamber to absorb excess chlorine.

$$Ca(OH)_2 + Cl_2 \longrightarrow Ca(OCl)Cl + H_2O$$

The above reaction is somewhat complex. The first products are the basic chloride $CaCl_2Ca(OH)_2$. $H_2O$ and the basic hypochlorite $Ca(OCl)_2$, then the basic hypo chlorite is converted by the further action of chlorine in to substance consisting of calcium chloro hypochlorite.

***Physical properties:*** It is a dull white powder, which slowly undergo decomposition on exposure to air due to the absorption of carbon dioxide and moisture. It is partially soluble in water and alcohol. The aqueous solutions are strongly alkaline in nature.

***Chemical properties:***

1. *Reactions with acids:* Chlorinated lime reacts with dilute acids and evolves hypochlorous acid which acts as bleaching and oxidizing agent. Further treatment with excess of dilute acid or carbon dioxide, the total chlorine is liberated. This amount of chlorine is called as available chlorine. The good quality sample contains 35.38% of available chlorine.
2. *Auto oxidation:* Chlorinated lime itself gets oxidized and gives calcium chloride.

***Test for identification:***

1. When hydrochloric acid is treated with chlorinated lime, evolves chlorine gas. The resulting solution gives the characteristic reactions of calcium and chloride ions.

***Test for purity:*** It should be tested for stability and available chlorine.

***Stability:*** Heat the required amount of sample at 100 °C for 2 hours. The loss of available chlorine is not more than 3% w/w.

**Assay**

***Principle:*** It is assayed by **iodometry method of titration (also called redox titration)** to find out the "available chlorine".

In this assay the substance is treated with acetic acid in presence of excess of potassium iodide and titrated with sodium thiosulphate, using starch mucilage as an indicator. End point is the disappearance of blue colour.

In this assay when the substance is reacted with acetic acid in presence of excess of potassium iodide, available chlorine is liberated from chlorinated lime and it displaces equal amount of iodine from potassium iodide. The liberated iodine is determined by titrating with N/10 sodium thiosulphate using starch mucilage as an indicator. End point is the disappearance of blue colour.

During this titration iodine is reduced to sodium iodide and sodium thiosulphate is oxidized to sodium tetrathionate. As the oxidation and reduction takes place simultaneously this is called Redox titration. The chemical reactions of this assay are shown below.

$$\underset{\text{(Chlorinated lime)}}{Ca(OCl)Cl} + 2\,CH_3COOH \longrightarrow (CH_3COO)_2Ca + HOCl + HCl$$

$$HOCl + HCl \rightleftharpoons Cl_2 + H_2O$$

$$Cl_2 + 2KI \longrightarrow I_2 + 2\,KCl$$

$$I_2 + \underset{\text{Sodium thiosulphate}}{2\,Na_2S_2O_3} \longrightarrow 2\,NaI + \underset{\text{Sodium tetrathionate}}{Na_2S_4O_6}$$

***Procedure***: Triturate 4 gm with successive small quantities of water, dilute to 1000 ml with water and shake thoroughly. Mix 100 ml of the resulting suspension with a solution containing 3 gm of potassium iodide in 100 ml of water, acidify with 5 ml of 6M acetic acid and titrate the liberated iodine with 0.1M sodium thiosulphate, using starch mucilage as an indicator.

***Uses:***

1. Chlorinated lime is used for its rapid bactericidal action and bleaching properties.
2. It is used for the chlorination treatment of municipal supply water and swimming pools.
3. It is used as a cleansing agent for lavatories, drains and effluents.
4. It is used for the preparation of Dakin's solution (surgical chlorinated soda) for cleaning of wounds.
5. It kills most of bacteria, fungi, yeasts, algae, virus and protozoa.
6. Eusol solution (mixture of chlorinated lime and boric acid) is used as a disinfectant in lotion and wet dressings.

***Storage:*** It should be stored in well closed containers and kept in a cool place, protected from heat and moisture.

***Adverse effects:***

1. Ingestion of bleaching powder leads to irritation and corrosion of mucous membranes with pain and vomiting.
2. Inhalation of fumes causes pulmonary edema, pulmonary irritation and death.

## Iodine Preparations

## Iodine I.P.

**Mol. Formula:** $I_2$ **Mol. Weight:** 126

It contains not less than 99.5% and not more than 100.5 % of iodine.

Iodine compounds are commonly distributed in nature but are not found in workable amounts. Sea water contains minute quantity of iodine which is absorbed by some marine plants like *Fucus vesiculosus* (fewer amounts). Iodine also occurs in chile saltpetre (0.2%) in the form of sodium iodate.

***Preparation:*** Most of the iodine is manufactured from sea weeds, chile saltpetre mother liquor and from different types of brines.

1. *From sea weeds:* Dried sea weeds are burned and the resulting kelp is extracted with water. To the above solution add small quantities of sulphuric acid to remove sulphides and thio sulphate and sulphur.

   The resulting solution is concentrated, crystallized; the chlorides and sulphates of potassium and sodium ions are removed. Now the acid solution contains the freely soluble iodides with small amount of bromides and chlorides are treated with the correct proportion of chlorine. The precipitated iodine is collected and purified by sublimation process.

   $$2\ NaI + 3\ H_2SO_4 + MnO_2 \longrightarrow I_2 + MnSO_4 + 2NaHSO_4 + 2\ H_2O$$

   Impurities like ICl and IBr are also present along with iodine which can be removed by sublimation with potassium iodide.

   $$ICl + KI \longrightarrow KCl + I_2$$

   $$IBr + KI \longrightarrow KBr + I_2$$

2. *From chile saltpetre:* The concentrated solutions of chile saltpetre is treated with sodium nitrate, crystallizes the solution which leaves mother liquor containing sodium iodate. Mother liquor is treated with sodium hydrogen sulphite. The iodine is collected and purified by sublimation.

   $$2\ NaIO_3 + 5\ NaHSO_3 \longrightarrow I_2 + 2\ Na_2SO_4 + 3\ NaHSO_4 + H_2O$$

***Physical properties***: Iodine is a greenish violet brittle plates or heavy bluish black rhombic prisms with a metallic sheen, peculiar odour. It volatilizes slowly at room temperature. The melting point is 114 °C, at higher temperatures it dissociates due to decreasing its density.

$$I_2 \rightleftharpoons 2\ I$$

It is soluble in alcohol, chloroform and freely soluble in ether, completely soluble in potassium iodide but insoluble in water.

***Chemical properties:***

1. *Reaction with metals and non metals*: Iodine is a halogen but it is less active than chlorine and bromine, it readily reacts with metals and non metals to yield the respective iodides.

   $$Fe + I_2 \longrightarrow FeI_2$$

   $$Hg + I_2 \longrightarrow HgI_2$$

   $$4\ P + 6\ I_2 \longrightarrow 4\ PI_3$$

2. *Oxidizing property*: In aqueous medium iodine acts as a oxidizing agent. It oxidizes the reducing agents.

$$H_3AsO_3 + I_2 + H_2O \longrightarrow 2\,HI + H_3AsO_4$$

$$H_2S + I_2 \longrightarrow 2\,HI + S\downarrow$$

$$2\,Na_2S_2O_3 + I_2 \longrightarrow 2\,NaI + Na_2S_4O_6$$

3. *Reaction with cold sodium hydroxide*: Iodine reacts with cold alkali solution, it forms sodium hypo iodide which on further hydrolysis gives hypoiodous acid.

$$2\,NaOH + I_2 + O_2 \xrightarrow[-\,H_2O]{-\,NaI} NaIO_3 \xrightarrow{H_2O} HIO_3 + NaOH$$

4. *Reaction with hot alkalis*: Iodine reacts with hot sodium hydroxide solution to form sodium iodate and ammonium iodate respectively.

$$6NaOH + 3I_2 \xrightarrow{\Delta} NaIO_3 + 5NaI + 3H_2O$$

$$6\,NH_4OH + 3\,I_2 \longrightarrow NH_4IO_3 + 5\,NH_4I + 3\,H_2O$$

5. *Reaction with liquor ammonia*: Iodine reacts with ammonia liquor and yields explosive powder of nitrogen triiodide.

$$6\,I_2 + 2\,NH_3 \longrightarrow 2\,NI_3 + 6\,HI$$

6. *Reaction with potassium chlorate*: Iodine reacts with concentrated solution of potassium chlorate in the presence of nitric acid on heating to form potassium iodate.

$$2KClO_3 + I_2 \xrightarrow{HNO_3} 2KIO_3 + Cl_2$$

7. *Reaction with unsaturated acids:* Addition reaction: Iodine undergoes addition reaction with unsaturated acids which are present in the oils.

$$R\text{-}CH{=}CH\text{-}COOH + I_2 \longrightarrow R\text{-}CHI\text{-}CHI\text{-}COOH$$

8. *Reaction with oxidizing agents*: Iodine reacts with oxidizing agents like excess chlorine and gets reduced.

$$I_2 + 5\,Cl_2\,(\text{excess}) + 6\,H_2O \longrightarrow 2\,HIO_3 + 10\,HCl$$

$$3\,I_2 + 5\,KClO_3 + 3\,H_2O \longrightarrow 6\,HIO_3 + 5\,KCl$$

***Test for identification***: When heated gently iodine forms violet color vapours which condenses and forming a bluish black sublimate.

To the saturated solution of iodine in potassium iodide, add starch solution, produces blue color which disappears on heating and reappears on cooling.

***Test for purity:*** It should be tested for bromides, chlorides, non volatile matter and cyanogens.

***Test for cyanogens*:** To the clear colorless solution of iodine, add few drops of ferrous sulphate solution and one or two drops of sodium hydroxide solution, warmed and acidified with hydrochloric acid. No Prussian blue color is produced.

**Assay**

***Principle:*** It is assayed by **iodimetry method of titration** (also called redox titration).

In this assay the substance is dissolved in a solution of Pottasium iodide in an iodine flask. The solution is made acidic by treating with acetic acid and titrated with N/10 sodium thiosulphate using starch mucilage as an indicator. End point is the disappearance of blue colour. During this titration iodine is reduced to sodium iodide and sodium thiosulphate is oxidised to sodium tetrathionate. As the oxidation and reduction takes place simultaneously this is called Redox titration. The chemical reactions of this assay are shown below.

$$I_2 + \underset{\text{Sodium thiosulphate}}{2Na_2S_2O_3} \longrightarrow 2\,NaI + \underset{\text{Sodium tetrathionate}}{Na_2S_4O_6}$$

***Procedure*:** Weigh accurately about 0.2 gm, transfer to a flask containing 1 gm of potassium iodide and 2 ml of water, add 1 ml of 2M acetic acid, dissolve completely and add 50 ml of water. Titrate with 0.1M sodium thiosulphate using starch solution as indicator.

***Uses*:**

1. Iodine is mainly used in the treatment of thyroid deficiency which should be supplied in the form of elemental iodine or sodium potassium iodide.
2. It also used as a disinfectant, counter irritant and local germicide.
3. Elemental iodine is highly toxic in nature. Sodium thiosulphate and starch are used as an antidote for iodine poisoning.

***Storage*:** It should be stored in ground glass stoppered bottles since the vapors affects the cork and rubber stoppers or earthenware containers with waxed bungs.

## Weak Iodine Solution

**(Synonym: Tincture of iodine or Iodine tincture)**

It is having 2% w/v of iodine (limit 1.9 - 2.1%) and 2.5% w/v of potassium iodide (limit 2.4-2.6%).

**Composition:**

Iodine = 20 gm

Potassium iodide = 25 gm

Alcohol (50%) quantity sufficient to produce = 1000 ml.

***Preparation***: Required quantity of iodine is dissolved in an aqueous solution of potassium iodide and add sufficient volume of 90% alcohol to make up to 1000 ml.

The amount of potassium iodide is more than that required for the compound potassium iodate which is the main constituent of the solution.

***Physical properties:*** It is a brown, transparent liquid with the smell of iodine.

***Test for identification:*** To the solution of iodine add starch solution. It gives a blue color.

The residue obtained after evaporation and ignition yields the characteristic reactions of potassium and iodine.

**Assay**

The assay of iodine solutions are carried out for iodine and potassium iodide after the suitable dilution.

***For Iodine:*** It is assayed by **iodimetry method of titration** (also called **redox titration**).

In this assay the iodine solution diluted with water and and titrated with N/10 sodium thiosulphate using starch mucilage as an indicator. End point is the disappearance of blue colour. During this titration iodine is reduced to sodium iodide and sodium thiosulphate is oxidized to sodium tetrathionate. As the oxidation and reduction takes place simultaneously this is called Redox titration. The chemical reactions of this assay are shown below.

$$\underset{\text{Sodium thiosulphate}}{I_2 + 2Na_2S_2O_3} \longrightarrow \underset{\text{Sodium tetrathionate}}{2NaI + Na_2S_4O_6}$$

***For Potassium iodide:*** It is assayed by **Andrew's method of titration** (also called **iodometry method, redox titration**).

In this assay the diluted solution was acidified by treating with hydrochloric acid and titrated with standard potassium iodate solution until the brown colour turns into light brown. At this stage a small amount of chloroform is added to it and the titration continued until the disappearance of colour in chloroform layer and the supernatant layer becomes clear yellow, Starch mucilage cannot be used as an indicator due to the use of high concentration of hydrochloric acid, which prevents the hydrolysis of iodine monochloride (ICl). As the oxidation and reduction takes place simultaneously this is called redox titration. In this assay, potassium iodide is oxidised to iodine by potassium iodate in presence of HCl. This liberated iodine is converted to iodine monochloride.

Iodine is more soluble in chloroform than water. After the reaction of free iodine at aqueous layer the iodine may be available at chloroform layer. Hence upon each addition after the aqueous layer becomes colourless, the flask should be shaken well to allow iodine in chloroform layer to react with potassium iodate.

$$2\,KIO_3 + 6\,HCl + KI \longrightarrow 3\,KCl + 3\,ICl + 3\,H_2O + 3(O)$$

***Procedure:***

*Assay for iodine:* Transfer 10 ml of the solution and dilute with 20 ml of water. Then the solution is titrated with 0.1N sodium thiosulphate solution using starch solution as an indicator.

*Assay for potassium iodide:* Transfer 10 ml of weak iodine solution in to a conical flask, and add 40 ml of water, 16 ml of hydrochloric acid. Then it is titrated with 0.05M potassium iodate solution, shaking vigorously until dark brown color of the solution becomes fade. Then add 5 ml of chloroform and continue the titration until the chloroform layer becomes colorless and the supernatant liquid becomes yellow color. Then add starch solution and continue the titration until the solution becomes colorless. From the number of ml of 0.05M potassium iodate is subtracted half the number of ml of 0.1N sodium thiosulphate which is needed for the assay of iodine.

***Uses:***

1. When it is taken internally, acts as a good source of iodine.
2. It used as a germicide and fungicide.
3. It also acts as a good antiseptic for cuts and wounds.

***Storage:*** It should be stored in tightly closed plastic or glass containers which are resistant to iodine. It should not be stored in metal containers since iodine attacks metals.

## Strong Iodine Solution

It contains 10% w/v of iodine (Limit 9.5-10%) and 6% w/v of potassium iodide.

**Composition:**

| | | |
|---|---|---|
| Iodine | = | 100 gm |
| Potassium iodide | = | 60 gm |
| Purified water | = | 100 ml |

Alcohol (90%) quantity sufficient to produce -1000 ml

***Preparation:*** Iodine and potassium iodide are first of all dissolved in required quantity of water. Then add alcohol to produce 1000 ml.

***Physical properties:*** It is a brown, transparent liquid with the smell of iodine.

***Test for identification:*** To the sample solution of iodine add starch solution, it gives a blue color.

The residue obtained after evaporation and ignition yields the characteristic reactions of potassium and iodine.

**Assay**

***Principle:*** The assay of iodine solutions is carried out for iodine and potassium iodide after the suitable dilution.

*For Iodine:* It is assayed by **iodimetry method of titration (also called redox titration)**.

In this assay the iodine solution diluted with water and and titrated with N/10 sodium thiosulphate using starch mucilage as an indicator. End point is the disappearance of blue colour. During this titration iodine is reduced to sodium iodide and sodium thiosulphate is oxidized to sodium tetrathionate. As the oxidation and reduction takes place simultaneously this is called Redox titration. The chemical reactions of this assay are shown below.

$$\underset{\text{Sodium thiosulphate}}{I_2 + 2Na_2S_2O_3} \longrightarrow \underset{\text{Sodium tetrathionate}}{2NaI + Na_2S_4O_6}$$

*For Potassium iodide:* It is assayed by **Andrew's method of titration** (also called iodometry method, redox titration).

In this assay the diluted solution was acidified by treating with hydrochloric acid and titrated with standard potassium iodate solution until the brown colour turns into light brown. At this stage a small amount of amaranth is added to it and the titration continued until the disappearance of colour in chloroform layer and the supernatant layer becomes clear yellow, Starch mucilage cannot be used as an indicator due to the use of high concentration of hydrochloric acid, which prevents the hydrolysis of iodine monochloride (ICl). As the oxidation and reduction takes place simultaneously this is called redox titration. In this assay, Potassium iodide is oxidised to iodine by potassium iodate in presence of HCl. This liberated iodine is converted to iodine monochloride.

Iodine is more soluble in chloroform than water. After the reaction of free iodine at aqueous layer the iodine may be available at chloroform layer. Hence upon each addition after the aqueous layer becomes colourless, the flask should be shaken well to allow iodine in chloroform layer to react with potassium iodate.

$$2\,KIO_3 + 6\,HCl + KI \longrightarrow 3\,KCl + 3\,ICl + 3\,H_2O + 3(O)$$

***Procedure:***

*For iodine*: Transfer 10 ml of solution in to a glass stoppered flask , add 10 ml of water, and titrate with 0.1N sodium thiosulphate, adding 3ml of starch as the end point is reached.

*For potassium iodide*: Transfer 10 ml of solution in to a glass stoppered flask, add 30 ml of water and 50 ml of hydrochloric acid, cool to room temperature, and titrate 0.05M potassium iodate until the dark brown solution that is produced becomes pale brown. Add 1 ml of amaranth and continue the titration slowly until the red color changes to yellow. The difference between the number of ml of 0.05M potassium iodate used and half the number of ml of 0.1N sodium thiosulphate used in the assay for iodine, multiplied by 16.6, represents the number of mg of KI in the volume of the solution taken.

***Uses:***

1. When it is taken internally, acts as a good source of iodine.
2. It used as a germicide and fungicide.
3. It also acts as a good antiseptic for cuts and wounds.

***Storage:*** It should be stored in tightly closed plastic or glass containers which are resistant to iodine. It should not be stored in metal containers since iodine attacks metals.

## Aqueous Iodine Solution

**(Synonym: Lugol's solution)**

It contains 5% w/w of iodine and 10% w/w of potassium iodide. It is the only official iodine solution without alcohol.

**Composition:**

Iodine = 50 gm

Potassium iodide = 100 gm

Purified water, quantity sufficient to produce = 1000 ml

***Preparation:*** Iodine and potassium iodide are first of all completely dissolved in water by trituration or by frequent shaking. Then the volume is makeup to 1000 ml with purified water.

***Physical properties:*** It is a brown, transparent liquid with the smell of iodine.

***Test for identification:*** To the aqueous solution of iodine add starch solution. Its gives a blue color.

The residue obtained after evaporation and ignition yields the characteristic reactions of potassium and iodine.

**Assay**

***Principle:*** The assay of iodine solutions are carried out for iodine and potassium iodide after the suitable dilution.

*For Iodine:* It is assayed by **iodimetry method of titration** (also called **redox titration**).

In this assay the iodine solution diluted with water and and titrated with N/10 sodium thiosulphate using starch mucilage as an indicator. End point is the disappearance of blue colour. During this titration iodine is reduced to sodium iodide and sodium thiosulphate is oxidised to sodium tetrathionate. As the oxidation and reduction takes place simultaneously this is called Redox titration. The chemical reactions of this assay are shown below.

$$\underset{\text{Sodium thiosulphate}}{I_2 + 2Na_2S_2O_3} \longrightarrow \underset{\text{Sodium tetrathionate}}{2NaI + Na_2S_4O_6}$$

*For Potassium iodide:* It is assayed by **Andrew's method of titration** (also called **iodometry method, redox titration**).

In this assay the diluted solution was acidified by treating with hydrochloric acid and titrated with standard potassium iodate solution until the brown colour turns into light brown. At this stage a small amount of chloroform is added to it and the titration continued until the disappearance of colour in chloroform layer and the supernatant layer becomes clear yellow, Starch mucilage cannot be used as an indicator due to the use of high concentration of hydrochloric acid, which prevents the hydrolysis of iodine monochloride (ICl). As the oxidation and reduction takes place simultaneously this is called redox titration. In this assay, potassium iodide is oxidised to iodine by potassium iodate in presence of HCl. This liberated iodine is converted to iodine monochloride.

Iodine is more soluble in chloroform than water. After the reaction of free iodine at aqueous layer the iodine may be available at chloroform layer. Hence upon each addition after the aqueous layer becomes colourless, the flask should be shaken well to allow iodine in chloroform layer to react with potassium iodate.

$$2\,KIO_3 + 6\,HCl + KI \longrightarrow 3\,KCl + 3\,ICl + 3\,H_2O + 3(O)$$

***Procedure:***

*For iodine*: Transfer 20 ml of the solution and dilute with 10 ml of water. Then the solution is titrated with 0.1N sodium thiosulphate solution using starch solution as an indicator.

*For potassium iodide*: Transfer 10 ml of aqueous iodine solution in to a conical flask, and add 20 ml of water, 16 ml of hydrochloric acid. Then it is titrated with 0.05M potassium iodate solution, shaking vigorously until dark brown color of the solution becomes fade. Then add 5 ml of chloroform and continue the titration until the chloroform layer becomes colorless and the supernatant liquid becomes yellow color. The number of ml of 0.05M potassium iodate is subtracted half the number of ml of 0.1N sodium thiosulphate which is needed for the assay of iodine. Subtract one quarter of the number of 0.1N sodium thiosulphate needed in the assay for iodine from the number of ml of 0.05N potassium iodate used in the titration.

***Uses***

1. When it is taken internally, it acts as a good source of iodine.
2. It is used as germicide and fungicide.

***Storage:*** It should be stored in tightly closed plastic or glass containers which are resistant to iodine. It should not be stored in metal containers since iodine attacks metals.

## Povidone-Iodine Solution I.P., U.S.P.

Povidone iodine solution is an aqueous solution of povidone iodine. It is an iodophoric complex produced by the interaction between iodine and poly (2-oxo pyrrolidin-1-yl-ethylene). It may contain small amount of ethanol.

It contains not less than 9% and not more than 12% of the stated amount of iodine.

***Properties:*** It is a yellowish brown or deep brown liquid or amorphous powder with characteristic odour. It is soluble in alcohol and water. The aqueous solution is acidic in nature.

***Test for identification:***

1. To the dilute solution of sample, add one or two drops of starch solution; a deep blue color is produced.

2. Take the required amount of the solution and transferred to a small flask and cover the mouth of the flask with filter paper soaked in starch solution, no blue color is produced on the paper within 60 seconds.
3. To the dilute solution of sample add required quantity of 0.1M sodium thio sulphate until the color disappears. To this solution add required amount of 2M hydrochloric acid and small volume of potassium dichromate solution, a red color precipitate is produced.

***Test for purity:*** It should be tested for pH of the solution, ethanol.

**Assay**

***Principle:*** It is assayed by **iodimetry method of titration** (also called **redox titration**).

In this assay the substance is dissolved in water by stirring. The solution is titrated with N/10 sodium thiosulphate using starch mucilage as an indicator. End point is the disappearance of blue colour. During this titration iodine is reduced to sodium iodide and sodium thiosulphate is oxidised to sodium tetrathionate. As the oxidation and reduction takes place simultaneously this is called Redox titration. The chemical reactions of this assay are shown below.

$$\underset{\text{Sodium thiosulphate}}{I_2 + 2Na_2S_2O_3} \longrightarrow \underset{\text{Sodium tetrathionate}}{2NaI + Na_2S_4O_6}$$

***Procedure*:** To an accurately measured volume containing about 50 mg of iodine add sufficient water to produce not less than 30 ml and titrate immediately with 0.02M sodium thiosulphate, using 3 ml of starch solution, added towards the end of the titration, as indicator. Carry out a blank titration.

***Uses:***

1. The free iodine content of 10% solution is only 0.001%. When this solution is diluted to 0.1% the free iodine content increases and acts as a powerful bactericidal agent. So it should be diluted before use.
2. It is also used as a disinfectant at various concentrations mainly for cuts, wounds, burns of skin and mouth.
3. It contains antiseptic activity against bacteria due to the slow release of iodine.

***Advantages of povidone Iodine solution:***

1. Good water solubility.
2. Non irritant to the skin.
3. Less toxic and has non staining property. It is easily removed from skin and clothes by washing.

***Storage*:** It should be stored in well closed containers and protected from light.

***Official formulations*:**

Aqueous solution (0.1-1% iodine)

Aerosol (0.5% Iodine)

Surgical scrub (0.75 to 1%)

## Tincture of Iodine U.S.P.

It is having 2% w/v of iodine (limit 1.8 to 2.2) and 2.4% w/v of sodium iodide (limits 2.1-2.6 of NaI). In all aspects it is similar to that weak iodine solution but contain a very less amount of alcohol.

**Assay**

***Assay for iodine:***

***Procedure:*** As directed in the assay for iodine under iodine topical solution, using 10 ml of iodine tincture.

***Assay of potassium iodide:***

***Procedure***: As directed in the assay for sodium iodide under iodine topical solution, using 10 ml of iodine tincture. The difference between the number of ml of 0.05M potassium iodate used and half the number of ml of 0.1N sodium thiosulphate used in the assay for iodine, multiplied by 14.99, represents the number of mg of NaI in the volume of the solution taken.

## Iodised Oil Injection U.S.P.

It is a sterile preparation dispensed in single dose container.

It contains not less than 38% and not more than 41% of combined iodine.

***Preparation:*** It is obtained by the reaction between ethyl ester of fatty acids with hydroiodic acid. The complete saturation of double bonds are takes place by the addition of hydrogen iodide, usually fatty acids obtained from the poppy seeds oils are used. The ethyl esters of oils are commonly used because it provides less viscous preparation when compared with the use of oil.

***Tests for purity:*** It should be tested for specific gravity, acidity, chloro compounds and free iodine.

***Uses:*** It is used for certain X-ray diagnosis.

## Boric Acid I.P., U.S.P.

**(Synonym: Boracic acid)**

**Mol. Formula:** $H_3BO_3$ **Mol. Weight:** 61.83

It contains not less than 99.5% and not more than 100.5% of $H_3BO_3$ with reference to the dried basis.

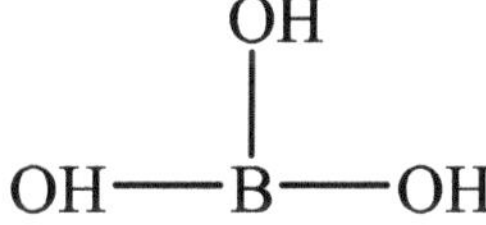


***Preparation:***

1. *From natural sources:* Boric acid naturally occurs in volcanic jets of steam (soffioni) which is from the ground in Tuscany. The steam is condensed in natural lagoons or

artificial lagoons and the resulting liquid is concentrated by using steam. Crude boric acid crystallizes out on cooling and purified by recrystallisation.

2. *Laboratory process:* Boric acid is prepared by the decomposition of native borax and from native borates with hydrochloric acid or sulphuric acid.

   A mixture of concentrated sulphuric acid and water (12:60 ml) is added to a boiling solution of borax in water (60 gm in 160 ml water).

$$Na_2B_4O_7 + H_2SO_4 + 5\,H_2O \longrightarrow 4\,H_3BO_3 + Na_2SO_4$$

$$Na_2B_4O_7 + 2HCl + 5\,H_2O \longrightarrow 4\,H_3BO_3 + 2\,NaCl$$

   The above solution is filtered in hot condition and set aside for crystallization. The boric acid is then filtered off, washed until free from sulphate and allowed to dry at room temperature.

3. *Commercial preparation:* Boric acid is prepared by the decomposition of colemanite, resonite and borax (natural borates).

   A. *From colemanite:* The powdered colemanite is suspended in boiling water; sulphur dioxide gas is passed through the suspension. Crystals of boric acid separates out on cooling.

$$Ca_2B_6O_{11}.5\,H_2O + 2\,SO_2 + 4\,H_2O \longrightarrow 6\,H_3BO_3 + 2\,CaSO_3$$

   B. *From borax:* A high grade medicinally used boric acid is prepared from the treatment of borax solution with hydrochloric acid.

$$Na_2B_4O_7.10\,H_2O + 2\,HCl \longrightarrow 4\,H_3BO_3 + 2\,NaCl + 5\,H_2O$$

***Physical properties:*** Boric acid is present or available in three forms.

1. Colorless pearly scales.
2. Six sided triclinic crystals.
3. White, odorless powder, unctuous to touch with slightly acidic and bitter taste. It is soluble in 25 parts of cold water and 4 parts of glycerol. It is stable in air, the density is 1.46, the crystal and the scale forms are suitable for the preparation of aqueous solution because the powder form is float on the surface of water. The powder form is mainly useful in dusting powders and ointments.

***Chemical properties:***

*Action of heat on boric acid:* Boric acid is a weak acid with a pKa value of 9.19 for the ionization of first proton at 25 °C.

When heated to 100 °C, it loses one molecule of water to give meta boric acid. Further heating up to 160 °C gives tetra boric acid still heating at more than 160 °C it gives anhydride of boric acid called boron trioxide which is a glassy appearing solid.

$$\underset{\text{Boric acid}}{4H_3BO_3} \xrightarrow[-4H_2O \; \Delta]{100\ ^\circ C} \underset{\text{Meta Boric acid}}{4HBO_2} \xrightarrow[-H_2O \; \Delta]{160\ ^\circ C} \underset{\text{Tetra Boric acid}}{H_2B_4O_7} \xrightarrow[-H_2O \; \Delta]{>160\ ^\circ C} \underset{\text{anhydride form}}{2B_2O_3}$$

It is weakly acidic than carbonic acid, the solution gives slightly dull claret red color in litmus paper.

It reacts with turmeric paper and turns the paper brown which in turns blackish when dipped in sodium hydroxide solution.

Boric acid reacts with ethyl alcohol and gives green color flame due to the formation of ethyl borate.

*Reaction with glycerin*: Boric acid is reacts with the equimolar quantity of glycerin at 140 °C and 150 °C and produce a compound known as boroglycerin glycerite ($C_3H_5BO_3$), which acts as a suppository base.

***Test for identification:***

1. A small quantity of sample is dissolved in methanol (5 ml) by gently warming the solution to which a few drops of sulphuric acid is added. Ignite the solution; the flame is tinged with green owing to the formation of ethyl borate.
2. A small amount of boric acid is dissolved in sufficient quantity of boiled water the resulting solution is faintly acidic.

***Test for purity:*** It should be tested for appearance of solution, pH and solubility in ethanol, arsenic, heavy metals, sulphates and loss on drying.

***Test for pH:*** It should be within the range of 3.8 to 4.8.

***Test for solubility in ethanol:*** 1 gm of sample is dissolve in 10 ml of boiling ethanol (95%) the solution is not more opalescence than that of standard solution which is prepared as per the monograph.

**Assay**

***Principle:*** It is assayed by **acidimetry-alkalimetry method of titration** (also called **neutralization method**).

In this assay the substance is dissolved in water and mixed with glycerol or mannitol and titrated with sodium hydroxide, using phenolphthalein as an indicator. End point is the appearance of permanent pale pink colour.

Boric acid is a weak acid, it cannot be titrated directly with sodium hydroxide to get a sharp end point. Hence in this assay polyhydroxy alcohol (glycerol or mannitol) added to the boric acid and hence the boric acid is converted into strong monobasic acid (glyceryl boric acid or mannityl boric acid). The glyceryl boric acid or mannityl boric acid reacts readily with sodium hydroxide (the base) and gives sharp end point. The indicator is colourless in acid medium and it changes to pink in alkali medium which is the end point.

As the acid and alkali involved in this assay, it is called as acidimetry-alkalimetry method of titration and the neutralization takes place in this assay during titration hence this assay is also called as Neutralization method. The chemical reactions of this assay are shown below.

$$2\ \begin{matrix} CH_2OH \\ | \\ CH\text{-}OH \\ | \\ CH_2OH \end{matrix} + \begin{matrix} HO \\ HO - B \\ HO \end{matrix} \longrightarrow \left[ \begin{matrix} CH_2-OH \quad HO-CH_2 \\ CH-O \quad O-CH \\ \quad B \quad \\ CH_2-O \quad O-CH_2 \end{matrix} \right] + H_3O^+ + 2\,H_2O$$

$$2\ \begin{matrix} CH_2\text{-}OH \\ | \\ (CHOH)_2 \\ | \\ CH\text{-}OH \\ | \\ CH\text{-}OH \\ | \\ CH_2\text{-}OH \end{matrix} + \begin{matrix} HO \\ HO - B \\ HO \end{matrix} \longrightarrow \left[ \begin{matrix} CH_2OH \qquad CH_2OH \\ (CHOH)_2 \quad (CHOH)_2 \\ CH-O \quad O-CH \\ \quad B \quad \\ CH-O \quad O-CH \\ CH_2OH \qquad CH_2OH \end{matrix} \right] + H_3O^+ + 2\,H_2O \ \text{(Srong acid)}$$

$$H_3\overset{+}{O} + NaOH \longrightarrow Na^+ + 2\,H_2O$$

***Procedure:*** Weigh accurately about 2.0 gm, dissolve in a mixture of 50 ml of water and 100 ml of glycerin, previously neutralized to phenolphthalein solution. Titrate with 1M sodium hydroxide using phenolphthalein solution as an indicator.

***Uses:***

1. Boric acid is a weak bacteriostatic and fungistatic.
2. It is local anti-infective agent and it is used in local antiseptic creams, lotions, ointments and dusting powders which are used to apply to the skin or mucous or eye.
3. It is also used as an insecticide for cockroaches and black carpet beetles.
4. Aqueous solutions have been used as mouth washes, eye lotions and skin lotions.
5. It is also used in dusting powder after triturating with some other inert material due to its smooth unctuous property.
6. The aqueous solutions are used in the form of douches for irrigating the bladder and vagina and hot fermentation of boils, whitlows and carbuncles.
7. The 1.9% solution in water is iso osmotic with serum.
8. Boroglycerin glycerite is used for the preparation of suppository base.
9. If it is taken internally, it leads to toxic effects more over no specific and satisfactory antidote for boric acid poisoning available. Therefore it has been largely replaced by some better and safer drugs. If ingested, boric acid produces diarrhoea, vomiting, abdominal cramps, erythmatous rash, circulatory collapse and coma etc.

10. Boric acid is used in buffer systems such as aluminium acetate and aluminium sub acetate solution, ephedrine bitartarate ophthalmic solution.
11. It should not be applied to ruptured skin.

***Storage***: It should be stored in well closed container.

***Labelling***: It is very dangerous if ingested, so the label should states that it is not meant for internal use.

## Sodium Carbonate

This compound is discussed under **acidifiers and alkalinising agents**.

## Sodium Hypochlorite Solution U.S.P.

**(Synonym: Chlorinated soda)**

**Mol. Formula:** NaOCl **Mol. Weight:** 74.44

The sodium hypochlorite salt (solid state) is highly unstable. Hence the solution form of sodium hypochlorite is used for the practical purpose.

It contains not less than 4% and not more than 6% by weight of NaOCl.

***Preparation:*** It is prepared by passing required quantity of chlorine gas into a cold solution of sodium hydroxide or sodium carbonate.

$$NaOH + Cl_2 \longrightarrow NaOCl + HCl$$

$$Na_2CO_3 + Cl_2 \longrightarrow 2NaOCl + CO_2\uparrow$$

***Properties:*** It is a pale greenish liquid with a smell of chlorine. It turns red litmus to blue and bleaches it.

***Test for identification:***

1. Addition of 3N hydrochloric acid to the sample solution causes an evolution of chlorine gas.
2. The above solution burns with yellow flame when ignited.

***Test for purity:*** It should be tested for alkalinity, sulphate, iron, heavy metals, and arsenic

**Assay**

***Principle:*** It is assayed by **iodometry method of titration** (also called **redox titration**) to find out the "available chlorine".

In this assay the substance is treated with acetic acid in presence of excess of potassium iodide and titrated with sodium thiosulphate, using starch mucilage as an indicator. End point is the disappearance of blue colour.

In this assay the substance is treated with acetic acid in presence of excess of potassium iodide whereby the available chlorine is liberated from sodium hypochlorite and it displaces equal amount of iodine from potassium iodide. The liberated iodine is determined by titrating with N/10 sodium thiosulphate using starch mucilage as an indicator. End point is the disappearance of blue colour.

During this titration iodine is reduced to sodium iodide and sodium thiosulphate is oxidised to sodium tetrathionate. As the oxidation and reduction takes place simultaneously this is called redox titration. The chemical reactions of this assay are shown below.

$$\underset{\text{(Sodium hypochlorite)}}{2NaOCl} + 2\,CH_3COOH \longrightarrow 2\,CH_3COONa + HOCl + HCl$$

$$HOCl + HCl \rightleftharpoons Cl_2 + H_2O$$

$$Cl_2 + 2KI \longrightarrow I_2 + 2\,KCl$$

$$I_2 + \underset{\text{Sodium thiosulphate}}{2\,Na_2S_2O_3} \longrightarrow 2\,NaI + \underset{\text{Sodium tetrathionate}}{Na_2S_4O_6}$$

***Procedure:*** Measure accurately about 3 ml of solution, transferred it to glass stoppered flask, and dilute it with 50 ml of water. Add 2 gm of potassium iodide and 10 ml of 6N acetic acid, and titrate the liberated iodine with 0.1N sodium thiosulphate, adding 3 ml of starch as the indicator which is added at the end of titration. Perform the blank titration also.

***Uses:*** It is mixed with boric acid solution known as Dakin's solution and is used for skin infection. It is also used as an antiseptic.

***Caution:*** The solution is not suitable for application to wounds.

***Storage:*** It is easily affected by light, so it should be stored in tight, light resistant containers at a temperature not exceeding 25 °C.

## Dilute Sodium Hypochlorite Solution

***Definition:*** It is an aqueous solution of sodium hypochlorite containing 0.9-1% of available chlorine, with suitable stabilizing agents and sodium chloride.

***Preparation:*** It is prepared from sodium hypochlorite solution by diluting 5 times with purified water. The pH of the solution is adjusted with 5% sodium bicarbonate such that it does not give color with phenolphthalein.

***Properties:*** It is colorless or slight yellow color solution with slight odour of chlorine. It is easily affected by light.

***Test for identification:*** Similar to that of sodium hypochlorite solution.

***Test for purity:*** Similar to that of sodium hypochlorite solution.

***Mechanism of action:*** The sodium hypochlorite solution is too strong to be used on tissues due to its alkalinity and oxidizing action. The dilute solution is mainly used for disinfectant and antibacterial action due the liberation of chlorine when contact with acid and partly to oxidizing action due to liberation of oxygen. The dilute solution is having less alkalinity and increases the effectiveness of hypochlorite.

***Disadvantage:*** The dilute solution dissolves blood clot, delays clotting time which leads to hemorrhage.

**Assay:** Similar to that of sodium hypochlorite solution.

***Uses:***

1. Sodium hypochlorite solution is mainly used as a disinfectant for utensils.
2. It is also used as a deodorant.
3. Dilute solution of sodium hypochlorite solution acts as a germicidal agents due to its irrigation action.
4. The diluted solution is also used to prevent fungal infection in foot bath.

***Storage*:** It should be stored in well closed light resistant container and protected from sunlight at a temperature not exceeding 20 °C and away from acids.

***Labelling*:** The label should state that

(i) The expiry date.
(ii) Storage condition.
(iii) It is indicated in the pharmaceutical form as "cutaneous solution".

**Other formulations:**

Strong sodium hypochlorite solution B.P.

Sodium Hypochlorite topical solution U.S.P.

Chlorinated lime and boric acid solution B.P. (Eusol solution).

### 6.2.5 Protein Precipitant Antimicrobials

#### Silver Nitrate I.P., B.P.

**Mol. Formula:** $AgNO_3$ **Mol. Weight:** 169.9

Silver nitrate contains not less than 99% and not more than 100.5% of $AgNO_3$.

***Preparation:*** Silver nitrate is prepared by dissolving metallic silver in hot and fairly concentrated nitric acid.

$$Ag + 2HNO_3 \longrightarrow AgNO_3 + NO_2 + H_2O$$

By this method 3 parts of silver is mixed to a 25% solution of nitric acid (about 10 parts) and warmed. Then the mixture is heated to remove the nitrous oxide fumes, filtered and evaporated until it become dry. Then the mass is fused, so that copper nitrate present gets converted into insoluble oxide. The products so obtained gets dissolved in hot water, filtered and kept undisturbed in a dark place for crystallization. The crystals are collected on a sintered glass crucible and dried at about 50 °C. Purification of silver nitrate has been costly process; it becomes necessary to use pure silver and nitric acid which are free from halogen.

***Physical properties:*** Silver nitrate occurs as colorless or white crystalline plates or crystalline powder, odorless. It is a bitter and metallic taste. It is very soluble in water, more soluble in boiling water, one part is soluble in 50 ml of alcohol or about 7 ml of boiling alcohol and slightly soluble in ether, melting point is 212 °C. It slowly decomposes in light, turning black. So both the solid and its solution should be protected from light.

***Chemical properties:***

1. *Decomposition Reaction:* Silver nitrate when heated at 209 °C, it melts to a liquid yellowish color without decomposition. When heated to red hot, gets decomposed in to metallic silver residue along with the evolution of $NO_2$ and $O_2$.

$$2AgNO_3 \xrightarrow{\Delta} 2Ag + 2NO_2 + O_2$$

2. *Reaction with hydrochloric acid:* The neutral or acidic solution of silver nitrate is added to hydrochloric acid or soluble chlorides, a curdy white precipitate of silver chloride is formed which is insoluble in dilute acids but soluble in dilute ammonia solution yields cations.

   In potassium cyanide or sodium thiosulphate solution the precipitate gives cations.

$$AgNO_3 + HCl \longrightarrow AgCl + HNO_3$$

$$AgCl + 2NH_3 \longrightarrow [Ag(NH_3)_2]^+ + Cl^-$$

$$AgCl + 2CN^- \longrightarrow [Ag(CN)_2]^+ + Cl^-$$

$$AgCl + 2S_2O_3^{2-} \longrightarrow [Ag(S_2O_3)_2]^{3+} + Cl^-$$

3. *Reaction with sodium carbonate:* If sodium carbonate is added to silver nitrate, silver carbonate is formed which upon boiling, yields silver oxide.

$$2AgNO_3 + Na_2CO_3 \longrightarrow Ag_2CO_3 + 2NaNO_3$$

$$Ag_2CO_3 \xrightarrow{\Delta} \underset{\text{Silver oxide}}{Ag_2O} + CO_2\uparrow$$

4. *Reaction with alkali hydroxides:*

   (a) If silver nitrate is added to sodium hydroxide, gives silver hydroxide which decomposes to yield brown silver oxide.

$$AgNO_3 + NaOH \longrightarrow \underset{\text{Silver hydroxide}}{Ag(OH)\downarrow} + NaNO_3$$

$$2AgOH \longrightarrow \underset{\substack{\text{Silver oxide} \\ \text{(brown color)}}}{Ag_2O} + H_2O$$

(b) If ammonium hydroxide is added to silver nitrate solution, maximum amount of silver ions are get converted into silver ammonium complex and few silver ions are present in solution. If any reducing agents are added to this (like formaldehyde, glucose) the free silver ions are get reduced to metallic silver and forms silver mirror.

$$AgNO_3 + 3NH_4OH \longrightarrow \underset{\text{Silver-ammonium complex}}{Ag(NH_3)_2OH} + NH_4NO_3 + 2H_2O$$

$$2Ag(NH_3)_2OH + HCHO \longrightarrow HCOONH_4 + \underset{\text{Silver mirror}}{2Ag\downarrow} + 3NH_3 + H_2O$$

(c) If any phosphate or borate reagents are added to silver nitrate it yields silver phosphates and silver borate respectively.

(d) It reacts with proteins to yield a heavy precipitate of silver protein complex.

***Test for identification*:** It gives the characteristic reactions of silver and nitrate ions.

***Test for purity*:** It should be tested for pH, appearance of solution, acidity or alkalinity, aluminium, bismuth, copper, lead and foreign salts.

***Test for pH*:** The pH of 4% w/v solution of silver nitrate is in between 5.4 - 6.4.

***Test for acidity or alkalinity*:** To the required amount of sample solution add bromocresol green solution, the solution becomes blue. To the small amount of sample solution add phenol red solution, the solution becomes yellow.

***Test for Aluminium, Bismuth, Copper and Lead*:** A small quantity of sample is dissolved in a mixture of 4 ml of strong ammonia solution and water (excess of dilute ammonia solution). The resulting solution should be clear and colorless.

**Assay**

***Principle:*** It is assayed by **precipitation method of titration**.

In this assay the substance is dissolved in water and acidified with nitric acid and titrated against 0.1N ammonium thiocyanate. Ferric ammonium sulphate (Ferric alum) is used as an indicator. End point is the appearance of brick red colour.

During this assay, silver ions nitrate reacts with ammonium thiocyanate and silver thiocyanate precipitate is formed. After the completion of this reaction, further addition of ammonium thiocyanate reacts with the indicator ferric ammonium sulphate and yield brick red colour ferric thiocyanate, which is the end point. As the test substance is converted to a precipitate during this assay, this is called precipitation method. The chemical reactions of this assay are shown below.

$$AgNO_3 + NH_4SCN \longrightarrow AgSCN\downarrow + NH_4NO_3$$

$$3\,NH_4SCN + Fe(SO_4)_3(NH_4)_2SO_4 \longrightarrow \underset{\text{Brick Red colour}}{Fe(SCN)_3} + 2\,(NH_4)_2SO_4$$

***Procedure*:** Dissolve 0.300 gm in 50 ml of water; add 2 ml of dilute nitric acid and 2 ml of ferric ammonium sulphate solution. Titrate with 0.1M ammonium thiocyanate until a reddish yellow colour is obtained.

***Uses:***

1. Silver nitrate is used as a germicide, astringent and disinfectant.
2. 0.01 - 10% solution is act as mild antiseptic.
3. A 10% solution is also used to treat infected ulcers in mouth.
4. A 1% solution of silver nitrate finds use for ophthalmic purposes as installation to the eyes of the new born babies for the prevention of ophthalmia neonatorum.
5. Ammonical silver nitrate solution is used for dentistry.
6. Stick form of silver nitrate is used as a caustic to destroy warts and skin growths.
7. In cosmetics it is used to dye eye brows, eyelashes and as a hair dye.
8. It also used in homoeopathic medicine.
9. Silver nitrate is specially used for the treatment of gonococcal infections in new borns.
10. It is also very successfully used to treat severly burnt patients.

***Mechanism of action of silver nitrate*:** The antibacterial action is due to the binding or combination of silver ions with tissue proteins, so astringent, caustic and perhaps the germicidal activity attributed to it.

***Adverse effects*:** It includes diarrohoea, vomiting, pain in the mouth, coma and convulsions.

***Storage*:** It should be stored in non-metallic, amber colored bottles, protected from light and moisture.

## Mild Silver Protein

It is a preparation containing colloidal silver by the presence of proteins or in combination with it. It contains not less than 19.0% and not more than 23% of Ag.

***Preparation:*** It is prepared by treating silver oxide with gelatin in the presence of alkali or treating silver salts with excess of denatured protein or silver oxide with serum albumin or by suspending moist silver oxide in a solution of casein. The mixture is heated until no precipitate is formed on the addition of sodium chloride, the mixture is then evaporated and dried.

***Properties:*** It is a brown or dark brown or almost black, odorless, lustrous granules or scales and hygroscopic in nature. It is freely soluble in water and forming a colloidal solution, insoluble in alcohol, chloroform and ether. Solution should be freshly prepared and protected from light.

A solution in nitric acid is treated with dilute hydrochloric acid gives silver chloride precipitate. The aqueous solutions are containing 10 mg/ml of disodium EDTA as a stabilizing agent.

***Test for identification:***

*Test 1:* 1 gm of silver protein is heated until charring takes place. It is incinerated completely, a greyish white residue is formed. Then add nitric acid and neutralize, it gives the characteristic reaction of silver ions.

*Test 2:* To the 1% of solution, add ferric chloride solution when the dark color is disappeared and the solution becomes cloudy.

*Test 3:* To the 1% of solution, add mercuric chloride solution, no white precipitate is produced. (Distinction from strong silver protein)

***Test for purity:*** It should be tested for silver salt, distinction from silver protein.

***Silver salt:*** To the small amount of sample is treated with 10 ml of 90% alcohol and filtered. To the filtrate add dilute hydrochloric acid. No opalescence produced.

***Uses:***

1. The mild silver protein is non-irritant and hence is used for application on mucous membrane.
2. It also finds use in the treatment of gonococcal eye infections.
3. It posses mild antibacterial activity.

**Assay**

***Principle:*** It is assayed by **precipitation method of titration**.

In this assay the substance is dissolved in water by gentle heating and ignited to remove carbonaceous matter. The residue is dissolved in nitric acid, diluted with water and titrated against 0.1N ammonium thiocyanate. Ferric ammonium sulphate (Ferric alum) is used as an indicator. End point is the appearance of brick red colour.

During this assay, silver ions reacts with ammonium thiocyanate and silver thiocyanate precipitate is formed. After the completion of this reaction, further addition of ammonium thiocyanate reacts with the indicator ferric ammonium sulphate and yield brick red colour ferric thiocyanate, which is the end point. As the test substance is converted to a precipitate during this assay it is called precipitation method. The chemical reactions of this assay are shown below.

$$Ag^+ + NH_4SCN \longrightarrow AgSCN\downarrow + NH_4^+$$

$$6\,NH_4SCN + Fe(SO_4)_3(NH_4)_2SO_4 \longrightarrow \underset{\text{Brick Red colour}}{2\,Fe(SCN)_3} + 4\,(NH_4)_2SO_4$$

***Storage:*** It should be stored in tightly closed, amber colored glass containers, protected from light and moisture.

## Strong Silver Protein

It is a compound of silver and protein.

It contains not less than 7.5% and not more than 8.5% of silver.

It is prepared by adding silver nitrate solution to peptone solution. The precipitate obtained is digested with protalbumose until a solution is obtained which is then evaporated in a moderate vacuum.

Instead of the silver nitrate solution, sometimes silver oxide may be suspended in the peptone solution. The suspension is shaken until the silver peptone has formed. The digested and dried product obtained is similar to that of product obtained from silver nitrate.

***Physical properties:*** It occurs as a pale yellowish orange to brownish black, odorless, hygroscopic powder. It slowly dissolves in water and forms a dark brown solution. It is almost insoluble in alcohol, ether and chloroform.

***Test for identification:*** It gives the reactions similar to that of test (1) and (2) in mild silver protein and gives the following additional tests. (3) To a small quantity of 2% w/v of sample solution, add required amount of sodium hydroxide solution (5 ml), add water and 2% w/v of copper sulphate solution. The solution is allowed to stand for 5 minutes, a violet color is produced. (4) To the 1% w/v of sample solution, add mercuric chloride solution, a white precipitate is formed and the supernatant is colorless or almost colorless.

***Test for purity:*** It should be tested for silver salt, foreign protein.

***Test for silver salt:*** To the sample solution, add 10 ml of 90% alcohol and then filtered. To the filtrate add 20 ml of dilute hydrochloric acid. No opalescence is produced.

***Uses:***

1. Due to the presence of low concentration of ionized silver, it is used on mucous membranes in the nose, throat and conjunctiva of eyes.
2. It is mainly used as local antibacterial agent.
3. The solutions are employed to irritate the bladder and urethra, to treat gonococcal infections i.e., Gonococcal conjunctivitis.
4. It is also used in nasal solutions, respiratory tract infections (Prophylactic medication).

**Assay**

***Principle:*** It is assayed by **precipitation method of titration**.

In this assay the substance is dissolved in water by gentle heating and ignited to remove carbonaceous matter. The residue is dissolved in nitric acid, diluted with water and titrated against 0.1N ammonium thiocyanate. Ferric ammonium sulphate (Ferric alum) is used as an indicator. End point is the appearance of brick red colour.

During this assay, silver ions reacts with ammonium thiocyanate and silver thiocyanate precipitate is formed. After the completion of this reaction, further addition of ammonium thiocyanate reacts with the indicator ferric ammonium sulphate and yield brick red colour ferric thiocyanate, which is the end point. As the test substance is converted to a precipitate during this assay it is called precipitation method. The chemical reactions of this assay are shown below.

$$Ag^+ + NH_4SCN \longrightarrow AgSCN\downarrow + NH_4^+$$

$$3\,NH_4SCN + Fe(SO_4)_3(NH_4)_2SO_4 \longrightarrow \underset{\text{Brick Red colour}}{Fe(SCN)_3} + 2\,(NH_4)_2SO_4$$

***Storage:*** It should be stored in well closed containers and protected from sunlight. The solutions should be freshly prepared in cold water and dispensed in amber colored glass bottles.

## Toughened Silver Nitrate

***Preparation:*** This is prepared by melting silver nitrate with small amount of potassium nitrate or with about 4% of hydrochloric acid and the resulting fused mass is poured into conical or cylindrical silver or platinum moulds.

***Properties:*** It is having the caustic properties like silver nitrate.

## Mercury Compounds

### Yellow Mercuric Oxide B.P., U.S.P.

**Mol. Formula:** HgO **Mol. Weight:** 216.6

It contains not less than 99.5% of HgO calculated with reference to the substance on dried basis.

***Preparation:***

*Method 1:* It is prepared by precipitation reaction method using mercuric salt solution and alkali hydroxide.

Example: Mercuric chloride and sodium hydroxide. By pouring a concentrated solution of mercuric chloride into a dilute solution of sodium hydroxide with constant agitation and allow to stand for an hour. The yellow precipitate of mercuric oxide is settled down and the supernatant is decanted off.

The precipitate is transferred to the calico filter and it is washed several times with water until the washings are free from alkali and chloride. It is then allowed to dry at room temperature.

$$HgCl_2 + 2NaOH \longrightarrow Hg(OH)_2 + 2NaCl$$

$$Hg(OH)_2 \longrightarrow HgO + H_2O$$

*Method 2: From mercuric nitrate:* Mercuric nitrate undergoes decomposition to yields yellow mercuric oxide.

$$2Hg(NO_3)_2 \xrightarrow{O_2} 2HgO + 4NO_3$$

*Method 3: From mercury:* For long term heating of mercury in air at 300 °C gives yellow mercuric oxide.

$$2Hg + O_2 \longrightarrow 2HgO$$

***Physical properties:*** Yellow mercuric oxide is yellow or orange yellow, heavy amorphous powder, the color variation depends upon the temperature at which it is precipitated and also the differences in the particle size, it is stable in air but becomes discolored on exposure to light. It is practically insoluble in water and alcohol. Soluble in dilute hydrochloric acid or nitric acid and soluble in alkali cyanide solutions or iodides forming colorless solutions. It is slowly soluble in alkali solutions.

$$HgO + 2HCl \longrightarrow HgCl_2 + H_2O$$

$$HgO + 2HNO_3 \longrightarrow Hg(NO_3)_2 + H_2O$$

***Chemical properties:*** When it is heated the yellow mercuric oxide is converted into red oxide and when it is heated at high temperature it decomposes into oxygen and metallic mercury vapour.

$$2\,HgO \longrightarrow O_2\uparrow + 2\,Hg$$

*Reaction with oleic acid:* It reacts with oleic acid, forms mercuric oleate.

$$2CH_3(CH_2)_7CH{=}CH(CH_2)_7COOH + HgO$$

$$\downarrow$$

$$[CH_3(CH_2)_7CH{=}CH(CH_2)_7COO]_2Hg + H_2O$$

***Test for identification:***

1. When it is heated gently it gives red color and when it is heated at high temperature it decomposes into oxygen and mercury.
2. The acidic solution of mercuric oxide gives the characteristic reactions of mercuric ion.

***Test for purity:*** It should be tested for mercurous salt, chloride, sulphated residue and loss on drying.

1. *Test for mercurous salt:* The aqueous suspension of sample is allowed to settle, the supernatant liquid is neutral to litmus.
2. *Test for mercurous chloride:* To the sample add alcohol and filtered. To the filtrate $H_2S$ gas is passed. The color produced should not be more than that of the color produced in the standard which is prepared as per the monograph.
3. *Test for lead:* To the sample solution add dilute $H_2SO_4$, no cloudiness is produced if lead is absent.
4. *Test for copper:* To the sample solution, the slight excess of dilute ammonia solution is added. A white precipitate is formed, but the supernatant liquid does not show any bluish tint.
5. *Test for silver:* To the sample solution add HCl, no precipitate is formed.
6. *Tests for foreign protein:* (a) The 1% of sample solution gives no deposits within 10 min. (b) To the 2% of sample solution, equal quantity of sodium chloride is added, no turbidity is produced.

### Assay

***Principle:*** It is assayed by **precipitation method of titration.**

In this assay the substance is dissolved in a mixture of water and nitric acid and titrated against 0.1N ammonium thiocyanate. Ferric ammonium sulphate (Ferric alum) is used as an indicator. End point is the appearance of brick red colour.

During this assay, mercury ions reacts with nitric acid and the mercuric nitrate so formed reacts with ammonium thiocyanate whereby mercuric thiocyanate precipitate is formed. After the completion of this reaction, further addition of ammonium thiocyanate reacts with the indicator ferric ammonium sulphate and yield red colour mercuric thiocyanate, which is the end point. As the test substance is converted to a precipitate during this assay it is called precipitation method. The chemical reactions of this assay are shown below.

$$HgO + 2\ HNO_3 \longrightarrow Hg(NO_3)_2 + H_2O$$

$$Hg(NO_3)_2 + 2\ NH_4SCN \longrightarrow 2\ NH_4NO_3 + Hg(SCN)_2$$

***Procedure:*** Weigh accurately about 0.4 gm of sample and dissolve in 5 ml of nitric acid and 10 ml of water and dilute with 150 ml of water and titrate with 0.1N ammonium thiocyanate solution using ferric alum as an indicator.

***Uses:***

1. It is used for some mild infections and inflammations of the eye including conjunctivitis and eradication of crab lices from the eye lashes.
2. 1% yellow mercuric oxide ointment is used for the local antibacterial properties, due to its insolubility and slow release of $Hg^{2+}$ ions.

***Storage:*** It should be stored in well closed container and protected from sunlight.

## Mercuric Oxide Eye Ointment

It contains not less than 0.9% and not more than 1.1% w/w of yellow mercuric oxide.

***Preparation:*** It is prepared by triturating finely powdered yellow mercuric oxide with less quantity of melted base until to get smooth mixture. Then gradually add sufficient quantity of melted base to get the required weight. Trituration is continued until the ointment reaches room temperature. All of the above operations are carried out under aseptic areas.

***Test for identification:*** The residue obtained after treatment with chloroform is used for the following tests.

1. When the residue is heated it shows red color and when heated at higher temperature, it dissociates to give mercury and oxygen.
2. The solution of the residue in mineral acid gives the characteristic reactions of mercuric ion.

### Assay

It is assayed by **oxidation reduction method of titration**. Similar to yellow mercuric oxide.

*Uses:*

1. It is mainly used in ophthalmology.
2. A 1% ointment is used for the treatment of mild inflammatory conditions like conjunctivitis.
3. A 2% ointment is used for the treatment of various types of skin infections.

## Calomel or Mercurous Chloride B.P., U.S.P.

This compound is discussed under **purgatives**.

## Ammoniated Mercury U.S.P.

**(Synonym: White precipitate, amino chloride of mercury)**

**Mol. Formula:** $NH_2HgCl$ **Mol. Weight:** 252.1

It is the mercuric chloride, in which one chlorine atom has been replaced by the univalent amino group. It is the most common important member of mercurammines with varying composition.

$$\text{Cl-Hg-Cl} \xrightarrow[+NH_2]{-Cl} NH_2\text{-Hg-Cl}$$

It contains not less than 98.0% of $NH_2HgCl$.

***Preparation:*** It is prepared by adding a 5% solution of mercuric chloride (3 parts in 60 ml water) to a diluted ammonia solution (4 parts) and 20 parts of water with constant stirring.

$$HgCl_2 + 2\,NH_3 \longrightarrow NH_2HgCl + NH_4Cl$$

The precipitated ammoniated mercury is collected in a filter paper, washed with cold water and dried at a temperature not exceeding 30 °C. The washing should not continue long enough to remove all the ammonium chloride. If washed for long time the product undergo decomposition to yield yellow basic compound.

$$HgCl_2 + 2NH_3 \longrightarrow NH_2HgCl + NH_4Cl$$

$$2\,HgNH_2Cl + H_2O \longrightarrow NH_4Cl + \underset{\text{Yellow basic compound}}{NH_2(HgO)HgCl}$$

***Physical properties:*** It is a white, heavy amorphous powder, odorless, tasteless, insoluble in water, ether and alcohol, but readily soluble in warm acetic acid.

***Chemical properties:***

*Decomposition reaction:* In cold water it gradually decomposes. However in boiling water it is hydrolyzed to yield yellow basic compound ($NH_2HgCl.HgO$). In boiling alkalis it is completely decomposed as ammonia and mercuric oxide.

$$NH_2HgCl + NaOH \longrightarrow NH_3 + HgO + NaCl$$

*Reaction with ammonium carbonate:* It reacts with ammonium carbonate to yield mercuric chloride.

$$2\,HgNH_2Cl + (NH_4)_2CO_3 \longrightarrow HgCl_2 + HgO\downarrow + 4\,NH_3 + CO_2\uparrow$$

*Reaction with ammonium chloride:* Ammoniated mercury reacts with warm solution of ammonium chloride to give mercuric chloride.

$$HgNH_2Cl + NH_4Cl \longrightarrow HgCl_2 + 2\,NH_3\uparrow$$

*Reaction with nitric acid:* Ammoniated mercury reacts with nitric acid and gives mercuric nitrate and ammonium chloride.

$$HgNH_2Cl + 2\,HNO_3 \longrightarrow Hg(NO_3)_2 + NH_4Cl$$

***Test for identification:***

1. Solution in acetic acid gives the characteristic reactions of mercuric ion and chloride ion.
2. When it is heating, it volatilizes without involving fusion.
3. When it is heated with sodium hydroxide it yields yellow mercuric oxide and ammonia.

$$HgNH_2Cl + NaOH \longrightarrow HgO\downarrow + NH_3\uparrow + NaCl$$

4. To the sample solution add small amount of aqueous solution of sodium thiosulphate (sample is completely soluble) which evolves of ammonia, when this solution is heated gently a rust colored mixture is formed which upon centrifugation a red color precipitate is obtained. If the solution is strongly heated a black mixture is formed.

***Test for purity:*** It should be tested for mercurous chloride, carbonates and sulphated residue (ash).

***Test for mercurous chloride and carbonate:*** The small quantity of sample is triturated with 10 ml of acetic acid followed by heating to 70 °C with occasional shaking; a clear solution is formed without evolution of carbon dioxide (no effervescence). A small amount of ammonium chloride is also present in the commercial product.

**Assay**

***Principle:*** It is assayed by **acidimetry-alkalimetry method of titration** (also called **neutralization method**).

In this assay the substance is dissolved in solvent ether and petroleum ether and potassium iodide is added. The liberated alkali is then titrated against 0.1N hydrochloric acid, using methyl red as an indicator. End point is the red colour. In this assay the base reacts with hydrochloric acid and neutralization takes place during the titration. The indicator is yellow colour in alkali medium and it changes to red colour upon neutralization which is the end point.

*Uses:*

1. It is mainly used topically as an anti infective agent.
2. It is used for the treatment of impetigo (skin infection), other staphylococcal skin infections.
3. It is also used in psoriasis, dermatomycoses and crab infestations.

***Adverse reactions:*** Mercury poisoning, acrordynia and allergic reactions.

***Official preparations:*** Ammoniated mercury ointment B.P.

## Sulphur and Sulphur Compounds
## Sulphur U.S.P.

**Atomic symbol:** S **Atomic weight:** 32.064

In nature, sulphur occurs as free or in combined form of sulphates of barium, calcium and magnesium and the sulphides of iron, copper, zinc and mercury.

The important minerals of sulphur are zinc blend (ZnS), iron pyrites ($FeS_2$), gypsum ($CaSO_4 . 2H_2O$), barytes ($BaSO_4$) and galena (PbS) etc. Among all these iron pyrites is very important mineral.

In the regions of volcanos e.g., Sicily and Italy and in parts of North America more amount of sulphur is present in free state and with native calcium sulphate and carbonate.

It is suggested that the deposits are formed by the interaction of hydrogen sulphide and sulphur dioxide.

$$2\,H_2S + SO_2 \longrightarrow 3\,S + 2\,H_2O$$

***Preparation:*** The crude Sicilian sulphur is obtained from earthy or siliceous matter by melting and running of the liquid sulphur. The product obtained is purified by distillation.

*Marseilles process:* By this method, from the iron retorts, sulphur is distilled and the vapour is received in brick chambers. The chambers are made cold, the sulphur condenses as yellow powder (flowers of sulphur, sublimed sulphur) which also consists of masses of minute rhombic crystals mixed with a little amount of amorphous particles. The air and the walls of the chamber become sufficiently hot, the sulphur collects as a liquid passed into cylindrical moulds to yield the roll sulphur containing a mass of rhombic crystals.

*Commercial preparation:* Most of the sulphur is obtained from deposits in texas. The sulphur is forced up to the borings in the molten state by means of super heated water, and the product is solidified and the pure sulphur is obtained.

***Physical properties:*** There are two important forms of sulphur available. One is rhombic or $\alpha$–sulphur and monoclinic or $\beta$-sulphur. Some other allotropes are also recognized. Rhombic crystals are stable at ordinary room temperature. It is insoluble in water, sparingly soluble in alcohol and ether, soluble in carbon disulphide, toluene and benzene.

***Chemical properties:***

1. *Reaction with alkalis:* Sulphur reacts with alkalis, on heating it gives sulphides and thiosulphates.

$$12\,S + 3\,Ca(OH)_2 \longrightarrow 2\,CaS_5 + CaS_2O_3 + 3\,H_2O$$

$$8\,S + 6\,NaOH \longrightarrow Na_2S + Na_2S_2O_3 + Na_2S_5 + 3\,H_2O$$

2. Reaction with metals and non metals: Sulphur reacts with elements like potassium, mercury, copper (metals) and carbon, chlorine, fluorine and hydrogen (non metals).

$$2\,S + C \longrightarrow CS_2$$

$$S + H_2 \longrightarrow H_2S$$

$$S + 2\,K \longrightarrow K_2S$$

$$Cl_2 + 2\,S \longrightarrow S_2Cl_2$$

$$Fe + S \longrightarrow FeS$$

3. Reduction Reaction: Sulphur reduces hot concentrated nitric acid and concentrated sulphuric acid.

$$6\,HNO_3 + S \longrightarrow H_2SO_4 + 6\,NO_2 + 2\,H_2O$$

$$2\,H_2SO_4 + S \longrightarrow 3\,SO_2 + 2\,H_2O$$

4. Sulphur burns in air at 250 °C with pale blue flame, giving sulphur dioxide and sulphur trioxide.

$$3S + 4O_2 \xrightarrow[\Delta]{250\ ^{\circ}C} SO_2 + 2SO_3$$

5. Sulphur reacts with oxidizing agents (e.g., potassium nitrate) and forms explosive mixtures.

***Test for purity:*** It should be tested for arsenic, acidity, insoluble matter in carbon disulphide, ash content and water content.

***Uses:***

1. Sulphur and its compounds are widely used in pharmaceutical and medicinal purpose.
2. Elemental sulphur is topically used as an antibacterial agent.
3. Elemental sulphur is internally used as a cathartic.
4. It is acts as fungicide, parasiticide and in the treatment of various skin diseases.
5. It is also used for fumigation or insecticide purpose and scabicide.
6. Sulphide in the form of various elements also used in depilatory purpose (In alkaline solution sulphides broken the disulphide bond of the amino acid cysteine in hair. This leads to softening of hair and thus acts as depilatory.

7. A large number of easily available sulphur salts (sodium bisulphite, sodium meta bisulphite etc.) are used as antioxidants, stabilizing agents and preservatives.
8. Sodium thiosulphate is used as an antidote for iodine and cyanide poisoning.
9. The organic compounds of sulphur like thiazide derivatives are used as a diuretic agent.
10. Sulpha drugs (sulphonamides) and sulphones are also important compounds of sulphur which are used as antibacterial.

***Storage:*** It should be stored in well closed containers.

## Sublimed Sulphur U.S.P.

**(Synonym: Flowers of sulphur)**

**Symbol:** S **At. Weight:** 32.064

It contains not less than 99.0% and not more than 100.5%of sulphur.

***Preparation:*** The sulphur obtained from various kilns containing about 3% earthy materials. It is used after refining.

***Refining process:*** The refinery is having large stone chambers which are attached with safety valves. The molten sulphur is kept in iron retorts which contact with the stone chambers. When sulphur vapors enter the stone chamber, they ignite and the subsequent vapors are allowed to pass through relatively cold. These are condensed on the walls and floors of the chamber in a fine crystalline form called sublimed sulphur or flower of sulphur. This sulphur after collection can be sieved.

***Properties:*** It is a fine crystalline, gritty powder with faint characteristic odour, tasteless. It is insoluble in water and 40% alcohol, but dissolves slowly and incompletely in carbon disulphide.

***Test for identification:***

1. It burns with air, converts into sulphur dioxide, which is identified by its characteristic odour.
2. When heated at 115 °C, it melts to yellow mobile liquid; on further heating at about 160 °C the liquid becomes dark and visible.
3. Under microscope, it consists of opaque rounded amorphous particles or aggregates.

***Test for purity:*** It is should be tested for arsenic, acidity, carbon disulphide, insoluble matters and sulphated ash.

***Test for acidity:*** Agitating required quantity of sample with 50 ml of freshly boiled and cooled water and the resulting solution is titrated with 0.1N sodium hydroxide using phenolphthalein solution as an indicator. Not more than 1 ml of 0.1N sodium hydroxide is consumed. The acidity is due to the presence of sulphurous and sulphuric acids which are formed due to oxidation of sulphur during its conversion in to sublimed sulphur.

***Test for matter insoluble carbon disulphide:*** 1 gm of sample is agitated with 20 ml of carbon disulphide and allows the solution to stand for 10 minutes. Then filter it and wash the residue with carbon disulfide, dried and weighed. The weight of the residue should not be less than 0.2 gm (Not less than 20% of insoluble sublimed sulphur).

***Test for sulphated ash:*** It should not be more than 0.2% w/w.

***Uses:***

1. It is used as a dermatological agent in the form of lotions or liniments for the treatment of psoriasis, ring worm, dandruff, seborrhoeic conditions and scabies.
2. It is also used in a *Lupus erythmatosus.*
3. Lotions of sulphur with lead acetate are used to darken the grey hair.
4. Seborrhoeic effects of sulphur are due to its conversion into hydrogen sulphide and parathionic acid.
5. Sulphur is taken by mouth; it is converted into alkali sulphides in small intestine, which produce irritant effect leads to mild laxative effect.
6. It is also used in homeopathic medicine.

***Storage:*** It should be stored in well closed containers.

## Precipitated Sulphur U.S.P.

**Symbol:** S **At. Weight:** 32.064

It contains not less than 99.5% and not more than 100.5% of S calculated on anhydrous basis.

***Preparation:***

*Small scale preparation:* It is prepared by acidification of thiosulphate solution with dilute mineral acid, the unstable thiosulphuric acid is first liberated which rapidly decomposes with the formation of precipitated sulphur.

$$Na_2S_2O_3 + 2\,HCl \longrightarrow H_2S_2O_3 + 2\,NaCl$$

$$H_2S_2O_3 \longrightarrow S + SO_2 + H_2O$$

Thiosulphates are too expensive to use on the large scale.

*Commercial preparation:* By using this method 5 parts of quick lime is slaked and the product is mixed with 50 parts of water. To this added 10 parts of powdered sulphur or roll sulphur and a further 100 parts of water. The resulting mixture is boiled for one hour with occasional shaking. Then the liquid is filtered and the filtrate which contains a mixture of calcium thiosulphate and calcium polysulphides are treated with hydrochloric acid with required quantity, to leave supernatant liquid which is slightly alkaline. Then the precipitated sulphur is collected, washed on filter paper until the washings give no reaction for calcium and then dried.

The chemical reactions takes place in these processes are complex one, the following equations are represented only some of the chemical reactions involved.

$$3\,Ca(OH)_2 + 6\,S \longrightarrow 2\,CaS_2 + CaS_2O_3 + 3\,H_2O$$

$$2\,CaS_2 + CaS_2O_3 + 6\,HCl \longrightarrow 3\,CaCl_2 + 6\,S + 3\,H_2O$$

The yield of the above process is about two third of theoretical yield since much amount of sulphur gets lost as hydrogen sulphide and sulphurdioxide gases which are formed in the initial stages of the process.

***Physical Properties:*** Precipitated sulphur is a greenish yellow or greyish yellow powder, which is completely amorphous, free from grittiness, odorless, tasteless. It is almost completely soluble in carbon disulphide (1 gm in 2 ml of $CS_2$). It is insoluble in water and 90% alcohol. Under a microscope it shows grouped amorphous sub globular particles free from crystals. It burns in the air with blue flame by the production of sulphurdioxide.

$$S + O_2 \longrightarrow SO_2$$

***Chemical properties:***

1. *Reaction with metals and non metals:* Sulphur is a very active element reacts with most metals and non metals forming sulphides

$$2\,Cu + S \longrightarrow Cu_2S$$
$$C + 2\,S \longrightarrow CS_2$$

2. *Reaction with alkali hydroxides:* Sulphur is soluble in alkali hydroxides.

$$3\,Ca(OH)_2 + 12\,S \longrightarrow 2\,CaS_5 + CaS_2O_3 + 3\,H_2O$$
$$6\,KOH + 6\,S \longrightarrow 2\,K_2S_2 + K_2S_2O_3 + 3\,H_2O$$

3. *Reactions with alkali sulphides:* Sulphur is also soluble with alkali sulphides.

$$Na_2S + S \longrightarrow Na_2S_2$$
$$Na_2S + 4\,S \longrightarrow Na_2S_5$$

***Test for identification:*** Similar to sublimed sulphur.

***Test for purity:*** It should be tested for acidity, arsenic, and matter insoluble in carbon disulfide, ash content, water content and microscopical appearance.

***Test for water content:*** Water is determined by Karl Fischer method using pyridine instead of methanol in which sulphur is insoluble.

***Test for ash content:*** It should not be more than 0.25 %.

***Test for microscopical appearance:*** Under microscope no crystalline particles are seen.

Apart from the above pharmacopoeial standards, an aqueous extract should not be alkaline to litmus and the hydrochloric acid extract should not give more than slight reactions for calcium.

**Assay**

***Principle:*** It is assayed by **acidimetry-alkalimetry method of titration** (also called **neutralization method**).

In this assay the substance is burned to form sulphur dioxide and it is absorbed in water containing hydrogen peroxide, diluted with water, boiled and cooled and the solution is titrated against sodium hydroxide using phenolphthalein as an indicator. Titration is continued until the disappearance of pink colour. As the acid and alkali involved in this assay, it is called as acidimetry-alkalimetry method of titration and the neutralization takes place in this assay during titration hence this assay is also called as neutralization method. The chemical reactions of this assay are shown below.

$$S + O_2 \longrightarrow SO_2$$

$$SO_2 + H_2O_2 \longrightarrow H_2SO_4$$

$$2\,NaOH + H_2SO_4 \longrightarrow Na_2SO_4 + 2\,H_2O$$

***Uses:***

1. It acts as a good scabicide and also it is the important constituent in sulphur ointment.
2. It also finds used as an active parasiticide.

***Dose:*** 1 to 4 gm.

## Other Allotropic Varieties of Sulphur

**Plastic sulphur:** If sulphur is heated to its boiling point and poured in to water, it forms a soft amorphous mass called as plastic sulphur, which slowly reverts to rhombic form.

**Monoclinic sulphur:** If sulphur is melted in a dish and allowed to cool until a crust forms on the surface and the liquid is then poured out through one of two holes made in the crust, amber colored needles of monoclinic sulphur is formed.

These also revert slowly to rhombic crystals. Monoclinic form is stable at high temperatures.

The transition temperature is 95.5 °C.

A lot of oxides of sulphur have been described, but the two important oxides are sulphur dioxide ($SO_2$) and sulphur trioxide ($SO_3$).

## Sulphur Ointment U.S.P.

It contains 10% of precipitated sulphur (limits 9.5 to 10.5% of S).

***Preparation:***

*Ingredients:*

Precipitated sulphur = 100 gm

Simple ointment prepared with white soft paraffin = 900 gm

***Procedure:*** All the precipitated sulphur is triturated with small amount of simple ointment until a smooth cream is formed. Then the remaining simple ointment is added and mixed thoroughly to get sulphur ointment.

***Extraction procedure:*** 20 gm of the ointment is refluxed with 25 ml of petroleum ether (40 °C - 60 °C) in 250 ml conical flask for one hour. The petroleum layer gets rejected. The residue in the flask is again refluxed with 25 ml of light petroleum for one hour. Then the petroleum layer is rejected and dried the residue i.e., the sulphur obtained has been used for the identification tests which are as follows.

***Test for identification:*** The tests are only performed after extracting sulphur from the ointment using petroleum ether and the extract is tested for tests similar to that of sublimed sulphur.

*Test:* 1 and 2 is similar to that of sublimed sulphur.

*Test 3:* It burns with air, converts into sulphur dioxide, which is identified by its characteristic odour.

*Test 4:* When heated at 115 °C, it melts to yellow mobile liquid on further heating at about 160 °C the liquid becomes dark and visible.

*Test 5:* A small quantity of residue is dissolved in hot pyridine. To this add sodium bicarbonate solution and the mixture is boiled. A blue or green color is produced.

**Assay:** Similar to that of precipitated sulphur.

***Use:*** It is used as a scabicide.

***Storage:*** It should be kept in a well closed container preferable in cool place.

## Boric Acid I.P.

This compound is discussed under **oxidative antimicrobials.**

## Borax I.P., B.P, U.S.P.

**(Synonym: Sodium tetra borate, Sodium borate)**

**Mol. Formula:** $Na_2B_4O_7$ (anhydrous ) **Mol. Weight:** 201.2
$Na_2B_4O_7$. 10 $H_2O$(decahydrate) 381.3

Borax is the sodium salt of pyroboric acid which is mainly occurs naturally in lakes of Tibet, Sri Lanka, India and California.

It contains not less than 99% and not more than 103% of $Na_2B_4O_7.10H_2O$ (di sodium tetra borate decahydrate).

***Preparation:***

*From crude borax (Tincal):* The naturally occurs crude borax is dissolved in water, filtered. The filtrate is concentrated and cooled. The crude borax crystallizes out.

*From calcium borate:* The mineral borate is boiled with concentrated solution of sodium carbonate. The resulting solution is filtered, concentrated and cooled to crystallize borax.

$$Ca_2B_6O_{11} + 2Na_2CO_3 \longrightarrow Na_2B_4O_7 + 2CaCO_3 + \underset{\text{Sodium metaborate}}{2NaBO_2}$$

To the above solution (mother liquor), a current of carbon dioxide gas is passed, metaborate is converted into borax.

$$4\,NaBO_2 + CO_2 \longrightarrow Na_2B_4O_7 + Na_2CO_3$$

***Physical properties:*** It is a white crystalline powder or colorless crystals or crystalline masses, efflorescent in dry air. It is soluble in water (1 in 20), very soluble in boiling water (1:1) and glycerol (1:1) and practically insoluble in alcohol. The pH of the aqueous solution is 9.5.

***Chemical properties:*** In concentrated solution, it is hydrolyzed partially.

$$Na_2B_4O_7 + 3\,H_2O \rightleftharpoons 2\,NaBO_2 + 2\,H_3BO_3$$

But in dilute solutions, the metaborate itself largely hydrolysed.

$$NaBO_2 + 2\,H_2O \rightleftharpoons NaOH + H_3BO_3$$

Borax has emulsifying action on oils due to the presence of free alkali formed by hydrolysis.

When heated on a platinum wire in Bunsen flame, borax fuses, swells, loses water and finally forms a clear bead of the anhydrous salt.

Fused borax dissolve compounds of certain metals, forming characteristically colored beads. The color depends on the nature of metal and on whether the bead is heated in the oxidizing or reducing part of the flame.

***Test for identification:***

*Test 1:* Similar to boric acid.

*Test 2:* To the sample solution add one or two drops of phenolphthalein solution. The red color produces. On the addition of 5 ml of 8% glycerol the colour disappears.

*Test 3:* The aqueous solution of the sample gives the characteristic reactions of sodium salt.

***Test for purity:*** It should be tested for clarity of solution, pH, Ammonium, sulphates, arsenic, calcium and heavy metals.

**Assay**

***Principle:*** It is assayed by **acidimetry-alkalimetry method of titration** (also called **neutralization method**).

In this assay the substance is dissolved in water and titrated with 0.5N hydrochloric acid, using methyl red as an indicator. End point is the appearance of red colour. In this assay borax (the base) reacts with hydrochloric acid and forms sodium chloride and ortho boric acid with the neutralization during the titration. The indicator is yellow colour in alkali medium and it changes to red colour upon neutralization which is the end point.

As the acid and alkali involved in this assay, it is called as acidimetry-alkalimetry method of titration and the neutralization takes place in this assay during titration hence this assay is also called as Neutralization method. The chemical reactions of this assay are shown below.

$$Na_2B_4O_7.10\ H_2O + 2\ HCl \longrightarrow 2\ NaCl + 4\ H_3BO_3 + 5\ H_2O$$

***Procedure:*** Dissolve about 3 gm of borax, accurately weighed, in 50 ml of water, add methyl red, and titrate with 0.5N hydrochloric acid. (NOTE: Heating on a steam bath may be required initially to effect solution).

***Uses:***

1. Borax is used as alkalinizing agent (Pharmaceutical aid).
2. It is also used as an antiseptic, detergent and astringent for mucous membranes.
3. 1 to 2% solution is externally used as an eye wash and as a wet dressings for wounds.

***Caution:*** Ingestion of borax leads to vomiting, nausea, diarrhoea, shock and death.

## Antimony Potassium Tartarate U.S.P.

This compound is discussed under the topic **emetics**.

## Selenium

**Atomic symbol:** Se **Atomic weight:** 78.96

Selenium mainly occurs in the form of sulphide ores and sulphur. In the form of selenides, it is mainly obtained from the flue dust of pyrite burners and also from the electrolytic refining of copper.

## Selenium Sulphide B.P., U.S.P.

**(Synonym: Selum)**

**Mol. Formula:** $SeS_2$ **Mol. Weight:** 143.09

Selenium sulphide contains not less than 52% and not more than 55.5% of selenium (Se).

***Preparation:*** It is prepared by adding selenous acid solution to aluminium chloride solution saturated with hydrogen sulphide and continuing the passage of the gas.

$$H_2SeO_3 + 2\ H_2S \longrightarrow SeS_2 + 3\ H_2O$$

The aluminium chloride acts as a coagulant, the precipitated selenium sulphide is filtered off, washed and dried.

***Properties:*** It is a bright orange powder, practically insoluble in water. It dissolves in nitric acid and gives the formation of selenous acid and sulphuric acid.

$$SeS_2 + 16\ HNO_3 \longrightarrow H_2SeO_3 + 2\ H_2SO_4 + 16\ NO_2\uparrow + 5\ H_2O$$

***Test for identification:***

*Test 1:* Urea is added to the above test which inactivates excess nitric acid by forming urea nitrate and destroys nitrous acid.

$$2\,HNO_2 + NH_2\text{-}\overset{\overset{\displaystyle O}{||}}{C}\text{-}NH_2 \longrightarrow CO_2 + 2\,N_2 + 3\,H_2O$$

*Test 2: Test for selenium:* To the above sample solution add potassium iodide solution which liberates iodine and selenium which forms a yellowish orange to orange color and it darkens rapidly.

$$H_2SeO_3 + 4\,HI \longrightarrow 2\,I_2 + Se + 3\,H_2O$$

*Test 3:* To the sample solution add 10 ml of barium chloride; the solution becomes turbid (presence of sulphur).

***Test for purity:*** It should be tested for residue on ignition and soluble selenium compounds.

**Assay**

***Principle:*** It is assayed by **iodometry method of titration** (also called **redox titration**).

In this assay the substance is dissolved in fuming nitric acid by heating. After cooling to room temperature, the solution was diluted with water and treated with potassium iodide solution. In this reaction potassium iodide is oxidized to iodine. The liberated iodine is determined by titrating with N/10 sodium thiosulphate using starch mucilage as an indicator. End point is the disappearance of blue colour. During this titration iodine is reduced to sodium iodide and sodium thiosulphate is oxidized to sodium tetrathionate. As the oxidation and reduction takes place simultaneously this is called redox titration.

$$I_2 + \underset{\text{Sodium thiosulphate}}{2Na_2S_2O_3} \longrightarrow 2\,NaI + \underset{\text{Sodium tetrathionate}}{Na_2S_4O_6}$$

***Procedure:*** To 0.100 gm add 25 ml of fuming nitric acid and heat on a water-bath for 1 hr; a small insoluble residue may remain. Cool and dilute to 100 ml with water. To 25 ml of this solution add 50 ml of water and 5 gm of urea and heat to boiling. Cool, add 7 ml of potassium iodide solution and 3 ml of starch solution. Titrate immediately with 0.1M sodium thiosulphate. Carry out a blank titration.

***Uses:***

1. It is mainly used topically as antidandruff agent.
2. 1 to 2.5% of selenium sulphide is added to the shampoos as antiseborrheic.
3. The usual treatment is 5 – 10 ml of 2.5% shampoo which is to be applied on the scalp. It is allowed to remain in contact for five minutes and then it gets washed off.
4. Lotion is used in the treatment of *Pityriasis versicolour*.

***Caution:***

1. For longer exposure leads to skin irritation.
2. While using as a shampoo, care should be taken and it should not be introduced into the eyes or mouth since the compound is highly toxic, the hands and finger nails should be thoroughly washed after using the compound.
3. It should not be administered internally.
4. It leads to scalp oiliness; hair discoloration and hair loss have been reported.

***Storage:*** It should be preserved in tightly closed containers.

***Other official formulations:*** Selenium sulfide detergent suspension.

## PROBABLE QUESTIONS

1. Define the following terms
   (a) Adsorbents (b) Protectives (c) Demulcents
   (d) Emollients (e) Caustics (f) Antiseptics
   (g) Astringents
2. Write about the preparation, properties, test for purity and test for identification, assay and uses of purified talc.
3. Write in detail about zinc oxide and its official formulations.
4. How does zinc oxide is assayed. Explain the method with chemical equations.
5. Describe the preparation, test for purity, assay and uses of zinc undecylenate.
6. Briefly explain about calamine and its formulations.
7. Write a note on zinc stearate.
8. Explain about the preparation, properties, assay and uses of titanium dioxide.
9. Write a brief note on topical protective agents.
10. Define the following terms
    (a) Bacteriostatic (b) Disinfectant (c) Antiseptic
    (d) Sanitizers (e) Astringent
11. Enumerate the ideal characteristics of antimicrobial agents.
12. Explain about the various mechanism of action of antimicrobial agents with suitable examples.
13. Explain the preparation, properties, assay and uses of alum.
14. Explain the aluminium compounds which are used as an astringent. How do these compounds are assayed.
15. Describe the preparation, properties (both physical and chemical), assay and uses of the following compounds
    (a) Zinc sulphate (b) Zinc chloride (c) Zinc peroxide
16. Write a preparation, properties, test for identification and mechanism of action, assay and uses of calcium hydroxide.

17. Explain the pharmaceutical aspects of silicone polymers as protective agents.
18. Explain in detail about the mode of action of inorganic antimicrobial agents.
19. Explain the pharmaceutical aspects of following compounds.
    (a) Boric acid (b) Iodine solution
    (c) Hydrogen peroxide (d) Potassium permanganate
    (e) Selenium sulfide
20. Write a short note on:
    (a) Potassium permanganate.
    (b) Silver nitrate as antimicrobial agents.
    (c) Iodine preparations as topical agents.
21. Enumerate the compounds of aluminium as astringents. Explain their assay method.
22. Define activated dimethicone I.P.? Write in detail about its composition, properties and uses.
23. Explain about the assay of boric acid with chemical equations.
24. What are the chlorine compounds used as anti-infective agents? Briefly write their preparation and properties.
25. Define oxidative antimicrobials with examples.
26. Describe the mechanism of action of oxidative anti microbials.
27. Write the preparation, properties, and test for purity, assay and uses of sodium perborate.
28. Write a note on iodine with respect to pharmaceutical aspects.
29. How does povidone iodine is assayed.
30. Explain briefly about iodized oil injection.
31. Describe sodium hypochlorite solution and dilute sodium hypochlorite solution.
32. Briefly explain about protein precipitant anti microbials with their mechanism of action. Write the preparation and assay of any one of them.
33. Write a short note on the following.
    (a) Strong silver protein (b) Mild silver protein
34. Write the preparation, properties, test for identification, test for purity, assay and uses of mercuric compounds as antimicrobials.
35. Explain the following.
    (a) Aluminium compound as antimicrobials
    (b) Minor topical agents
36. Write in detail about the following compounds.
    (a) Sulphur (b) Sublimed sulphur
    (c) Precipitated sulphur (d) Sulphur ointment
37. Write the preparation, properties, assay and uses of borax.
38. Describe the pharmaceutical aspects of selenium and selenium sulphide.

## 6.3 DENTAL PRODUCTS

**Introduction:** A large number of inorganic compounds and their formulations are used as dental product to clean, polish and removes the dental caries. This chapter deals about the agents used in the prevention of dental caries (dentifrices, fluoxides), polishing and desensitizing agents.

Dental hygiene is an important one, inorder to maintain the oral hygiene number of dental products are available in market. Various factors are involved in tooth decay and oral hygiene. As they are used in human body they are considered as drugs and pharmaceuticals. Dental products include

(i) Anticaries agents

(ii) Cleansing and polishing agents.

### 6.3.1 Anticaries Agents

**Introduction:** These are chemical compounds used to prevent the dental caries produced by the action of microorganism in the mouth leads to bad mouth odour.

The three main types of anticaries agents are

1. Topical anticaries agents
2. Immunologic anticaries agents
3. Systemic anticaries agents

The main 5 constituents of anticaries agents are

1. Chemicals
2. Fluorides
3. Mechanical tooth brush
4. Antimicrobial
5. Cellular

The main three targets of anticaries agents are 1. Host 2. Diet or substrate 3. Plaque.

Dental caries is defined as a progressive irreversible microbial disease affecting the hard parts of tooth leads to demineralization of inorganic constituents and dissolution of organic constituent there by producing dental cavity. The word caries arises from latin means "rot" or "decay".

$$\text{Bacterial enzymes} + \text{Fermentable carbohydrates}$$
$$\downarrow$$
$$\text{Acid} + \text{enamel} \Longrightarrow \text{Dental caries}$$

**Requirements for ideal of anticaries agents**

1. It should have an acceptable taste.
2. It should have degree of specificity.

3. It should not produce local irritation.
4. It should be destroyed or inactivated by GIT.
5. It should be able to penetrate dense microbial plaque.
6. Agents used for topical application should not be produce toxic effect if swallowed accidently.
7. It should be a bactericidal as contact time is less.

**Types of anticaries agents**

1. Substances which alters the tooth structure or tooth surface. Chemicals coming under this categories include:

   Fluorides, iodides, bisbiguanides, silver nitrate, zinc chloride and potassium ferrocyanates.
2. Substances which interfere with carbohydrate degradation through enzymatic alteration which includes: sarecoside, vitamin K
3. Substances which interfere with bacterial growth and metabolism. Antibiotics, caries vaccine.

**Role of fluorides as anticaries agents:** Fluoride as a trace element occurs in our body and is obtained from food and water. In some places, where it lacks fluoride, drinking water must be fluorinated by the process called fluoridation. Fluoride is administered in to body by oral and topical routes either by mixing in drinking water, juice etc. and also as sodium fluoride tablets (2.2 mg /day) or as 2% fluoride solution that can be applied topically on teeth.

**Role of fluoride to prevent tooth decay:**

1. Fluoride occurs naturally, but it does not need it for growth and normal development. It is mainly used to prevent tooth decay.
2. During tooth formation, fluoride is taken up in to the enamel which helps to reduce tooth decay later.
3. Fluoride also helps maintain bone structure, very low doses of fluoride salts may be used to treat conditions that cause faster bone loss than normal.

***Sources of fluoride:*** Fluoridated water is the most commonly used source. Natural sodium fluoride is present in the ocean, so most of the seafood contains fluoride.

***Dietary intake of fluoride:*** The food and nutrition board recommends the following dietary intake for fluoride.

Infants 6 months-12 months 0.01 mg/day – 0.5 mg/day

Children 1-13 years – 0.7 mg/day -2 mg/day

Adolescents and adults - males 14-18 - 3 mg/day –4 mg/day

Females over 14 years –3 mg/day

## Sodium Fluoride I.P., B.P., U.S.P.

**Mol. Formula:** NaF **Mol. Weight:** 42

It contains not less than 98.5% and not more than 100.5% of sodium fluoride with reference to the dried substance.

***Preparation:***

*Method 1: From sodium carbonate:* This is manufactured by neutralization of sodium carbonate solution with hydrogen fluoride.

$$Na_2CO_3 + 2HF \longrightarrow 2NaF + H_2O + CO_2 \uparrow$$

This salt is sparingly soluble in nature, so it is precipitated out, as the reaction proceeds leaving some of the impurities in solution. The precipitate is contaminated with fluorosilicate and acid salt. It is rendered alkaline to phenolphthalein with sodium carbonate and then heated to neutralize the acid salt and decompose the fluorosilicate.

$$Na_2SiF_6 + 2H_2O \longrightarrow 2NaF + 4HF + SiO_2$$

The crystal size depends upon pH, but too much hydrogen fluoride gives sodium bifluoride.

*Method 2: Double decomposition reaction:* This method involves the double decomposition of calcium fluoride with sodium carbonate. The precipitated insoluble calcium carbonate is removed by filtration.

$$CaF_2 + Na_2CO_3 \longrightarrow 2NaF + CaCO_3$$

*Method 3: From cryolite ($AlF_3.3NaF$):* The mineral cryolite is treated with excess of sodium hydroxide. The insoluble sodium fluoride formed is extracted with hot water, whereas the aluminium fluoride is soluble in the alkaline solution.

$$2AlF_3 \,.\, 3NaF + 2NaOH \longrightarrow 8NaF + 2AlF_2 + H_2O_2$$

***Physical properties:*** It occurs as a white powder or colorless crystals, odorless and tasteless. It is soluble in water (1:25), practically insoluble in alcohol. The aqueous solution of sodium fluoride corrodes glass containers hence its solution should be prepared in distilled water and stored in dark colored, pyrex bottles.

***Chemical properties:***

*Reaction with concentrated sulphuric acid:* Sodium fluoride reacts with concentrated sulphuric acid yield hydrogen fluoride. This gas attacks the silicates and glass.

$$2NaF + H_2SO_4 \longrightarrow 2HF + Na_2SO_4$$

$$Na_2SiO_3 + 6HF \longrightarrow Na_2SiF_6 + 3H_2O$$

***Test for identification:***

1. The required quantity of sample is dissolved in sufficient amount of carbon dioxide free water, make up to 100 ml. To the 2 ml of above solution, add small amount of calcium chloride solution, a gelatinous white precipitate is formed which dissolves in ferric chloride solution.

$$2NaF + 2\,CaCl_2 \longrightarrow 2CaF + 2NaCl$$

2. To the small amount of sample solution, add a mixture of alizarin red S solution and zirconyl nitrate solution and mix. The yellow color is formed.
3. The aqueous solution of sample gives the characteristic reactions of sodium salts.

***Test for purity:*** It should be tested for appearance of solution, acidity or alkalinity, lead, chlorides, fluorosilicate, sulphates and loss on drying.

***Test for fluorosilicate:*** The neutral solution of sodium fluoride is titrated with 0.1M sodium hydroxide until a red color is produced. The titer value should not be more than that of 1.5 ml.

**Assay *Principle:***

*Method 1:* It is assayed by **complexometry method of (Back) titration**.

In this assay the substance is dissolved in water, add alcohol, boil, to this added Known Excess Standard (KES) lead nitrate. To this solution xylenol orange added as an indicator and titrated against disodium EDTA. End point is the appearance of violet colour due to the formation of lead-xylenol orange complex.

In this assay sodium fluoride reacts with lead nitrate, whereby the lead fluoride is formed, after this reaction, the Excess Unreacted (EUR) lead nitrate is determined by titrating with disodium EDTA. The indicator is colourless before complexation and change into violet colour due to the formation of lead-xylenol orange complex. As the acid lead ions forms complex with disodium EDTA in this assay, it is called as complexometry method of titration. The chemical reactions of this assay are shown below.

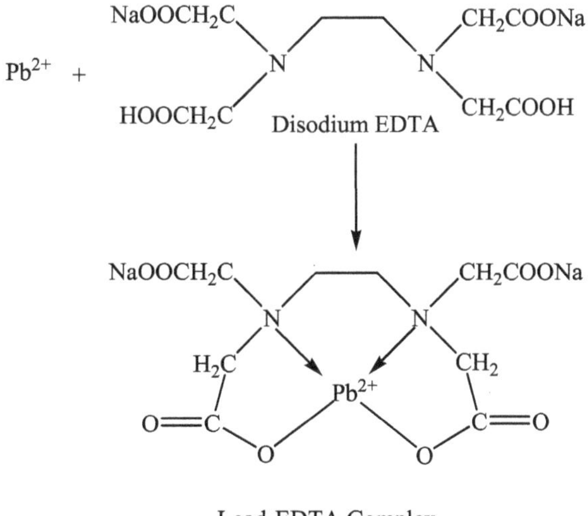

$Pb^{2+}$ + $(NaOOCH_2C)(HOOCH_2C)N-CH_2CH_2-N(CH_2COONa)(CH_2COOH)$

Disodium EDTA

↓

$NaOOCH_2C$, $CH_2COONa$, N, N, $H_2C$, $CH_2$, $Pb^{2+}$, O=C, C=O, O, O

Lead-EDTA Complex

*Method 2:* Sodium fluoride is a very weak base hence it can also be assayed by **non-aqueous method** of titration.

***Procedure:*** Weigh accurately about 80 mg add a mixture of 5 ml of acetic anhydride and 20 ml of anhydrous glacial acetic acid and heat to dissolve. Cool, add 20 ml of dioxan. Titrate with 0.1M perchloric acid, using crystal violet solution as indicator.

*Uses:*

1. Due to the presence of fluoride ion, it is an important agent in dental practice for retarding or preventing dental caries.
2. It may render enamel of teeth more resistant to acid to promote remineralization or prevent microbial acid production.
3. The 2% aqueous solution is widely used as a topical agent.
4. A 2% aqueous solution of sodium fluoride may be applied to children's teeth, after preliminary cleansing, 3 times at the interval of one week of 3,7,10 and 13 years of age correspond with the tooth eruption.
5. Sodium fluoride paste containing 75% of sodium fluoride and 25% glycerol is applied to the teeth, rubbed for 1 minute and removed by a mouth wash.
6. It is also used as an insecticide mainly for cockroaches, ants and in other pesticide formulations.
7. It is also used for the fluoridation of drinking water.

The 2.2 mg of sodium fluoride approximately contains 1 mg of fluoride ion. Each gram of sodium fluoride is equivalent to 23.8 mmols of sodium and fluoride. Sodium fluoride and all other soluble fluorides are readily absorbed from gastro intestinal tract.

***Dose:***

1. 2.2 mg once in a day or 1 mg of fluoride per day.
2. Fluoridation in drinking water purpose 1.5 to 3 ppm.
3. For topical application to the teeth 2%.

***Caution:*** Larger doses of sodium fluoride are poisonous. Fluoride content of water is more than 3 ppm leads to mottling of teeth, nausea, vomiting, diarrhoea, abdominal distress, stupor, weakness, tremors, convulsion, collapse, dyspnea, respiratory and cardiac failure. It is also used as an insecticide, so great precaution is to be taken to prevent children getting accurse to such preparations.

***Storage:*** It should be stored in well closed containers and protected from moisture.

---

## Sodium Monofluorophosphate U.S.P.

**(Synonym: SMFP)**

**Mol. Formula:** $Na_2PO_3F$ **Mol. Weight:** 143.9

***Physical properties:*** It is colorless, odorless powder, completely soluble in water.

*Uses:*

1. It is used for the fluoridation of water and also used as fluoride supplements for diets.
2. It is the one of the ingredient of mouthwashes and dentifrices.
3. It is also used to decreases the demineralisation of dental enamel due to its better fluoridation capacity (less sodium fluoride).

---

## Stannous Fluoride B.P.

**Mol. Formula:** $SnF_2$ **Mol. Weight:** 156.7

It contains not more than 71.2% of stannous ($Sn^{2+}$) ions and not less than 22.3% and not more than 25.5% of fluoride with reference to the dried basis.

***Preparation:***

1. *From Stannous oxide:* It is prepared by evaporating a solution of stannous oxide in hydrofluoric acid in the absence of air or oxygen.

$$SnO + 2HF \longrightarrow SnF_2 + H_2O$$

2. *From Tin (stannous):* The stannous fluoride is also prepared by reaction between stannous (Tin) with hydrogen fluoride in the absence of oxygen.

$$Sn + 2HF \longrightarrow SnF_2 + H_2$$

The solution of stannous fluoride is prepared by dissolving tin fluoride capsules in water. The 8% solution in water is used in dentistry.

***Physical properties:*** It is a white or colorless crystalline powder with unpleasant, astringent and salty taste. It is soluble in water but insoluble in alcohol and other organic solvents. An aqueous solution of stannous fluoride deteriorates quickly on standing due to the oxidation of stannous cation to stannic which produces turbidity. The pH of freshly prepared 0.4% solution is in between 2.8 to 3.5.

***Test for identification:***

1. To the small amount of sample solution, add calcium chloride solution, a white color precipitate of calcium fluoride is formed.

$$SnF_2 + CaCl_2 \longrightarrow SnCl_2 + \underset{\text{White ppt}}{CaF_2\downarrow}$$

2. An aqueous solution of stannous fluoride is mixed with silver nitrate on a spot plate; a brownish black precipitate is formed.

$$SnF_2 + AgNO_3 \longrightarrow \underset{\text{Brownish black precipitate}}{AgF_2\downarrow} + SnNO_3$$

3. When the sample solution is added to mercuric chloride solution, a white, silky precipitate is formed. On further addition of the solution, a brown-black precipitate is produced.

$$SnF_2 + HgCl_2 \longrightarrow \underset{\text{Silky white ppt}}{HgF_2} + SnCl_2$$

**Assay**

***Assay for stannous ion:***

***Principle:*** It is assayed by **iodometry method of titration** (also called **redox titration**). In this assay the substance is dissolved in hot dilute hydrochloric acid, cooled and to this a known volume of potassium iodide added and the solution is titrated with potassium iodate using starch mucilage as an indicator. End point is the disappearance of blue colour. During this titration potassium iodide is oxidized and potassium iodate is reduced. As the oxidation and reduction takes place simultaneously this is called Redox titration.

***Procedure:*** Transfer about 250 mg of stannous fluoride in to a 500 ml conical flask, and add 300 ml of hot, recently boiled 3N hydrochloric acid. While passing a stream of an oxygen-free inert gas over the surface of the liquid, swirl the flask to dissolve the stannous fluoride, and cool to room temperature. Add 5 ml of potassium iodide, and titrate in inert atmosphere with 0.1N potassium iodide-iodate, adding 3 ml of as the indicator which is added at the end of the titration.

***Assay for fluoride ion:*** It is assayed by **potentiometric method of titration**.

***Uses:***

1. It is used to treat or prevent dental caries, similar to sodium fluoride in the form of solution, gel, mouthwash or tooth paste.
2. It contains an unpleasant taste and may cause discoloration of teeth on over usage.
3. Due to the instability of the solution, it should be prepared at the time of application.
4. A freshly prepared 8% solution of stannous fluoride is used to clean dry teeth. A single application is sufficient for 6-12 months.

## 6.3.2 Dentifrices

**Introduction:** These are agents used to clean and polish the natural teeth. They are used along with tooth brush. They are available as powder, paste, gel or liquid form in the market, these are used to removes the debris and dental plaque.

***Types of dentifrices:*** There are four types of dentifrices

1. Tooth paste
2. Tooth powder
3. Mouth wash
4. Tooth soap

***Tooth paste:*** It is a dentifrice used in conjunction with tooth brush to remove debris and plaque. The main ingredients of tooth paste are abrasive, humectants, surfactant and fluorides. (Non fluorinated tooth pastes are also available)

***Tooth powder:*** It is an alternative for tooth powder. It was generally used among Romans with variety of substances such as bones, hoofs, horns and egg shells in powdered forms. Tooth powders are used to clean and whitening of teeth fix them when loose, strengthening the gums and prevent toothache.

***Mouth wash:*** It is liquid preparation used to kills the bacteria that produce plaque and gives fresh breath.

***Tooth soap:*** It is available in hard liquid and gel form used to cleanse gums as well as pit and fissures.

## Calcium Carbonate I.P. B.P., U.S.P.

**(Synonym: Precipitated chalk)**

**Mol. Formula:** $CaCO_3$ **Mol.Weight:** 100.1

It contains not less than 98% and not more than 100.5% calcium carbonate. Which is calculated on dried the sample at 105 °C.

In nature it is widely distributed in chalk, lime stone, marble, aragonite and calcite. It is the one of the main constituents of corals, pearls and shells.

***Preparation:*** For commercial process, the boiling solutions of calcium chloride and sodium carbonate are mixed and allow the resulting precipitate to settle down. The precipitated calcium carbonate is filtered through a calico filter, washed and dried.

$$CaCl_2 + Na_2CO_3 \longrightarrow CaCO_3\downarrow + 2\,NaCl$$

***Physical properties:*** Calcium carbonate is a fine, white, micro crystalline powder, odorless and tasteless. It is insoluble in water but soluble in $CO_2$ free water (boiling water) and ammonium salts due to the formation of calcium carbonate and free calcium ions respectively.

$$CaCO_3 + H_2CO_3 \longrightarrow Ca(HCO_3)_2$$

$$CaCO_3 + 2\,NH_4^+ \longrightarrow Ca^{2+} + 2\,NH_3 + H_2O + CO_2\uparrow$$

***Chemical properties:*** It reacts with mineral acids and produce effervescence due to the elimination of carbon dioxide. (neutralization reaction).

$$CaCO_3 + 2HCl \longrightarrow CaCl_2 + H_2O + CO_2$$

***Test for identification:*** The solution in acetic acid gives the characteristic reactions of calcium salts and carbonates.

***Test for purity:*** It should be tested for arsenic, heavy metals, aluminium, iron, phosphate, insoluble matter in acetic acid, barium, magnesium, alkali metals, chlorides, sulphates and loss on drying.

**Assay**

***Principle:*** It is assayed by **complexometry method of (Direct) titration**.

In this assay the substance is dissolved in hydrochloric acid, to this 1N sodium hydroxide added until the pH reaches to 12. The solution is then titrated against 0.05M disodium Ethylene Diamine Tetra Acetate (EDTA) using murexide and naphthol green as indicator. End point is the appearance of deep blue colour.

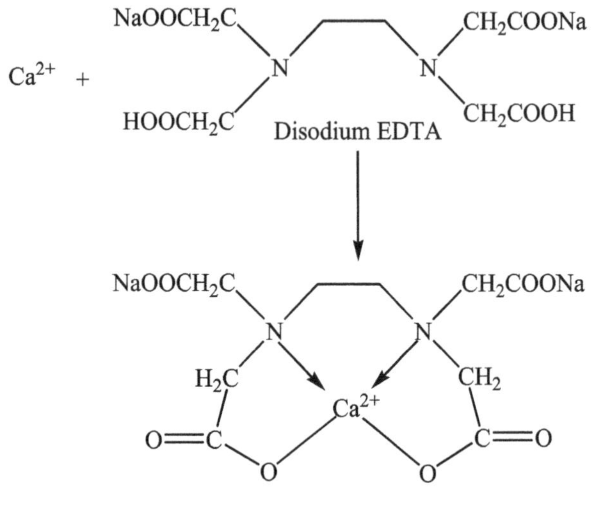

$NaOOCH_2C$ $CH_2COONa$

$Ca^{2+}$ + N N

$HOOCH_2C$ $CH_2COOH$

Disodium EDTA

↓

$NaOOCH_2C$ $CH_2COONa$

N N

$H_2C$ $CH_2$

$Ca^{2+}$

O=C C=O

O O

Calcium-EDTA Complex

In this assay calcium ions of calcium carbonate reacts with disodium EDTA, whereby the complexation takes place. Naphthol green is non-chelating dye. Therefore murexide is used with it to get a sharp end pint. As the calcium ions forms complex with disodium EDTA in this assay, it is called as complexometry method of titration. The chemical reactions of this assay are shown above.

***Uses:***

1. It is traditionally used as a dental cleaning, polishing agent for most of the tooth pastes and tooth powders.
2. The precipitated chalk is dried at 200 °C for 4 hours, it contains calcium equivalent to not less than 98% of $CaCO_3$. This preparation is externally used as a dentifrice, due to its mild abrasive quality because of its microcrystalline structure.
3. It is a common ingredient of tooth powder and tooth paste. It produces both antacid and abrasive effect in the mouth. The fine powdery texture is used in dentifrices both in powders and paste.

***Dose:*** 1 to 5 gm.

## Calcium Phosphate I.P., B.P., U.S.P.

This compound is discussed under **antacids**.

## Dibasic Calcium Phosphate I.P., B.P.

**(Synonym: Dicalcium phosphate, Dicalcium orthophosphate, Calcium hydrogen phosphate)**

**Mol. Formula:** $CaHPO_4$ (anhydrous) **Mol. Weight:** 136.7

$CaHPO_4.\ 2H_2O$ (dihydrate) 172.1

Dibasic calcium phosphate is in anhydrous form or contains two molecules of water of hydration.

It contains not less than 98% and not more than 105% of $CaHPO_4$ (for anhydrous material) or of $CaHPO_4 .2H_2O$ (for the dihydrate)

***Preparation:***

*From Disodium hydrogen phosphate:* It is manufactured by the interaction between neutral calcium chloride solution and disodium hydrogen phosphate.

$$CaCl_2 + Na_2HPO_4 \longrightarrow CaHPO_4 + 2NaCl$$

The white, flocculent precipitate of dibasic calcium phosphate is filtered off, washed and dried. The solution must be neutral; in the presence of alkali, tribasic calcium phosphate is formed.

***Physical properties:*** A white crystalline powder or very fine powder, odorless, having good flow properties, tasteless.

***Test for identification:*** The aqueous solution of the sample gives the characteristic reactions of calcium and phosphates.

***Test for purity:*** It should be tested for acid insoluble substances, arsenic, heavy metals, barium, iron, carbonate, sulphates, chlorides, nitrates, nitrite, reducing substances, protineous impurities, mono calcium and tri calcium phosphates and loss on ignition.

***Test for carbonate:*** To the small amount of sample solution, add hydrochloric acid, no effervescence is produced.

***Test for nitrate:*** To the sample solution, add required amount of nitrogen free sulphuric acid and add small amount of indigo carmine solution and heat to boil, the blue colour does not disappear.

***Test for protineous impurities:*** Heat gently a small quantity of sample in a dry test tube, no color change and no unpleasant odour is emitted.

**Assay**

***Principle:*** It is assayed by **complexometry method of (Back) titration**.The assay is for the calcium content and not for dibasic calcium phosphate.

In this assay the substance is dissolved in a mixture of water and hydrochloric acid; add Known Excess Standard 0.1M disodium edetate. Neutralize with strong ammonia solution, add ammonia buffer pH 10.0 and mordant black II mixture and titrate the excess of disodium edetate with 0.1M zinc sulphate.

In this assay, calcium ions of calcium phosphate react with disodium EDTA, whereby the complexation takes place. As the calcium ions forms complex with disodium EDTA in this assay, it is called as complexometry method of titration. The chemical reactions of this assay are shown below.

$Ca^{2+}$ + $NaOOCH_2C$ / $CH_2COONa$ N—N $HOOCH_2C$ / $CH_2COOH$

Disodium EDTA

↓

$NaOOCH_2C$ / $CH_2COONa$ N—N $H_2C$ / $CH_2$ $Ca^{2+}$ O=C–O / O–C=O

Calcium-EDTA Complex

***Procedure:*** Weigh accurately about 0.3 gm and dissolve in a mixture of 5 ml of water and 1 ml of 7M hydrochloric acid, add 25.0 ml of 0.1M disodium edetate and dilute to 200 ml with water. Neutralize with strong ammonia solution, add 10 ml of ammonia buffer pH 10.0 and 50 mg of mordant black II mixture and titrate the excess of disodium edetate with 0.1M zinc sulphate.

***Uses:***

It contains 1:1 ratio of calcium and phosphorous.

1. Externally it is used as a dentifrice having cleaning action.
2. Due to its moderate abrasive quality, it is suitable for tooth powders and tooth pastes.
3. It is one of the ingredients of fluoride dentifrice (sodium monofluorophosphate)
4. It is also used as an oral electrolyte replenisher.
5. It is a good source of calcium and phosphorous for growing children, pregnant woman and lactating mothers.

***Dose:*** 1 to 5 gm daily in oral route.

### 6.3.3 Desensitizing Agents

**Introduction:** These are used to reduce the sensitivity of teeth to heat and cold. Usually, sensitivity of teeth is caused due to tooth decay. The local anesthetic action of these desensitizing agents is used for its action. Example: Strontium chloride and Zinc chloride.

#### Strontium Chloride U.S.P.

**Mol. Formula:** $SrCl_2$ **Mol. Weight:** 158.52

$SrCl_2 . 6H_2O$ 266.6

It is not official in any pharmacopoeia.

***Physical properties:*** Strontium chloride hexahydrate occurs as colorless, odorless crystals or white granules. It is soluble in water and alcohol. The aqueous solution is neutral. It effloresces in air and deliquesces in moist air.

When it is heated up to 100 °C, it loses 5 molecules of water. At 150 °C, it loses its all water molecule and forms anhydrous salt.

$$SrCl_2.\,6H_2O \xrightarrow{100^\circ C} \underset{\text{Strontiummono chloride}}{SrCl_2.\,H_2O} + 5H_2O$$

$$SrCl_2.\,6H_2O \xrightarrow[\Delta]{150^\circ C} \underset{\text{Anhydrous salt}}{SrCl_2} + 6H_2O$$

When rapidly heated, the anhydrous salt melted at 868 °C.

***Uses:***

1. Usually it is used in the range of 10% w/w tooth paste for the relief of dental hypersensitivity or dentifrice as a tooth desensitizing agent.
2. It is used in medicated dentifrices occasionally.
3. It is also used for replacement in bone formation, promotes bone remineralization in diseases (osteoporosis).

---

## Zinc Chloride I.P.

**Mol. Formula:** $ZnCl_2$ **Mol. Weight:** 136.3

It contains not less than 95% and not more than 100.5% of $ZnCl_2$.

***Preparation:***

*Method 1:* It is prepared by heating metallic or granular zinc with moderately concentrated hydrochloric acid.

$$Zn + 2HCl \longrightarrow ZnCl_2 + H_2$$

The slight excess quantity of zinc is used; the evolution of hydrogen ceases, the solution is filtered and evaporated to dryness.

*Method 2:* It is also prepared by treating zinc oxide or zinc carbonate with appropriate amount of hydrochloric acid.

$$ZnO + 2HCl \longrightarrow ZnCl_2 + H_2O$$

$$ZnCO_3 + 2HCl \longrightarrow ZnCl_2 + H_2O + CO_2\uparrow$$

*Method 3: From mercuric chloride:* Zinc chloride is prepared by distilling zinc with mercuric chloride.

$$Zn + HgCl_2 \longrightarrow ZnCl_2 + Hg$$

***Physical properties:*** It is a white or practically white, crystalline powder or granules or opaque white masses or sticks, odorless, very deliquescent in nature. It is very soluble in water, freely soluble in alcohol, and glycerol. The aqueous solution is acidic to litmus (pH =4). It always contain small amount of zinc oxy chloride, (Zn(OH)Cl) due to hydrolysis, which produces a slightly turbid aqueous solution. The turbid solutions may be cleared by gradual addition of small amount of dilute HCl.

Solutions of zinc chloride should be filtered through asbestos (or) sintered glass, because they dissolve paper cotton wool.

$$ZnCl_2 + H_2O \longrightarrow Zn(OH)Cl + H^+ + Cl^-$$

***Test for identification:***

1. The solution of sample in carbon dioxide free water gives the characteristic reactions of zinc.
2. The 5% w/v solution of sample in nitric acid gives the characteristic reactions of chloride ions.

***Test for purity:*** It should be tested for pH, aluminium, calcium, heavy metals, iron and magnesium, ammonium salts, oxychlorides and sulphates.

**Assay**

***Principle:*** It is assayed by **complexometry method of (Direct) titration**.

In this assay the substance is dissolved in water, to this ammonia-ammonium chloride solution is added as buffer solution and it is then titrated against 0.05M disodium Ethylene Diamine Tetra Acetate (EDTA) using eriochrome black T as an indicator. End point is the appearance of deep blue colour.

$Zn^{2+}$ + $(NaOOCH_2C)(HOOCH_2C)N-CH_2CH_2-N(CH_2COONa)(CH_2COOH)$

Disodium EDTA

↓

$(NaOOCH_2C)N(CH_2COO)-CH_2CH_2-N(CH_2COO)(CH_2COONa) \cdot Zn^{2+}$

Zinc-EDTA Complex

In this assay zinc ions of zinc chloride reacts with disodium EDTA, whereby the complexation takes place. As the zinc ions forms complex with disodium EDTA in this assay, it is called as complexometry method of titration. The chemical reactions of this assay are shown above.

***Procedure:*** Weigh accurately about 3.0 gm, dissolve in 125 ml of water, add 3 gm of ammonium chloride and add sufficient water to produce 250.0 ml. To 25.0 ml of the resulting solution add 100 ml of water and 10 ml of strong ammonia-ammonium chloride solution. Titrate with 0.1M disodium edetate, using eriochrome black T solution as indicator until a deep blue colour is obtained.

***Uses:***

1. Zinc chloride acts as a powerful caustic, antiseptic and astringent.
2. The mechanism of antiseptic action is due to interaction of the zinc metal with certain microbial enzymes.
3. It is used as an injection for zinc replacement.
4. It is also used as an obtundent in dentistry, as deodorant, disinfectant, embalming material.
5. It is also used in mouth washes, in ulcers, fistulas and pododermatitis
6. 10% solution of zinc chloride is used as a desensitizing agent.

## Sodium Meta Phosphate BPC

**(Synonym: Sodium hexaphosphate, Maddrell's salt)**

**Mol. Formula:** $(NaPO_3)_6$ **Mol. Weight:** 611.83

This salt is not official in any pharmacopoeia but it was official in BPC 1973. It usually occurs in more complex polymerized form and is known as sodium polymetaphosphate.

***Preparation:*** It is prepared by dehydration of sodium phosphates.

*Example:* $Na_2H_2P_2O_7$, $NaH_2PO_4$, $Na_2HPO_4$.

$$n\,NaH_2PO_4 \rightleftharpoons n\,NaPO_3 + H_2O$$

***Physical properties:*** It occurs as a white or colorless powder, soluble in water. But sodium poly metaphoshate is insoluble in water.

***Uses***

1. In very fine powder form it is used in dentifrices as an abrasive.
2. 5% sample is used as a dusting powder in bromhidrosis and hyperhidrosis.
3. It is also used as a prophylactic agent against athlete's foot.

### Pumice U.S.P.

It is a substance of volcanoic origin, which consists of complex aluminium, potassium and sodium silicates.

***Physical properties:*** It occurs as a very light, hard, rough, porous, grey masses, grey colored powder, insoluble in water and dilute acids. Powdered pumice meets the following requirements.

***Pumice flour or super fine pumice:*** It should not be less than 97% of pumice, passes through sieve number 200.

***Fine pumice:*** It should not be less than 95% fine pumice passes through 150 mesh size and not more than 50% passes through sieve number 200.

***Coarse pumice:*** It should not be less than 95% coarse pumice passes through a sieve number 60 and not more than 5% passes through standard sieve number 200.

***Use:*** It is used as dentifrice.

## 6.3.4 Dentifrices with Desensitizing Agent

### Zinc Chloride

This compound is discussed under **dentifrices.**

---

### Ammoniacal Silver Nitrate Solution N.F.

**Mol. Formula:** $Ag(NH_3)_2NO_3$ **Mol. Weight:** 159

It is official in National Formulary.

***Uses:***

1. It is used as a dental protective and desensitizing agent.
2. It is mixed with 10% formaldehyde solution and then applied to the small lesions and exposed dentin.

## 6.3.5 Oral Antiseptics and Astringents

**Introduction:** Substances like hydrogen peroxide, sodium peroxide and zinc peroxide are having antiseptic properties on teeth. When they are used, acts by evolving oxygen which is able for the mechanical cleaning between the teeth.

### Hydrogen Peroxide

This compound is discussed under **oxidative antimicrobials**.

---

## Sodium Peroxide N.F.

**Mol. Formula:** $Na_2O_2$ **Mol. Weight:** 78

It is rarely used as a dental product due to its antimicrobial activity.

## Magnesium Peroxide N.F.

**Mol. Formula:** $MgO_2$ **Mol. Weight:** 56.3

It is rarely used as a dental product due to its antimicrobial activity.

**Assay**

***Principle:*** It is assayed by **permanganometry method of titration** (also called **redox titration**).

In this assay the substance is dissolved in a mixture of water and dilute sulphuric acid and the solution is titrated against 0.1N potassium permanganate. Potassium permanganate is acting as a self indicator. End point is the appearance of permanent pale pink colour.

During this assay, sulphuric acid first reacts with potassium permanganate and liberate nascent oxygen. Thus the liberated nascent oxygen oxidizes magnesium peroxide. After the completion of this reaction, addition of potassium permanganate remains in the flask and its colour is retained i.e., permanent pale pink colour. As the oxidation and reduction takes place simultaneously this is called Redox titration. The chemical reactions of this assay are shown below.

$$2\,KMnO_4 + 3\,H_2SO_4 \longrightarrow K_2SO_4 + 2\,MnSO_4 + 3\,H_2O + 5(O)$$

$$5MgO_2 + 5(O) \longrightarrow 5MgO + 5\,O_2$$

These equations can also be written as

$$2\,KMnO_4 + 3\,H_2SO_4 + 5\,MgO_2 \longrightarrow K_2SO_4 + 2\,MnSO_4 + 3\,H_2O + 5MgO + 5\,O_2$$

***Procedure:*** Dissolve 80.0 mg, shaking cautiously, in a mixture, previously cooled to 20 °C, of 10 ml of sulphuric acid and 90 ml of water. Titrate with 0.02M potassium permanganate until a pink colour is obtained.

## Zinc Peroxide

**(Synonym: Medicinal Zinc peroxide)**

**Mol. Formula:** $ZnO_2$ **Mol. Weight:** 97.39

***Preparation:*** It is prepared by treating concentrated hydrogen peroxide with very pure zinc oxide.

$$ZnO + H_2O_2 \longrightarrow ZnO_2 + H_2O$$

The final product contains zinc hydroxide ($Zn(OH)_2$) and zinc carbonate ($ZnCO_3$) due to unchanged zinc oxide and carbon dioxide. The composition of the particular compound is varying according to the conditions of the preparation.

***Physical properties:*** It is a white or slightly white powder.

***Test for identification:*** Similar to that of hydrogen peroxide.

***Test for purity:*** It should be tested for chloride, sulphate, alkali and alkaline earth metals.

***Test for alkali and alkaline earth metals:*** A small amount of sample solution is prepared by using dilute hydrochloric acid (zinc is converted into $ZnCl_2$). To this add ammoniacal ammonium sulphide solution. The zinc sulphide is filtered, acidified with dilute sulphuric acid, evaporated, ignited and the residue is weighed.

**Assay:** Similar to that of hydrogen peroxide.

*Uses:*

1. It is used as an astringent, antiseptic and protective.
2. Due to its oxidative properties it is used in the treatment of infected wounds and dressings in post operative treatment.

---

## Sodium Perborate

This compound is discussed under **oxidative antimicrobials**.

---

### 6.3.6 Mouth Washes

The following inorganic compounds are used as mouth washes due to their medicinal properties.

1. Zinc sulphate - Mild astringent and antiseptic
2. Zinc Chloride - Deodorant and antiseptic
3. Potassium Permanganate - Anti infective and astringent
4. Sodium bicarbonate - Antacid property
5. Sodium Chloride - Irrigating property
6. Ammoniacal silver nitrate solution - Decreases the hypersensitivity of teeth and gum, astringent

### 6.3.7 Cements and Fillers

**Introduction:** The 'Dental cements' are used to temporarily covers and protect the areas that have undergone operation as dental surgery. The cementing material is applied as a paste, and this gets hardened in a short time and acts as a protective layer. This can be easily removed after its projection is over. Noble metals like gold and silver can be used as filling materials.

## Zinc Oxide

This compound is discussed under **topical agents.**

## PROBABLE QUESTIONS

1. Define anticaries agents. Explain the role of fluorides as anticaries agent?
2. Explain the method of preparation, properties, uses and assay of
   (a) Sodium fluoride (b) Sodium mono fluoro phosphate
3. Enumerate the fluoride compounds used in dental products and highlight their relative efficacies, advantages and limitations.
4. Explain briefly about various inorganic compounds used as mouth wash; mention their chemistry and specific applications in oral hygiene products.
5. Describe the method of preparation, properties, assay and uses of stannous fluoride.
6. Define dentifrices. List out the official dentifrices
7. Explain about the preparation, properties, test for identification, test for purity, assay and uses of the following compounds
   (a) Calcium carbonate (b) Calcium phosphate
   (c) Dibasic calcium phosphate
8. What is meant by desensitizing agents.
9. Write a note on strontium chloride.
10. Write the preparation, properties, assay and uses of the following compounds.
    (a) Zinc chloride (b) Maddrell's salt
    (c) Pumice
11. Explain about the dentifrices containing desensitizing agents
12. Define oral antiseptics and astringents with examples.
13. Write a note on
    (a) Sodium peroxide (b) Magnesium peroxide
    (c) Zinc peroxide
14. Define cements and fillers. Describe the preparation, test for purity, assay and uses of zinc oxide.

## 6.4 MAJOR INTRA AND EXTRA CELLULAR ELECTROLYTES

**Introduction:** In our body most of the chemicals exist in the form of compounds. These compounds have been divided as organic compounds and inorganic compounds. Water, salts, acid and bases are inorganic compounds where as the concentration of these organic and inorganic compounds have been balanced in such a way that the body cells and the tissues have same environment. In our body the ionic balance, osmotic balance, pH are maintained by several regulatory mechanisms, in order to maintain the concentration of solutes (inorganic compounds) in various body fluids. All these inorganic compounds are present in solutes in the form of ions/electrolytes.

In the human body, there are three body fluid compartments with different electrolytic concentrations. They are

1. **Intracellular fluid:** Fluid present inside the cell (cytoplasm).
2. **Interstitial fluid:** Fluid present between the cells.
3. **Vascular fluid:** Fluid present within the blood vascular system.

Interstitial fluid and vascular fluid are collectively called as extra-cellular fluid (ECF).

The concentration of dissolved ion (electrolytes) in each compartment gives rise to the osmotic pressure that holds water in the appropriate space. The normal osmolarity of three compartments is 280 -310 mOsm/L.

Sodium and chloride is more in extracellular fluid, potassium and phosphate are rich in intracellular fluid. Other osmotically active substances are glucose, urea, phospholipids, cholesterol and neutral fats. These are in either anionic or cationic form (e.g.: $HCO_3^-$, $Cl^-$, $Na^+$ etc.)

These three fluid compartments are demarcated/separated from each other by membranes which are permeable to water and certain organic and inorganic compounds present in the body fluids. These membranes do not permit protein like molecules, but are permeable to these cations and anions of inorganic compounds, so there is a change existing on the membrane due to the presence and transfer of ions between the membranes. This change is called as "Resting membrane potential" (-90 mV) and it establishes an "Electrical gradient" to the plasma membrane. The membrane has certain "Ion channels" for the movement of ions through it.

The transport mechanism involved in the passage of these ions between the membranes will be two types.

1. Passive process by Diffusion and Osmosis.
2. Active process by $Na^+$ - $K^+$ pump (ATP mediated).

The main role played by these cations and anions is to propagate the impulses all along the neurons of the body. This helps to conduct the nerve impulses from brain (integrating centre) to different parts of the body; which is the basis for all the physiological and biological processes of the body. This process is called as "action potential". It can be defined as "the series of events which eventually decrease or reverse the membrane potential values thereby, restoring it to the normal". The change in the membrane potential value is due to movement of ions through the ion channels of the plasma membrane.

Action potential based on the movement of ions consists of two phases, depolarization and repolarization. In the beginning of action process, an impulse is generated on the neuron received by its dendrite and transmitted to axon. During this process the impulse activates initially voltage-gated sodium channels ($Na^+$) on the membrane causing its opening. As the $Na^+$ concentration is rich extracellularly, the sodium ions diffuses from outside to inside the cell (cytoplasm). This changes the negative membrane potential to zero, then to positive (+30 mV). This phase is called as "depolarization". Then the sodium channels are closed and potassium channels are opened leading to outward flow of $K^+$ concentration is more in cytoplasm. This leads to change of membrane potential to negative (–70 mV). This is called as "Repolarization" phases Fig. 6.4.

So, by these two phases the impulse gets conduction in the neurons. After a "resting stage" or "refractory period" next action potential begins. So, we can understand the key role of cations and anions of inorganic compounds in action potential; in turn, this action potential plays a key role in all the vital processes like contraction of heart muscles, stimulation of nerves, muscle contractions etc.

**Physiological Role of Ions and Electrolytes**

Physiological ions or electrolytes are released through the dissociation of inorganic compounds, they are so named because they can conduct electrical current in a solution. Electrolytes play a vital role in maintaining homeostasis within the body. They help to regulate myocardial and neurological functions, fluid balance, oxygen delivery, acid base balance. Sodium, potassium, calcium, magnesium, chloride, phosphate and bicarbonate are major electrolytes.

1. **Chlorides:** The chloride ion is formed when the element chlorine picks up one electron to anion $Cl^-$. Chloride is the major extra cellular anion and is principally responsible for maintain proper hydration, osmotic pressure and normal cation-anion balance in the vascular and intestinal fluid components. The total concentration of Na in human body is 50 meq/kg. Best food sources include animal foods, table salt. The daily requirement is 5 to 10 gm as NaCl. Chloride balance has important physiological roles. In CNS, the inhibitory action of glycine and GABA's action relies on the entry of $Cl^-$ in to specific neurons.

   The other important functions of chloride ions are

   1. $Cl^-$ along with sodium maintains the osmotic balance of the body fluids.
   2. It maintains the membrane potential (change) between intracellular and extracellular fluids.

Chloride imbalance causes:

**(a)** ***Hypochloremia:*** An electrolyte disturbance where there is an abnormal depleted level of $Cl^-$ in body.

Causes are - Chronic polynephritis - leads to salt loss, metabolic acidosis in diabetes mellitus, renal failure, prolonged vomiting, hypoventilation.

**(b)** ***Hyperchloremia:*** An electrolyte disturbance where there is an abnormally elevated level of $Cl^-$ in the blood.

Causes are - Diarrhoea, over activity of parathyroid gland.

2. **Phosphate:** About 1 gm of phosphate is ingested daily. Approximately 70% (700 mg) is absorbed from the intestine; rest (300 mg) 50% is eliminated in feces.

Phosphate functions to store and release energy *via* high energy phosphates and is an integral to the structure of proteins lipids and bones. It occurs in organic and inorganic forms. Plasma contains lipid phosphates, organic ester phosphates and inorganic divalent ($HPO_4^{-2}$) and monovalent ($H_2PO_4^-$) phosphate. Inorganic phosphate is maintained between 3 to 4.5 mg/100 ml in adults and 4 - 5 ml/100 ml in children. Parathyroid hormone inhibits proximal tubular inorganic phosphate reabsorption and increases inorganic phosphate excretion.

In hyperparathyroid patients, as parathyroid hormone is elevated, phosphate levels are low (Hypophosphatemia). Also prolonged respiratory alkalosis, poor dietary intake also causes it. Hyperphosphatemia caused by tissue damage or cell death, renal failure, liver failure.

3. **Bicarbonate ($HCO_3^-$):** It is an intermediate form in deprotonation of carbonic acid. Bicarbonate serves a crucial biochemical role in physiological pH buffering system. As it is alkaline in nature, it plays a role in maintaining acid base homeostasis. 70 - 75% of $CO_2$ in body is converted to carbonic acid ($H_2CO_3$), which can quickly turn in to $HCO_3^-$. This $HCO_3^-$ with water, $H_2$ and $CO_2$ forms a buffer system and provide a resistance to drastic pH changes in body. $HCO_3^-$ also acts to regulate pH in small intestine, as it is released from the pancreas and neutralize the acidic chyme which enters duodenum from stomach.

$$HCO_3 + H_2O \longrightarrow CO_2 + H_2O$$

The most common salt form of $HCO_3^-$ is sodium bicarbonate ($Na_2CO_3$) called as baking soda. This also releases $CO_2$ when heated, so used in baking. It also plays a role in digestion process by raising internal pH of stomach after digestion process is over.

4. **Sodium:** It is the critical ion in determining the extra cellular and intra cellular osmolarity. Its necessity or utilization in infants is 3 meq/kg/day and during growth process it is 0.5 meq/kg/day, in adults 1.5 meq/kg/day. The renin angiotensin system (RAS) plays an important role in sodium homeostasis. Mainly sodium is obtained as a

part of diet and water through NaCl (sodium chloride), used as common salt. The human body contains 1.3 gm of sodium and among this $1/3^{rd}$ is present in bones and rest is in body fluids. Sodium helps in water retention and pH balances. It plays a role in nerve functions i.e., stimulation of neurons (action potential) and also in muscle contraction. It also plays a major role in controlling heart beat. The other important functions of sodium include

1. Sodium is an important component of extracellular fluid, where it is associated with chloride and bicarbonate in regulating acid-base equilibrium.
2. It helps in the maintenance of osmotic pressure of various body fluids and thereby protecting the body against excessive fluid loss.

Food sources of sodium include NaCl (common salt), pickled or refined food, bread and tomato sauce. Dietary requirement is 3-5 gm/day.

**(a)** ***Hyponatremia:*** Plasma sodium less than 135 meq/L; due to excess loss of sodium due to excessive sweating, burns, vomiting, diarrhea, diabetes insipidus (excess urination).

**(b)** ***Hypernatremia:*** Defined as an increase in extra cellular sodium concentration caused due to lack of anti diuretic hormone, inadequate water intake, water or excess salt (sodium) intake, cushing's syndrome.

**5. Potassium:** Potassium is the most abundant exchangeable cation in the body. It is 140-150 meq/lit concentration intra cellularly and as 3.5 -5 meq/lit in extra cellular fluid. So, around 120 gm of potassium is found in the body. It is obtained in whole grains, vegetables (lettuce, beans, spinach), fruits (citrus, banana and tomato) and helps to maintain normal blood pressures and sometimes lower the elevated blood pressure. Body consists of more potassium than sodium. Potassium is well absorbed from intestine and distribution is wide. Its elimination by kidney is regulated by aldosterone. In body, along with sodium, potassium regulates the water balance and acid base balance in tissues and blood. In nerves, sodium potassium flux (Na - $K^+$ pump) generates action potential for conduction of nerve impulses. Potassium is also very important in energy metabolism like glycogen, glucose metabolism, synthesis of proteins in cells and also in growth and development of muscles.

**(a)** ***Hypokalemia:*** Occurs when $K^+$ concentration is low in blood, caused due to inadequate potassium intake, urinary loss in diabetic ketoacidosis and on usage of diureties, vomiting, diarrhea etc.

**(b)** ***Hyperkalemia:*** Refers to condition in which concentration of $K^+$ in blood is elevated.

Causes include excessive intake of $K^+$, hereditary factors, medication with diuretics, ACE inhibitors etc. and due to excess of $K^+$ release from cells.

6. **Calcium:** It plays an important role in physiology and biochemistry of organism and the cell. Calcium levels in the body are regulated by parathyroid hormone. This hormone regulates resorption of $Ca^{+2}$ from bone, reabsorption in the kidney back into circulation and increase the activation of vitamin $D_3$ to calcitriol. Calcitriol promotes the absorption in calcium from intestine and the mobilization of calcium ion from bone matrix. Calcitionin (from thyroid gland) also effects $Ca^{2+}$ levels in the body by opposing parathormone. The dietary sources of $Ca^{2+}$ include chese, almonds, milk, molasses, lentils, wheat germs etc. Daily requirement of $Ca^{2+}$ if 748-908 mg/day for females and 871-1266 mg/day for males. Calcium is required for vascular contraction and vasodilation, muscle function, nerve transmission, hormone secretion and fertilization.

   Decrease in extra cellular $Ca^{2+}$ concentration results in 'hypocalcemic tetany', marked by spontaneous motor discharge and affects signal transduction and blood coagulation.

   Chronically elevated plasma levels of $Ca^{2+}$ results in 'Hypercalcaemia'. It leads to cardiac arrhythmias, decreased neuromuscular excitability. Excess $Ca^{2+}$ ions will damage cells, seen in neurodegenerative diseases. Excessive entry of $Ca^{2+}$ into a cell may even leads to apoptosis or necrosis.

7. **Magnesium:** It is an essential mineral nutrient for life and is present in every cell type in every organism. For example, ATP must bound to $Mg^{2+}$ in order to be biologically active (i.e., for $Na^+$-$K^+$ ATP are pump system) over 300 enzymes require $Mg^{2+}$ for their biological and catalytic roles. Green vegetables like spinach, peas, milk, oats, bread, peanut, butter are rich in magnesium. The daily requirement is 80 mg/day (1-3 years age); and 310 to 320 mg (females), 350-400 mg (pregnancy) and 400-420 (males).

   Magnesium plays an important role in signal mechanism of cells, enzyme activation and catalysis and transport mechanisms of cells.

   **(a)** ***Hypomagnesemia:*** Deficiency of $Mg^{2+}$ leads to sleepiness, muscle weakness and hyper excitability.

   ***Causes:*** Burns, alcohol abuse, low blood levels of $Ca^{2+}$, malabsorptic.

   **(b)** ***Hypermagnesemia:*** Excess $Mg^{2+}$ in plasma.

   Symptoms –apathy, confusion, insomnia, muscle twitching and poor memory.

   ***Causes:*** Rapid heartbeat, muscle contraction increases, hallucinations, delirium and numbness.

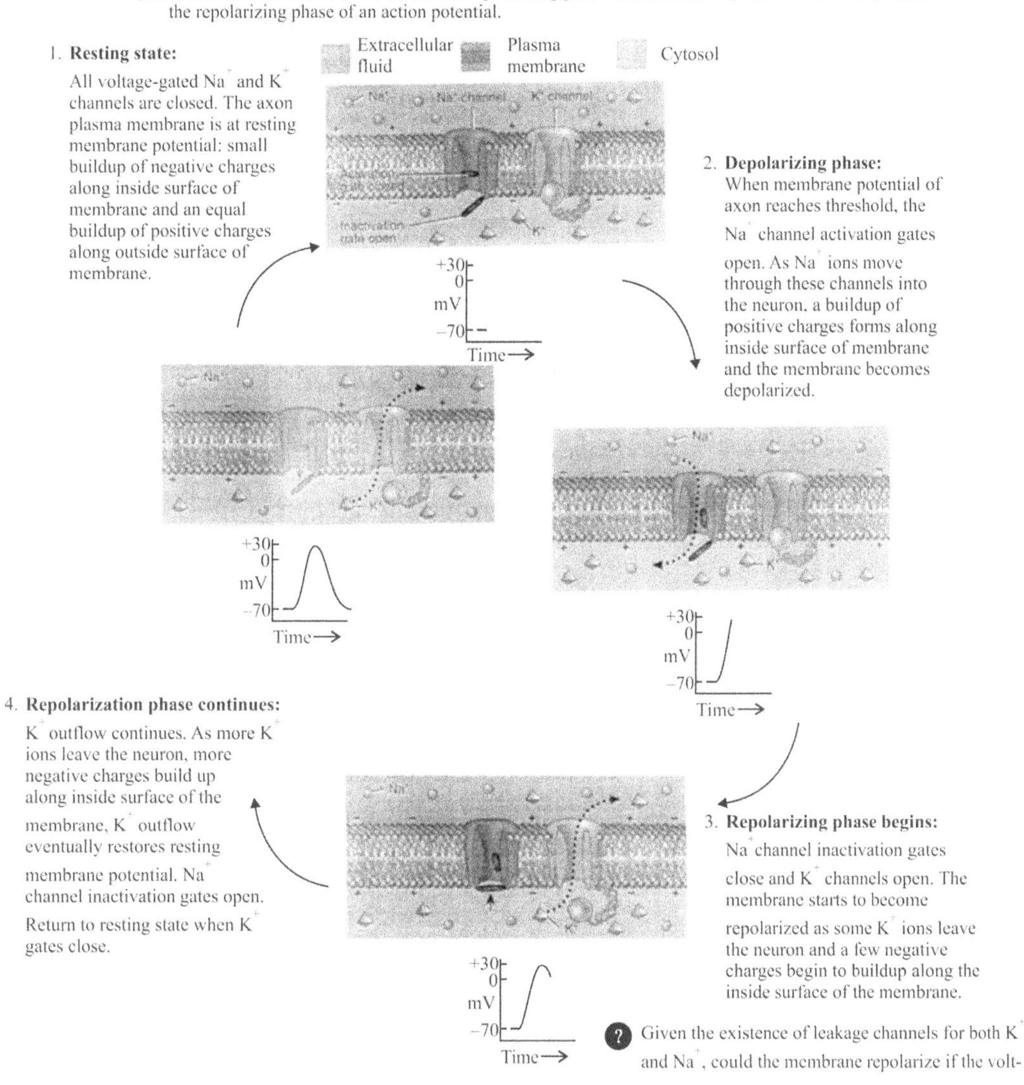


Fig. 6.4 Sodium and potassium channels

## Electrolytes used for Replacement Therapy

**Introduction:** Normally, the body is able to adjust the electrolyte balance by its own mechanisms. But, in some conditions like severe vomiting, diarrhea, severe burns, prolonged fever etc. there will be loss of water and electrolytes from the body. In such conditions, it is essential to administer the lost electrolytes in appropriate concentrations to compensate the loss. For this, the electrolyte, preparations are available in two types.

(a) ***Electrolytes for rapid initial replacement:*** These resemble to the concentration of electrolyte in extracellular fluid. The concentrations of electrolytes are Sodium: 130

– 150 meq/l; Chlorine: 98-110 meq/l; Bicarbonate: 28-55 meq/l; Potassium: 4-12 meq/l; Calcium: 3-5 meq/l; magnesium: 3 meq/l.

(b) ***Electrolytes for subsequent replacement:*** The concentration of electrolyte is Na: 40-120 meq/l; Cl: 30-105; $HCO_3$: 16-53 meq/l; K: 16-35 meq/l; Ca: 10-15 meq/l; Mg: 3-6 meq/l; Phosphorus: 0-13 meq/l.

***Sodium replenishers:*** Sodium chloride- tablets, injections.

***Potassium replenishers:*** Potassium chloride injection, Potassium gluconate tablets.

***Calcium replenishers:*** Calcium chloride injection, Calcium gluconate tablets, Calcium lactate tablets.

## 6.4.1 Sodium Replenishers

### Sodium Chloride I.P., B.P., U.S.P.

**(Synonym: Common salt)**

**Mol. Formula:** NaCl **Mol. Weight:** 58.4

It contains not less than 99.0% and not more than 100.5% of NaCl calculated on the dried basis.

***Preparation:*** Common salt has been manufactured from hundreds of years by evaporation of sea water in shallow pans. In England, the pure salt is manufactured from underground rock salt deposits, mainly in Cheshire.

*Method 1:* Boreholes are drilled through the marlstone beds and water either percolates naturally or is run down to the rock salt strata. The clear, saturated brine is pumped to the surface and evaporated in a triple effect evaporator and purified by special lime soda process.

*Method 2:* A very pure analytical grade sodium chloride is prepared by passing hydrogen chloride into a concentrated solution of the salt. The sodium chloride formed is insoluble in concentrated HCl than water, is crystallizes out leaving the impurities in solution.

***Physical properties:*** It occurs as white or colorless crystals or white crystalline powder, odorless, transparent or translucent when in large crystals. It is soluble in water, slightly soluble in alcohol and insoluble in HCl. A 0.9% w/v solution is iso osmotic with human serum.

***Chemical properties:*** Sodium chloride oxidizes chemically and liberates chlorine gas.

$$2\,Cl^- + MnO_2 + 2\,H_2SO_4 \longrightarrow Mn^{2+} + 2\,SO_4^{2-} + 2\,H_2O + Cl_2\uparrow$$

*Reaction with silver nitrate solution:* Sodium chloride reacts with silver nitrate and gives a white precipitate of silver chloride which is soluble in ammonia solution.

$$NaCl + AgNO_3 \longrightarrow AgCl\downarrow + NaNO_3$$

***Test for identification:*** The solution in water gives the characteristic reactions of sodium and chloride ions.

***Test for purity:*** It has to be tested for clarity, color of the solution, acidity or alkalinity, arsenic, barium, bromide, calcium and magnesium, heavy metals, ferrocyanide, iodides, iron, sulphates and loss on drying.

**Assay**

***Principle:*** It is assayed by **precipitation method of (Back) titration (Modified Volhard's method**).

In this assay the substance is dissolved in water and acidified with nitric acid and to this a Known Excess Standard (KES) silver nitrate and nitrobenzene added and the Excess Unreacted (EUR) silver nitrate is back titrated against 0.1N ammonium thiocyanate. Ferric ammonium sulphate (Ferric alum) is used as an indicator. End point is the appearance of brick red colour.

During this assay, sodium chloride reacts with silver nitrate and silver chloride is formed. After completion of this reaction, the Excess Unreacted silver nitrate is determined by titrating against ammonium thiocyanate. After the completion of this reaction, further addition of ammonium thiocyanate reacts with the indicator ferric ammonium sulphate and yield brick red colour ferric thiocyanate, which is the end point. As the test substance is converted to a precipitate during this assay this is called precipitation method. The chemical reactions of this assay are shown below.

$$NaCl + AgNO_3 \longrightarrow AgCl\downarrow + NaNO_3$$

$$AgNO_3 + NH_4SCN \longrightarrow AgSCN + NH_4NO_3$$

***Procedure:*** Weigh accurately about 0.1 gm and dissolve in 50 ml of water in a glass-stoppered flask. Add 50.0 ml of 0.1M silver nitrate, 5 ml of 2M nitric acid and 2 ml of dibutyl phthalate, shake well and titrate with 0.1M ammonium thiocyanate using 2 ml of ferric ammonium sulphate solution as indicator, until the colour becomes reddish yellow.

***Uses:***

1. 0.9% solution of sodium chloride is used for wet dressings and irrigating body cavities or tissues.
2. It is mainly used as an electrolyte replenisher, emetic and topical inflammatory agent.
3. 0.9% solution is also used as a nasal drop to relieve nasal congestion and as a mouthwash to remove debris to treat throat infection.
4. In dermatological preparation it is used as a hydrating agent.
5. It is also used for the treatment of extra cellular volume depletion, dehydration and sodium depletion due to excessive diuresis (diabetes insipidus).
6. Hypertonic solutions are used to excessive loss of sodium along with water. When hypertonic solutions are given orally, it induces vomiting and thus it can be used in case of poisoning as a first aid.
7. It is the major source of sodium and chloride ions.

8. Sodium chloride is an important constituent of Ringer's solution, ringer lactate solution, ringer's injection, sodium chloride and potassium chloride intravenous infusions and oral rehydration salt (ORS).

***Oficial preparations:*** Sodium chloride tablets I.P., sodium chloride solutions I.P. and sodium chloride parenetral preparations I.P., B.P.

***Storage:*** It should be stored in tightly closed containers and protected from light.

***Labelling:*** The label indicates that whether the solution is used for the manufacture of parenetral preparation or for the preparation of dialysis solution.

## Sodium Chloride Solution B.P.

It contains 0.9% w/v of NaCl.

**Composition:**

| | | |
|---|---|---|
| NaCl | = | 0.9 gm |
| Purified water (q.s) | = | 100 ml. |

***Preparation:*** The required amount of sodium chloride is dissolved in purified water and clarified by filtration. When normal saline is prescribed and then the above solution is dispensed. The label states that it is a solution and then it should comply for its sterility.

## Compound Sodium Chloride Solution I.P.

**(Ringer's solution)**

It contains not less than 0.82% and not more than 0.9% w/v of sodium chloride, not less than 0.025% and not more than 0.035% w/v of potassium chloride, not less than 0.03% w/v and not more than 0.036% w/v of calcium chloride.

**Composition:** It is a sterile solution containing

| | | |
|---|---|---|
| Sodium chloride | = | 0.82 gm |
| Potassium chloride | = | 0.03 gm |
| Calcium chloride | = | 0.033 gm |
| Purified water (q.s) | = | 100 ml. |

All the ingredients are dissolved in purified water and clarified by filtration.

***Physical properties:*** It occurs as a clear, colorless solution.

***Test for identification:*** The sample solution gives the characteristic reactions of sodium, potassium, calcium and chloride ions.

***Test for purity:*** It should be tested for pH, heavy metals and it should comply with the test for sterility.

**Assay**

***For sodium chloride:*** It assayed by **flame photometry** measuring at **589 nm.**

***For potassium chloride:*** It assayed by **flame photometry** measuring at **767 nm**.

***For calcium chloride:*** It assayed by **complexometry method** of titration.

***Uses:*** It is mainly used as an irrigation solution.

***Storage:*** It should be stored in well closed container and protected from moisture.

## Sodium Chloride Injection I.P., B.P., U.S.P.

**(Synonym: Sodium chloride intravenous infusion)**

It is a sterile isotonic solution of sodium chloride in water for injection. It contains no antimicrobial agents. It contains not less than 0.85% w/v and not more than 0.95% w/v of sodium chloride.

**Composition:**

Sodium chloride = 0.9 gm

Water for injection q.s = 100 ml.

***Preparation:*** The required quantity of sodium chloride is dissolved in required quantity of water for injection, filtered and immediately sterilized by heating in an autoclave or by filtration.

***Physical properties:*** It is a clear, colorless solution.

***Test for identification:*** The pH of the solution is 4.5 to 7.0. The solution gives the characteristic reactions of sodium and chloride ions.

***Test for purity:*** It should be tested for pH, heavy metals, bacterial endotoxin and other tests for parenetral preparations.

**Assay**

***Principle:*** Similar to that of sodium chloride.

***Procedure:*** To an accurately measured volume containing about 0.16 gm of sodium chloride in a glass-stoppered flask, add 50 ml of water and 50.0 ml of 0.1M silver nitrate, 5 ml of 2M nitric acid and 2 ml of dibutyl phthalate. Shake well and titrate with 0.1M ammonium thiocyanate using 2 ml of ferric ammonium sulphate solution as indicator, until the colour becomes reddish yellow.

***Storage:*** It should be stored in single dose glass or plastic containers. When stored in glass containers a small solid particles may separate out which must not be used.

***Labelling:*** The label should states that

1. The strength as the per the % w/v of NaCl.
2. A solution containing visible particles must not be used. When the preparation is intended for IV infusion, the label states that the injection contains approximately 150 millimoles of sodium ions and chloride ions/L.

***Use:*** It is used as an electrolyte replenisher.

## Sodium Chloride Tablets B.P.

The average content of sodium chloride in each tablet is not less than 95% and not more than 105% of sodium chloride.

***Preparation:*** The tablets are prepared by compression.

***Test for identification:*** It gives the characteristic reactions of sodium and chloride ions.

***Test for purity:*** It should be tested for color and clarity of solution, disintegration time and it also complies with the tests for tablets.

***Test for clarity of solution:*** The tablet powder equivalent to 0.65 gm of sodium chloride is dissolved in water. The resulting solution should be clear.

**Assay**

***Principle:*** Similar to sodium chloride.

***Procedure:*** Weigh twenty tablets and then powdered. Take the weight of the powder equivalent to 0.25 gm sodium chloride. Remaining procedure is similar to that of sodium chloride.

***Uses:*** It is mainly used as an electrolyte replenisher.

***Dose:*** 0.3 gm. The tablet should be dissolved in water before administration.

***Storage:*** It should be stored in well closed container.

---

## Compound Sodium Chloride Injection I.P., B.P.

**(Synonym: Ringer's Injection)**

Compound sodium chloride injection contains not less than 0.82% w/v and not more than 0.90% w/v of sodium chloride, not less than 0.0285% w/v and not more than 0.0315% w/v of potassium chloride and not less than 0.03% w/v and not more than 0.036% w/v of calcium chloride ($CaCl_2.2H_2O$).

It is a sterile solution does not contain the antimicrobial agents.

**Composition:**

| | | |
|---|---|---|
| Sodium chloride | = | 8.6 gm |
| Potassium chloride | = | 0.03gm |
| Calcium chloride | = | 0.033 gm |
| Purified water (q.s) | = | 1000 ml (water for injection) |

***Preparation:*** All the above ingredients are dissolved in water for injection. The solution is filtered until it becomes clear. Finally, the solution is sterilized by heating in an autoclave.

***Physical Properties:*** It is a clear, colorless solution with pH of 5 to 7.5.

***Test for identification:*** The solution gives the characteristic reactions of sodium and chloride ions. When concentrated to one half of its original volume gives the characteristic reactions of potassium and calcium ions.

***Test for purity:*** It should be tested for pH, heavy metals, bacterial endotoxin and other tests for parenetral preparations.

**Assay**

***Principle:*** It is assayed for its total chlorides, calcium chloride and potassium chloride by the methods adopting mentioned herein.

*Test for total chlorides:* It is assayed by **precipitation method of titration (Modified Volhard's method)**.

In this assay the substance is diluted with water and acidified with nitric acid and to this a Known Excess Standard (KES) silver nitrate and nitrobenzene are added whereby silver chloride is precipitated. The Excess Unreacted (EUR) Silver nitrate is back titrated against 0.1N ammonium thiocyanate. Ferric ammonium sulphate (Ferric alum) is used as an indicator. End point is the appearance of brick red colour.

During this assay, chlorides react with silver nitrate and forms silver chloride. After completion of this reaction, the excess unreacted silver nitrate is determined by titrating against ammonium thiocyanate. After the completion of this reaction, further addition of ammonium thiocyanate reacts with the indicator ferric ammonium sulphate and yield brick red colour ferric thiocyanate, which is the end point. Nitrobenzene used in this assay prevents interaction of silver chloride with ferric thiocyanate. As the test substance is converted to a precipitate during this assay this is called precipitation method. The chemical reactions of this assay are shown below.

$$NaCl + AgNO_3 \longrightarrow AgCl\downarrow + NaNO_3$$

$$AgNO_3 + NH_4SCN \longrightarrow AgSCN\downarrow + NH_4NO_3$$

*For calcium chloride:* It is assayed by **complexometry method of (Direct) titration**.

In this assay the substance is diluted and to this add known excess standard magnesium sulphate added. Ammonia-ammonium chloride solution is added as buffer to the solution and it is then titrated against 0.05M disodium Ethylene Diamine Tetra Acetate (EDTA) using mordant black II mixture as an indicator. End point is the disappearance of pink colour.

In this assay magnesium ion of magnesium sulphate acts as replacement for calcium ions of ringer lactate. The magnesium ions then react with disodium EDTA, whereby the complexation takes place. As the magnesium ions forms complex with disodium EDTA in this assay, it is called as complexometry method of titration. The chemical reactions of this assay are shown below.

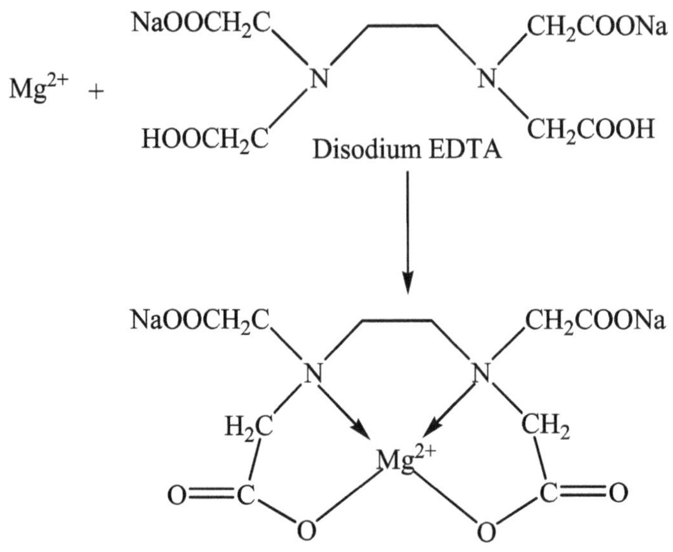

$Mg^{2+}$ + $NaOOCH_2C$ / $HOOCH_2C$ N–$CH_2$–$CH_2$–N $CH_2COONa$ / $CH_2COOH$

Disodium EDTA

↓

$NaOOCH_2C$ N–$CH_2$–$CH_2$–N $CH_2COONa$

$H_2C$ $CH_2$

$Mg^{2+}$

O=C–O O–C=O

Magnesium-EDTA Complex

*For Potassium chloride:* It is assayed by **ceriometry method of titration**.

In this assay, to the substance sodium cobalt nitrate is added. The precipitate is centrifuged and Known Excess standard (KES) ceric sulphate added. The Excess Unreacted (EUR) ceric sulphate is titrated against ferrous ammonium sulphate using orthophenanthroline complex as an indicator.

After finding the total chlorides the volume equivalent to potassium chloride and calcium chloride are subtracted from the total volume and the content for sodium chloride is found out.

***Storage:*** It should be stored in single dose glass or plastic containers. When stored in glass containers a small solid particles may separate out which must not be used.

***Labelling:*** The label should states that

1. The strength as the % w/v of NaCl, KCl and $CaCl_2$.
2. A solution containing visible particles must not be used.

## Sodium Chloride Eye Lotion B.P.

It contains 0.85 to 0.95% w/v of NaCl.

It is prepared by dissolving sodium chloride in purified water, filtered and transferred to a final container. Avoid the entry of microbes and sterilized by heating in an autoclave.

## Hypertonic Saline I.P.

This compound is discussed under **sclerosing agents**.

## Sodium Chloride and Dextrose Injection I.P.

**(Synonym: Sodium chloride and dextrose intravenous infusion, sodium chloride and glucose injection, sodium chloride and glucose intravenous injection)**

It is a sterile solution of sodium chloride and dextrose in water for injection.

It contains not less than 95% and not more than 105% of the stated amount of sodium chloride (NaCl) and dextrose ($C_6H_{12}O_6$).

***Preparation:*** The calculated quantities of sodium chloride and dextrose are dissolved in water for injection. Then it is sterilized immediately by autoclaving or by filtration.

***Physical properties:*** It is a clear, colorless or faintly straw colored solution. pH of the solution is 3.5 to 6.5.

***Test for identification:***

1. The solution gives the characteristic reaction of sodium ion and chloride ion.
2. To the sample solution add one or two drops of potassium cupric tartarate solution (PCT), the solution becomes blue color and clear. When heated to boiling, a copious red color precipitate is formed.

***Test for purity:*** It should be tested for pH, 5-hydroxy methyl furfural and related substances and bacterial endotoxins.

***5-hydroxy methyl furfural:*** A dilute solution of sample containing dextrose equivalent to 1 gm is diluted to 500 ml with water and the absorbance of the solution is measured maximum at 284 nm, which is not more than 0.25.

***Other tests:*** It should be complies with the test for parenetral preparations.

**Assay:** It should be assayed

***For sodium chloride:*** Similar to that of sodium chloride.

***For dextrose:*** It is determined by measuring optical rotation using **optical rotatory dispersion method.**

***Uses:*** It is used as a fluid nutrient and electrolyte replenisher.

***Storage:*** It should be stored in single dose glass or plastic containers. When stored in glass containers a small solid particles may separate out which must not be used.

***Labelling:*** When the preparation is intended for intravenous infusion, the label indicates the approximate concentrations in millimoles/L of sodium and chloride ions and number of grams/L of dextrose.

---

## Sodium Chloride and Fructose Injection I.P.

**(Synonym: Sodium chloride and fructose intravenous infusion, Sodium chloride and fructose infusion, Fructose and sodium chloride injection)**

It contains not less than 95% and not more than 105.0% of sodium chloride, fructose. It does not contain any antimicrobial agents.

It is a sterile solution of sodium chloride and fructose in water for injections.

***Physical properties:*** It is a clear, colorless or faintly straw colored solution.

***Test for identification:***

1. To the small amount of sample solution, add one drop of potassium cupric tartarate solution, heat it, a brownish red precipitate is obtained.
2. It gives the characteristic reactions of sodium and chloride ions.

***Test for purity, assay, uses and storage:*** Similar to that of sodium and dextrose injection.

## Compound Sodium Chloride and Dextrose Injection I.P.

**(Synonym: Compound sodium chloride and dextrose infusion)**

It is a sterile solution containing

| | | |
|---|---|---|
| Sodium chloride | = | 0.86 gm |
| Potassium chloride | = | 0.03 gm |
| Calcium chloride | = | 0.033 gm |
| Dextrose | = | 5 gm |
| Water for injection (q.s.) | = | 100 ml |

It does not contain any antimicrobial agent.

***Physical properties:*** It is a clear, colorless or faintly straw colored solution

***Test for identification:***

1. To the small amount of sample solution, add one drop of potassium cupric tartarate solution, heat it, a brownish red precipitate is obtained.
2. It gives the characteristic reactions of sodium and chloride ions.

***Test for purity, assay, uses and storage:*** Similar to that of sodium and dextrose injection.

## Sodium Chloride Irrigation Solution I.P.

It is a sterile solution containing

| | | |
|---|---|---|
| NaCl | = | 0.9 gm |
| Water for injection (q.s) | = | 100 ml |

It contains not less than 0.85% w/v and not more than 0.95% w/v of sodium chloride. No antimicrobial agent is added to this solution.

***Physical properties:*** It occurs as a clear, colorless solution.

***Test for identification:*** It gives the characteristic reactions of sodium and chlorides.

***Test for purity:*** It should be tested for pH, heavy metals, bacterial endotoxins and other usual tests for parenterals.

***Assay:*** Similar to sodium chloride.

***Labelling:*** The label should be stated that "For irrigation only or not for injection". Once the container is opened, the unused portion should be discarded.

## Sodium Lactate Injection I.P.

**(Synonym: Sodium lactate intravenous infusion)**

It contains not less than 1.75% and not more than 1.95% w/v of sodium lactate, $C_3H_5NaO_3$.

**Ingredients:**

| | | |
|---|---|---|
| Sodium lactate | = | 1.85 gm. |
| Water for injection (q.s) | = | 100 ml |

It is prepared by dissolving sodium lactate in water for injection with the aid of sufficient quantity of sodium hydroxide and sufficient amount of dilute hydrochloric acid to adjust the pH of the injection.

***Physical properties:*** It occurs as a clear, colorless solution.

***Test for identification:***

1. Heated with potassium permanganate gives acetaldehyde which is recognized by its odour.
2. The residue obtained after evaporation is moistened with hydrochloric acid and introduced on a platinum wire in to a flame which gives yellow color to the flame.

***Test for purity:*** It should be tested for pH (4 to 6.5), bacterial endotoxins and complies with the tests for parenterals.

**Assay**

***Principle:*** It is assayed by **acidimetry-alkalimetry method of (Back) titration** (also called **neutralization method**).

In this assay the substance is dissolved in Known Excess Standard (KES) 1N sulphuric acid and the excess unreacted sulphuric acid is titrated with 1N sodium hydroxide using methyl orange as an indicator. End point is the yellow colour.

As the acid and alkali involved in this assay, it is called as acidimetry-alkalimetry method of titration and the neutralization takes place in this assay during titration hence this assay is also called as Neutralization method. The chemical reactions of this assay are shown below.

***Procedure:*** Measure accurately 10 ml, evaporate to dryness in a platinum dish and ignite very gently until completely carbonized. Boil the residue with 25.0 ml of 0.05M sulphuric acid, filter and wash thoroughly with hot water. Titrate the excess of acid in the combined filtrate and washings with 0.1M sodium hydroxide using methyl orange solution as indicator.

***Uses:*** It is used as fluid and electrolyte replenisher.

***Storage:*** It should be stored in single dose glass or plastic containers.

## Compound Sodium Lactate Injection I.P.

**(Synonym: Compound Sodium Lactate IV infusion, Ringer lactate solution for injection, Hartmann's solution of injection)**

It contains not less than 0.27% w/v and not more than 0.32% w/v of sodium, not less than 0.019% and not more than 0.022% w/v of Potassium, not less than 0.37% and not more than 0.42% w/v of total chloride, not less than 0.025% and not more than 0.029% w/v of calcium chloride and not less than 0.23% and not more than 0.28% w/v of lactate as lactic acid.

It is a sterile solution containing

| | | |
|---|---|---|
| Lactic acid | = | 0.24 ml |
| Sodium Chloride | = | 0.6 gm |
| Potassium Chloride | = | 0.04 gm |
| Calcium Chloride | = | 0.02 gm |
| Water for injection (q.s) | = | 100 ml |

***Preparation:*** Dissolve all the ingredients in water for injection and immediately sterilized.

***Physical properties:*** It occurs as a clear, colorless or faintly straw colored solution

***Test for identification:***

1. To the prescribed amount of sample solution add one drop of potassium cupric tartarate solution, boil it. A brown red precipitate is obtained.
2. Heated with potassium permanganate gives acetaldehyde which is recognized by its odour.
3. The residue obtained after evaporation is moistened with hydrochloric acid and introduced on a platinum wire in to a flame which gives yellow color to the flame.
4. The solution gives the characteristic reactions of calcium and chlorides.

***Test for purity:*** It should be tested for pH (4 to 6.5), 5–hydorxy furfural and related substances, heavy metals, bacterial endotoxin and it complies with the other tests for parenterals.

**Assay**

***For sodium:*** It is determined by **flame photometry**.

***For potassium:*** It is assayed **flame photometry** or **atomic absorption spectrophotometry**.

***For total chlorides:*** It is determined by **precipitation method of titration**.

***For calcium chloride:*** It is determined by **complexometry method of titration**.

***For lactate:*** It is determined by **HPLC**.

***For dextrose:*** It is determined by **ORD Method**.

***Uses:*** It is used as a fluid and electrolyte replenisher.

## Compound Sodium Lactate and Dextrose Injection I.P.

**(Synonym: Compound sodium lactate with Dextrose IV infusion, Ringer Lactate solution with Dextrose for injection, Hartmann's solution with dextrose for injection)**

It contains not less than 0.27% and not more than 0.32% w/v of Na, Not less than 0.019% and not more than 0.022% w/v of K, not less than 0.37% and not more than 0.42% w/v of total chloride, Not less than 0.02% and not more than 0.029% w/v $CaCl_2$, Not less than 0.23% w/v and not more than 0.28% w/v lactate, not less than 4.5% and not more than 5.25% w/v of dextrose.

**Ingredients:**

| | | |
|---|---|---|
| Lactic acid | = | 0.24 gm |
| NaCl | = | 0.6 gm |
| KCl | = | 0.04 gm |
| $CaCl_2$ | = | 0.027 gm |

Dextrose in water for injection- 5 gm

***Preparation:*** Dissolve all the ingredients in water for injection and immediately sterilized. It does not contain any anti microbial agents.

***Physical properties:*** It occurs as a clear, colorless or faintly straw colored solution

***Test for identification:***

1. To the prescribed amount of sample solution add one drop of potassium cupric tartarate solution, boil it; a brown red precipitate is obtained.
2. Heated with potassium permanganate gives acetaldehyde which is recognized by its odour.
3. The residue obtained after evaporation is moistened with hydrochloric acid and introduced on a platinum wire in to a flame which gives yellow color to the flame.
4. The solution gives the characteristic reactions of calcium and chlorides.

***Test for purity:*** It should be tested for pH (4 to 6.5), 5–hydorxy furfural and related substances, heavy metals, bacterial endotoxin and it complies with the other tests for parenterals.

**Assay**

***For sodium:*** It is determined by **flame photometry**.

***For potassium:*** It is assayed **flame photometry** or **atomic absorption spectrophotometry**.

***For total chlorides:*** It is determined by **precipitation of titration method.**

***For calcium chloride:*** It is determined by **complexometry method of titration**.

***For lactate:*** It is determined by **HPLC**.

***For dextrose:*** It is determined by **ORD Method**.

*Uses:* It is used as a fluid and electrolyte replenisher.

***Storage:*** It should be stored in single dose containers of glass or plastic at a temperature below 30 °C.

## Half Strength Compound Sodium Lactate and Dextrose Injection I.P.

**(Half strength compound Sodium Lactate with Dextrose IV Infusion: Half strength Ringer-Lactate solution with Dextrose Injection)**

It is a sterile solution containing.

| | | |
|---|---|---|
| Lactic acid | = | 0.12 gm |
| NaCl | = | 0.3 gm |
| KCl | = | 0.02 gm |
| $CaCl_2$ | = | 0.0135 gm |
| Dextrose | = | 5 gm |
| Water for injection (q.s) | = | 100ml |

***Preparation:*** Dissolve all the ingredients in water for injection and immediately sterilize.

Remaining all other aspects are similar to compound sodium lactate and dextrose injection.

---

## Modified Compound Sodium Lactate and Dextrose Injection I.P.

It is a sterile solution containing

| | | |
|---|---|---|
| Lactic acid | = | 0.048 gm |
| NaCl | = | 0.12 gm |
| KCl | = | 0.008 gm |
| $CaCl_2$ | = | 0.0054 gm |
| Dextrose | = | 5 gm |
| Water for injection (q.s) | = | 100 ml |

***Preparation:*** Dissolve all the ingredients in water for injection and immediately sterilize.

Remaining all other aspects are similar to compound sodium lactate and dextrose injection.

---

## Compound Sodium Lactate Solution for Irrigation I.P.

**(Synonym: Ringer lactate solution for irrigation, Hartmann's solution for irrigation)**

It is a sterile solution containing

| | | |
|---|---|---|
| Lactic acid | = | 0.24 gm |
| NaCl | = | 0.6 gm |
| KCl | = | 0.04 gm |
| Calcium Chloride | = | 0.027 gm |
| Water for injection (q.s) | = | 100 ml |

***Test for identification:*** Similar to that of previous compound.

***Test for purity:*** It should be tested for pH and it also complies with the other usual tests for parenterals.

***Uses:*** It is used as an irrigation fluid.

***Storage:*** It should be stored in glass or plastic containers.

***Labelling:*** The label should be stated that "For irrigation only or not for injection". Once the container is opened, the unused portion should be discarded.

---

## Sodium Chloride and Mannitol Injection U.S.P

**Composition:**

| | | |
|---|---|---|
| NaCl | = | 0.3 gm |
| Mannitol | = | 5 gm |
| Water for Injection (q.s) | = | 100 ml |

***Uses:*** It is used as an electrolyte replenisher and diuretic.

***Dose:*** 50 – 200 gm/day by intravenous infusion.

---

### 6.4.2 Potassium Replenishers

## Potassium Chloride I.P., B.P., U.S.P.

**Mol. Formula:** KCl **Mol. Weight:** 74.6

It contains not less than 99% and not more than 100.5% of KCl calculated on the dried basis.

***Preparation:***

*Method 1: Fusion process:* Potassium chloride is mainly obtained from the mineral carnallite (KCl, $MgCl_2$ .6 $H_2O$) by fusion process. The raw mineral carnallite is grounded and treated with hot water. Then the resulting solution is cooled, the less soluble potassium crystallizes out. The process is repeated until the complete removal of potassium chloride from the mother liquor, washed with water and dried.

*Method 2: Laboratory preparation:* It is also prepared by the action of HCl on potassium carbonate or potassium bicarbonate.

$$K_2CO_3 + 2HCl \longrightarrow 2KCl\downarrow + CO_2 + H_2O$$

$$KHCO_3 + HCl \longrightarrow KCl + CO_2 + H_2O$$

***Physical properties:*** It is a colorless crystals or white crystalline powder, odorless, saline taste. It is soluble in water, insoluble in alcohol and ether. m.p. 772 °C. The aqueous solution of KCl is neutral to litmus. $Ag^{2+}$, $Hg^{2+}$, $Pb^{2+}$ etc. diminishes its solubility in water. It is incompatible with amikacin sulphate, dobutamine HCl, amphotericin and fixed oil emulsions.

***Test for identification:*** A solution of potassium chloride in carbondioxide free water gives the characteristic reactions of potassium and chloride ions.

***Test for purity:*** It should be tested for acidity or alkalinity, arsenic, heavy metals, barium, calcium, magnesium, iron, bromides, iodides, sulphates and loss on drying.

### Assay

***Principle:***

*1st method:* It is assayed by **precipitation method of (Back) titration (Modified Volhard's method)**.

In this assay the substance is dissolved in water and acidified with nitric acid and to this a Known Excess Standard (KES) silver nitrate and nitrobenzene added and the Excess Unreacted (EUR) silvernitrate is back titrated against 0.1N ammonium thiocyanate. Ferric ammonium sulphate (Ferric alum) is used as an indicator. End point is the appearance of brick red colour.

During this assay, sodium chloride reacts with silver nitrate and silver chloride is formed. After completion of this reaction, the Excess Unreacted silver nitrate is determined by titrating against ammonium thiocyanate. After the completion of this reaction, further addition of ammonium thiocyanate reacts with the indicator ferric ammonium sulphate and yield brick red colour ferric thiocyanate, which is the end point. As the test substance is converted to a precipitate during this assay this is called precipitation method. The chemical reactions of this assay are shown below.

$$KCl + AgNO_3 \longrightarrow AgCl\downarrow + KNO_3$$

$$AgNO_3 + NH_4SCN \longrightarrow AgSCN + NH_4NO_3$$

*2nd Method:* It is assayed by **Argentometric titration** called **Mohr's method**.

In this assay the substance is dissolved in water and titrated against 0.1N silver nitrate using potassium chromate solutions as an indicator. During this assay, potassium chloride reacts with silver nitrate and forms silver chloride. After the completion of this reaction, further addition of silver nitrate reacts with the indicator potassium chromate and yield brick red colour, which is the end point.

$$KCl + AgNO_3 \longrightarrow AgCl + KNO_3$$

***Procedure:*** Weigh accurately about 0.15 gm, dissolve in 50 ml of water and titrate with 0.1M silver nitrate using potassium chromate solution as indicator.

***Uses:***

1. Potassium chloride and its preparations are mainly used as electrolyte replenishers.
2. It is also used for the treatment of potassium deficiency.
3. It is also used in the condition of hypochloremic alkalosis.
4. It is used for the treatment of myasthenia gravis (muscle weakness), familial paralysis meniere's syndrome (Inner ear disease).
5. It is an antidote for digitalis intoxication.
6. It is the one of the constituent of oral rehydration powder, sodium chloride and potassium chloride intravenous infusion, sodium chloride and potassium chloride and glucose intra venous infusion, Ringer's injection and Ringer's solution.

7. It is used intravenously, if person can't take it orally or incase of severe hypo potassemia.

***Dose:*** Therapeutic use = 10 to 15 gm/day.

Prophylactic use = 2 to 4 gm/day.

## Potassium Chloride and Dextrose Injection I.P.

**(Synonym: Potassium chloride in dextrose injection, potassium chloride and dextrose intravenous infusion, potassium chloride and glucose intravenous infusion.)**

It is a sterile solution of potassium chloride and dextrose in water for injections. It does not contain any antimicrobial agents.

It contains not less than 95% and not more than 110% of potassium chloride, not less than 95% and not more than 105% of dextrose.

***Physical properties:*** It is clear, colorless or faintly straw colored solution.

***Test for identification:*** It gives the characteristic reactions of potassium and chloride ions.

***Test for purity:*** It should be tested for acidity or alkalinity, arsenic, heavy metals, barium, calcium, magnesium, iron, bromides, iodides, sulphates and loss on drying.

**Assay**

***Principle:***

*For potassium chloride:* Similar to potassium chloride.

*For dextrose:* By measuring optical rotation using **optical rotatory dispersion method**.

***Uses:*** It is mainly used as electrolyte replenisher.

## Potassium Chloride, Sodium Chloride and Dextrose Injection I.P.

**(Synonym: Potassium chloride in dextrose and sodium chloride injection; potassium chloride, sodium chloride and dextrose intra venous infusion; potassium chloride, sodium chloride and glucose Intravenous Infusion.)**

It is a sterile solution of potassium chloride, sodium chloride and dextrose in water for injections.

It contains not less than 95% and not more than 110% sodium, potassium and chloride and not less than 95% and 105% of the stated amount of dextrose.

***Physical properties:*** It is clear, colorless or faintly straw colored solution.

***Test for identification:*** It gives the characteristic reactions of potassium and chloride ions.

***Test for purity:*** It should be tested for acidity or alkalinity, arsenic, heavy metals, barium, calcium, magnesium, iron, bromides, iodides, sulphates and loss on drying.

**Assay**

***For sodium:*** It is determined by **flame photometry** or **atomic absorption spectro photometry** at **589 nm**.

***For potassium:*** It is determined by **flame photometry** or **atomic absorption spectro photometry** at **767 nm**.

***For total chlorides:*** It is determined by **Volhard's method**.

***For dextrose:*** By measuring optical rotation using **optical rotatory dispersion method**.

***Uses:*** It is mainly used as electrolyte replenisher.

### 6.4.3 Calcium Replenishers

**Calcium Chloride I.P., B.P.**

**(Synonym: Calcium chloride dihydrate)**

**Mol. Formula:** $CaCl_2 . 2H_2O$ **Mol.Weight:** 147

It contains not less than 97.0% and not more than 103.0% of $CaCl_2 . 2H_2O$.

***Preparation:***

*Method 1: Ammonia soda or Solvay process:* It is obtained as a byproduct of Solvay process for the manufacture of sodium carbonate.

$$NaCl + CO_2 + NH_3 + H_2O \longrightarrow NH_4Cl + NaHCO_3$$

$$2\,NH_4Cl + Ca(OH)_2 \longrightarrow CaCl_2 + 2\,NH_4OH$$

The product obtained by the Solvay process is used for pharmaceutical purpose.

*Method 2:* It is also prepared by the addition of pure calcium carbonate in slight excess to the hot dilute hydrochloric acid. After the completion of reaction the solution is filtered and the filtrate is evaporated, concentrated and cooled at 10 °C, with refrigeration if necessary. The crystals are separated by suction and immediately transferred to a stoppered bottle.

$$CaCO_3 + 2\,HCl \longrightarrow CaCl_2 + CO_2\uparrow + H_2O$$

***Physical properties:*** It occurs as a white crystalline powder or fragments or granules, odorless. The crystals are deliquescence in moist air, effloresce in dry air. It is freely soluble in water (exothermic reaction) and alcohol, and very soluble in boiling water. The pH of the 5% solution is 4.5 to 9.2. It is insoluble in organic solvents. 42.5 gm of $CaCl_2$/100 gm of water freezes at -55 °C and hence it is used as refrigerant.

***Chemical properties:*** It combines with eight molecules of ammonia to form $CaCl_2, 8NH_3$.

$$CaCl_2 + 8\,NH_3 \longrightarrow CaCl_2 .8NH_3$$

*Reaction with ethanol:* Calcium chloride reacts with ethanol gives $CaCl_2.C_2H_5OH$.

$$CaCl_2 + C_2H_5OH \longrightarrow CaCl_2.C_2H_5OH$$

When the aqueous solutions are evaporated, it gives hexahydrates. When hydrates are heated, they lose some of their hydration and porous mass results, which finds use for drying gases and liquids. While heating, some calcium oxide is formed as follows.

$$CaCl_2 + 2\,H_2O \rightleftharpoons Ca(OH)_2 + 2\,HCl$$

$$Ca(OH)_2 \xrightarrow{\Delta} CaO + H_2O$$

***Test for identification:***

1. When it is heated in a dry test tube, it melts and droplets are formed in the inner walls of the test tube.
2. The sample solution in boiling water gives the characteristic reactions of calcium and chloride.

***Test for purity:*** It should be tested for appearance of solution, acidity or alkalinity, arsenic, aluminium and phosphate, barium, heavy metals, iron, magnesium and alkali salts and sulphates.

**Assay**

***Principle:*** It is assayed by **complexometry method of titration**.

In this assay the substances is diluted and to this add known excess standard magnesium sulphate added. Ammonia-ammonium chloride solution added as buffer to the solution and it is then titrated against 0.05M disodium Ethylene Diamine Tetra Acetate (EDTA) using calcon mixture as an indicator. End point is the change of colour from pink to a full blue colour

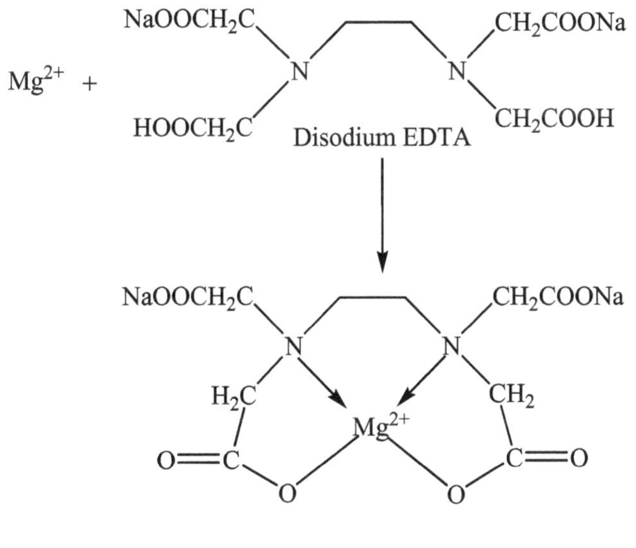

$Mg^{2+}$ +
$NaOOCH_2C$, $CH_2COONa$, N, N, $HOOCH_2C$, $CH_2COOH$
Disodium EDTA

$NaOOCH_2C$, $CH_2COONa$, N, N, $H_2C$, $CH_2$, $Mg^{2+}$, O=C, C=O, O, O

Magnesium-EDTA Complex

In this assay magnesium ions of magnesium sulphate acts as replacement for calcium ions of ringer lactate. The magnesium ions then react with disodium EDTA, whereby the complexation takes place. As the calcium and magnesium ions forms complex with disodium EDTA in this assay, it is called as complexometry method of titration. The chemical reactions of this assay are shown above.

***Procedure:*** Weigh accurately about 0.15 gm, 5 ml of 0.05M magnesium sulphate and dissolve in 50 ml of water. Titrate with 0.05M disodium edetate to within a few ml of the expected end-point, add 8 ml of sodium hydroxide solution and 0.1 gm of calcon mixture and continue the titration until the colour of the solution changes from pink to a full blue colour.

***Uses:***

1. Calcium chloride is mainly used as calcium replenisher (calcium deficiency).
2. It is also used for diuretic, urinary acidifier and anti allergic agent.
3. It is used for producing an acidic urine or definite acidosis (treatment of calcium tetany).
4. The anhydrous form of the salt is used as desiccant for organic compounds.
5. It is used as an ingredient of compound sodium lactate injection.
6. It also acts as an antispasmodic agent, for the treatment colic and lead poisoning.

For oral administration of calcium chloride can cause constipation and GIT replenishers.

***Adverse effects:*** Over usage of calcium salts leads to hypercalcaemia with the symptoms of anorexia, nausea, vomiting, constipation, abdominal pain, muscle weakness, mental disturbances, polydipsia, polyuria, bone pain, renal calculi, cardiac arrythmiasis and coma.

For IV injection, it is irritating veins, it should be injected slowly. Rapid administrations may leads to burning sensation, peripheral vasodilation and fall in BP.

***Dose:*** For oral route 1 to 2 gm.

For IV injection 5 to 10 ml of 10% w/v solution.

***Storage:*** It should be stored in well closed container and protected from moisture.

***Official preparations:*** Calcium chloride injection I.P.

## Calcium Gluconate I.P., B.P.

**Mol. Formula:** $C_{12}H_{22}CaO_{14}.\ H_2O$ **Mol. Weight:** 448.4

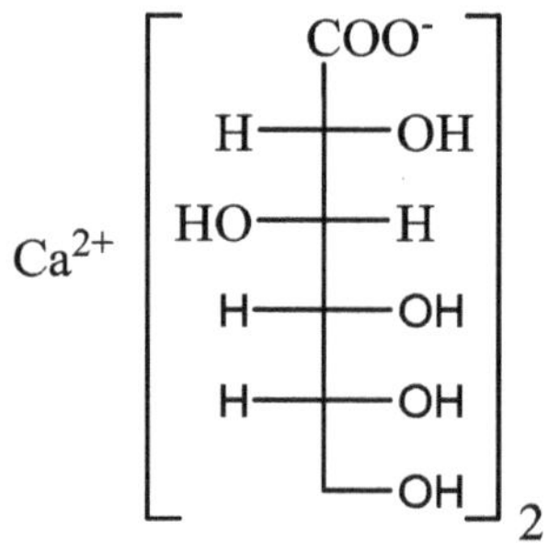

$Ca^{2+}$ [ $COO^-$ ; H–C–OH ; HO–C–H ; H–C–OH ; H–C–OH ; $CH_2$–OH ]$_2$

It is calcium - D- gluconate monohydrate.

It contains not less than 98.5% and not more than 102% of $C_{12}H_{22}CaO_{14}.\ H_2O$.

***Preparation:*** It is prepared by boiling a solution of slight excess of calcium carbonate with gluconic acid, filtered and crystallizes the product from the filtrate.

$$\underset{\text{Gluconic acid}}{CH_2OH.(CHOH)_4.COOH} + CaCO_3 \longrightarrow [CH_2OH.(CHOH)_4.COO]_2Ca + CO_2 + H_2O$$

The gluconic acid used for the above preparation is obtained by the oxidation of glucose with either bromine or iodine or electrolytic oxidation with sodium bromide or action of various *acetobacter* bacteria on glucose.

***Physical properties:*** A white crystalline powder or granules. It is odorless and tasteless. It is less soluble in water, soluble in boiling water, insoluble in organic solvents. The pH of the aqueous solution is 6 to 7.

***Chemical properties:*** When it is heated up to 100 °C, it loses its water for crystallization. It is incompatible with oxalates and borates.

*Reaction with Hydrochloric acid:* When hydrochloric acid is added to the solution of calcium gluconate, gluconic acid is formed, which is easily converted in to d-glucono lactone.

$$\underset{\text{Solution}}{\text{Calcium Gluconate}} + 2\,HCl \longrightarrow 2\,CH_2OH\text{–}(CHOH)_4\text{–}COOH + CaCl_2$$

$$\downarrow -H_2O$$

$$H_2COH\text{–}CH(OH)\text{–}CH\text{–}CH(OH)\text{–}CH(OH)\text{–}C{=}O \quad (\text{ring through } O)$$

d-glucanolactone

***Test for identification:***

1. It gives the characteristic reactions of calcium ions.
2. To the aqueous solution of the sample, add ferric chloride solution, a yellow color is produced.
3. To the sample solution, add glacial acetic acid and phenyl hydrazine, heat the mixture. A white crystalline precipitate of phenyl hydrazone is produced. (m.p. 200 °C to 202 °C)
4. It is also identified by thin layer chromatography using water, ethanol, strong ammonia solution and ethyl acetate as a mobile phase.

***Test for purity:*** It should be tested for color, clarity of the solution, acidity, alkalinity, arsenic, heavy metals, chlorides, sulphates, sucrose, dextrose and reducing substances.

***Test for sucrose, dextrose and reducing sugars:*** The sucrose and dextrose are tested by treating the sample solution with Fehling's reagent. After hydrolyzing the sucrose with dilute hydrochloric acid, no red precipitate is formed.

**Assay**

***Principle:*** It is assayed by **complexometry method of (Direct) titration**.

In this assay the substance is dissolved in water by heating, to this add known excess standard magnesium sulphate and ammonia-ammonium chloride solution is added as buffer solution and it is then titrated against 0.05M disodium Ethylene Diamine Tetra Acetate

(EDTA) using mordant black II mixture as an indicator. End point is the color change from red to blue.

In this assay, magnesium ions of magnesium sulphate act as replacement for calcium ions of calcium gluconate. The magnesium ions then react with disodium EDTA, whereby the complexation takes place. As the calcium and magnesium ions forms complex with disodium EDTA in this assay, it is called as complexometry method of titration. The chemical reactions of this assay are shown below.

$Mg^{2+}$ + $NaOOCH_2C$ $CH_2COONa$ N N $HOOCH_2C$ $CH_2COOH$

Disodium EDTA

↓

$NaOOCH_2C$ $CH_2COONa$ N N $H_2C$ $CH_2$ $Mg^{2+}$ O=C C=O O O

Magnesium-EDTA Complex

***Procedure:*** Weigh accurately about 0.5 gm and dissolve in 50 ml of warm water; cool, add 5.0 ml of 0.05M magnesium sulphate and 10 ml of strong ammonia solution and titrate with 0.05M disodium edetate using mordant black II mixture as indicator. From the volume of 0.05M disodium edetate required subtract the volume of the magnesium sulphate solution added.

***Uses:***

1. It is mainly used as a source of calcium ion for treating hypocalcaemia, tetany or calcium deficiency.
2. It is also used as diuretic, urinary acidifier and anti allergic agent.
3. It is used for producing an acidic urine or definite acidosis (treatment of calcium tetany).
4. The anhydrous form of the salt is used as desiccant for organic compounds.

5. It is used as an ingredient of compound sodium lactate injection.
6. It also acts as an antispasmodic agent, for the treatment colic and lead poison

***Dose:***

2 to 10 gm/day orally in divided doses.

1 to 2 gm/day Intramuscular injection/slow intravenous infusion.

***Advantage:***

1. When it is compared to calcium chloride, it is less irritating and it can be administered orally or parenterally.
2. It is considered the best of all calcium salts, so it can be administered intravenously.

***Official formulations:***

Calcium gluconate injection I.P.

Calcium gluconate tablets I.P.

Calcium gluconate effervescent tablets B.P.

---

## Calcium Gluconate Injection I.P.

Calcium gluconate injection is a sterile solution of calcium gluconate in water for injection. It contains a quantity of calcium equivalent to not less than 8.5% and not more than 9.4% of the stated amount of calcium gluconate.

***Preparation:*** Not more than 5% of calcium gluconate is made to replace Calcium D-saccharate, which acts as stabilizing agent.

Calcium-D-saccharate is used as a sequestering agent, increases the solubility and prevents precipitation of calcium gluconate. The solution is sterilized by an autoclaving.

***Test for identification:*** It reacts with Fehling's solution an intense yellow color is formed. Remaining tests are similar to calcium gluconate.

***Test for purity:*** It should be tested for pH, bacteria endotoxins and other tests under parenteral preparations.

**Assay**

***Principle:*** Similar to that of calcium gluconate.

***Procedure:*** To an accurately measured volume equivalent to 0.5 gm of calcium gluconate add 50 ml of water; cool, add 5.0 ml of 0.05M magnesium sulphate and 10 ml of strong ammonia solution and titrate with 0.05M disodium edetate using mordant black II mixture as indicator. From the volume of 0.05M disodium edetate required subtract the volume of the magnesium sulphate solution added.

***Labelling:*** The label on the container should state that

1. The strength of the calcium gluconate equivalent to the total amount of calcium in % w/v.

2. The solutions containing visible solid particles must not be used.
3. The percentage of any added stabilizing agents.

*Uses:*

1. It is mainly used as a source of calcium ion for treating hypocalcaemia tetany or calcium deficiency.
2. Other uses are similar to that of calcium gluconate.

## Calcium Gluconate Tablets I.P.

It contains not less than 95.0% and not more than 105.0% of the stated amount of calcium gluconate. These tablets are generally intended to be chewed before swallowing and are generally prepared in suitably flavored base.

***Test for identification:*** Similar to calcium gluconate injection.

***Test for purity:*** It should be tested for dissolution, other tests for tablets, hardness test and disintegration test etc.

**Assay**

***Principle:*** Similar to calcium gluconate.

***Procedure:*** Weigh and powder 20 tablets. Weigh accurately a quantity of the powder containing about 0.5 gm of calcium gluconate and ignite, gently at first, until free from carbon. Cool, add 10 ml of water and sufficient dilute hydrochloric acid, drop wise, to effect complete solution of the residue. Neutralize with dilute ammonia solution, add 5.0 ml of 0.05M magnesium sulphate and 10 ml of strong ammonia solution and titrate with 0.05M disodium edetate using mordant black II mixture as indicator. From the volume of 0.05 M disodium edetate required subtract the volume of the magnesium sulphate solution added.

*Uses:*

1. It is the drug of choice for severe hypocalcemic tetany.
2. It is also used as a supplementary diet for expectant mothers and diet of convalescent mothers.
3. It is administered orally, does not produce any gastro intestinal tract irritation.
4. The injections are given by intravenous route; the intramuscular (IM) route should not be used essentially in children as it is responsible for the abscess at the injection site.

## Calcium Gluconate Effervescent Tablet B.P

It is prepared by using suitable effervescent base. It is used as an electrolyte replenisher.

## Dibasic Calcium Phosphate

This compound is discussed under **antacids**.

### 6.4.4 Electrolytes used in acid base Therapy

**Introduction**

Acids are constantly being produced during metabolism. i.e., carbonic acid from $CO_2$ and lactic acid from anaerobic metabolism, hence in order to maintain the acid-base balance by buffering these excess amount of acids, several buffer systems operated in our body like - bicarbonate/carbonic acid ($HCO_3^-/H_2CO_3$) in plasma and kidney; monohydrogen phosphate/dihydrogen phosphate ($HPO_4^{2-}/H_2PO_4^-$) in kidney cells; Haemoglobin buffer (Hb) in RBC. Maintenance of the acid - base balance by these buffers is very critical for the normal cellular function. So, the removal of $H^+$ from body fluids and its subsequent elimination from the body is carried by three mechanisms.

1. Buffer systems
2. Exhalation of $CO_2$
3. Excretion of $H^+$ through kidney

1. ***Buffer systems:*** This consists of a weak acid and the salt of that acid, which functions as a weak base. Buffers prevent rapid and drastic changes in the pH of body fluids by converting strong acids and strong bases to weak acids and weak bases in the fraction of second. Strong acids lower pH more than weak acids because strong acids release $H^+$ more readily, thus contribute more free hydrogen ions. Similarly strong bases raise pH more than weak ones.

   The principle buffer systems of our body fluids are Protein buffer system, Phosphate buffer system, Carbonic acid - bicarbonate buffer system.

2. ***Exhalation of $CO_2$:*** Breathing also plays an important role in maintain pH of body fluids.

   An increase in $CO_2$ concentration in body fluids, increases $H^+$ concentration and thus lowers pH conversely; a decrease in $CO_2$ concentration of body fluid raises the pH.

$$CO_2 + H_2O \rightleftharpoons H_2CO_3 \rightleftharpoons H^+ + HCO_3^-$$

   Changes in the rate and depth of breathing can alter pH of body fluids, with an increase in ventilation, $CO_2$ will be exhaled out and $H^+$ concentration decrease, leading to a rise in the blood pH.

3. ***Kidney excretion of $H^+$:*** Metabolic reactions produce nonvolatile acids such as sulphuric acid. The only way to eliminate these huge acids is to excrete $H^+$ in the urine. Or else, the problem of renal failure occurs, leading to death as there occurs an acid base imbalance.

The cells in collecting ducts and proximal convoluted tubules secrete $H^+$ into the tubular fluid. In proximal convoluted tubes (PCT), $Na^+/H^+$ antiportes secrete $H^+$. The apical membrane of intercalated cells has proton pumps that secrete $H^+$ into tubular fluid. Some other intercalated cells have "$Cl^-$/ $HCO_3$ antiportes" will help the dissociation of $H_2CO_3$ into $H^+$, $HCO_3$, this $HCO_3$ enters into peritubular capillaries and $H^+$ is reabsorbed the way by which buffering mechanism occurs.

That is, the buffers like $HPO_4^{2-}$, $NH_3$ etc. will combine to $H^+$ present in tubular forms $H_2PO_4^-$ and $NH_4^+$ respectively which one excreted in the urine as these cannot be diffuse back into the tubules.

1. ***Respiratory acidosis:*** Caused by inadequate exhalation of $CO_2$ -blood pH drops- leads to emphysema, pulmonary edema, injury to respiratory tract, airway obstruction.

   In this, there is abnormally high $pCO_2$ in systemic arterial blood (above 45 mmHg).

   Treatment is by increasing $CO_2$ exhalation; i.v administration of $HCO_3^-$
2. ***Respiratory alkalosis:*** Systemic arterial blood $pCO_2$ falls below 35mmHg.

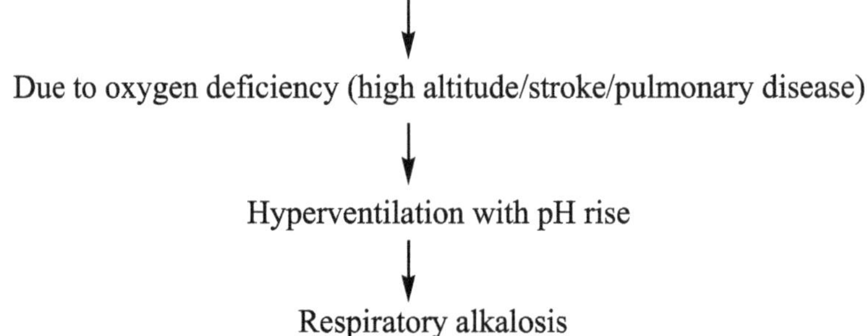


   Treatment: Increasing the levels of $CO_2$ in body.
3. ***Metabolic acidosis:*** In this, the systemic arterial blood $HCO_3^-$ levels drop below 22 mEq/litre - blood pH decreases to 7.35

   Reasons for $HCO_3^-$ drop is diarrhea, renal dysfunction, kidney failure to excrete $H^+$

   Treatment includes: administration of IV sodium bicarbonate solution.
4. ***Metabolic alkalosis:*** Systemic arterial blood $HCO_3^-$ concentration is above 26 mEq/litre and the pH of blood is above 7.45.

It is caused by excess intake of alkaline drug like antacids, use of diuretics etc. Treated by hypoventilation.

---

## Sodium Acetate I.P., B.P.

**Mol. Formula:** $CH_3COONa.\ 3H_2O$ **Mol. Weight:** 136.1

It contains not less than 99.9% and not more than 101.0% of sodium acetate calculated on the dried substance. It is a sodium salt of acetic acid.

***Preparation:*** It is prepared by the neutralization reaction between acetic acid and sodium carbonate or sodium bicarbonate. The solution is filtered, concentrated and crystallized.

$$2\,CH_3COOH + Na_2CO_3 \longrightarrow 2\,CH_3COONa + CO_2\uparrow + H_2O$$

$$CH_3COOH + NaHCO_3 \longrightarrow CH_3COONa + CO_2\uparrow + H_2O$$

*From wood vinegar:* Sodium acetate is prepared by neutralizing the wood vinegar with sodium carbonate. Then the impurities are removed by various processes, evaporate the solution and collect the crystals.

$$2\ CH_3COOH + Na_2CO_3 \longrightarrow 2\ CH_3COONa + CO_2\uparrow + H_2O$$

***Physical properties:*** It occurs as a white or colorless crystals or white granular crystalline powder, odorless. It is having slightly saline and bitter taste. It is soluble in water and alcohol. The aqueous solutions are alkaline in nature. It effloresces in warm dry air, m.p 58 °C. It is incompatible with sodium metabisulphite.

***Chemical properties:***

*Decomposition reaction:* When it is heated to 120 °C, it converted into anhydrous form. Heating at higher temperature leads to decomposition.

$$CH_3COONa.\ 3\ H_2O \xrightarrow[\Delta \atop -3H_2O]{120\ ^\circ C} CH_3COONa$$

***Test for identification:*** The aqueous solution of sample in boiling water gives the characteristic reactions of sodium and acetate ions.

***Test for purity:*** It should be tested for appearance of solution, pH, arsenic, calcium, magnesium, heavy metals, iron, chlorides, reducing substances and loss on drying.

**Assay**

***Principle:*** As the sodium acetate is very weak base, it cannot be assayed by the usual acid-base titration and hence it is assayed by **non-aqueous method of titration**. In this assay the substance is dissolved in a mixture of glacial acetic acid and acetic anhydride and the solution is titrated against 0.01M perchloric acid, using 1-naphthol benzein as an indicator. End point is the appearance of green colour. As the assay is carried out in a non-aqueous medium it is called nonaqueous assay.

***Procedure:*** Weigh accurately the equivalent of about 200 mg of anhydrous sodium acetate, and dissolve in 25 ml of glacial acetic acid, warming gently if necessary to effect complete solution. Add 2 drops of p-naphthol benzein, and titrate with 0.1N perchloric acid.

***Uses:***

1. It is the main ingredient of intra peritoneal dialysis fluid.
2. It is used as pharmaceutical aid and acts as an acidulant in flood.
3. It is an effective buffer in metabolic acidosis.
4. It acts as an alkalinising agent due to the conversion of sodium acetate into to sodium bicarbonate by body tissues.

---

## Potassium Acetate I.P., B.P.

**Mol. Formula:** $CH_3COOK$ **Mol. Weight:** 98.14

It contains 99% and not more than equivalent of 101% of potassium acetate which is calculated with reference to the ignited basis.

***Preparation:*** It is obtained by neutralization of acetic acid with potassium carbonate or potassium bicarbonate until the effervescence ceases. The neutralization is carried out carefully to avoid an excess of carbonate solution. The solution is filtered.

$$2\,CH_3COOH + K_2CO_3 \xrightarrow{\Delta} 2CH_3COOK + CO_2\uparrow + H_2O$$

The filtrate is evaporated to dryness, the residue is fused and solidified. At warm condition, it is quickly powdered and stored in bottles.

If the crystalline potassium acetate is needed, the solution of potassium acetate is stirred continuously during evaporation. The crystalline mass obtained is separated, centrifuged and dried in a current of dry air. In this preparation potassium bicarbonate is preferred instead of potassium carbonate which gives pure quality of potassium acetate.

***Physical properties:*** It is colorless crystals or white crystalline powder or a fused mass, odorless. It is having a saline alkaline taste. It is deliquescent in moist air. It is soluble in water and alcohol, insoluble in ether. It is incompatible with Ag, Hg, iron salts and acids.

***Chemical properties:***

*Reaction with ethyl alcohol:*

When potassium acetate is warmed with ethanol and sulphuric acid, yields ethyl acetate with a pleasant smell.

$$2\,CH_3COOK + 2\,C_2H_5OH \xrightarrow[H_2SO_4]{\Delta} \underset{\text{Ethyl acetate}}{2\,CH_3COOC_2H_5} + 2\,H_2O + K_2SO_4$$

When potassium acetate is heated at 290 °C, it melts above 290 °C leaving a residue (potassium carbonate).

$$2\,CH_3COOK + 4O_2 \xrightarrow{290\ ^\circ C} K_2CO_3 + 3\,CO_2\uparrow + 3\,H_2O$$

*Hydrolysis of potassium acetate:* When it is hydrolysed in water gives an alkaline solution.

$$CH_3COOK + H_2O \longrightarrow CH_3COOH + KOH$$

$$CH_3COO^- + H_2O \longrightarrow CH_3COOH + OH^-$$

***Test for identification:*** The aqueous solution of the sample gives the characteristic reactions of potassium and acetate.

***Test for purity:*** It should be tested for arsenic, heavy metals, aluminium, calcium, sodium chloride, sulphate, nitrate, readily oxidisable substances, loss on drying and alkalinity.

***Test for nitrate:*** To the aqueous solution of sample, add sodium chloride, nitrogen free sulphuric acid and indigo carmine solution. A blue color appears which is stable for at least 10 minutes.

**Assay**

***Principle:***

*Method 1:* It is assayed by **acidimetry-alkalimetry method of (Back) titration** (also called **neutralization method**).

In this assay the substance is ignited and the residue is dissolved in Known Excess Standard (KES) 0.5N sulphuric acid and the Excess Unreacted (EUR) sulphuric acid is titrated with 0.5N sodium hydroxide using methyl orange as an indicator. End point is the appearance of yellow colour.

In this assay upon ignition of the potassium acetate, potassium carbonate is formed which when treated with sulphuric acid, the potassium carbonate (the base) goes into the solution in sulphuric acid and neutralization takes place, after this reaction the excess unreacted sulphuric acid is determined by titrating with sodium hydroxide. The indicator is orange colour in acid medium and it changes to yellow colour upon neutralization which is the end point.

As the acid and alkali involved in this assay, it is called as acidimetry-alkalimetry method of titration and the neutralization takes place in this assay during titration hence this assay is also called as neutralization method. The chemical reactions of this assay are shown below.

$$2\,CH_3COOK \xrightarrow{\Delta} K_2CO_3$$

$$K_2CO_3 + H_2SO_4 \longrightarrow K_2SO_4 + H_2O + CO_2$$

$$2NaOH + H_2SO_4 \longrightarrow Na_2SO_4 + 2\,H_2O$$

*Method 2:* It can also be assayed by **non-aqueous titration**. Potassium acetate is a very weak base, hence it is assayed by dissolving in acetic anhydride and glacial acetic acid and titrating against perchloric acid using crystal violet solution as indicator end point is the appearance of green colour.

***Procedure:*** Dissolve 200 mg of potassium acetate, previously dried and accurately weighed, in 25 ml of glacial acetic acid, add two drops of crystal violet, and titrate with 0.1N perchloric acid. End point is the appearance of green colour. Perform a blank determination also.

*Uses:*

1. It is used in solutions form for haemodialysis and peritoneal dialysis and as an urinary alkaliser.
2. It is mainly used as a diuretic.
3. The acetate ion binds with hydrogen atoms in the stomach, by this way it acts as an antacid.

4. It decomposes in the body and converts into potassium bicarbonate, which acts as a systemic alkaliser.

$$CH_3COOK + 2\,O_2 \longrightarrow KHCO_3 + CO_2 + H_2O$$

## Sodium Bicarbonate, Sodium Bicarbonate Injection, Compound Sodium Bicarbonate Tablets, Sodium Phosphate, Dried Sodium Phosphate, Sodium Citrate

All of these compounds are discussed under **antacids**.

## Sodium Citrate Tablets B.P.

The average content of the each tablet is not less than 95% and not more than 105% of sodium citrate.

***Preparation:*** The tablets are prepared by compression.

***Test for identification:*** The tablet powder gives the characteristic reactions of sodium and citrate ions.

***Test for purity:*** It should be tested for color and clarity of solution and it also complies with the quality control tests for tablets.

***Assay:*** Weigh twenty tablets and then powdered. Remaining procedure is similar to that of sodium citrate.

***Uses:*** It is used as acid base regulator.

***Dose:*** 1 to 4 gm

***Storage:*** It should be stored in well closed container.

## Sodium Citrate Anticoagulant Injection

It contains not less than 3.8% and not more than 4.2% of sodium citrate.

**Ingredients:**

| | | |
|---|---|---|
| Sodium citrate | = | 40 gm |
| Water for injection (q.s.) | = | 1000ml |

***Preparation:*** Sodium citrate is dissolved in water for injection, filtered and immediately sterilized by filtration or autoclave.

***Test for identification:*** It gives the characteristic reactions of sodium and citrate ions.

***Test for purity:*** It should be tested for color and clarity of solution and it also complies with the tests for parenterals.

***Uses:*** It is used as an anticoagulant.

***Storage:*** It should be stored in well closed container with cotton wool and the injection should be used within one month.

***Labelling:*** The label should state that "If any visible particles are seen, it must not be used".

## Potassium Bicarbonate U.S.P.

**Mol. Formula:** $KHCO_3$ **Mol. Weight:** 100.12

***Physical properties:*** It occurs as a colorless, transparent prisms or granular powder, odorless. The solutions are neutral. It is freely soluble in water and practically insoluble in alcohol.

***Test for identification:*** The sample solution gives the characteristic reactions of potassium and bicarbonate ions.

***Test for purity:*** Similar to that of sodium bicarbonate.

***Assay:*** Similar to that of sodium bicarbonate.

***Uses:***

1. It is used for acid-base imbalance therapy.
2. It is used as an antacid for people who must restrict their sodium salts intake.

***Dose:*** 500 mg to 8 gm daily or 1 gm four times a day.

## Potassium Citrate, Sodium Lactate Injection, Ammonium Chloride, Ammonium Chloride Injection, Compound Sodium Chloride Injection

These compounds are discussed under **acid base therapy**.

## 6.4.5 Electrolytes Combination Therapy

***Introduction:*** In the short term treatment of electrolyte replacement therapy such as after surgery, the glucose and saline solution in the form of infusion may be adequate, however in severe conditions, solution containing extra electrolytes are needed. Hence the combination electrolyte preparations are marketed. Commercially the electrolyte infusion solutions with varying amounts of electrolytes are available. Any one of these preparations is normally used for the electrolyte needs of the patients. These combination electrolyte preparations are classified in to two major heads as mentioned below

1. Fluid maintenance therapy.
2. Electrolyte replacement therapy.

***Fluid maintenance therapy:*** Here the intravenous infusions are used to supply normal requirements of electrolytes for the patients those who are unable to take orally. All of the maintenance solution contains 5% dextrose.

General electrolyte composition of maintenance solutions:

| | | |
|---|---|---|
| Sodium | = | 25 - 30 mEq/l |
| Potassium | = | 15 - 20 mEq/l |
| Chlorine | = | 22 mEq/l |
| Bicarbonate | = | 20- 23 mEq/l |
| Magnesium | = | 3 mEq/l |
| Phosphorous | = | 3 mEq/l |

***Electrolyte replacement therapy:*** Electrolyte replacement therapy is needed for very severe loss of electrolytes and water due to severe vomiting, high fever, wounds due to burns and diarrhea. There are two types of solutions are used for this therapy, a solution for rapid initial replacement and a solution for subsequent replacement. The concentration of electrolytes in quick initial replacement solution is more or less similar to that of extra cellular fluids. Some solutions contain large amount of potassium.

General electrolyte composition of rapid initial replacement solution is as follows

| | | |
|---|---|---|
| Sodium | = | 130 - 150 mEq/l |
| Potassium | = | 4 - 12 mEq/l |
| Chlorine | = | 98- 109 mEq/l |
| Bicarbonate | = | 28- 55 mEq/l |
| Magnesium | = | 3 mEq/l |
| Calcium | = | 3 - 5 mEq/l |

General electrolyte composition of subsequent replacement solution is shown below

| | | |
|---|---|---|
| Sodium | = | 40 - 121mEq/l |
| Potassium | = | 16 - 35 mEq/l |
| Chlorine | = | 30 - 103 mEq/l |
| Bicarbonate | = | 16 - 53 mEq/l |
| Magnesium | = | 3 - 6 mEq/l |
| Phosphorous | = | 13 mEq/l |
| Calcium | = | 5 mEq/l |

## Oral Rehydration Salts (ORS)

**(Synonym: ORS Powder)**

It contains not less than 90% and not more that 110% of dextrose and the required amount of sodium, potassium, chloride and citrate.

These are dry, homogenously powdered mixture of dextrose, sodium chloride, potassium along with either sodium citrate or sodium bicarbonate used for oral electrolyte replacement therapy after being dissolved in the required quantity of water. Sometimes it may contain some flavouring agent and sweetening agent. But it not contains artificial sweetening agents. It also contains some diluents for increase the flow property.

Saccharin/aspartame are used as a sweetening agent for pediatric ORS preparation, the concentration of saccharin for daily intake is not more than 5 mg/kg of body weight daily intake of aspartame also not more than 40 mg/kg of body weight.

**Composition of the formulation is as follows**:

| | | |
|---|---|---|
| Sodium chloride | = | 2.6 gm |
| Dextrose (anhydrous) | = | 13.5 gm |

(Or)

| | | |
|---|---|---|
| Dextrose monohydrate | = | 14.85 gm |
| Potassium chloride | = | 1.5 gm |
| Sodium citrate | = | 2.9 gm |
| Water (q.s) | = | 1000 ml |

***Physical properties:*** It is a white or creamy white, crystalline or amorphous powder. It may or may not contain odour and taste.

***Test for identification:***

1. A small amount of sample is heated, melts and charring occurs with a smell of burnt sugar.
2. To a small volume of solution add potassium cupric tartarate solution, a red precipitate is obtained.
3. A small amount of solution gives the characteristics reactions of sodium, chloride and citrates.

***Test for purity:*** It should be tested for uniformity of weight, seal test and other tests of oral powders.

**Assay**

| | | |
|---|---|---|
| For total sodium | - | It is determined by **atomic absorption spectrophotometry**. |
| For potassium | - | It is determined by **flame photometry**. |
| For total chloride | - | It is determined by **Modified Volhard's method**. |
| For citrate | - | It is determined **Non-aqueous titration method**. |
| For dextrose | - | It is determined by **ORD method**. |

***Storage:*** It should be stored in sachets made up of aluminium foil for single dose or for a day's treatment. If glucose is used, sodium bicarbonate is packed separately.

***Uses:*** It is used as an oral electrolyte replacement therapy.

### 6.4.6 Dialysis Fluids

These are electrolyte solutions of concentrations similar to those of extracellular fluids. These are not administered internally, but are made to across the semi permeable membrane. Glucose or dextrose may be added as an osmotic agent. Dialysis solution is used for the management of renal failure and poisoning. It is also used to selective removal of toxic substances, electrolytes and excessive body fluids from the blood. There are two types of dialysis fluids commonly used in the hospitals.

1. Haemodialysis fluid.
2. Peritoneal dialysis Fluid.

***Haemodialysis:*** In this, the exchange of ions takes place between the dialysis fluid and the patient's blood through a synthetic semi permeable membrane.

***Peritoneal dialysis:*** The exchange of ions takes place between membranes of peritoneal cavity.

## Haemodialysis Fluid

These fluids are needed in large quantities and are used with artificial kidney machine. A haemodialysis fluid is kept in a tank which is constantly agitated from this tank, which is made to circulate across a semi synthetic membrane inside which the patient's blood is being circulated through a bypass system.

The exchange of ions and glucose are takes place by both ways and there also reaches equilibrium. At the same time the passage of waste products like urea and other excretory chemicals also occurs, when this process is carried out for few hours, the patient's blood become free from urea. The dialysis fluid is then discarded.

In order to carryout artificial dialysis, a large amount of haemodialysis fluid is needed. This need too many containers and storage space if prepared in the concentration used for dialysis. In order to avoid this, the concentrated solutions are usually stocked which are diluted just before use with good, clean but non-sterile water. The concentrated solutions are diluted to 10-20 times. So that, the final composition of haemodialysis fluid is as follows.

| | | |
|---|---|---|
| Sodium | = | 130 - 140 mmol/l |
| Potassium | = | 0 - 3 mmol/l |
| Calcium | = | 1- 2 mmol/l |
| Magnesium | = | 0.25 - 2 mmol/l |
| Acetate (or) Lactate | = | 32 - 4 mmol/l |
| (Expressed as $HCO_3$) | | |
| Chloride | = | 95-100 mmol/l |

The exact concentration of the diluted fluid is not possible to express. The concentration has to be varied according to the patient's need. Due to this reason, the haemodialysis concentrates are not usually marketed but are prepared in hospital pharmacies.

## Peritoneal Dialysis Fluid

**(Synonym: Intra peritoneal dialysis fluid)**

These are sterile preparations for intra peritoneal use containing electrolytes with a concentration close to the electrolyte composition of plasma and without any anti oxidants.

It contains not less than 97.5% and not more than 102.5% of the stated amount of sodium, not less than 95% and not more than 105% of the stated amount of potassium, calcium, magnesium, chloride, acetate, lactate, sodium bicarbonate, bicarbonate and dextrose.

| Composition | | Concentration in mmol/l |
|---|---|---|
| Sodium | = | 125 - 150 |
| Potassium | = | 0 - 4.5 |
| Calcium | = | 0 - 2.5 |

| | | |
|---|---|---|
| Magnesium | = | 0.25 - 1.5 |
| Acetate and / or | | |
| Lactate and /or | | |
| Bicarbonate | = | 3 - 60 |
| Chloride | = | 90 - 120 |
| Dextrose | = | 25 - 250 |

The above ingredients are dissolved in appropriate solvent and filtered, autoclaved and rapidly cooled to avoid caramelization of dextrose. When bicarbonate is present, the solution of sodium bicarbonate is supplied in a separate container and is added to the electrolyte solution immediately before use.

***Physical properties:***

1. To the sample solution, add sodium hydroxide solution, 0.05 ml of potassium cupric tartarate solution, the solution becomes blue and clear. Heat to boil, a copious red precipitate is formed.
2. The sample solution gives the characteristic reactions of sodium, potassium, chloride and calcium salts.
3. The distillate obtained after treatment with hydrochloric acid, gives the characteristic reactions of acetates.
4. To the sample solution, add one drop of titan yellow solution, water and 1ml of 1M sodium hydroxide, a pink colour is produced if magnesium salts are present.

***Test for purity:*** It should be tested for color and clarity of the solution, pH, 5-hydroxy furfural and related substances, aluminium, particulate contamination, other tests, bacterial endotoxin, pyrogen and sterility test.

**Assay**

For sodium – Determined by **flame photometry**.

For potassium, calcium – Determined by **flame photometry**.

For magnesium – Determined by **complexometry**.

For dextrose – Determined by **optical rotatory dispersion**.

***Storage:*** It should be stored in rigid or semi rigid plastic containers, in flexible plastic containers fitted with a special connecting device or in glass containers and the temperature not exceeding 30 °C. Do not freeze.

## PROBABLE QUESTIONS

1. Write in detail about the major intra and extra cellular electrolytes in our body.
2. Explain about the transport mechanism of ions in our body.
3. Describe the important functions of chloride ions.

4. Define the following terms.
5. (a) Hypochloremia (b) Hyperchloremia
6. Write a brief note on phosphate ions.
7. What is mean by hyponatremia and hypernatremia.
8. Explain about the essential role of potassium in our body and explain about hypokalemia and hyperkalemia.
9. Write the role of calcium in our body.
10. Define the following terms.
    (a) Hypercalcemia (b) Hypocalcemia
    (c) Hypermagnesia (d) Hypomagnesia
11. Enumerate the sodium compounds which are used as electrolyte replenishers.
12. Write the preparation, properties, and test for purity, assay and uses of sodium chloride.
13. Write in brief about the official formulations of sodium chloride.
14. Explain about the assay of sodium compounds.
15. Write in detail about Ringer's solution.
16. Write in detail about sodium chloride irrigation solution.
17. Write a short note on ringer lactate solution.
18. How potassium chloride does assay and explain it.
19. Explain about the official preparation of potassium chloride.
20. List out the calcium compounds which are used as electrolyte replenishers.
21. Write a note on the followings.
    (a) Calcium chloride (b) Calcium gluconate and its formulations.
22. Define the following metabolic disorders and how they are corrected.
23. (a) Respiratory acidosis (b) Respiratory alkalosis
    (c) Metabolic acidosis (d) Metabolic alkalosis
24. Explain about the preparation, properties, test for identification, test for purity, assay and uses of sodium acetate or potassium acetate.
25. Write a short note on the following.
    (a) Potassium carbonate (b) Sodium citrate and its formulations
26. Explain in detail about dialysis fluids and haemodialysis fluids.
27. Describe oral rehydration salts (ORS).
28. Write a note on peritoneal dialysis fluids.

## 6.5 MEDICINAL GASES (INHALANTS)

***Introduction:*** Inhalants or medicinal gases are defined as gases which are manufactured, packaged and intended for giving to a patient for diagnosis or therapy or to produce anaesthesia. These are considered as drugs because their use without knowledge of medical practitioner is unsafe. Three types of medicinal gases are there. They are

1. Therapeutic gases
2. Laboratory gases
3. Anaesthetic gases.

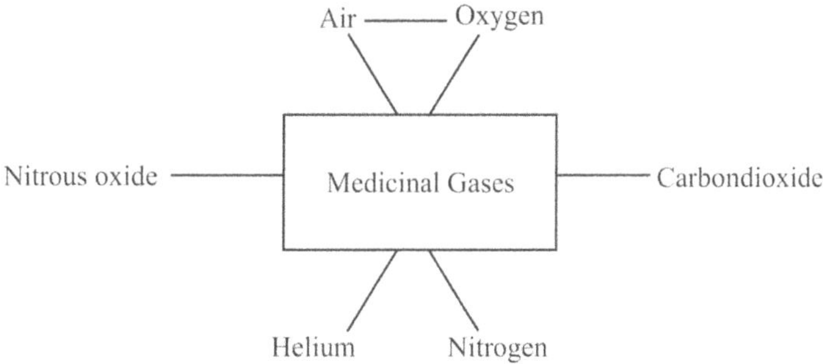


### Nitrous Oxide I.P., B.P., U.S.P.
**(Synonym: Laughing gas)**

**Mol. Formula:** $N_2O$ **Mol. Weight:** 44

It contains not less than 98.0% v/v of $N_2O$. It is otherwise called as "Laughing gas" due to its exhilarating effect when inhaled.

***Preparation:***

1. *Laboratory preparation:* It is manufactured by the thermal decomposition of ammonium nitrate. The ammonium salt decomposes at a temperature a little above its melting point and the reaction may be dangerously explosive, if the temperature is allowed to rise too high.

$$\underset{\text{ammonium nitrate}}{NH_4NO_3} \xrightarrow[170^{\circ}C]{\Delta} N_2O + 2H_2O$$

Small amount of nitrogen, higher oxides of nitrogen are obtained as a byproduct especially at the high temperature. The gas obtained is purified by washing with sodium dichromate, sodium hydroxide and water and finally filled in cylinders under pressure at 100 atm.

2. *From ammonium sulphate:* Laughing gas is also prepared by heating a mixture of sodium nitrate and ammonium sulphate.

$$2\,NaNO_3 + (NH_4)_2SO_4 \longrightarrow 2\,N_2O + Na_2SO_4 + 4H_2O$$

***Physical properties:*** It occurs as a colorless, odorless and tasteless gas, heavier than air, it support combustion. It is soluble in water (1 in 1.4 ml) at 20 °C & 760 mm. It is freely soluble in alcohol, soluble in organic solvents. It liquefies under 50 atm pressure at 15 °C.

At a higher temperature (500 °C), it gets decomposed. The liberated oxygen supports for burning.

$$N_2O \xrightarrow[500^\circ C]{\Delta} N_2 + (O)$$

***Chemical properties:***

1. Sulphur, carbon and phosphorous burns in nitrous oxide atmosphere.

$$S + 2\,N_2O \longrightarrow SO_2 + 2\,N_2$$

$$C + 2\,N_2O \longrightarrow CO_2 + 2\,N_2$$

$$P_4 + 10\,N_2O \longrightarrow P_4O_{10} + 10\,N_2$$

2. When it is passed over red hot copper, it is reduced to nitrogen.

$$Cu + N_2O \longrightarrow CuO + N_2$$

***Test for identification:***

1. A glowing splinter of wood bursts into flame on contact with the gas.
2. When shaken with pyrogallol solution, it does not absorbed by pyrogallol solution (No brown color).
3. When mixed with nitric oxide, no red color fumes are obtained.

***Test for purity:*** It should to be tested for acidity or alkalinity, carbon dioxide, carbon monoxide, arsine, phosphine, nitric oxide, nitrogen dioxide, halogens and hydrogen sulphide, oxidizing substances and water vapour.

**Assay**

Nitrous oxide is assayed by **gasometric method**. A special type of apparatus shown in Fig. 6.5 is used for this assay. The apparatus consists of a gas burette with 100 ml capacity which is connected to two capillaries such as A and B at its upper end through a two way tap.

The capillary "A" is used to pass the gas into the apparatus, the other one "B" is connected to a vertical capillary arm to form a four way junction. The right arm of the junction is attached to a mercury manometer (M). The descending arm of the four way tube is connected to a condenser with a capacity of 60 ml. Tap D is connected to the air (open one). The lower portion of the gas burette is attached to a one way tap which is connected to a mercury reservoir through a rubber tube. The upper part of the gas burette is calibrated from 0 to 5ml, and the lower part of the burette is calibrated from 99.5 to 100 ml, both in difference of 0.1ml.

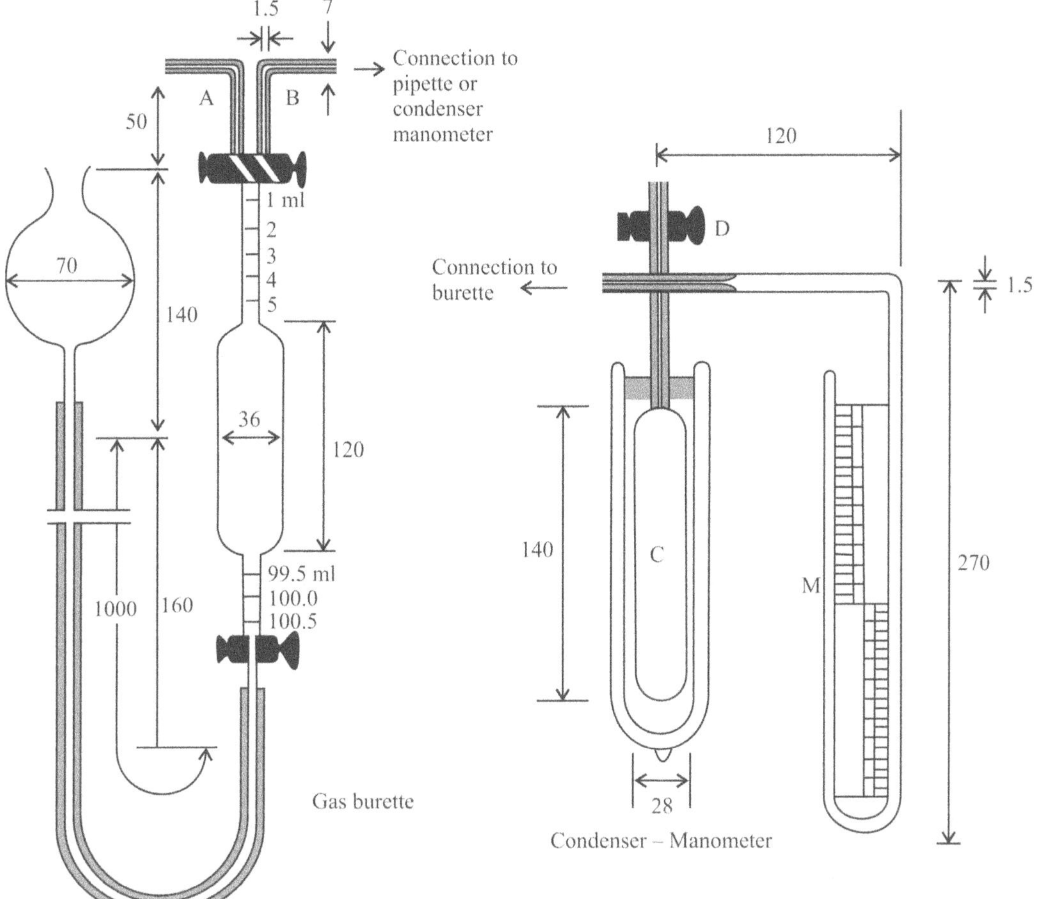


Fig. 6.5 Apparatus for assay of nitrous oxide

***Method:***

1. Tightly close the three taps immerse the condenser slightly above the upper of the condenser in liquid nitrogen.
2. Create a partial vacuum in the apparatus by adjusting the two way tap and the mobile reservoir (arbitrary pressure is 6.7 to 8 $KP_a^2$). Maintain this pressure up to 10 minutes to make the apparatus is gas tight.
3. Open the two way tube A, completely fill the burette and the tube A with mercury. Close the two way tube.
4. Then connect a rubber tube trough a pressure relieving device to the exit valve of the gas to be analyzed and pass the gas through the rubber tube for 1 minute, connect the rubber tube to the end of "A" tube, immediately open the two way tap to "A".
5. By lowering the mercury reservoir to allow the specified volume of gas to enter the burette.

6. Disconnect the rubber tube and allow removing the gas from the burette by slowly raising the mercury reservoir, above the capillary tube.
7. Pass the required volume of gas to be analyzed to enter the burette by lowering the mercury reservoir until the pressure of gas is equal to atmospheric pressure, then close the two way tube.
8. Then lower the liquid nitrogen to the middle of the condenser by raising the mercury reservoir slightly above tube A.
9. Slowly open the burette tap to connect the condenser and allow the mercury to rise in the burette until it reaches the tap.
10. Close the tap, increase the level of the liquid nitrogen so as to immerse the condenser. Note the pressure and remains constant for 2 minutes.
11. Move the mercury reservoir to down position, open the burette tap to connect with the condenser. Adjust the mercury reservoir until the manometer reading is similar to that of the initial pressure is $P_o$ close the burette tap and maintain that pressure is equal to atmospheric pressure. The volume of gas in ml indicates the volume of gas used.
12. Similarly take 10 determinations, remove the liquid nitrogen, and dry the condenser.

***Uses:***

1. It is mainly used as a general anesthetic for producing analgesia and anaesthesia.
2. A mixture of 1:1 ratio with oxygen is used for the relief of pain in child birth and myocardial infarction.
3. It is used in calming the excited mental patients and it is also used to induce anaesthesia, this is maintained by using other gaseous anaesthetics.
4. It is non toxic in nature, so frequently used in dental and obstetric practice.
5. It is very quickly absorbed by inhalation & it acts as a better analgesic and weak anaesthetic.
6. Nitrous oxide would produce deep anaesthesia in about 1minute but the symptoms of hypoxia.

***Dose:*** By inhalation 60 to 80 % is mixed with 20-40% of oxygen, as required.

***Storage:*** It should be stored and supplied in metal cylinders with the appropriate safety regulation and the temperature not exceeding to 37 °C.

***Labelling:*** The cylinder is painted with blue color with the name "Nitrous Oxide" and the symbol $N_2O$ or the name should be stenciled in paint on the shoulder of the cylinder.

## Oxygen I. P.

**Mol. Formula:** $O_2$ **Mol. Weight:** 32

It is important for all living cells oxygen in necessary for normal oxidative metabolism for the production of useful energy. Mitochondria of each cell containing tightly integrated enzymes that receives electrons from reduced nicotinamide adenine dinucleotide (NADH) and flavin adenine dinucleotide ($FADH_2$) and transport them in to chains of oxidation - reduction reactions leads to the reduction of atomic oxygen and formation of oxide anion which quickly combines with protons to gives water which in turn reacts with carbondioxide gives energy by combustion. This energy is used by the cell to synthesize ATP. When ATP gets hydrolysed, energy is released to drive. This process of release of energy from the electron transport system is called as oxidative phosphorylation. The transport of oxygen and other gases ($CO_2$) is takes place by haemoglobin in RBC. Oxygen is combined with haemoglobin and converted into oxy haemoglobin. This reaction is reversible one.

$$\underset{\text{Haemoglobin}}{Hb + O_2} \rightleftharpoons \underset{\text{Oxy haemoglobin}}{HbO_2}$$

This oxy haemoglobin easily dissociates and releases oxygen to the cell. This reaction depends upon various factors such as effect of carbon dioxide, carbon monoxide and pH of blood. Each gram of haemoglobin binds with 1.34 ml of oxygen.

Requirements of oxygen in body are classified in to four types.

1. Anoxic
2. Anaemic
3. Stagnant
4. Histotic

1. ***Anoxic:*** Inadequate supply of oxygen to the tissues. In these cases oxygen is administered by mask, nasal tubes or in tents.
2. ***Anaemic:*** Inadequate amount of haemoglobin to supply the oxygen to the tissues. This is due to hemorrhage, carbon monoxide poisoning etc. Carbon monoxide has more affinity to bind with haemoglobin than oxygen leads to the formation of carboxyhaemoglobin. Only oxygen administration is not effective for this condition a carbon dioxide oxygen mixture (Hyperbaric oxygen) is used for conditions. The hyperbaric oxygen dissociates carboxyhaemoglobin complex liberates carbon monoxide and increases the amount of oxygen dissolved in the plasma.
3. ***Stagnant:*** It occurs due to the inadequate general circulation or retardation of local circulation. Oxygen supply is not used in these cases whereas cardiotonic drugs are used to speed up the circulation.
4. ***Histotic:*** It occurs due to interferences of tissue cell oxidation or uncoupling of oxidative phosphorylation or cyanide poisoning.

Oxygen is the most abundant element on the earth and present 20.95% by volume of dry air and 46.6% of earth's crust. In combined state it is present in water (89% w/v) and plants and in animal tissues (50-70%).

Oxygen contains not less than 99% v/v of oxygen. The residue contain either of argon with trace amount of nitrogen and hydrogen. It is available and supplied in compressed form in metallic cylinders.

***Preparations:*** It is mostly manufactured by two methods.

1. Fractionation of liquid air.
2. Electrolysis of water.

1. *By fractionation of liquid air:* By this method oxygen is prepared by fractional distillation of liquid air.

   First of all, the air is purified by removing moisture, carbon dioxide, dust etc., and then it is compressed into a liquid air. Then the liquid air is fractioned by distillation, to get oxygen which is then filled under pressure in metallic cylinders. Nitrogen is more volatile and evaporates first, leaving behind oxygen. Argon present in the air is difficult to separate because its boiling point is only 3 °C higher than that of oxygen.

2. *By electrolysis of water:* In this method, a direct current is passed through the 1-20% of potassium or sodium hydroxide solution, which contains the iron or steel electrodes. Due to the electrolysis of the alkali solution, oxygen gets liberated at the anode and hydrogen at the cathode. The liberated oxygen is then filled under pressure in metallic cylinders.

   Oxygen is also prepared by heating some oxygen containing salts and metallic oxides. It is also prepared by the action of concentrated sulphuric acid with manganese dioxide, potassium permanganate or potassium dichromate.

$$2KClO_3 \xrightarrow{\Delta} 2KCl + 3O_2$$

$$2MnO_2 + 2H_2SO_4 \longrightarrow 2MnSO_4 + 2H_2O + O_2$$

***Physical properties:*** Oxygen occurs as a colorless, odorless, tasteless gas with the density of 1.105. One volume of oxygen is soluble in 32 ml of water, soluble in alcohol (1 in 3.6) at 1 atm pressure at 20 °C.

***Chemical properties:*** It combines with large number of element and this process is called as oxidation. For example:

$$S + O_2 \longrightarrow SO_2$$

$$P_4 + 5O_2 \longrightarrow P_4O_{10}$$

$$4Fe + 3O_2 \longrightarrow 2Fe_2O_3$$

$$4NH_3 + 5O_2 \longrightarrow 4NO + 6H_2O$$

***Test for identification:***

1. A glowing splinter of wood bursts into flame on contact with the gas.
2. The sample is shaken with pyrogallol solution; a dark color solution is obtained due to absorption of gas.

***Test for purity:*** It has to be tested for carbon dioxide, carbon monoxide and water vapour.

***Test for carbon dioxide:*** It is determined by using carbon dioxide detector tube (should not contain more than 300 ppm v/v).

***Test for carbon monoxide:*** It is determined by using carbon monoxide detector tube (should not contain more than 5 ppm v/v)

***Test for water vapour:*** It is determined by water vapour detector tube (should not contain more than 67 ppm v/v)

**Assay**

The apparatus used in this assay (Fig. 6.6) is similar to that of the assay of nitrous oxide, but here tube B is connected to a gas pipette containing two bulbs of suitable size. The absorbing gas used here is ammonium chloride and ammonium hydroxide and follow the all procedures similar to that of nitrous oxide. Measure the residual gas volume which is present in the burette. It should not be more than 1% v/v.

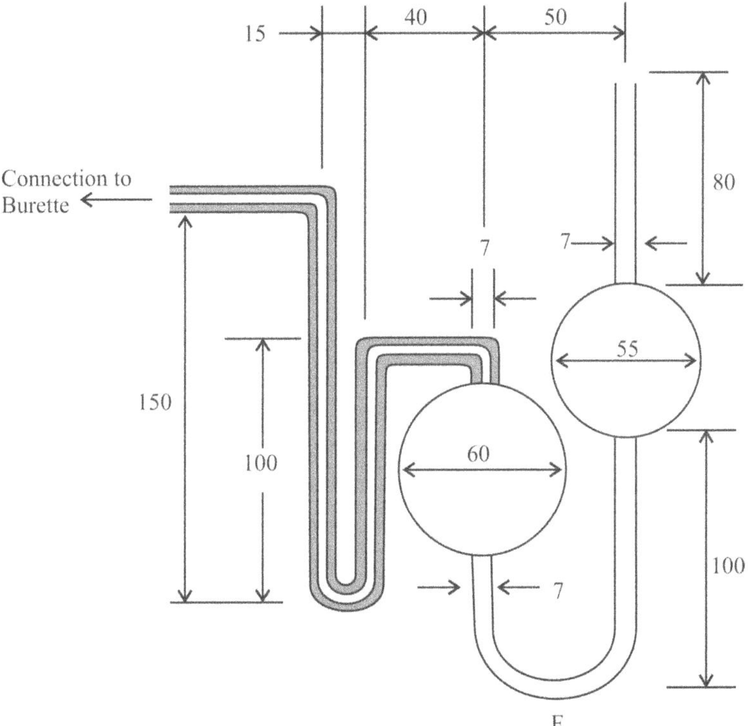


Fig. 6.6 Aparatus used for oxygen assay

*Uses:*

1. Oxygen is used as an inhalant (support respiration) in anesthesia, post operative condition, burns and wounds, asphyxia, asthmatic conditions, gaseous poisoning, shock, malignant type wounds and for artificial respiration for various hypoxia conditions.
2. It is mixed with 5-7% of carbondioxide which is used for stimulating respiratory centre.
3. The mixture of oxygen and helium (21:79) is used for patients with severe lung damage.

***Storage:*** It should be stored in the metal cylinders, with appropriate safety regulations. Valves and taps should not be lubricated with any oils or grease.

***Labelling:*** The shoulder of cylinder should be painted white and the remainder should be painted black. The cylinder should carry a label stating "Oxygen". Along with this, oxygen or the symbol $O_2$ should be stenciled in paint on the shoulder of the cylinder.

## Carbondioxide I.P.

**Mol. Formula:** $CO_2$ **Mol. Weight:** 44.01

It contains not less than 99.5% w/w of carbon dioxide.

Air contains 0.03% v/v of carbon dioxide. It is evolved from the following processes.

1. Volcanoes.
2. Dead bodies decay.
3. Respiration, combustion and fermentation process.

***Preparation:***

1. *By fermentation process:* On large scale process, it is prepared as a byproduct from fermentation industries (Fermentation of sugar molasses). Fermentation of sugar produces alcohol and carbon dioxide as bye products.

$$C_6H_{12}O_6 \longrightarrow 2C_2H_5OH + 2CO_2\uparrow$$

2. *Commercial scale preparation:* On commercial scale preparation carbon dioxide is obtained from fuel gases which are passed under pressure over potassium carbonate, which yields potassium bicarbonate and the carbon dioxide is liberated by releasing the pressure and compressed into metal cylinders or the potassium bicarbonate obtained is boiled at 100 °C to liberate pure carbon dioxide.

$$K_2CO_3 + CO_2 + H_2O \longrightarrow 2KHCO_3$$

$$2KHCO_3 \xrightarrow[\Delta]{100^\circ C} K_2CO_3 + CO_2 + H_2O$$

3. *From carbonates of heavy metals or bicarbonates of alkali metals:*

When calcium carbonate or sodium bicarbonate/carbonate are heated or treated with acids, gives carbon dioxide.

$$CaCO_3 \xrightarrow{\Delta} CaO + CO_2$$

$$2NaHCO_3 \xrightarrow{\Delta} Na_2CO_3 + CO_2 + H_2O$$

$$Na_2CO_3 + H_2SO_4 \longrightarrow Na_2SO_4 + CO_2 + H_2O$$

$$CaCO_3 + 2HCl \longrightarrow CaCl_2 + CO_2 + H_2O$$

Carbon dioxide under pressure may be dissolved in cold water, leads to the formation of carbonic acid ($H_2CO_3$) from which carbon dioxide is liberated when pressure gets released.

4. *From carbonaceous substances or carbon containing substances:*

Compounds having carbon like coal, coke etc. is burned with excess of oxygen to give carbon dioxide.

$$C + O_2 \xrightarrow{\text{Burning}} CO_2$$

***Physical properties:*** It is a heavy, colorless, odorless gas with faintly acidic taste. It can be liquefied under water and soluble in water at normal temperature and pressure. One liter of carbon dioxide at 0 °C temperature and at one atmospheric pressure weighs 1.977 gm.

***Chemical properties:***

1. *Reaction with metals:* Carbon dioxide is neither combustible nor a supporter of combustion. It reacts with active metals burn in the carbon dioxide atmosphere.

$$2Mg + CO_2 \longrightarrow 2MgO + C$$

$$4Na + CO_2 \longrightarrow 2Na_2O + C$$

2. *Reaction with water:* Carbon dioxide dissolves in water to form carbonic acid, which is unstable, turns blue litmus to red and neutralizes alkalis.

$$CO_2 + H_2O \longrightarrow H_2CO_3$$

$$2NaOH + CO_2 \longrightarrow Na_2CO_3 + H_2O$$

$$Na_2CO_3 + CO_2 + H_2O \longrightarrow 2NaHCO_3$$

The ratio of carbonic acid/bicarbonate determines the body fluid pH. A decrease level of carbon dioxide causes respiratory acidosis. An increased level of carbon dioxide causes respiratory alkalosis.

3. *Reaction with lime water ($Ca(OH)_2$):* When passed through lime water, it first turns milky and is again clear. On boiling the clear solution, milkiness reappears.

$$\underset{\text{Lime water}}{Ca(OH)_2} \xrightarrow[-H_2O]{CO_2} \underset{\text{(Insoluble milky)}}{CaCO_3} \xrightarrow[+H_2O]{CO_2} \underset{\text{Soluble}}{Ca(HCO_3)_2} \xrightarrow[-CO_2,\ -H_2O]{\Delta} \underset{\text{calcium carbonate}}{CaCO_3}$$

4. When passed through red-hot coke, it is reduced to carbon monoxide.

$$CO_2 + C \longrightarrow 2\,CO$$

***Test for identification:***

1. It extinguishes a flame.
2. When the gas is passes through barium hydroxide solution, a white precipitate of barium carbonate is formed which is dissolved in 2M acetic acid, with effervescence.

$$Ba(OH)_2 + CO_2 \longrightarrow BaCO_3 + H_2O$$

***Test for purity:*** Tests for acidity, sulphur dioxide, phosphine, hydrogen sulphide, organic reducing substances, carbon monoxide, ammonia, nitric oxide, nitrogen dioxide and sulphur dioxide.

***Test for acid and sulphur dioxide:*** It may be tested by comparing the color of a carbon dioxide free water having methyl orange through which a measured volume of carbon dioxide is passed, with that of a sample of carbon dioxide free water having 1ml of 0.01N hydrochloric acid and same amount of methyl orange. The color produced in the sample should not show deeper shade of red color than that of blank.

***Test for phosphine, hydrogen sulphide and organic reducing substance:*** The sample is allowed to pass through an ammonical silver nitrate solution. No turbidity is formed (due to the formation of silver phosphide or silver sulphide).

***Test for carbon monoxide:*** It is tested by treating a sample of dilute oxalated blood with pyrogallol and tannic acid and shaking the content and keeping the mixture undisturbed for 40 minutes. The greyish brown color precipitate is produced and no red color is produced (If carbon monoxide is present the content will get red color).

**Assay**

It is assayed by gasometry. The absorbing gas used is potassium hydroxide solution (50%). The decreased gas volume is measured at standard temperature and pressure. Not more than 1 ml of the gas is remaining in the tube if 100 ml of sample is used. Remaining all is similar to oxygen.

***Uses:***

1. It is mainly used as a respiratory stimulant.
2. It is added to the oxygen in certain types of pump oxygenators to maintain the carbon dioxide content of the flask.
3. The mixture of 95:5 ratios of carbon dioxide and oxygen is used in the treatment of carbon monoxide poisoning for increasing the ventilator exchange rate and dissociation rate of carbon monoxide from carboxy haemoglobin.
4. Carbonated vehicles are useful for masking the unpleasant taste of saline aperients.
5. Inhalation of carbon dioxide has been used for the relief of intractable hiccups.
6. It is also used for the detoxification of heroin addicts without the painful withdrawal syndrome.
7. Solid state of carbon dioxide or dry ice, has a temperature of 80 °C used to treat warts and naevi by cryotherapy, skin diseases like acne, angiomas, moles, psoriasis etc.

***Side effects:*** Above a concentration of 6% carbon dioxide leads to headache, mental confusion, palpitations, increase the depth and rate of respiration and depression of CNS.

***Storage:*** Carbon dioxide should be stored in metal cylinders under compression.

***Labelling:*** The shoulder of the cylinder should be painted grey and having the name and symbol of "$CO_2$" stenciled with paint on it.

## Helium B.P., U.S.P.

**Symbol:** He **Atomic weight:** 4

It contains not less than 99% by volume of He.

It is the second highest element in the periodic table. It is used as a diluent in oxygen administered during mucosal plug obstructions, laryngeal edema etc., which produces turbulent air flow. The density of this mixture is one third of the density of air since the diffusion of gas through the small orifice, by this way it penetrates the restricted respiratory passages with greater facility than air.

Due to less density than air, it changes or pitches or sounds uttered by the vocal cords to be increased leads to unintelligible speech like "Donald duck" sound.

***Preparation:*** Helium is obtained from either natural gas or fractional distillation of liquid air which is intended for medicinal gas.

***Physical properties:*** It occurs as a colorless, inert gas. It is the second lightest element in nature with the relative density of 7.16. It does not support combustion.

***Test for identification:*** It is identified by chromatography.

***Test for purity:*** It should be tested for methane, oxygen and water.

***Uses:***

1. Helium - oxygen mixtures are easier to breathe by patients with severe lung damage or with obstructions in upper respiratory tract.
2. Helium breathing may also influence vocal pattern and vocal pitch.

***Storage:*** It should be stored and supplied in brown colored metal cylinder under compression in 98% v/v purity. Mixtures of oxygen and helium in the ratio of 20-21% and 79-80% v/v are also supplied in cylinders which are painted black on the body and white and brown batches on the shoulders and neck.

---

## Nitrogen U.S.P.

**Mol. Formula:** $N_2$ **Mol. Weight:** 28.01

It is the important constituent of animal and plant tissues; largely present as amino acid as proteins. Animals and higher plants cannot able to fix the atmospheric nitrogen. It has a little therapeutic use. It is used as diluents for pure oxygen and also used as a pharmaceutical aid to remove air, by this way it is used as an antioxidant. The increased concentration of nitrogen in blood leads to narcosis.

It contains not less than 99.5% by volume of $N_2$.

***Preparation:*** It is mainly obtained by the fractional distillation of liquid air.

***Physical properties:*** It is a colorless, odorless and tasteless gas.

***Test for identification:***

1. Nitrogen gas extinguishes a burning wood splint.
2. It will not turn lime water milky.

***Test for purity:*** It should be tested for carbon dioxide.

***Assay:*** It is assayed by Gasometry.

***Uses:***

1. It is used as diluent for oxygen before administration.
2. It is also used to remove tumors (Cryoscopic surgery).

***Storage:*** It should be stored and supplied in metal cylinders painted grey with black on the neck and shoulders and the name or the symbol is stenciled on the body of the cylinder.

---

## Dilute Ammonia Solution I.P., B.P.

This compound is discussed under the topic **acidifiers and alkalinising agents**.

---

## Ammonium Carbonate B.P., U.S.P.

**(Synonym: Sal volatile, Preston's salt, Baker's ammonia, Ammonium sesqui carbonate)**

**Mol. Formula:** $(NH_4)_2CO_3$ **Mol. Weight:** 96.09

The official ammonium carbonate is a mixture of varying amounts of ammonium bicarbonate and anhydride of ammonium carbonate (ammonium carbamate).

It contains the equivalent of not less than 3% of $NH_3$.

***Preparation:*** It is prepared by sublimation of ammonium chloride or sulphate with calcium carbonate.

$$(NH_4)_2SO_4 + CaCO_3 \longrightarrow (NH_4)_2CO_3 + CaSO_4$$

$$2NH_4Cl + CaCO_3 \longrightarrow (NH_4)_2CO_3 + CaCl_2$$

The product obtained is resublimed with small quantity of water, to obtain a white semitransparent ammonium carbonate mass with an outer layer of white opaque powder of ammonium bicarbonate.

***Physical properties:*** It is a white powder or almost white translucent, hard, crystalline masses with strong ammoniacal odour and pungent taste.

***Chemical properties:***

1. When exposed to air, it dissociates partially, and loses ammonia and carbon dioxide leads to the formation of opaque substance and finally gives the porous lumps or a white powder of ammonium bicarbonate.

$$(NH_4)_2CO_3 \longrightarrow 2\,NH_3 + CO_2\uparrow + H_2O \longrightarrow NH_4HCO_3 + NH_3$$

2. *Solubility:* It is freely soluble in water, partly soluble in alcohol. It is easily decomposed by hot water. It volatilizes at 60 °C.

$$(NH_4)_2CO_3 \xrightarrow[\Delta]{60^\circ C} 2\,NH_3\uparrow + CO_2\uparrow + H_2O$$

The solution obtained is sharply alkaline to litmus and alkaline taste.

***Uses:***

1. Ammonium carbonate is mainly used as a respiratory stimulant, pharmaceutical aid and expectorant.
2. It is a source of both ammonia and carbon dioxide both are acts as a respiratory stimulant.
3. The evolution of the above gases are slow at ordinary temperatures, particularly in the presence of moisture, they are better suited as smelling salts than solutions of ammonia.
4. Ammonium carbonate is prescribed as reflux stimulant (smelling purpose) ammonium bicarbonate could be substituted.

***Storage:*** It should be stored in well closed containers at a temperature not exceed 30 °C and protected from light.

## PROBABLE QUESTIONS

1. Define inhalants? Enumerate the official inhalants.
2. Write any two large scale method of preparation for oxygen. Write its test for purity.
3. Write the preparation supply and storage conditions of nitrogen. What are its various uses?
4. Write in detail about preparation, properties and applications of ammonium carbonate in medicine. Highlight its advantage over dilute ammonia solution?
5. Write the methods of preparations, properties, uses and assay of following compounds.
   (a) Nitrous oxide (b) Oxygen
6. Write a note on helium gas and its importance.
7. Explain in detail about nitrous oxide. How does it assayed and mention the storage and supplied condition.
8. Write the method of preparation, properties, and test for purity, assay and uses of carbon dioxide.
9. What are the types of impurities should be included in nitrous oxide.

## 6.6 ESSENTIAL TRACE ELEMENTS

### 6.6.1 Haematinics

***Introduction:*** These are the compounds required in the formation of blood and are employed in the treatment of anemia. Haematinics include Iron, vitamin $B_{12}$ and folic acid.

#### Iron

Iron is an essential dietary mineral plays an important component of haemoglobin, myoglobin and a number of enzymes. About 60 to 70% of the total iron is present in haemoglobin. About 57% is stored as ferritin 3% as myoglobin and only about 0.1% is present in plasma as transferrin. The average dietary intake of iron is 18 to 20 mg/day. The absorption of iron is regulated by the amount of iron that is stored in the intestinal mucosa. Iron is highly absorbed or conserved by the body and only small amount of it is excreted through the intestinal tract.

The dietary requirement of iron per kilogram of body weight is highest in infants and pregnant women but somewhat lower in children and non pregnant women. If dietary intake is inadequate to support erythropoiesis, the body will utilize the stored iron to maintain erythropoiesis.

Most of the iron in food occurs in ferric ($Fe^{3+}$) state such as $Fe(OH)_3$ or as ferric organic compounds. The iron absorption is increased by low molecular weight proteins.

***Physiological importance of iron:*** Iron is an important mineral for the body being required for tissue respiration erythropoiesis and a number of enzyme reactions. Many of the iron compounds in the body are (i) haemoproteins (ii) iron transport and/or transport proteins.

***Haemoproteins:*** It includes haemoglobin, myoglobin and cytochromes.

***Haemoglobin:*** It contains four heme groups; each one is linked to a specific globin chain and ability of binding with four molecules of oxygen. The heme moiety is a complex of porphyrin and one atom of ferrous iron and molecule reversibly in ferrous state or oxygenated state.

***Myoglobin:*** A muscle haemoprotein consists of a single polypeptide chain attached to a heme molecule with higher affinity to oxygen than haemoglobin. It has the ability to accept oxygen from haemoglobin and acts as an oxygen store in muscle. Myoglobin releases oxygen by cytochrome oxidase when oxygen supply in limited.

***Transport proteins***

*Transferrin:* It is a specific iron binding protein in the blood. It is synthesized in the liver and transports iron through the plasma and extra vascular spaces. It increases during iron deficiency. Each transferrin molecule binds with two ferric ions. The ability of transferrin to binds with iron is called as iron binding capacity.

*Iron storage proteins:* The storage forms of iron in humans are ferritin and hemosiderin which are present in liver, spleen and bone marrow. If the level of stored iron or storage levels decreases, the serum level of iron also decreases, leads to anaemia.

***Anemia:*** Anemia is the reduction of the erythrocyte mass in the blood. In anemia the number of erythrocytes is reduced or erythrocytes are deficient in haemoglobin leads to the overall reduction in circulating haemoglobin. There are different types of anemias, due to chronic or acute blood loss, reduced erythrocyte production, increased erythrocyte destruction or combination of these.

***Iron deficiency:*** The main reason for iron deficiency is reduced absorption (presence of internal parasite, chronic diarrhea, acute or chronic inflammation) or increased absorption in certain conditions (Anoxia, pyridoxine deficiency, pregnancy). Other causes of iron deficiency includes pernicious anaemia, pica syndrome and atrophic gastritis).

Iron deficiency anaemia is produced by the decreased production of erythrocytes by the bone marrow due to the lack of available iron for haemoglobin synthesis.

***Treatment of iron deficiency:*** Iron deficiency can be treated by the administration of either oral or parenteral iron. Most of the iron therapy is given by oral route and very few situations only parenteral iron is selected.

The drugs which are used to treat anemia are called as haematinics.

The iron containing preparations are available as liquid oral forms or solid dosage forms (tablets and capsules) and parenteral preparations. Oral iron preparations are less readily available from sustained release preparations, due to high dosage care must be taken to calculate the doses, because each salt containing different amounts of elemental iron. Maximum absorption occurs when the drugs are taken before food. Large doses of haematinic leads to GIT irritation and diarrhea, continued administration sometimes leads to constipation.

***Drug interactions with oral iron:***

1. Concurrent use of penicillamine and tetracyclines reduces the absorption of iron.
2. Antacids containing carbonates and magnesium trisilicates decreases the bioavailability of iron.
3. A number of food stuffs can interact with iron.

*For example:* Foods like milk and milk products, tea, coffee, eggs, whole grain breads and foods contains oxalates, carbonates or phosphates reduces the oral absorption of iron. This is reduced by giving the iron supplements within one hour before or 2 hr after ingestion of above foods.

***Parenteral iron therapy:*** This is recommended for the following conditions like severe malabsorption, mentally defective patients and persons in poor society's. Parenteral iron preparations are available in a colloidal (non-ionic) form complexed with carbohydrate compounds. Example: Iron-dextran and Iron – sorbitol injections.

Iron therapy should not be used in hemochromatosis and hemosiderosis (iron overload). Iron is also used cautiously in alcoholism, peptic ulcer and inflammatory conditions of GIT.

***Iron-toxicity:*** It may be acute or chronic due to accidental poisoning or over dosage or thalassemia. Iron toxicity due to overload occurs by the excessive absorption of iron in the body than is excreted.

1. *Hemochromatosis:* It is a syndrome associated with increased amount of total iron. The symptoms are increased pigmentation, liver damage, hepatic cancer and cardiac damage etc.
2. Megaloplastic anaemia
3. Pernicious anaemia

Common Iron preparations

| Proprietary Name | Active ingredient | Elemental iron | (Iron %) |
|---|---|---|---|
| Ferrous sulphate tablet | Ferrous sulphate hepta hydrate | 60 mg/300 mg | 20 |
| Fergon | Ferrous gluconate | 39 mg/325 mg | 8.5 |
| Chel-Iron | Ferro cholinate | 39 mg/333 mg | 8.5 |
| Ferro drops | Ferrous lactate | 25 mg/ml | 25 |
| Mol-Iron liquid | Ferrous sulphate | 10 mg/ml | 10 |

## Vitamin $B_{12}$

It occurs in cyanocobalamin and hydroxycobalamin. Vitamin $B_{12}$ is a water soluble, thermostable red crystal. It is synthesized in nature only by micro-organism (*Streptomyces griseus*). The plants and animals acquire it from them. The daily requirement is 1-3 mg and 3-5 mg (during pregnancy and lactation). The dietary sources are kidney, liver, egg yolk, sea fish, meat, cheese etc.

***Functions of vitamin $B_{12}$:*** It is linked with folate metabolism by generating deoxy adenosyl-cobalamin ($DAB_{12}$) and melthyl - cobalamin (methyl $B_{12}$) coenzymes in the body.

Vitamin $B_{12}$ is present in food as protein conjugates and is released by cooking or by proteolysis in stomach facilitated by gastric acid. Intrinsic factor secreted by stomach forms a complex with $B_{12}$ gets attached to specific receptors present on the intestinal mucosal cells and is absorbed by an active carrier mediated transport. This mechanism is essential for absorption of vitamin $B_{12}$ ingested in physiological amounts.

Vitamin $B_{12}$ is transported in blood in combination with specific β–globin "Transcobalamin II" (TC II). Vitamin $B_{12}$ is taken up by liver cells and stored. It is degraded in the body; excreted mainly in bile (3 - 7 mg/day); but 0.5 mg/day is reabsorbed through enterohepatic circulation. So, in the absence of intrinsic factor, deficiency of $B_{12}$ develops and leads to pernicious anaemia.

***Deficiencies of vitamin $B_{12}$:***

1. Pernicious anaemia.
2. Mucosal damage due to gastrectomy, chronic gastritis.
3. Malabsorption.
4. Nutritional deficiency.
5. Increased demand (Pregnancy, lactation).

*Uses:*

1. It is used in the treatment of vitamin $B_{12}$ deficiencies.
2. High doses are used in psychiatric disorders, neuropathies.
3. It is used in the treatment of prophylaxis.

**Folic acid**

It exists as yellow crystals which are insoluble in water; but its sodium salt is freely water soluble. It is chemically "Pteroyl glutamic acid". The dietary sources include liver, spinach, egg, meat and milk. It is synthesized by gut flora. The daily requirement is 0.2 mg/day; during lactation and pregnancy - 0.8 mg/day. Folic acid is rapidly extracted by tissues and stored in cells as polyglutamates. Liver takes up a large part and secretes methyl tetrahydro folic acid (methyl-THFA), which undergoes enterohepatic circulation.

Folic acid is inactive as such and is reduced to the coenzyme form in 2 steps: By folate reductases and dihydro folate reductase into dihydro folate and tetrahydro folate.

***Deficiency:*** It occurs due to -

1. Inadequate dietary intake.
2. Increase demand during pregnancy, lactation.
3. Chronic alcoholism.
4. Malabsorption.

*Uses:*

1. Megaloblastic anemia
2. Prophylaxis
3. Methotrexate toxicity

## Ferrous Sulphate I.P.

**Mol. Formula:** $FeSO_4.7H_2O$ **Mol. Weight:** 278

It contains not less than 98% and not more than 105% of $FeSO_4.7H_2O$

***Preparation:*** Ferrous sulphate is prepared by adding slight excess amount of iron to dilute sulphuric acid.

$$Fe + H_2SO_4 \longrightarrow FeSO_4 + H_2\uparrow$$

After the effervescence ceases, concentrate the liquid by boiling. Then filter, allowed to cool and the crystals are separated and dried at room temperature. In all the above process, exposure of air is prevented since ferrous sulphate easily oxidized in air and converted into brownish yellow ferric oxide.

***Physical properties:*** It is a bluish green crystals or light green crystalline powder. It is in monoclinic crystals or rhombic, odorless. It effloresces in dry air. On exposure to moist air it gets oxidized, converted into brown color ferric sulphate. It is soluble in water but insoluble in alcohol.

***Chemical properties:***

1. *Decomposition reaction:* When heated, ferrous sulphate decomposes it gives ferric oxide, sulphur dioxide and sulphuric acid.

$$2(FeSO_4.7H_2O) \xrightarrow{\Delta} Fe_2O_3 + SO_2 + H_2SO_4 + 13H_2O$$

2. *Reducing property:* Ferrous sulphate is a reducing agent. It reduces silver salts and gold to their corresponding metals.

$$Ag^+ + Fe^{2+} \longrightarrow Ag + Fe^{3+}$$

$$Au^{3+} + 3Fe^{2+} \longrightarrow Au + 3Fe^{3+}$$

   It decolorizes acidified potassium permanganate and turns the acidified potassium dichromate into green.

   It reduces nitrous oxide to nitric oxide.

$$2FeSO_4 + H_2SO_4 + NO_2 \longrightarrow Fe_2(SO_4)_3 + H_2O + NO$$

   In presence of light, ferrous sulphate reduces mercuric chloride to mercurous chloride.

$$2HgCl_2 + 2Fe^+ \longrightarrow Hg_2Cl_2 + 2Fe^{3+} + 2Cl^-$$

3. *Reaction with sodium carbonate:* It reacts with sodium carbonate to yield $FeCO_3$ and $CO_2$ gas

$$FeSO_4 + Na_2CO_3 \longrightarrow FeCO_3 + Na_2SO_4$$

$$H_2O + FeCO_3 \longrightarrow Fe(OH)_2 + CO_2$$

4. *Oxidation:* Ferrous sulphate oxidized easily in moist air and converted into brown ferric sulphate.

$$4FeSO_4 + 2H_2O + O_2 \longrightarrow 4Fe(OH)SO_4$$

5. *Reaction with alkaline metal sulphate:* Ferrous sulphate reacts with sulphates of alkali metals, it forms double salts.

   *For Example:* It reacts with ammonium sulphate and yields ferrous ammonium sulphate (Mohr's salt).

$$FeSO_4.7H_2O + (NH_4)_2SO_4 \longrightarrow FeSO_4.(NH_4)_2SO_4.7H_2O$$

***Test for identification:*** It gives the characteristic reactions of ferrous salts and sulphate ions.

***Test for purity:*** It should be tested for color and clarity of the solution, pH, arsenic, copper, lead, zinc, manganese, ferric ions and chlorides.

**Assay**

***Principle:***

*1st method:* It is assayed by **permanganometry method of titration** (also called **redox titration**).

In this assay the substance is dissolved in dilute sulphuric acid and the solution is titrated against 0.1N potassium permanganate. Potassium permanganate is acting as a self indicator. End point is the appearance of permanent pale pink colour.

During this assay, sulphuric acid first reacts with potassium permanganate and liberate nascent oxygen. Thus the liberated nascent oxygen oxidizes the ferrous sulphate to ferric sulphate and the nascent oxygen is reduced to water. After the completion of this reaction, addition of potassium permanganate remains in the flask and its colour is retained i.e., permanent pale pink colour. As the oxidation and reduction takes place simultaneously this is called redox titration. The chemical reactions of this assay are shown below.

$$2\,KMnO_4 + 3\,H_2SO_4 \longrightarrow K_2SO_4 + 2\,MnSO_4 + 3\,H_2O + 5(O)$$

$$2\,FeSO_4 + (O) + H_2SO_4 \longrightarrow Fe_2(SO_4)_3 + H_2O$$

*These reactions can also be written as*

$$2\,KMnO_4 + 8\,H_2SO_4 + 10\,FeSO_4 \longrightarrow K_2SO_4 + 2\,MnSO_4 + 5\,Fe_2(SO_4)_3 + 8\,H_2O$$

*2nd Method:* It is assayed by **ceriometry method of titration** (also called **redox titration**).

In this assay sample is dissolved in water and 1M sulphuric acid and titrated a with 0.1M ceric ammonium nitrate using ferroin sulphate as indicator. End point is the disappearance of red colour.

***Procedure:*** Dissolve 2.5 gm of sodium bicarbonate in a mixture of 150 ml of water and 10 ml of sulphuric acid. When effervescence ceases, add about 0.5 gm of the substance under examination, accurately weighed, shake gently to dissolve and titrate with 0.1M ceric ammonium nitrate, using 0.1 ml of ferroin solution as indicator, until the red colour disappears.

***Uses:*** Ferrous sulphate is used as a haematinic (increases the haemoglobin content in iron deficiency anaemia).

***Dose:*** For prophylactic use 300 mg daily in divided doses.

For therapeutic use 600 to 900 mg daily in divided doses.

***Storage:*** It should be stored in tightly closed container.

***Official preparations:*** Ferrous sulphate tablets I.P., capsules and liquid preparations.

## Dried Ferrous Sulphate I.P., B.P., U.S.P.

**Mol. Formula:** $FeSO_4.2H_2O$ **Mol. Weight:** 188

It contains not less than 86% and not more than 90% of $FeSO_4$.

***Preparation:*** It is prepared by drying the ferrous sulphate crystals in oven at 40 °C until it loses the exact amount of water. The product obtained is a mixture but corresponds in composition with the formula $FeSO_4.2H_2O$.

***Physical properties:*** Dried ferrous sulphate is a greyish white to buff colored powder, slowly soluble in water with astringent taste. When used in dispensing, 3.5 parts of dried salt may be accepted as the equivalent of 5 parts of ferrous sulphate. It is completely soluble in carbon dioxide free water.

***Test for identification:*** Similar to ferrous sulphate.

***Test for purity:*** It should be tested for arsenic, copper, lead, zinc, manganese, ferric ion and basic sulphate.

**Assay**

***Principle:*** It is assayed by **ceriometry method of titration** (also called **redox titration**). In this assay sample is dissolved in water and 1M sulphuric acid and titrated a with 0.1M ceric ammonium nitrate using ferroin sulphate as an indicator. End point is the disappearance of red colour.

***Procedure:*** Weigh accurately about 0.5 gm, dissolve in a mixture of 30 ml of water and 20 ml of 1M sulphuric acid and titrate with 0.1M ceric ammonium sulphate using ferroin solution as an indicator.

***Uses:*** Dried ferrous sulphate is used as a haematinic (increases the haemoglobin content in iron deficiency anaemia).

***Dose:*** For prophylaxis use 200 mg.

For therapeutic use 400 to 600 mg daily in divided doses.

## Ferrous Sulphate Tablets I.P., B.P., U.S.P.

Ferrous sulphate tablet contains dried ferrous sulphate.

It contains not less than 80% and not more than 90% of the stated amount of dried ferrous sulphate.

***Preparation:*** Ferrous sulphate tablets are prepared from dried ferrous sulphate by compression method and sugar coated.

***Test for identification:***

1. The powdered tablets give the characteristic reactions of ferrous salts.
2. Extract of the tablet with hydrochloric acid gives the characteristic reactions of sulphates.

***Test for purity:*** Similar to ferrous sulphate and it also complies with the tests for tablets.

**Assay**

***Principle:***

*Method 1:* It is assayed by **iodometry method of titration** (also called **redox titration**).

In this assay the tablets are first digested with dilute sulphuric acid and filtered. To the filtrate was added strong iodine monochloride solution and concentrated hydrochloric acid. Iodine monochloride oxidizes the ferrous to the ferric ions and iodine is liberated. The liberated iodine is determined by titrating with standard potassium iodate solution until the colour turns into light brown. At this stage a small amount of chloroform is added to it and the titration continued until the disappearance of colour in chloroform layer, which indicates the complete removal of free iodine. As the oxidation and reduction takes place simultaneously this is called Redox titration. The chemical reactions of this assay are shown below.

$$2\,Fe^{2+} + 2\,ICl \longrightarrow 2\,Fe^{3+} + Cl_2 + I_2$$

$$KIO_3 + 2I_2 + 6\,HCl \longrightarrow KCl + 5\,ICl + 3\,H_2O$$

*Method 2:* It is assayed by **ceriometry method of titration** (also called **redox titration**). In this assay sample is dissolved in water and 1M sulphuric acid and titrated a with 0.1M ceric ammonium nitrate using ferroin sulphate as indicator. End point is the disappearance of red colour.

***Procedure:*** Weigh and powder 20 tablets. Weigh accurately a quantity of the powder containing about 0.5 gm of dried ferrous sulphate; dissolve in a mixture of 30 ml of water and 20 ml of 1M sulphuric acid and titrate with 0.1M ceric ammonium sulphate using ferroin solution as indicator.

***Uses:***

1. It is mainly used as a haematinic. Smaller size tablet are prepared due to use of dried ferrous sulphate.

***Dose:*** 200 mg/day in divided doses (20 mg of dried ferrous sulphate is equivalent to 60 mg of ferrous sulphate).

## Ferrous Sulphate Paediatric Mixture B.P.

This preparation is official in B.P only. It contains 1.10 to 1.30 percent of w/v of ferrous sulphate hepta hydrate ($FeSO_4.7H_2O$) with suitable antioxidant (ascorbic acid) in a suitable vehicle and a flavoring agent (orange flavor).

## Ferrous Fumarate I.P., B.P., U.S.P.

**(Synonym: Fersamal)**

**Mol. Formula:** $C_4H_2FeO_4$ **Mol. Weight:** 169.9

***Structure:***

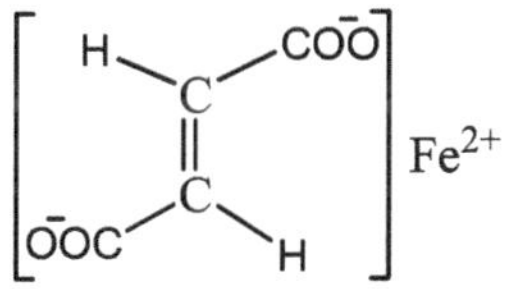

$$\left[ \begin{array}{c} H \diagdown \quad \diagup COO^- \\ C \\ \| \\ C \\ ^-OOC \diagup \quad \diagdown H \end{array} \right] Fe^{2+}$$

It contains not less than 93% and not more than 101% of $C_4H_2FeO_4$, calculated on dried basis.

***Preparation:*** It is prepared by double decomposition reaction between hot aqueous solutions of ferrous sulphate and solution of sodium fumarate, with constant stirring. The sparingly soluble ferrous fumarate is separated, filtered and dried.

$$\text{NaOOC–CH=CH–COONa} + FeSO_4 \xrightarrow{\Delta} \left[ {}^{-}\text{OOC–CH=CH–COO}^{-} \right] Fe^{2+} + Na_2SO_4$$

***Properties:*** It is a reddish orange to reddish brown fine powder. It may contain soft lumps that produce a yellow streak when crushed. Light odour with astringent taste. It is slightly soluble in water and alcohol.

***Test for identification:*** Heat small amount of sample with a mixture of equal volume of water and hydrochloric acid in a water bath for 15 minutes. Cool and filter.

1. The filtrate gives the characteristic reactions of ferrous salts.
2. The precipitate obtained from the above test is washed with 1 volume of dilute HCl and 9 volumes of water and dried at 105 °C. To the residue add small amount of sodium carbonate solution, add potassium permanganate solution drop wise, the brown color is obtained.
3. To the small amount of sample, add required quantity of resorcinol and sulphuric acid heated in a crucible, a deep red semisolid mass is obtained. To this add water and an orange yellow solution without any florescence is obtained.

***Test for purity:*** It should be tested for arsenic, heavy metals, sulphates, ferric ion and loss on drying.

**Assay**

***Principle:*** It is assayed by **ceriometry method of titration (redox titration)**.

In this assay the substance is dissolved in water and to this dilute sulphuric acid was added. The solution is kept aside for some time and titrated with N/10 ceric ammonium sulphate using ferroin sulphate as an indicator. End point is the change of colour from red to blue. During this titration ceric ammonium sulphate oxidizes ferrous ions of ferrous fumarate to ferric and ceric ions are reduced to cerous. As the oxidation and reduction takes place simultaneously this is called Redox titration. The chemical reactions of this assay are shown below.

$$2FeSO_4 + 2Ce(SO_4)_3.2\,(NH_4)_2SO_4 \longrightarrow Fe_2(SO_4)_3 + Ce_2(SO_4)_3 + 4(NH_4)_2SO_4$$

*It can be also written as*

$$Fe^{2+} + Ce^{4+} \longrightarrow Fe^{3+} + Ce^{3+}$$

***Procedure:*** Weigh accurately about 0.3 gm and dissolve in 15 ml of dilute sulphuric acid with the aid of gentle heat. Cool, add 50 ml of water and immediately titrate with 0.1M ceric ammonium sulphate using ferroin sulphate solution as indicator.

***Uses:***

1. It is used as a haematinic like other iron salts.
2. It is mainly used for the condition, when other preparations are not tolerated.

***Dose:*** Prophylactic dose = 200 mg.

Therapeutic dose = 400 - 600 mg daily in divided doses.

## Ferrous Fumarate Tablets I.P., B.P.

It contains not less than 90% and not more that 105% of stated amount of ferrous fumarate.

***Available strength:*** 20 mg (Equivalent to 65 mg).

***Test for identification:*** Similar to ferrous fumarate.

***Test for purity:*** Ferric ion, Disintegration test and it also complies with the tests for tablets.

**Assay**

***Principle:*** Similar to ferrous fumarate.

***Procedure:*** Weigh and powder 20 tablets. Weigh accurately a quantity of the powder containing about 0.3 gm of ferrous fumarate and dissolve in 15 ml of dilute sulphuric acid with the aid of gentle heat. Cool, add 50 ml of water and immediately titrate with 0.1M ceric ammonium sulphate using ferroin sulphate solution as indicatr.

***Use:*** It is used as haematinic.

## Ferrous Gluconate I.P., B.P.

**Mol. Formula:** $C_{12}H_{22}FeO_{14}. x H_2O$ **Mol. Weight:** 446.1

It is dihydrate of the ferrous salt of gluconic acid.

$Fe^{2+}$ [ $COO^-$ / H–C–OH / HO–C–H / H–C–OH / H–C–OH / $H_2C$–OH ]$_2$

It contains not less than 95% and not more than 102% of $C_{12}H_{22}FeO_{14}$, calculated on dried basis.

***Preparation:*** It is mainly prepared from gluconic acid. Gluconic acid is first prepared by oxidation of dextrose (D-glucose) by dilute nitric acid. Then to this add barium carbonate to get barium salt. This is further treated with ferrous sulphate, and the precipitated barium sulphate is removed and the filtrate is concentrated and cooled to get crystals of ferrous gluconate.

$$\underset{\text{Glucose}}{2\,CHO-(CHOH)_4-CH_2OH} \xrightarrow[\text{[O]}]{\text{Dil.}HNO_3} \underset{\text{Gluconic acid}}{2\,COOH-(CHOH)_4-CH_2OH} \xrightarrow[-H_2O,-CO_2]{BaCO_3} \underset{\text{Barium gluconate}}{[COO^{-}-(CHOH)_4-CH_2OH]_2\,Ba^{2+}}$$

$$\xrightarrow{FeSO_4} \underset{\text{Ferrous gluconate}}{[COO^{-}-(CHOH)_4-CH_2OH]_2\,Fe^{2+}} + BaSO_4\downarrow$$

*Double decomposition reaction:* Ferrous gluconate is also obtained by the double decomposition reaction between calcium gluconate and ferrous sulphate.

$$\underset{\text{Calcium gluconate}}{[COO^{-}-(CHOH)_4-CH_2OH]_2\,Ca^{2+}} + FeSO_4 \longrightarrow \underset{\text{Ferrous gluconate}}{[COO^{-}-(CHOH)_4-CH_2OH]_2\,Fe^{2+}} + CaSO_4$$

***Physical properties:*** It occurs as a yellowish grey or pale greenish yellow, fine powder or granules with slight odour similar to that of burnt sugar. It is soluble in water and almost insoluble in organic solvents. The aqueous solution is acidic to litmus.

***Test for identification:***

1. The sample in carbon dioxide free water or the aqueous solution of sample gives the characteristic reactions of ferrous salts.
2. To the small amount of sample, add required quantity of water, glacial acetic acid and 1 ml of phenyl hydrazine and heated the solution in water bath for half an hour. On cooling the solution, gluconic acid phenyl hydrazide crystallizes out. It is purified and the melting point is determined (200-202 °C) with decomposition.

$$[(CH_2OH).(CHOH)_4.COO]_2Fe + 2CH_3COOH$$

$$\downarrow$$

$$2CH_2OH(CHOH)_4COOH + (CH_3COO)_2Fe$$

$$CH_2OH.(CHOH)_4.COOH + \underset{\text{Phenyl hydrazine}}{C_6H_5NHNH_2}$$

$$\downarrow$$

$$CH_2OH.(CHOH)_4CO.NH.NH.C_6H_5 + H_2O$$

3. It is also identified by thin layer chromatography.

***Test for purity:*** It should be tested for pH, arsenic, heavy metals, chlorides, sulphates, barium, ferric ion, oxalic acid, reducing sugars, and loss on drying.

***Test for acidity:*** The 5% w/v solution is acidic to litmus.

***Test for ferric ion:*** It is determined by iodometric method by titrating the liberated iodine against standard sodium thiosulphate.

***Test for oxalic acid:*** It is done by precipitating the oxalate as calcium oxalate from the ether extract residue.

***Test for dextrose and sucrose:*** It is done by reduction of Fehling's solution after conversion of ferrous ion as ferrous sulphide, during which sucrose gets hydrolyzed.

**Assay**

***Principle:*** It is assayed by **ceriometry method of titration (redox titration)**.

In this assay the substance is dissolved in water and to this dilute sulphuric acid was added. The solution is kept aside for some time and titrated with N/10 ceric ammonium sulphate $Ce(NH_4)_2SO_4$ using ferroin sulphate as an indicator. End point is the change of colour from orange red to pale green. During this titration ceric ammonium sulphate oxidizes ferrous ions of ferrous gluconate to ferric and ceric ions are reduced to cerous. As the oxidation and reduction takes place simultaneously this is called Redox titration. The chemical reactions of this assay are shown below.

$$\underset{\text{Oxidised form}}{Ce^{4+}} + \underset{\text{Reduced form}}{Fe^{2+}} \longrightarrow Fe^{3+} + Ce^{3+}$$

***Procedure:*** Dissolve 0.5 gm of sodium bicarbonate in a mixture of 70 ml of water and 30 ml of 1M sulphuric acid. When effervescence ceases, add about 1.0 gm, accurately weighed, of the substance under examination, shake gently to dissolve and titrate with 0.1M ceric ammonium nitrate, using 0.1 ml of ferroin solution as indicator, until the red colour disappears.

***Uses:***

1. It is mainly used as haematinic.

2. Other uses are similar to that of other ferrous salts.
3. It is also used for the preparation ferrous gluconate tablets.

***Dose:*** For prophylactic treatment = 600 mg/daily.

For therapeutic treatment = 1.2 to 1.8 gm in divided doses.

***Dosage forms:*** It is mainly available in the form of tablets and elixir.

***Advantages:*** It causes fewer side effects when compared to other ferrous salts like ferrous sulphate.

***Storage:*** It should be stored in well closed containers and protected from light.

## Ferrous Gluconate Tablets I.P., B.P.

According to I.P. standard it contains not less than 90% and not more than 105% of the stated amount. According to B.P. standards the amount of ferrous gluconate in each tablet is average weight of salt 90 - 105% of the stated amount.

***Preparation:*** The ferrous gluconate tablets are prepared by compression method and they are sugar coated.

***Test for identification:***

1. Dissolve the required quantity of tablet powder equivalent to 1 gm of ferrous gluconate in water, and filter it. The filtrate gives the characteristic reactions of ferrous salts.
2. The filtrate also gives the reactions similar to that of ferrous gluconate.
3. Dissolve the required quantity of powdered tablet equivalent to 5 mg of ferrous gluconate with required amount of dilute hydrochloric acid and filter it. To the filtrate add barium chloride solution, an opalescence is produced but no precipitate is formed.

***Test for purity:*** It should be tested for ferric ion, comply with the other tests for tablets.

**Assay**

***Principle:*** Similar to ferrous gluconate

***Procedure:*** Weigh and powder 20 tablets. Weigh accurately a quantity of the powder containing about 1.0 gm of ferrous gluconate, dissolve in a mixture of 140 ml of water and 60 ml of 1M sulphuric acid and titrate with 0.1M ceric ammonium sulphate, using ferroin solution as indicator, until the red colour disappears.

***Use:*** It is used as haematinic.

***Storage:*** It should be stored in well closed container and protected from light.

***Usual strength:*** 300 mg (equivalent to 35 mg of ferrous ion).

## Ferrous Succinate

**(Synonym: Ferromyn)**

It is official in B.P. 1968. It contains not less than 34% and not more than 36% of $Fe^{2+}$, calculated with reference to the dried basis.

**Mol. Formula:** $C_4H_4FeO_4$. **Mol. Weight:** 172

***Structure:***

$$\begin{array}{l} CH_2COO \\ | \\ CH_2COO \end{array} \!\!> Fe$$

***Preparation:*** It is prepared by the reaction between boiled aqueous solutions of sodium succinate and ferrous sulphate. After cooling the solution the yellow to brown amorphous powder of ferrous succinate is obtained.

$$\underset{\text{Sodim Succinate}}{\begin{array}{l} CH_2COONa \\ | \\ CH_2COONa \end{array}} + FeSO_4 \longrightarrow \underset{\text{Ferrous Succinate}}{\begin{array}{l} CH_2COO \\ | \\ CH_2COO \end{array} \!\!> Fe} + Na_2SO_4$$

***Physical properties:*** It occurs as brownish yellow to brown color amorphous powder with slight odour. It is almost insoluble in water and alcohol, but soluble in dilute mineral acids.

**Assay**

***Principle:*** It is assayed by **ceriometry method of titration (redox titration)**.

In this assay the substance is dissolved in water and to this was added dilute sulphuric acid. The solution is kept aside for some time and titrated with N/10 ceric ammonium sulphate ($Ce(NH_4)_2SO_4$ ) using ferroin sulphate as an indicator. End point is the change of colour from orange red to pale green. During this titration ceric ammonium sulphate oxidizes ferrous ions of ferrous succinate to ferric and ceric ions are reduced to cerous. As the oxidation and reduction takes place simultaneously this is called Redox titration. The chemical reactions of this assay are shown below.

$$\underset{\substack{\text{Oxidised}\\\text{form}}}{Ce^{4+}} + \underset{\substack{\text{Reduced}\\\text{form}}}{Fe^{2+}} \longrightarrow Fe^{3+} + Ce^{3+}$$

***Official formulations:*** Ferrous succinate tablets and capsules B.P. The usual strength is 100 mg of the succinate which is equivalent to 35 mg of ferrous ion.

---

## Ferric Ammonium Citrate I.P., B.P.

**(Synonym: Iron ammonium citrate)**

It is a complex of ammonium ferric citrate. It contains not less than 20.5% and not more than 22.5% of iron (Fe). This preparation is known as "Scale preparations" of iron.

***Preparation:*** It is obtained by using ferric sulphate, sodium hydroxide, citric acid and ammonia.

**Step 1**

*Preparation of ferric hydroxide:* The freshly prepared ferric hydroxide is obtained by treating the ferric sulphate solution with sodium hydroxide by constant stirring and not vice versa, otherwise it prevents the formation of scales.

$$Fe_2(SO_4)_3 + 6NaOH \longrightarrow 2Fe(OH)_3 + 3Na_2SO_4$$

**Step 2**

*Preparation of ferric and ammonium citrate:* The ferric hydroxide precipitate obtained from the step1 is collected and washed until free from soluble ions. Then the precipitate is added by stirring into a solution of citric acid. Most of it goes into solution. Any undissolved ferric hydroxide is present, removed by the addition of slight excess of ammonia. The clear reddish brown filtrate obtained is evaporated to syrup (little ammonia has to be added during this process for compensating any loss during evaporation). Then the syrup is painted on glass plates and dried at 40 °C. The dried scale have been scrapped off and packed. It may also obtain as brownish red granular powder. The chemistry of final product is complicated and depends upon the conditions of preparations.

$$C_6H_8O_7 + xFe(OH)_3 \longrightarrow Fe(C_6H_5O_7).xFe(OH)_3 + 3H^+$$

The general formula for ferric ammonium - citrate complex is variable one and indicated by $Fe(C_6H_5O_7)$. X $Fe(OH)_3$. Where X is greater than one but less than two.

The hydrogen ion concentration reveals the following changes.

Decrease in $H^+$ ion concentration.

$$FeC_6H_5O_7 \rightleftharpoons FeC_6H_5O_7.xFe(OH)_3 \rightleftharpoons Fe(OH)_3$$

| $FeC_6H_5O_7$ | $FeC_6H_5O_7.xFe(OH)_3$ | $Fe(OH)_3$ |
|---|---|---|
| Yellow-green normal citrate | Brownish red basic complex | Brownish red colloidal ferric hydroxide |

There is no doubt some ferric hydroxide is associated with the product. Ammonia is able to maintain the amount of ferric hydroxide associated with each molecule of ferric citrate to about 2 moles. Stronger alkali is able to precipitate ferric hydroxide whereas large amount of citric acid reduces the ferric hydroxide content rendering the product green with decreased iron content.

***Physical properties:*** It is a thin, transparent, dark red scales or granules or a brownish red powder with slight astringent taste, odorless, deliquescent in moist air and is affected by light. It is freely soluble in water and insoluble in organic solvent. It is well absorbed and dispensed with alkali carbonates without involving the precipitation of ferric hydroxide.

***Test for identification:***

1. The residue on ignition is dissolved in required amount of hydrochloric acid and the resulting solution gives the characteristics reactions of ferric salt.
2. The sample is heated with sodium hydroxide, ammonia is evolved and the solution gives the characteristic reactions of citrates.

***Test for purity:*** It should be tested for arsenic, lead, zinc, free ferric compounds, chlorides and sulphates.

**Assay**

***Principle:*** It is assayed by **iodometry method of titration** (also called **redox titration**).

In this assay the substance is dissolved in water and acidified with sulphuric acid and warmed until the solution becomes yellow. Cool the solution and add potassium permanganate solution drop by drop to oxidize small amount of ferrous to ferric. When the pink colour persists add few drops of hydrochloric acid and potassium iodide. The liberated hydroiodic acid is oxidized by ferric salt and iodine is liberated. The amount of iodine liberated is determined by titrating with N/10 sodium thiosulphate using starch mucilage as an indicator. End point is the disappearance of blue colour. During this titration iodine is reduced to sodium iodide and sodium thiosulphate is oxidized to sodium tetrathionate. As the oxidation and reduction takes place simultaneously this is called Redox titration. The chemical reactions of this assay are shown below.

$$I_2 + 2\,Na_2S_2O_3 \longrightarrow 2\,NaI + Na_2S_4O_6$$

***Procedure:*** Weigh accurately about 0.5 gm, dissolve in a mixture of 15 ml of water and 1 ml of sulphuric acid and warm until the dark brown colour becomes yellow. After cooling the solution to 15 °C add 0.02 M potassium permanganate drop wise till a pink colour is obtained persisting for 5 seconds. Add 15 ml of hydrochloric acid and 2 gm of potassium iodide, allow it to stand for 3 minutes, add about 60 ml of water and titrate with 0.1M sodium thiosulphate using starch solution as indicator.

*Uses:*

1. It is used as a source of iron in the treatment of iron deficiency anemia (Haematinic).
2. When compared with ferrous sulphate and ferrous gluconate it is less irritant and has less constipating effect.

***Dose:*** 1 to 3 gm.

***Other complex scale preparation of iron salt:*** Quinine citrate scale preparation with ferric citrate and ferric hydroxide with green color and uses similar to ferric and ammonium citrate scale preparation.

## Iron and Dextran Injection I.P., B.P.

Iron and dextran injection is a sterile colloidal solution containing a complex of ferric hydroxide with dextran of average molecular weight between 5000 and 7500.

It contains not less than 4.75% and not more than 5.25% w/v of iron and not less than 17% and not more than 23% of dextran.

***Physical properties:*** It is a dark brown color solution.

***Test for identification:*** It does not give the reactions of ferric ions. But after hydrolysis with hydrochloric acid, gives ferric chloride which gives the characteristic reactions of ferric ion.

***Test for dextran:*** The sample is hydrolyzed with hydrochloric acid and the liberated ferric chloride is removed by the addition of hydrogen sulphide. Then the dextran is hydrolyzed to glucose which is identified by the reduction of Fehling's solution.

***Test for purity:*** It should be tested for pH of the solution, arsenic, heavy metals, copper, zinc, chloride, iron absorption capacity, abnormal toxicity, dextran, bacterial endotoxins and other tests.

**Assay**

It is assayed by **ceriometry method of titration** (also called **redox titration**).

It is assayed by dissolving the ferric ion in sulphuric acid and reducing the ferric to ferrous iron using zinc amalgam. Thus the reduced ferrous ion is determined by titrating with ceric ammonium sulphate using ferroin sulphate as an indicator.

***Uses:***

1. It is mainly used for patients whom oral administration is not possible.
2. It is used as a haematinic.
3. It is also given by intravenous infusion at a slow rate.

***Dose:*** 1-2 ml daily or it should be determined by the physician according to the patient's need and in accordance with the manufacturer's dosage schedules.

***Contraindications:*** Care should be taken for the patients with dextran allergy.

## Iron-Sorbitol Injection I.P., B.P.

This compound is official in B.P. 1968.

Iron-sorbitol injection is a sterile solution of complex of iron, sorbitol and citric acid that is stabilized with the aid of dextrin and excess sorbitol.

It contains not less than 94.0% and not more than 104.0% of the labeled amount of iron.

***Physical properties:*** It is a clear brown color solution.

***Test for identification:***

1. To a small amount of sample solution, add 5ml of water and add small amount of ammonium hydroxide. No precipitate is formed.
2. To the sample solution, add one drop of hydrochloric acid and one drop of potassium ferrocyanide solution, dark blue precipitate is formed.

***Test for purity:*** It should be tested for specific gravity, viscosity, pH of the solution (7.2 - 7.9), ferrous ion, bacterial endotoxin and it is meet the other requirements for injections.

**Assay**

***Principle:*** It is assayed by ceriometry method of titration (also called redox titration).

It is assayed by dissolving the ferric ion in sulphuric acid and reducing the ferric to ferrous iron using zinc amalgam as reducing agent. Thus the reduced ferrous ion is determined by titrating with ceric ammonium sulphate using ferroin sulphate as an indicator.

***Uses:***

1. It is mainly given to the patients those who are not responding to the oral iron and in case of anaemia in advanced pregnancy.
2. It is more rapidly adsorbed than iron dextran injection. It is given by intramuscular route.

***Storage:*** It should be preserved in single dose glass containers.

Other iron compounds

| Sr. No. | Compound name | Molecular formulae | Preparation | Properties | Uses |
|---|---|---|---|---|---|
| 1 | Ferrous carbonate | $FeCO_3$ | It contains small amount of ferric hydroxide and other iron oxide. **Preparation:** It is prepared by mixing of ferrous carbonate with liquid glucose. | Hygroscopic power. | Less astringent, less irritant than other compounds. |
| 2 | Ferrous iodide | FeI | Mixing of iron and iodine and made up to solution. | Its available in the form of clear solution (or) syrup. | Antioxidant. |
| 3 | Ferrous phosphate | $FeO_4P$ | It's a mixture of ferric phosphate and hydrated ferrous phosphate contains 16% of iron in ferrous form. | – | It is mainly used in compound syrups. (May be with quinine and strychnine to other mineral phosphate. |
| 4 | Ferrous lactate, ferrous succinate, ferrous tartarate and ferrous glycine sulphate | | These are some of the ferrous salts with organic acids. | – | Less astringent than other iron salts and used in iron deficiency anaemia. |
| 5 | Ferrous cholinate | | It is a ferric iron chelate, available in tablet form and pediatric drops. | | Less toxic than ferrous sulphate and gluconate. |
| 6 | Ferric cacodylate | $(Fe(CH_3)_2$ $(ASO_3)_3$ | | | It is mainly used in the treatment of leukemia due to the presence of arsenic |
| 7 | Ferric citrate | $C_6H_5FeO_7.$ $5H_2O$ | | Greenish and reddish brown powder. | Oral haematinic, dietary supplement, nutrient. |

***Contd...***

| Sr. No. | Compound name | Molecular formulae | Preparation | Properties | Uses |
|---|---|---|---|---|---|
| 8 | Ferric glycero phosphate | $C_9H_{21}Fe_2$ $O_{18}P_3$ | | Greenish brown to greenish yellow solid, sinks and mixes with water. | It is one of the ingredient of glycerol phosphate elixir. |
| 9 | Ferric hypophosphite | $Fe(H_2PO_2)_2$ | | A White or greyish white powder, odourless, tasteless. | It is one of the ingredients of some hypophosphite syrup. |

### 6.6.2 Other Essential Trace Elements

#### Iron

Iron is an essential metal to the elementary metabolic processes in the cell. In the process of respiration in higher animals, it functions as an electron carrier. It plays an important role for the transport of molecular oxygen in higher organisms. Both of the above functions are depends upon the ability of iron to exist in coordination in their oxidation states and bonding.

Iron content in body components is present in the following table

| Occurrence | Bounded iron nature | Mode of linkage | Function | Total iron content | Body iron % |
|---|---|---|---|---|---|
| Blood system | Hemoglobin plasma | Heme transferrin Heme ferritin | $O_2$ transport Fe transport | 4 mg -3 gm 650 mg - 1 gm | 0.1-65.4 |
| Tissues | Myoglobin storage iron | | Cell respiration iron pool | | 13.9-21.5 |

Most of the iron content present in the body is classified in two types.

1. Haemoproteins
2. Iron storage and/or transport proteins.

***Haemoproteins:*** These are iron containing proteins responsible for respiration and oxygen carriers. Example: Cytochrome C enzyme.

In the above enzyme iron is complexed in a porphyrin ring system which in turn covalently bonded to the proteins portion of the molecule. The iron is present in two forms one is ferrous ($Fe^{2+}$) and other is ferric ($Fe^{3+}$). Ferrous and ferric forms are used to pick up or donate the electron respectively, in the electron transfer process. The other iron containing oxidative enzymes are catalases and the peroxidases.

The other haemoprotein present in our body mainly in tissues are myoglobin and haemoglobin. Both are used as storing and/or transport of oxygen.

***Haemoglobin:*** It consists of four protein chains, each one contains heme unit of porphyrin ring and ferrous ion. The iron complexes with molecular oxygen by using a vacant orbital of the unpaired electrons from oxygen.

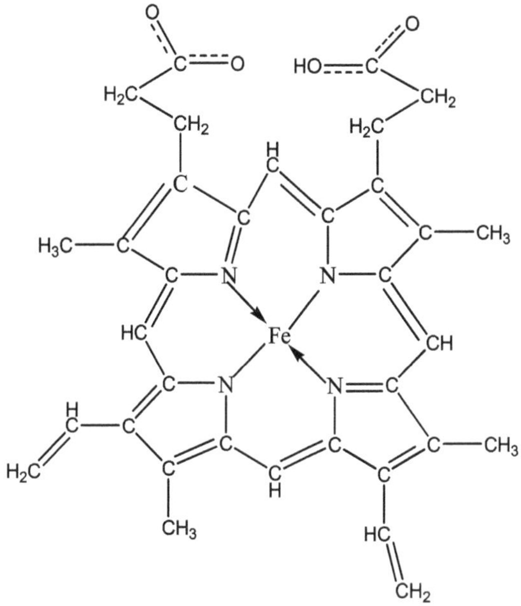

Haemoglobin

The uptake and release of oxygen are influenced by the following factors.

(a) Oxygen tension (b) pH

(c) Carbon dioxide concentration (d) 2,3-di phosphoglycerate

***Iron storage and/or transport proteins:*** Ferritin and hemosiderin are the two iron storage proteins present in the liver, spleen and bone narrow.

***Ferritin:*** It is water insoluble protein

***Transferrin:*** The major iron transport protein of plasma is transferrin. It binds tightly with two ferric atoms per molecule due to no free plasma iron is present.

***Functions:*** It releases iron into the red blood cell precursor by attaching to a receptor on the surface of the developing red blood cell.

The daily requirements of iron in male is 10-12 mg and for female is12-18 mg. The absorption of iron is controlled and regulated in our body by mucosal block hypothesis.

***Iron sulfur proteins:*** Rubredoxin and ferredoxins are the two important iron-sulphur proteins found in plants and photosynthetic bacteria which are being involved in nitrogen fixation.

The enzymes responsible for the nitrogen fixation which reduce nitro to ammonia are a *nitrogenase* and a *reductase* which is involves an iron sulfur protein.

## Copper

***Biological role of copper:*** Copper is essential metal in all animals and plants. It is mainly obtained from food water and cooking vessels. The adult human body contains 2 mg/kg of copper which is distributed in enzymes and other proteins. The average daily intake of copper is 2-5 mg/day.

***Distribution of copper in the body:*** Copper is solubilized in gastric juice and it absorbed from the stomach and upper small intestine. From the intestine, copper moves to blood serum as copper albumin complex.

Then it goes to liver as copper protein ceruloplasmin. The albumin copper complex distributes the copper to the liver, bone marrow, kidney, red blood cells and tissues.

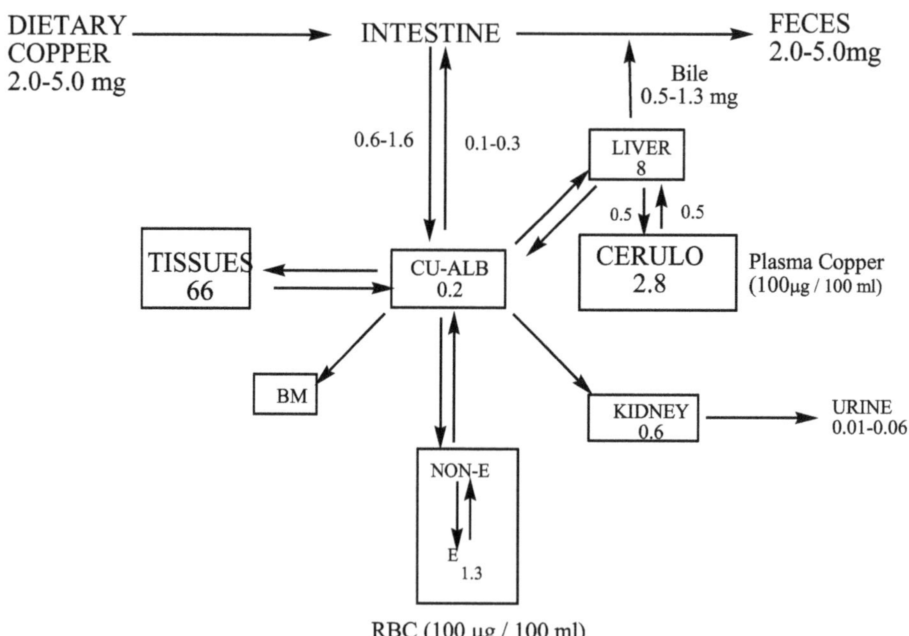


***Role of copper in the body***

(i) Copper facilitate iron absorption.

(ii) It stimulates the enzymes in the heme/globin biosynthetic pathways.

(iii) It involves, in the movement of stored iron, as haemoglobin.

(iv) Copper is important for the ATP production by cellular respiration (oxidative phosphorylation).

(v) It is the constituent of *cytochrome oxidase* (formation of higher energy phosphate bonds).

(vi) It is also involved in the formation of aortic elastin.

(vii) It is necessary for amine oxidase activity and plays an important role in the formation of cross linkages of elastin.

(viii) The blue copper proteins such as plastocyanin and azurin are involved in the electron transport mechanism.

(ix) It is also a component of *tyrosinase* enzyme, which is responsible for the conversion of tyrosine to melanine.

(x) Due to the capacity of copper to increase the iron uptake, copper deficiency produce some anaemia like symptoms.

(xi) The other biochemical role of copper includes bone developments, nucleic acid preparations, protein synthesis and pigmentation.

(xii) The major disease related to copper is Wilson's disease (condition of excess copper storage).

(xiii) Hepatic cirrhosis is another one copper related disease in which more amount of copper in liver, kidney, brain and cornea. Symptoms are brain damage and demyelination and kidney problems. The antidote for this condition is penicillamine or ammonium tetramolybdate. These are forming complex with copper and increases the excretion of copper.

There are no official copper preparations for administration during copper deficiency.

1. The only one copper salt official in national formulary is cupric sulfate which is used as an antidote for phosphorous poisoning. Copper preparation is used topically as fungicides and astringents.
2. It is also an essential ingredient of chemical reagents such as Fehling's solution and Benedict's solution. Both the solutions are used for qualitative determinations.

## Zinc

Zinc ion is widely distributed in the body. It is one of the important trace elements. It is associated with certain type of metallo enzymes such as *malate dehydrogenase*, *alcohol dehydrogenase*, *lactate dehydrogenase*, *carbonic anhydrase*, *aldolase*, *alkaline phosphatase*, *peptidase* and *neutral protease* etc. Zinc also found in RNA which is used to stabilize the secondary and tertiary structures. A maximum enzyme present in our body contains zinc. Prosthetic groups are one of this types which is called zinc finger. Most amount of zinc is present in bones and muscles.

***Sources of zinc:*** The main dietary source for zinc is meat, fish, eggs, milk beans and nuts. The total content of zinc required for human body is 10-15 mg/day; prostate gland is highly rich in zinc (100 mg/gm). The dietary requirement of zinc for male is 11 mg and for female is 8 mg after puberty. The higher concentration of zinc is needed during pregnancy and lactation.

***Biological role of zinc:***

1. It is an essential element of several enzymes, like *alcohol dehydrogenase*, *super oxide dismutase* etc.
2. Zinc is necessary to maintain the normal levels of vitamin A in serum.
3. It promotes the synthesis of retinol binding protein.
4. Zinc is important factor for red blood cell production.

5. It may be considered as an antioxidant since the superoxide dismutase enzyme protects the body against free radical damage.
6. The storage and secretion of insulin from the β-cells of pancreas require zinc.
7. Gustin, a zinc containing protein of the saliva is important for taste sensation.
8. Zinc ion is required for wound healing; it enhances the cell growth and division besides stabilizing bio-membranes.
9. The oral zinc sulphate is used for wound healing.
10. Zinc is absorbed in duodenum. Zinc from animal source is absorbed better than that of vegetable source. The enzyme responsible for zinc absorption is metallothionein.
11. Factors which increase the iron absorption are calcium, copper, iron, phytate, etc.

***Deficiency associated with zinc:***

1. Zinc deficiency is associated with impaired growth; poor wound healing, hair loss, loss of taste sensation, loss of appetite, impaired spermatogenesis.
2. Zinc deficiency also leads to depression, dementia and psychic disorders.
3. Acrodermatitis enteropathica: Inherited metabolic diseases caused by defect in zinc absorption.
4. Toxicity of zinc is resulted from acid food kept in galvanized container and from industrial workers inhaling zinc fumes. The symptoms included are fever, chillness, malaria, cough, salivation and headache.

## Chromium

Chromium is also a one of the essential trace element. It is necessary for the growth of animals. The levels of chromium are higher in infants than adults. The large quantity of chromium is toxic to body.

***Source:*** Brewer's yeast, cereals, grains, cheese and meat.

***Biochemical role:***

1. Chromium is used to improve or to normalize the impaired glucose tolerance of some diabetic, malnourished children and old people.
2. Chromium is a component of a protein namely chromodulin which facilitates the binding of insulin to cell receptor sites.
3. It participates in lipoprotein metabolism.

***Toxic effect:***

(i) They are commonly destructive to tissues when taken orally or applied topically.

(ii) When taken internally, produces nephritis and glycosuria.

(iii) Exposure of chromate dust leads to deep ulcers of skin and nasal mucosa.

## Manganese

Manganese is an essential trace element in human body. The total manganese content in the body is 10-20 mg. The highest concentration of manganese occurs in liver, bone, and pituitary, pineal and lactating mammary glands, it mainly present in nucleic acids.

***Biochemical functions of manganese:***

1. Manganese is one of the important co factors for several enzymes.

   For example: *Superoxide dismutase, pepetidase, arginase, pyruvate carboxylase* etc.
2. It is necessary for the synthesis of glycoproteins, mucopolysaccharides and hemoglobin.
3. It is also used for the bio synthesis of cholesterol.
4. Manganese is also important for the photo synthetic oxygen evolution of chloroplasts in plants. The metallo-enzymes responsible for the OEC (oxygen evolving complex) contain four manganese atoms. Due to this reason, most of the broad spectrum fertilizers contain manganese.
5. Manganese is required for the bone formation, proper reproduction and normal functioning of nervous system.
6. It also plays a role in oxidative phosphorylation, fatty acid metabolism.

***Dietary sources:*** Cereals, nuts, leafy vegetables, tea leaves and fruits.

Manganese is mainly absorbed in small intestine. Iron inhibits manganese absorption. The daily requirement of manganese is 3-9 mg. Serum manganese is bound to a specific carrier protein β-globulin.

***Deficiency:*** No deficiency is found in humans. In other mammals, manganese deficiency produces defective growth, CNS malfunctions, bone abnormalities, accumulation of fat in liver, reproductive dysfunctions etc.

The official preparations for manganese are Manganese citrate, glycerophosphate and a hypophosphate.

---

## Molybdenum

The one important trace element present in living organisms is molybdenum. It is present in the active site in some type of enzymes. For example, Nitrogenase enzyme (*Nitrite reductase*) which is used for nitrogen fixation in bacteria contains molybdenum. It is a constituent of the enzymes like *xanthine oxidase, aldehyde oxidase* and *sulfide oxidase*.

***Dietary source:*** It is widely distributed in natural foods. It is effectively absorbed by small intestine. It interferes with utilization of copper in the body.

***Disease condition:***

*Molybdenosis:* It is a rare disorder caused by excessive consumption of molybdenum. The symptoms include growth disorder anaemia and diarrhoea. Copper absorption is depleted.

***Uses and official preparations:*** Molybdenum oxide is used along with ferrous sulphate as a haematinic.

Molybdenum 99 is the parent isotope for technetium 99 radio isotope which is having many medicinal uses.

## Sulphur

Sulphur is widely distributed in the body. It is present in the form of amino acids (methionine, cysteine and cystine).

***Biochemical functions:***

1. Some of the vitamins and coenzymes contain sulfur as a one of a constituent.

   *Example:* Thiamine, lipoic acid and biotin. A cofactor containing sulfur is pantothenic acid.
2. The other important sulfur containing compounds are heparin, chondroitin sulfate, tauracholic acid, and glutathione.
3. The enzyme phosphoradenosine phosphorsulphate (PAPS) is used for the synthesis of glycosaminoglycans and detoxification mechanism.
4. The amino acid methionine is involved in trans methylation reactions.

***Dietary requirements and sources:*** Protein rich food containing methionine and cysteine are the major source of sulfur. The minimum daily requirement of sulfur is 2 - 3 gm.

***Therapeutic uses of sulphur:***

1. Sulphur contains catharatic action and depilatory action.
2. It is used as parasiticide in scabies.
3. It is also used as stimulant in alopecia, fumigation purposes and miscellaneous skin diseases.

## Iodine

Iodine is another one important trace element in human body. It is an essential ion necessary for the two thyroid hormones (Tri iodo thyronine and thyroxin). The total body contains 20 gm iodine, most of the iodine is present in thyroid gland. It is also present in other organs like muscles and salivary glands.

***Biochemical functions:***

1. The main function of iodine is the synthesis of thyroid hormones.
2. It is also used as a fibrinolytic agent and expectorant.

***Sources:*** Vegetables, fruits, sea foods and drinking water.

***Dietary requirements:*** The dietary requirements of iodine for adults is 100-150 mg/day and in pregnant women is 200 mg/day.

***Toxicity:***

1. Excess iodine in the body produces toxicity like that of iodine deficiency.
2. Exposure of radioactive iodine causes thyroid cancer.

3. Elemental iodine is highly toxic in nature when it comes into contact with skin causes lesions. Iodine vapor is very irritating to eyes and mucous membranes.

***Official Iodine preparations:*** Iodine I.P., Various iodine solutions, Potassium iodide I.P., Iodine Tincture I.P., Sodium iodide etc.

---

## Selenium

Originally selenium has been identified as an element that produce toxicity when taken internally and the metabolic products also too toxic for systemic uses. However a very small amount of selenium is needed for animals and humans.

***Biochemical function:***

1. It prevents liver necrosis in rats.
2. Selenium along with vitamin E prevents the development of muscular dystrophy
3. Selenium is bind with some heavy metals like mercury and calcium and protects the body form their toxic effects.
4. It involves in maintaining structural integrity of biological membranes.
5. It prevents lipid peroxidation, by this way it protects the cell against free radicals.
6. Selenium is a component of some enzymes. Selenocysteine is an essential component of *glutathione peroxidases*, which protects the cell damage against hydrogen peroxide. *5′-Deiodinase* a selenium containing enzyme which converts thyroxin to triiodothyronine in the thyroid gland. *Thioredoxin reductase* which is a selenoprotein involved in purine metabolism.
7. It is also used for the treatment of kwashiorkor (a protein deficiency present in children and infants).
8. In children the increased content of selenium produces dental cavities.

***Sources:*** The high selenium content is present in meat (liver, kidney) and sea foods. The daily requirement of selenium for adults is 50-200 mg.

***Diseases:***

*Keshan disease:* An endemic cardiomyopathy in human is associated with selenium deficiency.

Lower selenium level leads to cardiovascular diseases and various cancers.

***Toxicity:***

*Selenosis:* A very high intake of selenium. The selenium toxicity includes emotional disturbances, hair loss, diarrhoea and garlic odour in breath (Due to the formation of dimethyl selenide).

---

## Phosphates
### Sodium Acid Phosphate

This compound is discussed under **saline cathartics.**

### Sodium Phosphate

This compound is discussed under **saline cathartics.**

## Halogens
### Iodine and its Solutions

These are discussed under **oxidative antimicrobials.**

### Fluorides

These are discussed under **anti-caries agents.**

## PROBABLE QUESTIONS

1. Define haematinics. Enumerate the official haematinics.
2. Write the source and biological role of iron, vitamin $B_{12}$ and folic acid.
3. Explain the method of preparation, properties, purity tests, assay and uses of scale preparation of iron salt.
4. Explain about the ferrous and ferric compounds which are used in iron deficiency.
5. Explain in detail about the preparation, properties, assay and uses of the following iron compounds.
   (a) Ferrous sulphate (b) Dried ferrous sulphate
   (c) Ferrous gluconate (d) Ferrous fumarate
   (e) Ferrous succinate (f) Ferrous sulphate tablets
6. Write short notes on the followings:
   (a) Iron and dextran injection (b) Iron and sorbitol injection
7. Explain the distribution of iron in body proteins.
8. Define metallic and trace elements and explain its biological role.
9. Describe the distribution and biological importance of copper.
10. Write a note on the following.
    (a) Chromium (b) Manganese
    (c) Molybdenum (d) Sulphur (e) Selenium
11. Explain about the source, daily requirements, biological role and deficiency of zinc in the body.
12. Write a note on iodine compounds.
13. Define the followings.
    (a) Keshan disease (b) Selenosis (c) Molypdenosis

## 6.7 PHARMACEUTICAL AIDS

### 6.7.1 Adsorbents and Absorbents

#### Activated Charcoal

This compound is discussed under **adsorbents and protectives.**

---

#### Aluminium Sulphate B.P., U.S.P.

**Mol. Formula:** $Al_2(SO_4)_3.XH_2O$ **Mol. Weight:** 342.12

It contains not less than 51% and not more than 59% of aluminium sulphate with varying amount of water for crystallization.

***Preparation:*** It is prepared by reacting freshly prepared aluminium hydroxide with sulphuric acid. The resulting solution is concentrated and the salt crystallized when octadecahydrate is crystallizes out.

$$2Al(OH)_3 + 3H_2SO_4 \longrightarrow Al_2(SO_4)_3 + 6H_2O$$

***Physical properties:*** It occurs as white or colorless crystals, odorless, sweet astringent taste. It is very soluble in water. The crystals are efflorescence in atmospheric moisture, it loses its water. Due to hydrolysis, the solution is acidic, the pH of 2% solution is low as 3.

***Test for identification:*** The aqueous solution of sample gives the characteristic reactions of aluminium and sulphate ions.

***Test for purity:*** It has to be tested for clarity and color of the solution, alkali and alkaline earth metals, ammonium salts, arsenic, heavy metals and iron.

**Assay**

***Principle:*** It is assayed by **complexometry method of (Back) titration.**

In this assay the substance is dissolved in 1N hydrochloric acid by warming, to this Known Excess Standard (KES) 0.05N disodium Ethylene Diamine Tetra Acetate (EDTA) is added and the solution is neutralized with 1N sodium hydroxide using methyl red as an indicator (colour change from red to yellow). To this solution hexamine added as a buffer and xylenol orange as an indicator and titrated against 0.05M lead nitrate. End point is the appearance of violet colour due to the formation of lead-xylenol orange complex.

In this assay Aluminium ions of aluminium sulphate reacts with EDTA, whereby the complexation takes place, after this reaction, the excess unreacted disodium EDTA is determined by titrating with lead nitrate. The indicator is colourless before complexation and change into violet colour due to the formation of lead-xylenol orange complex. As the aluminium ions forms complex with disodium EDTA in this assay, it is called as complexometry method of titration. The chemical reactions of this assay are shown below.

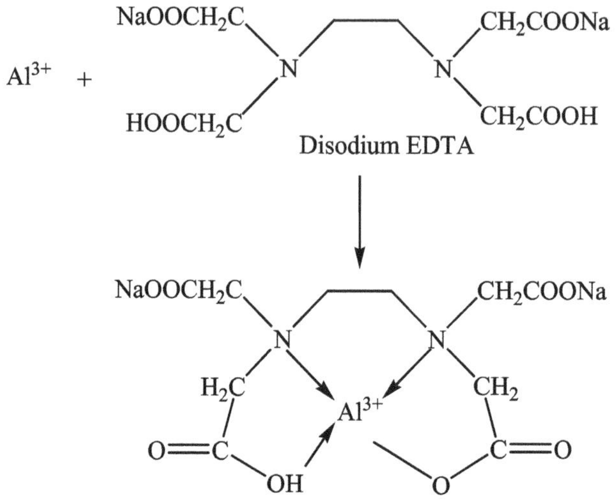

$Al^{3+}$ + $NaOOCH_2C$, $HOOCH_2C$ N–N $CH_2COONa$, $CH_2COOH$

Disodium EDTA

↓

$NaOOCH_2C$, $CH_2COONa$, N, N, $H_2C$, $CH_2$, $Al^{3+}$, O=C, OH, C=O, O

Aluminium-EDTA Complex

***Procedure:*** Weigh accurately about 0.6 gm sample and dissolve in 2 ml of 1M hydrochloric acid and 50 ml of water. Add 50.0 ml of 0.05M disodium edetate and neutralize to methyl red solution with 1M sodium hydroxide. Heat the solution to boiling, leave on a water-bath for 10 minutes, cool rapidly and add about 50 mg of xylenol orange mixture and 5 gm of hexamine. Titrate with 0.05M lead nitrate. Carry out a blank titration.

***Uses:***

1. Aluminium sulphate is mainly used as pharmaceutical aid in adsorbed bacterial toxoids (vaccines).
2. It acts as a powerful astringent.
3. It is also used as an antiperspirant.
4. It is used for the purification of water by flocculation methods.

---

### Aluminium Phosphate B.P., U.S.P.

This compound is discussed under **antacids**.

***Uses:*** It is mainly used as both antacid and also a pharmaceutical aid for absorbing bacterial toxoids in the preparation of vaccines.

---

## 6.7.2 Anti Oxidants

**Introduction:** An 'antioxidant' is a molecule that inhibits the oxidation of others molecule. During 'Oxidation process' there will be transfer of electron or hydrogen from a substance into an oxidizing agent, resulting in the formation of free radicals. This may lead to deterioration of the substance. So the 'Antioxidants' are added to the pharmaceutical preparations containing easily oxidizable substances. Chemically, these are reducing agents which prevent the oxidation either by getting oxidize themselves in place of active component as they undergo oxidation more easily than the active component. So, the mechanism of an antioxidant is based on oxidation – reduction reaction in which the oxidant itself gents oxidized. Example: Sulphur dioxide, hypophosphorous acid ($H_2PO_3$) etc.

## Sodium Sulphite B.P., U.S.P.

**Mol. Formula:** $Na_2SO_3.7H_2O$ **Mol. Weight:** 252.15

It is a colorless, odorless, efflorescent crystal and highly soluble in water.

**Assay**

***Procedure:*** Introduce 0.5 gm into a 500 ml conical flask containing 50.0 ml of 0.05M iodine. Shake until completely dissolved. Add 1 ml of starch solution and titrate the excess of iodine with 0.1M sodium thiosulphate. Carry out a blank titration.

***Uses:***

1. It is mainly used as an antioxidant and preservative.
2. It is used as the main immediate source of sulphur dioxide and acts as a reducing agent.

## Sodium Bisulphite

**(Synonym: Sodium hydrogen sulphite, Sodium acid sulphite, Sodium pyrosulphate)**

**Mol. Formula:** $NaHSO_3$ **Mol. Weight:** 104.06

It contains not less than 61.1% and not more than 67.4% of $SO_2$.

It consists of sodium bisulphite ($NaHSO_3$) and sodium metabisulphite ($Na_2S_2O_5$) in varying proportions.

***Preparation***: Sodium bisulphite is prepared by passing sulphur dioxide into a solution of sodium carbonate until the solution is saturated. Then the resulting solution is evaporated to yield a mixture of sodium bisulphite and metabisulphite.

$$Na_2CO_3 + 2SO_2 + H_2O \longrightarrow 2NaHSO_3 + CO_2\uparrow$$

***Physical properties***: It is a white or yellowish white crystalline powder, pungent odour of burning sulphur, disagreeable taste. It is unstable in air, loses some $SO_2$ and gradually oxidized to sulphate. It is soluble in cold water and alcohol. The aqueous solution is acidic. It is kept in a cool place and stored in well closed containers.

***Chemical properties:***

*Reaction with hydrochloric acid*: The sodium bisulphite reacts with hydrochloric acid, yields sulphurous acid which is actually the solution of sulphur dioxide in water.

$$NaHSO_3 + HCl \longrightarrow \underset{\text{Sulphurous acid}}{NaCl + H_2SO_3}$$

$$H_2SO_3 \rightleftharpoons H_2O + SO_2\uparrow$$

Sodium bisulphite form water soluble, stable compounds with aldehydes and ketones, so it is used to prepare their derivatives (carbonyl compounds containing formulations).

***Test for purity*:** It should be tested for heavy metals, iron and arsenic.

***Uses*:** 0.1% of sodium bisulphite is commonly used for all purposes.

1. It is used as a stabilizing agent and antioxidant.
2. It converts the water insoluble menadione (synthetic analogue of vitamin K) into very soluble menadione sodium bisulphite compound without the loss of significant biological activity (increasing the water solubility).
3. Externally used to treat parasitic skin disease.
4. It is also used to solubilize kidney stones.
5. 0.3 to 0.6 gm dose is used as an antiseptic in gastric fermentation.
6. It is also used in ephedrine hydrochloride, phenylephrine hydrochloride and ascorbic acid injections.

## Sodium Metabisulphite I.P., B.P., U.S.P.

**(Synonym: Sodium pyrosulphite, Sodium acid pyrosulphite, Sodium hydrogen sulphite)**

**Mol. Formula:** $Na_2S_2O_5$ **Mol. Weight:** 190.1

It contains not less than 95% of $Na_2S_2O_5$ equivalent to not less than 100.5% $Na_2S_2O_5$.

***Preparation:*** It is obtained by saturating, hot concentrated solution of sodium hydroxide with $SO_2$ and allowing the salt to crystallize by cooling. The $NaHSO_3$ first formed is not stable in the solid state, and the solid which separates is the metabisulphite (sometimes called as pyrosulphite).

$$NaOH + SO_{2\,(g)} \longrightarrow NaHSO_3$$

$$2NaHSO_3 \longrightarrow Na_2S_2O_5 + H_2O$$

***Physical properties*:** It occurs as white, light yellow crystals or colorless crystalline powder, with the smell of $SO_2$, acidic saline taste. It is freely soluble in water, glycerin and slightly soluble in alcohol. The aqueous solution is acidic to litmus. On exposure to air it effloresces and slowly oxidized to sulphate.

***Chemical properties:*** Sodium metabisulphite when dissolved in water is immediately converted to bisulphate, which upon reaction with aqueous acid yields sulphurous acid (essentially a solution of $SO_2$ in water).

$$Na_2S_2O_5 + H_2O \longrightarrow 2NaHSO_3$$

$$NaHSO_3 + HCl \longrightarrow NaCl + H_2SO_3$$

$$H_2SO_3 \rightleftharpoons H_2O + SO_2\uparrow$$

It is incompatible with compounds which are easily reducing in nature.

***Test for identification:***

1. To the sample solution, add iodine solution, decolorization occurs and the resulting solution gives the characteristic reactions of sulphates.
2. The sample solution in water gives the characteristic reaction of sodium.

***Test for purity***: It should be tested for acids, lead, arsenic, heavy metals and thiosulphate.

***Test for thiosulphate***: When the sample is heated with hydrochloric acid, an opalescence or turbidity of sulphur is formed.

$$Na_2S_2O_3 + 2HCl \longrightarrow 2NaCl + SO_2 + S + H_2O$$

$$Na_2S_2O_5 + 2HCl \longrightarrow 2NaCl + 2SO_2 + H_2O$$

***Assay:*** It is assayed by **iodimetry method of titration** (also called **redox titration**).

In this assay a the substance is dissolved in water and to this added a Known Excess Standard (KES) iodine solution. The solution is kept aside, whereby the sodium metabisulphite is oxidized by iodine to sulphate. After the completion of this reaction, the excess unreacted iodine is determined by titrating with N/10 sodium thiosulphate using starch mucilage as an indicator. End point is the disappearance of blue colour.

$$2\ I_2 + 2\ Na_2S_2O_3 \longrightarrow 2\ NaI + Na_2S_4O_6$$

***Procedure:*** Weigh accurately about 0.1 gm and dissolve in 50.0 ml 0.05M iodine, add 1 ml of hydrochloric acid and titrate the excess of iodine with 0.1M sodium thiosulphate using starch solution, added towards the end of the titration, as indicator.

***Uses:***

1. It is mainly used as an antioxidant and reducing agent, especially compounds containing substances which are readily oxidized to form colored decomposition products.
2. It is used as a stabilizing agent for injections containing adrenaline, apomorphine and sodium salicylate (phenol or catechol nucleus).
3. In ascorbic acid injection, sodium metabisulphite is used as a reducing agent.
4. It prevents the oxidation of quinine like compounds.
5. It is also acts as a preservative for acidic solutions and syrups.

***Storage:*** It should be stored in tightly closed container.

***Side effects:***

1. Oral ingestion of metabisulphite leads to gastric irritation.
2. Large doses leads to GIT upset, respiratory or circulatory failure and CNS disturbances.

## Sodium Thiosulphate I.P., B.P.

**(Synonym: Sodium hypo sulphite)**

**Mol. Formula:** $Na_2S_2O_3.\ 5H_2O$ **Mol. Weight:** 248.2

It contains not less than 99% and not more than 101% of $Na_2S_2O_3.5H_2O$.

***Preparation:***

1. *From sodium hydroxide:* Sodium thiosulphate is prepared by treating sodium hydroxide with sulphur.

$$6NaOH + 4S \longrightarrow Na_2S_2O_3 + 2Na_2S + 3H_2O$$

2. *From sodium sulphite:* It is obtained by treating sodium sulphite with powdered sulphur.

   Sodium sulphite is prepared by the reaction between sodium carbonate solution and sulphur dioxide.

$$Na_2CO_3 + 2SO_2 + H_2O \longrightarrow \underset{\text{Sodium bisulphite}}{2NaHSO_3} + CO_2\uparrow$$

$$2NaHSO_3 + Na_2CO_3 \longrightarrow \underset{\text{Sodium sulphite}}{2Na_2SO_3} + H_2O + CO_2\uparrow$$

$$Na_2SO_3 + S \longrightarrow Na_2S_2O_3$$

The excess of sulphur present is removed by filtration; the filtrate is concentrated and crystallized.

***Physical properties:*** It occurs as white or colorless large crystals or a coarse, crystalline powder, odorless, deliquescent in moist air and effloresces in dry air at 33 °C. It dissolves in its water of crystallization at about 49 °C. It is soluble in water, practically insoluble in alcohol. The solution is neutral or alkaline to litmus.

***Chemical properties:*** The sulphur atom present in sodium thiosulphate occurs in two different oxidation state (Oxidized state +6 and zero). Due to this property the compound acts as a reducing agent or as an antioxidant.

1. *Effect of heat or decomposition reaction:*
   (i) Sodium thiosulphate is heated up to 100 °C and it loses its all water yield anhydrous sodium thiosulphate.

$$Na_2S_2O_3.\ 5H_2O \xrightarrow[\Delta]{100^oC} Na_2S_2O_3 + 5H_2O$$

   (ii) When it is heated at higher temperature; it gets decomposed and yields sodium sulphide and sulphur.

$$4Na_2S_2O_3 \xrightarrow[\Delta]{>100^oC} 3Na_2SO_4 + Na_2S_5$$

$$Na_2S_5 \longrightarrow Na_2S + 4S$$

2. *Reaction with dilute acids:* Dilute mineral acids convert sodium thiosulphate in to thio sulphuric acid which decomposes to yield $SO_2$ and sulphur.

$$Na_2S_2O_3 + 2HCl \longrightarrow \underset{\text{Thio sulphuric acid}}{H_2S_2O_3} + 2NaCl$$

$$H_2S_2O_3 \longrightarrow SO_2 + S + H_2O$$

3. *Reaction with silver nitrate:* With dilute solution of sodium thiosulphate, silver nitrate gives a white precipitate, changing to yellow, brown and finally black, due to the formation of silver sulphide.

$$Na_2S_2O_3 + 2AgNO_3 \longrightarrow Ag_2S_2O_3 + 2NaNO_3$$

$$Ag_2S_2O_3 + H_2O \longrightarrow \underset{\substack{\text{Silver sulphide} \\ \text{(Black ppt)}}}{Ag_2S} + H_2SO_4$$

The concentrated solution of sodium thiosulphate solution, does not give precipitate with silver nitrate due to the high solubility of silver thiosulphate.

4. *Reaction with chlorine or halogens:*

Chlorine reacts with sodium thiosulphate to form sodium sulphate.

$$Na_2S_2O_3 + Cl_2 + H_2O \longrightarrow Na_2SO_4 + 2HCl + S$$

Sodium thiosulphate reacts with iodine to give tetrathionate. The color of iodine gets decolorized due to the formation of tetrathionate.

$$2Na_2S_2O_3 + I_2 \longrightarrow Na_2S_4O_6 + 2NaI$$

5. *Reaction with barium chloride or calcium chloride:* Sodium thiosulphate reacts with barium chloride and yields white precipitate of barium thio sulphate.

$$Na_2S_2O_3 + BaCl_2 \longrightarrow BaS_2O_3 + 2NaCl$$

It reacts with calcium chloride, forms calcium thiosulphate which is soluble in water.

$$Na_2S_2O_3 + CaCl_2 \longrightarrow CaS_2O_3 + 2NaCl$$

6. Sodium thiosulphate dissolves silver halides, so it is used in photography known as "hypo".

$$2Na_2S_2O_3 + AgBr \longrightarrow \underset{\substack{\text{Sodium argento} \\ \text{thio sulphate}}}{Na_3[Ag(S_2O_3)_2]} + NaBr$$

7. *Reaction with reducing agents:* Sodium thiosulphate acts as a reducing agent. It reduces ferric chloride solution to form a dark violet color solution, the colour disappears quickly.

$$3Na_2S_2O_3 + 2FeCl_3 \rightleftharpoons 2\,Fe(S_2O_3)_3 + 6\,NaCl$$

$$2FeCl_3 + \underset{\text{Neutral solution}}{2Na_2S_2O_3} \longrightarrow 2FeCl_2 + Na_2S_4O_6 + 2NaCl$$

***Test for identification:***

1. The aqueous solution of sample gives the characteristic reactions of sodium.
2. To the sample solution, add few drops of iodine solution. The color disappears.
3. To the sample solution, add small amount of 0.1M silver nitrate solution, gives a black precipitate of silver sulphide.

$$Na_2S_2O_3 + 2AgNO_3 \longrightarrow Ag_2S_2O_3 + 2NaNO_3$$

$$Ag_2S_2O_3 + H_2O \longrightarrow \underset{\substack{\text{Silver sulphide} \\ \text{(Black ppt)}}}{Ag_2S} + H_2SO_4$$

4. The dilute solution of sample is treated with one ml of hydrochloric acid, a gas is evolved which turns starch iodide paper blue and sulphur is precipitated.

***Test for purity:*** It should be tested for pH, arsenic, chlorides, heavy metals, sulphates, sulphites and sulphides.

**Assay**

It is assayed by **iodimetry method of titration** (also called **redox titration**).

In this assay the substance is dissolved in water in an iodine flask and titrated with 0.05M iodine solution using starch solution as an indicator which is added towards the end of the titration. End point is the appearance of blue colour. During this titration iodine is reduced to sodium iodide and sodium thiosulphate is oxidized to sodium tetrathionate. As the oxidation and reduction takes place simultaneously this is called Redox titration. The chemical reactions of this assay are shown below.

$$I_2 + \underset{\text{Sodium thiosulphate}}{2Na_2S_2O_3} \longrightarrow 2NaI + \underset{\text{Sodium tetrathionate}}{Na_2S_4O_6}$$

***Procedure***: Weigh accurately about 0.5 gm, dissolve in 20 ml of water and titrate with 0.05M iodine using starch solution, added towards the end of the titration, as an indicator.

***Uses:***

1. Sodium thiosulphate is mainly used as antidote in cyanide poisoning in combination with sodium nitrite.
2. It is a standard titrant in iodimetry and iodimetric titrations and acts as an important reducing agent.
3. Externally, along with acids it is used to treat dermatological diseases. For example: Mange, ring worm.
4. It has antifungal property, so it is used to treat pityriasis versicolour.

***Dose***: By IV/IM injection = 300 mg to 1 gm.

***Storage***: It should be stored in air tight containers, protected from moisture and light.

## Sodium Thiosulphate Injection I.P.

**(Sodium Hyposulphite Injection)**

It is a sterile solution of sodium thiosulphate in water for injection. It contains not less than 95% and not more than 105% of the stated amount of sodium thiosulphate.

***Preparation*:** A corrected quantity of sodium thiosulphate is dissolved in required quantity of water for injection and immediately sterilized by autoclave or filtration. It is covered with nitrogen, to prevent degradation by oxidation during autoclave.

***Physical properties*:** A clear, colorless solution.

***Test for identification*:**

1. The aqueous solution of sample gives the characteristic reactions of sodium.
2. To the sample solution, add few drops of iodine solution. The color disappears.
3. To the sample solution, add small amount of 0.1M silver nitrate solution, a black precipitate is formed.

$$Na_2S_2O_3 + 2AgNO_3 \longrightarrow Ag_2S_2O_3 + 2NaNO_3$$

$$Ag_2S_2O_3 + H_2O \longrightarrow Ag_2S + H_2SO_4$$

Silver sulphide
(Black precipitate)

4. The dilute solution of sample is treated with one ml of hydrochloric acid, a gas is evolved which turns starch iodide paper as blue and sulphur gets precipitated.

***Test for purity*:** It should be tested for pH, it also complies the tests stated under parenteral preparations (Injections).

**Assay**

***Principle*:** Similar to sodium thiosulphate.

***Procedure*:** To an accurately measured volume containing about 0.5 gm of sodium thiosulphate add about 20 ml of water and titrate with 0.05M iodine, using 3 ml of starch solution, added towards the end of the titration, as indicator.

***Uses*:** Sodium thiosulphate injection is mainly used in cyanide poisoning in combination with sodium nitrite.

***Dose*:** The dose of injection is equivalent to 100 mg/ml given by IV/IM route. The injection is for direct use, but it is not adjunction with prior administration of sodium nitrite, so low dose is enough.

***Storage*:** It should be stored in single dose container.

## Hypo Phosphorous Acid

This compound is discussed under **acidifiers and alkalinising agents**.

## Sodium Nitrite U.S.P.

**Mol. Formula:** $NaNO_2$ **Mol. Weight:** 68.99

It contains not less than 97% and not more than 101% $NaNO_2$ with reference to the dried basis.

***Preparation:***

*Method 1:* Sodium nitrite is prepared by heating sodium nitrate.

$$2NaNO_3 \xrightarrow{\Delta} 2NaNO_2 + O_2$$

*Method 2:* It is also prepared by heating sodium nitrate with metallic lead (lead metal) or carbon which reduces it at lower temperature.

$$NaNO_3 + Pb \longrightarrow NaNO_2 + PbO$$

$$2\,NaNO_3 + C \longrightarrow 2\,NaNO_2 + CO_2$$

The reaction mixture obtained is cooled and the product is extracted with water. The insoluble lead oxide is filtered; the filtrate is concentrated and crystallized, dried.

*Method 3:* The absorption of gases obtained from the catalytic oxidation of ammonia in sodium carbonate solution.

$$4NH_3 + 5\,O_2 \longrightarrow 4NO + 6H_2O$$

$$2Na_2CO_3 + 4NO + O_2 \longrightarrow 4NaNO_2 + 2CO_2\uparrow$$

The sodium nitrite crystals obtained by the any one of the above method is often fused and poured into moulds, which may be stick shaped.

*Method 4:* It is also obtained by heating a mixture of sodium nitrate and quicklime, passing the sulphur dioxide through the solution.

$$NaNO_3 + CaO + SO_2 \longrightarrow NaNO_2 + CaSO_4$$

***Physical properties:*** Sodium nitrite occurs as white or colorless granular powder or as a white crystal or fused mass or stick in nature. Odorless having saline taste. It is soluble in water, sparingly soluble in alcohol. Deliquescent on exposed to air, slowly oxidized and converted into sodium nitrate. The aqueous solutions are alkaline to litmus. It is incompatible with caffeine, iodides, sulphites, tannic acid, vegetable astringents and mercury.

***Chemical properties:***

1. *Reaction with metals*: Sodium nitrite reacts with metals like $Co^{3+}$, $Fe^{2+}$, $Cr^{3+}$ and $Pt^{2+}$ etc., to forms metal complexes.

For example:

$$Co^{3+} + NaNO_2 \longrightarrow Na[Co(NO_2)_6]^{3-}$$

2. Sodium nitrite solution is easily reacts with sulphuric acid and forms nitrous acid.

   (Evolution of brown fumes due to instability of liberated acid)

$$2NaNO_2 + H_2SO_4 \longrightarrow Na_2SO_4 + 2HNO_2 \longrightarrow NO + H_2O + HNO_3$$

3. Sodium nitrite acts as a reducing agent and gets oxidized in acidic medium ($KMnO_4$ or $KClO_3$).

4. *Reaction with aniline hydrochloride*: Sodium nitrite reacts with aniline hydrochloric acid at less than 15 °C and gives diazonium salt.

$$C_6H_5NH_2.HCl + NaNO_2 \longrightarrow C_6H_5N_2Cl + H_2O + NaOH$$

***Test for identification***: The solution of sample in water gives the characteristic reactions of sodium and nitrite ions.

***Test for purity***: It should be tested for chloride, sulphate, heavy metals and loss on drying.

**Assay**

***Principle***:

*Method 1:* It is assayed by **permanganometry method** of titration (also called **redox titration**).

In this assay sodium nitrite is dissolved in water and acidified with dilute sulphuric acid and potassium permanganate solution is added. Sodium nitrite reacts with sulphuric acid and forms nitrous acid, which undergo oxidation immediately by potassium permanganate. To the mixture add known excess of oxalic acid and warm up to 80 °C and the excess unreacted oxalic is determined by titrating against 0.1N potassium permanganate. Potassium permanganate is acting as a self indicator. End point is the appearance of permanent pale pink colour. As the oxidation and reduction takes place simultaneously this is called Redox titration. The chemical reactions of this assay are shown below.

$$2NaNO_2 + H_2SO_4 \longrightarrow Na_2SO_4 + HNO_2$$

$$2\ KMnO_4 + 3\ H_2SO_4 \longrightarrow K_2SO_4 + 2\ MnSO_4 + 3\ H_2O + 5(O)$$

$$5\ \begin{matrix} COOH \\ | \\ COOH \end{matrix} + 5(O) \longrightarrow 10\ CO_2 + 5\ H_2O$$

*These reactions can also be written as*

$$2\,KMnO_4 + 3\,H_2SO_4 + 5\begin{array}{c}COOH\\|\\COOH\end{array} \longrightarrow K_2SO_4 + 2\,MnSO_4 + 8\,H_2O + 10\,CO_2$$

*Method 2:* It is assayed by **iodometry method of titration** (also called **redox titration**). In this assay the substance is treated with potassium iodide and the liberated iodine is titrated with sodium thiosulphate, using starch mucilage as an indicator. End point is the disappearance of blue colour.

During this titration iodine is reduced to sodium iodide and sodium thiosulphate is oxidized to sodium tetrathionate. As the oxidation and reduction takes place simultaneously this is called Redox titration. The chemical reactions of this assay are shown below.

$$I_2 + 2Na_2S_2O_3 \longrightarrow 2\,NaI + Na_2S_4O_6$$

***Procedure*:** Dissolve 0.400 gm of sample in 100.0 ml of water. Introduce 20.0 ml of the solution, while stirring continuously and keeping the tip of the pipette below the surface of the liquid, into a conical flask containing 30.0 ml of 0.1M cerium sulphate. Immediately stopper the flask and allow to stand for 2 min. Add 10 ml of a 200 gm/l solution of potassium iodide and 2 ml of starch solution. While stirring continuously, titrate with 0.1M sodium thiosulphate until the blue colour disappears. Carry out a blank titration.

***Uses*:**

1. Sodium nitrite is mainly used for the treatment for cyanide poisoning (Antidote for cyanide poisoning) in conjugation with sodium thiosulphate.
2. It has a smooth muscle relaxant property and produce hypotensive effect.
3. It acts as a vasodilator but now a day's largely replaced by organic nitrites and nitrates i.e., nitroglycerin, isosorbide dinitrate.
4. It is also acts as a rust inhibitor for surgical instruments by immersing the instruments in dilute solution of sodium nitrite.
5. It is used as a preservative in foods such as meat.
6. Nitrites are used in urine solutions for the curing of meats and fish.

***Mechanism of action of sodium nitrite as an antidote:*** Sodium nitrite converts haemoglobin in to methaemoglobin (haemoglobin incapable of oxygen transport) and the cyanide ion combines with methaemoglobin to produce cyanomethaemoglobin which is slowly dissociates the cyanide and is converted into relatively nontoxic thiocyanate by sodium thiosulphate and excreted through kidney. Hence it is given along with sodium thiosulphate.

***Dose*:** For cyanide poisoning, 3% w/v of sodium nitrite solution is slowly infused intravenously, until 10 ml (300 mg) over a period of 3 min has been administered. Then this is followed by 25 to 50% w/v sodium thiosulphate (12.5 gm) solution is infused over a period of 10 min.

***Side effects*:** Sodium nitrite may produce nausea, vomiting, dizziness, cyanosis, headache and dyspnoea (Difficult to breathe).

***Storage*:** It should be stored in well closed container and protected from moisture.

## Nitrogen and Carbon Dioxide

These compounds are discussed under **medicinal gases**.

### 6.7.3 Desiccants

## Silica Gel

The anhydrous form of the silicic acid is called as silica gel.

***Preparation*:** This is prepared from silicic acid. Silicic acid is not obtained directly from silicon dioxide. A suitable form of silica is dissolve in hot alkali from which silicic acid gets precipitated with mineral acid. Silicic acid may be regarded as hydrated silicon dioxide. Depending on the conditions of precipitation different silicic acids are formed.

$$Na_4SiO_4 + 4HCl \longrightarrow 4NaCl + \underset{\text{Silicic acid}}{H_4SiO_4}$$

$$2H_4SiO_4 \longrightarrow \underset{\text{Disilicic acid}}{H_6Si_2O_7} + H_2O$$

$$H_4SiO_4 \longrightarrow \underset{\text{Meta silicic acid}}{H_2SiO_3} + H_2O$$

The disilicic acid and polysilicic acids are obtained by elimination of water for each additional silicic acid. These are called as silica gels.

***Properties*:** These are having large capacity for absorbing water, without loss of its amorphous structure. These are available in different grades of hydration and porosity.

***Uses:***

1. Silica gel is mainly used as desiccant, absorbent for gases, thickening and gelling agents.
2. Activated silica gel powders of desirable particle size are used extensively as stationary phases in column chromatography and thin layer chromatography (TLC).
3. It is also used as flocculating agent.
4. Desiccant grades used in laboratory may be having a trace of indicator that changes color when the gel is fully hydrated. This can be regenerated by drying for a few hours at high temperature.

### 6.7.4 Excipients

## Dibasic Calcium Phosphate I.P.

**(Synonym: Calcium hydrogen phosphate)**

**Mol. Formula:** $CaHPO_4$ (anhydrous) **Mol. Weight:** 136.1

$CaHPO_4\ 2H_2O$ (dihydrate) 172.1

It is anhydrous salt or the dihydrate form of calcium salt (contains two water molecules).

It contains not less than 98% and not more than 105% of $CaHPO_4$ for either anhydrous or dihydrate salt.

***Preparation*:**

*Method 1 (From calcium chloride)*: Dibasic calcium phosphate is prepared by the reaction between a neutral solution of calcium chloride and disodium hydrogen phosphate.

$$CaCl_2 + Na_2HPO_4 \longrightarrow CaHPO_4 + 2NaCl$$

The pH of the solution must be neutral because in the presence of alkali, tribasic calcium phosphate [$Ca_3(PO_4)_2$] is produced. Then the white, flocculant precipitate of dibasic calcium phosphate is filtered off, washed and dried.

*Method 2 (From mineral apatite)*: It is prepared by the digestion of the phosphate mineral apatite with sulphuric acid; phosphoric acid and calcium sulphate are produced. The precipitated calcium sulphate is removed by filtration. To the filtrate calculated amount of calcium hydroxide is added to give dibasic calcium phosphate.

$$\underset{\text{Phosphoric acid}}{H_3PO_4} + Ca(OH)_2 \longrightarrow CaHPO_4 \cdot 2H_2O$$

***Physical properties*:** It is a white, crystalline powder, odorless, with saline taste (slight) and stable in hydrochloric acid.

***Test for identification*:** A solution of sample in dilute nitric acid or dilute hydrochloric acid gives the characteristic reactions of calcium and phosphate ions.

***Test for purity*:** It should be tested for acid insoluble substances, arsenic, heavy metals, barium, iron, carbonates, chlorides, sulphates, nitrates, reducing substances, protineous impurities, mono calcium and tri calcium phosphate and loss on ignition.

***Test for nitrate*:** To the small amount of sample, add required amount of nitrogen free sulphuric acid, one or two drops of indigo carmine solution and boiled. There is no disappearance of blue color.

**Assay**

***Principle*:** It is assayed by **complexometry method of (Direct) titration**. For the calcium content and not for dibasic calcium phosphate.

In this assay the substance is dissolved in hydrochloric acid, triethanolamine added and the solution is then titrated against 0.05M disodium Ethylene Diamine Tetra Acetate (EDTA) using hydroxyl naphthol blue as indicator. Near the end point 1N sodium hydroxide added to adjust the pH until colour of indicator changes from red to blue. Titration continued until the colour changes to violet and then blue which persists for one minute.

In this assay calcium ions of dibasic calcium phosphate reacts with disodium EDTA, whereby the complexation takes place. As the calcium ions forms complex with disodium EDTA in this assay, it is called as complexometry method of titration. The chemical reactions of this assay are shown below.

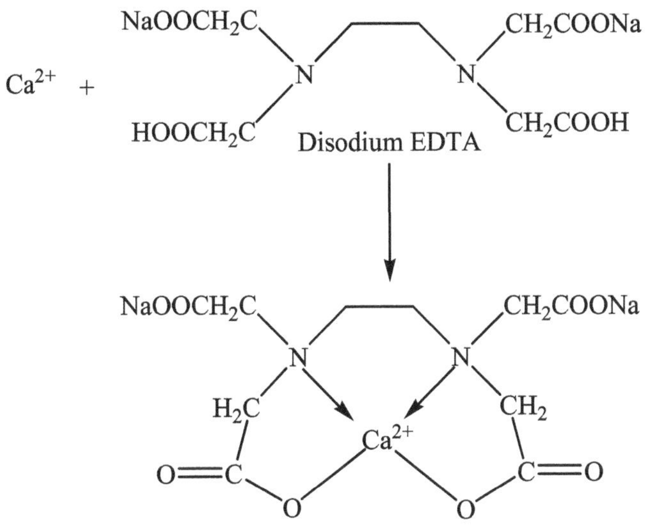

$$Ca^{2+} + \text{Disodium EDTA } [(NaOOCH_2C)(HOOCH_2C)N-CH_2-CH_2-N(CH_2COONa)(CH_2COOH)] \longrightarrow \text{Calcium-EDTA Complex}$$

Calcium-EDTA Complex

***Uses:***

1. The salt contains 1:1 ratio of calcium to phosphorous, so it is mostly recommended for calcium supplement.
2. It supplies both calcium and phosphorous, so it is useful for bone growth in children, pregnant women and lactating mothers.
3. It is also used as a pharmaceutical aid (Excipients).

***Dose:*** 1-5 gm in divided doses – as calcium supplement.

***Storage:*** It should be stored in tightly closed containers.

---

## Tribasic Calcium Phosphate I.P.

This compound is discussed under the topic **antacids**.

---

## Magnesium Stearate I.P., B.P.

Magnesium stearate mainly consists of magnesium stearate $(C_{17}H_{35}COO)_2Mg$ with variable proportions of magnesium palmitate $(C_{15}H_{31}COO)_2Mg$ and magnesium oleate $(C_{17}H_{33}COO)Mg$.

It contains not less than 3.8% and not more than 5% of Mg calculated on dried basis.

The fatty acid fraction contains not less than 40% of stearic acid and the sum of stearic acid and palmitic acid is not less than 90%.

***Preparation:*** Magnesium stearate is a mixture of magnesium salts prepared from commercial stearic acid.

*Step-1: Preparation of stearic acid:* Stearic acid required for this preparation is prepared by hydrolysis of fat and purified by separation from the low melting point fatty acids which are produced along with stearic acid.

$$C_{17}H_{35}COONa + HCl \longrightarrow C_{17}H_{35}COOH + NaCl$$

*Step-2: Preparation of sodium stearate:* A calculated quantity of stearic acid is added gradually to a hot solution of sodium hydroxide with constant stirring. The solution of sodium stearate obtained is cooled.

$$NaOH + C_{17}H_{35}COOH \longrightarrow C_{17}H_{35}COONa + H_2O$$

*Step-3: Preparation of magnesium stearate:* To the above sodium stearate solution, a calculated amount of magnesium sulphate or any other magnesium salts are added, the magnesium stearate is precipitated out, collected washed and dried.

$$2\ C_{17}H_{35}COONa + MgSO_4 \longrightarrow [C_{17}H_{35}COO]_2Mg + Na_2SO_4$$

***Physical properties*:** It is a very fine, light, white powder, odorless or with a faint odour of stearic acid, unctuous to touch and free from grittiness.

***Test for identification*:**

1. The residue obtained from peroxide free ether extract is dissolved in water, and the solution gives the characteristic reaction of magnesium ions.
2. The residue obtained from peroxide free ether extract has the freezing point not less than 53 °C.
3. The acid value of the fatty acid is in between 195 to 210.
4. It is also identified by chromatography.

***Test for purity*:** It should be tested for clarity of the solution, appearance of solution of the fatty acids, acidity or alkalinity, acid value of the fatty acids, free stearic acid, zinc stearate, heavy metals, chlorides, sulphates, iron and loss on drying.

***Test for appearance of solution of fatty acids:*** Dissolve the small amount of sample in required quantity of chloroform. The solution is clear and not more intensely colored than standard solution.

***Test for zinc stearate*:** The sample solution, or the filtrate obtained after boiling the sample with water and dilute sulphuric acid is treated with ammonium mercury thiocyanate solution and one to two drops of copper sulphate solution. Scratch the walls of the test tube with a glass rod and allow to stand for 15 minutes. No violet color precipitate is formed.

**Assay**

***Principle*:** It is assayed by **complexometry method of (Back) titration.**

In this assay the substance is dissolved in a mixture of 1-butanol, ethanol and strong ammonia solution, to this ammonia-ammonium chloride solution is added as buffer solution and Known Excess Standard (KES) 0.05N disodium Ethylene Diamine Tetra Acetate (EDTA) added to react with magnesium stearate and the excess unreacted EDTA is titrated against zinc sulphate using mordant black II as an indicator.

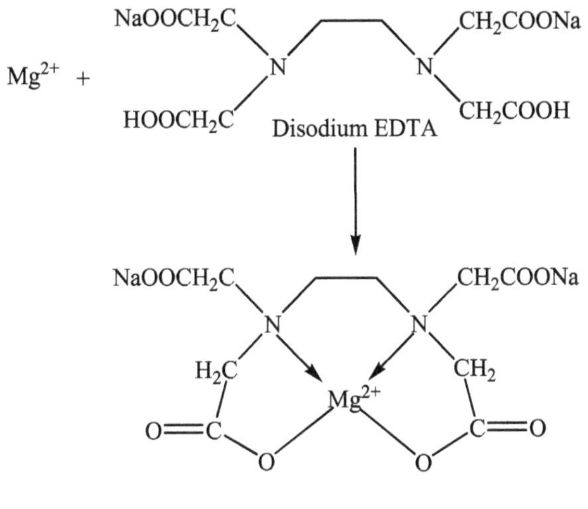

$Mg^{2+}$ + Disodium EDTA → Magnesium-EDTA Complex

Disodium EDTA

Magnesium-EDTA Complex

*Uses*:

1. It is used as dusting powder in cosmetics for skin creams, including barrier creams.
2. It is used as a lubricant for tablet manufacturing (Pharmaceutical aid).

## Talc

This compound is discussed under **topical agents (protectives)**.

## Precipitated Chalk

This compound is discussed under **antacids**.

### 6.7.5 Suspending Agents

These are otherwise called as viscosity imparting suspending agents. These agents prevent the settling and agglomeration of the particles in emulsions or suspensions by working as an energy barrier which minimizes inter particle attraction and agglomeration. Variety of inorganic substances is used as suspending agents. These agents acts as surfactants (alter the surface phenomena of solvents or protective colloids viscosity inducing agents or dispersing agents for getting the desired rheological properties Combinations of different types may be used).

## Bentonite I.P., B.P.

**(Synonym: Wilkinite)**

**Mol. Formula:** $Al_2O_3. 6SiO_2. XH_2O$

The name bentonite derives from benton formation in Wyoming, where it was first found. It is a natural, colloidal, hydrated aluminium silicate that has been processed to remove grit and non-swelling components of the ore.

It may contain calcium, iron and magnesium. The silica content is less than shown, and the water content depends upon the treatment to which the natural substance has been subjected. The most common type is volclay bentonite contains 90% montomorillonite ($Al_2Si_4O_{10}$ $(OH)_2$. $nH_2O$)

***Physical properties*:** A very fine, pale buff or cream colored to greyish white powder, free or almost free from gritty particles. It is odorless, slightly earthy taste. Insoluble in water but swells to about 12 times its volume when added to water. It neither dissolves nor swells in organic solvents.

When the bentonite is subjected to analysis, it contains small amount of ferric oxide, calcium oxide, magnesium oxide and some sodium and potassium. In an acid solution, the metallic ions are converted into hydrogen ions. Due to this reason bentonite could not be readily maintained in an acidic medium.

***Test for identification:***

1. When a sample of bentonite is fused with anhydrous sodium carbonate and extracted with water followed by repeated extractions with dilute hydrochloric acid, yields residue and the acid solution which on further neutralization gives the characteristic reaction of aluminium.
2. To the filtrate, add dilute hydrochloric acid, gelatinous precipitate is produced.

***Test for purity*:** It should be tested for pH, heavy metals, sedimentation volume, swelling power, coarse particles, microbial contamination and loss on drying.

***Test for microbial contamination*:** 1 gm of the sample is free from *E. coli.*

***Test for swelling power*:** Add required amount of sample (2 gm) in twenty portions at intervals of 2 minutes to a 100 ml of a 1% w/v solution of sodium lauryl sulphate in a 100 ml graduated cylinder about 3 cm in diameter. Allow each portion to settle by adding the next and let test for it by stand for 2 hours. The sedimentation volume is not less than 24 ml.

***Uses*:**

1. It is mainly used as a pharmaceutical aid (suspending agent).
2. It is used as a protective colloid to stabilize emulsions and emulsifier for oil in water emulsions (stabilizing agent).
3. It is the one of the ingredient of calamine lotion.
4. It is also used as a base for many preparations including plasters and ointments.

---

## Colloidal Silica B.P.

**(Synonym: Colloidal silicondioxide, Collodial anhydrous silica)**

**Mol. Formula:** $SiO_2$ **Mol. Weight:** 60.1

Colloidal silicon dioxide is submicroscopic silica prepared by the vapour phase hydrolysis of silicon compound.

It contains not less than 99% and not more than 100.5% of $SiO_2$, calculated on ignition of sample.

***Physical properties***: It is a white, fine, amorphous powder, with particle size of 15 mm. Non-gritty in nature, insoluble in water and dilute acids. It may soluble in hot dilute alkalis and yield silicates.

***Test for identification***: The required quantity of sample gives the characteristic reactions of silicates.

***Test for purity***: It should be tested for pH, arsenic, heavy metals, chlorides and loss on ignition.

**Assay**

***Principle***: It is assayed by **gravimetric method** of titration.

The residue obtained after the loss on ignition of sample is treated with one drop of sulphuric acid and ethanol. Add required amount of hydrofluoric acid, evaporate to dryness. Then add same quantity of hydrofluoric acid equal to previous one, evaporate and ignite at 1000 °C, allow cooling and weighing the residue. It should be within the limit.

***Procedure***: To the residue obtained in the test for loss on ignition add 0.2 ml of sulphuric acid and sufficient alcohol to moisten the residue completely. Add 6 ml of hydrofluoric acid and evaporate to dryness on a hot-plate at 95 °C to 105 °C, taking care to avoid loss from sputtering. Wash down the sides of the dish with 6 ml of hydrofluoric acid and evaporate to dryness. Ignite at 900 ± 50 °C, allow to cool in a desiccator and weigh. The difference between the mass of the final residue and the mass of the residue obtained in the test for loss on ignition gives the amount of $SiO_2$ in the quantity of the substance to be examined used.

***Uses***:

1. It is mainly used as tablet excipient (pharmaceutical aid), diluent or lubricant.
2. It is also used as a suspending or thickening agent for suspensions, stabilizers for some emulsions and granulating agent for some tablet formulations.
3. It is used as an anti-caking agent for granules and hygroscopic powder.

***Storage***: It should be stored in well closed containers and protected from light.

---

## Aluminium Stearate B.P., U.S.P.

**(Synonym: Aluminium monostearate)**

It consists of a mixture of aluminium mono stearate $(C_{17}H_{35}COO)_2$ Al and aluminium mono palmitate $(C_{15}H_{31}COO)_2Al$ with the aluminium content of 14.5 – 16.5% as $Al_2O_3$.

***Preparation***: Aluminium stearate is a mixture of aluminium salts prepared from commercial stearic acid.

*Step-1: Preparation of stearic acid:* Stearic acid required for this preparation is prepared by hydrolysis of fat and purified by separation from the low melting point fatty acids which are produced along with stearic acid.

$$C_{17}H_{35}COONa + HCl \longrightarrow C_{17}H_{35}COOH + NaCl$$

*Step-2: Preparation of sodium stearate:* A calculated quantity of stearic acid is added gradually to a hot solution of sodium hydroxide with constant stirring. The solution of sodium stearate obtained is cooled.

$$NaOH + C_{17}H_{35}COOH \longrightarrow C_{17}H_{35}COONa + H_2O$$

*Step-3: Preparation of aluminium stearate:* To the above sodium stearate solution, a calculated amount of aluminium sulphate or any other aluminium salts are added, the magnesium stearate is precipitated out, collected, washed and dried.

$$6C_{17}H_{35}COONa + 2Al(SO_4)_3 \longrightarrow 2[C_{17}H_{35}COO]_3Al + 3Na_2SO_4 + 3SO_2 + 3O_2$$

***Physical properties***: It occurs as a fine, white bulky powder with characteristic odour, insoluble in water and organic solvents. It is easily undergo decomposition with heat and leads to the formation of stearic and palmitic acid.

***Test for identification***: The small quantity of sample solution gives the characteristic reactions of aluminium ion.

***Test for purity***: It should be tested for arsenic, heavy metals and loss on drying.

***Assay***: Similar to that of magnesium stearate.

***Uses***:

1. When heated with fixed oils and mineral acids, it forms gel. This property is used for preparing oily gels containing medicaments.
2. It is used as gelling agents for the preparation of sterile procaine penicillin G with aluminium suspension (slow release depot preparation).

***Storage***: It should be stored in well closed containers.

## 6.7.6 Colourants

Colorants are substances that are used to provide distinct color and elegance appearance to a dosage form.

### Titanium Dioxide

This compound is discussed under **topical agents (protectives)**.

### Ferric Oxide

Two varieties of ferric oxides are commercially available. They are red and yellow ferric oxides. Both varieties are used as tinting agents or coloring agents for calamine.

***Red ferric oxide***: It is a fine powder contains 90% w/w $Fe_2O_3$.

***Preparation***: It is mainly prepared from a native, pure form of ferric oxide or from pure ferric hydroxide which are heated to a high temperature in laboratories.

***Yellow ferric oxide***: It contains 97.5% w/w of $Fe_2O_3$.

***Preparation*:** It is also obtained by heating ferrous hydroxide or ferrous carbonate.

The color or tint of the color is most possibly controlled by heating temperature, time and presence of trace substances like manganese or aluminium oxides. Sometimes the particle size also attributes the fine color. Most cosmetic manufactures prefers the red oxide for tinting calamine lotions.

---

### 6.7.7 Solvents and Vehicles

#### Purified Water I.P.

**Mol. Formula:** $H_2O$ **Mol. Weight:** 18

Purified water is prepared by ion exchange method or any other methods from suitable potable water and that it comply with all necessary requirements for the various pharmacopoeias. According to I.P. purified water is mainly used for washing purposes.

Water occurs naturally in different forms such as aerated waters, mineral water, sulphur containing water, etc. are commonly used as therapeutically. Some of the natural waters with slight curative properties are also available.

Natural water with sub-soil contains various undesirable impurities as mentioned below.

1. Dissolved minerals
2. Dissolved gases
3. Microbes and its metabolites
4. Finely suspended particles of minerals

Water obtained from rivers and lakes especially from the nearby areas of animals and human habitation gets further contamination with organic pollutants and industrial waste pollutants.

Water from municipal supply (potable water) is free from this above impurities which are removed by filtration process and this water is free from micro organism by killing them with adding chlorine to this water. In some part of earth, the water is hard due to the presence of dissolved calcium and magnesium salts which can be further converted into soft water by boiling or chemical methods or demineralization. Soft water is needed for the purpose of washing all the things.

Large amount of water is needed for hospitals and pharmaceuticals for the following purpose.

1. Washing of containers, bottles, clothes and others.
2. Preparation of drugs for internal (oral and parenterals) and external administration.

Containers and bottles for oral or external preparations are washed with potable water. But this process leaves some dissolved minerals as very fine layer during drying. This is not desirable for containers of parenteral preparations, so only purified water has to be used for washing of ampoule, vials and bottles that are used to store the parenteral preparations.

***Preparation*:** Purified water is mainly prepared from treated water (potable water or municipal water).

Three methods are used for preparing the purified water. In all these methods, the main principle is to remove all the volatile and non-volatile impurities from the potable water and kill the micro organisms which are harmful in nature. The microorganisms are eliminated by another method called sterilization.

The three methods are as follows.

1. Distillation
2. Ion exchange method
3. Reverse osmosis

1. ***Distillation*:** This process mainly eliminates the dissolved gases. Ammonia or any other alkaline gases are fixed by the addition of small quantity of dilute sulphuric acid. The still made up of natural glass or stainless steel is used for distillation. This distillation process retains some non-volatile impurities and metabolic products of micro organisms (pyrogens) in the remaining water present in the still. But these pyrogens are distilled by mechanically carried small droplets of water in the distilling steam. For preventing this, the stills are attached with traps and barriers on which water droplets are get retained and fall back in to the still. Only pure gaseous steam will pass through it.

   The initial portion of the distillate is discarded because it contains some dissolved volatile impurities and other impurities from condenser, connecting tubes, and the receiver which should be discarded.

   The freshly prepared distilled water is pure; free from microbes is stored for few hours. After about 8 to 12 hours it is not advisable to use for parenteral preparations, but could be used for oral preparations.

2. ***Ion exchange method (Deionization or Demineralization)*:** This method is suitable for large scale production of purified water. This process is done by using column which is packed with some synthetic ion exchange resins. It involves two stages,

   In first stage, by using cation exchangers, cations like calcium, magnesium, sodium are retained on the column, releases hydrogen ions from the exchanger, now the water becomes acidic.

$$CaSO_4 + H_2R \xrightarrow[\text{Resin}]{\text{Cation exchange}} Ca—R + H_2SO_4$$

   In second stage, this acidic water is passes through another one column which is packed with anionic exchanger, which is able to retains the anions and releases the hydroxyl ions.

$$\underset{\text{(acidic water)}}{H_2SO_4} + 2\,BOH \xrightarrow[\text{Resin}]{\text{Anionic exchange}} B_2SO_4 + 2\,H_2O$$

   Some strong anionic exchangers are having the ability to retains the acid and not release the hydroxyl ions. Water obtained from this column is free from ions which are controlled by checking the electrical conductivity of the water. Due to the presence of microbes and non volatile impurities in the deionized water, to remove this, the further purification process is essential. Further the exchanges are renewed or regenerated from time to time.

3. ***Reverse osmosis***: Osmosis is defined as a process by which water diffuses from the lower concentration to the high concentration region through a semi permeable membrane by osmotic pressure. If any positive pressure is applied or maintained on the high concentration region, the diffusion of water can be stopped. By increasing such pressure, the solution could be made to lose more water and across the membrane to the pure water, leaving the original solution more concentrated than previous. This is known as reverse osmosis.

   This process is mainly used for large scale production of purified water. The efficiency of the process depends upon the quality of the membrane used. These membranes are used to remove the dissolved organic impurities and pyrogens. The total equipment is properly sterilized and enclosed to eliminate further contamination; practically purified, sterile water can be obtained.

   Purified water used for the parenteral preparations can be sterilized by heat or filtration or radiation.

***Physical properties***: Purified water is a clear, colorless and odorless liquid.

***Test for purity***: It should be tested for acidity or alkalinity, ammonium, calcium and magnesium, heavy metals, chlorides, nitrates, sulphates, oxidisable substances and residue on evaporation.

***Test for acidity or alkalinity***: To the freshly boiled and cooled water separately add one or two drops of methyl red solution and bromothymol blue. No red color and no blue color are formed respectively.

***Test for ammonium***: To small amount of water, add 1 ml of alkaline potassium mercuric iodide solution, keep aside for 5 minutes. The sample is not more intense color than that of standard which is prepared as per the monograph.

***Test for calcium and magnesium***: To the required quantity of sample add ammonium chloride buffer, one drop of mordant black-II mixture and one of drop of standard EDTA solution, a pure blue color is produced.

***Test for chlorides***: The opalescence produced does not change for 15 minutes.

***Test for nitrates***: To the ice cold solution of purified water add 10% w/v of solution of potassium chloride, one drop of diphenylamine solution, and add sulphuric acid. Mix well. Blue colour produced in the test solution is not more intense than that of standard solution which is prepared as per the monograph.

***Test for oxidisable substances***: To the sample solution add sulphuric acid, one drop of potassium permanganate and allow it to boil. The solution becomes slightly pink.

***Test for residue on evaporation***: The weight of residue is not more than 1 mg.

Purified water when used for dialysis purpose and then it complies with following additional requirements.

***Test for aluminium and bacterial endotoxins*:** It should not be more than 0.25 endotoxin unit per ml.

***Uses*:**

1. Purified water is mainly used as solvent for many of the pharmaceutical preparationS.
2. It is used for the preparation of test reagents for chemical analysis and other uses.
3. It has been the water of choice for various types of extemporaneous preparations in compounding.
4. When distilled water is demanded, purified water shall be supplied or dispensed, which is not intended for parenteral preparations.

---

## Water for Injection I.P., B.P., U.S.P.

**Mol. Formula:** $H_2O$ **Mol. Weight:** 18

Water for injection is intended for use in the preparation of medicines for parenteral administration when water is used as a vehicle (water for injection in bulk) and for dissolving or diluting substances or preparations of injectables (sterile water for injections).

### Water for Injections in Bulk

***Production*:** It is produced by distilling potable water or purified water by using a neutral glass, quartz or suitable metal still fitted with an effective device for preventing the entrapment of droplets (The still must maintain the production of apyrogenic water). The first portion of the distillate is discarded as it may contain volatile impurities and the remainder is collected and stored in containers, which prevents the growth of microorganisms and other contaminations.

During the storage and production, it is recommended that adequate measures are taken to ensure that the microbial quality is controlled and monitored.

When water for injection free from carbon dioxide is needed, the distillate is boiled for 10 minutes with a little exposure to air, cooled and stored in final container and sterilized by heating in an autoclave.

***Physical properties*:** It occurs as a clear, colorless and odorless solution.

***Test for purity*:** It should be tested for acidity or alkalinity, calcium, magnesium, ammonium, chloride, heavy metals, sulphates, nitrates, aluminium and bacterial endotoxins.

***Storage and labeling*:** It should be stored in designed containers to prevent the growth of microbes. The label on the container should shows that the content is not been sterilized.

## Sterile Water for Injection I.P.

It is water for injections in bulk that is distributed in suitable containers of glass or any other materials, sealed and sterilized by heating in an autoclave or filtration method to ensure that the water complies with the test for bacterial endotoxins. It should free from any added substances.

***Physical properties***: It is a clear, colorless, odorless liquid.

***Test for purity***: It should be tested for appearance of solution, acidity or alkalinity, ammonium, calcium and magnesium, heavy metals, chlorides, sulphate, nitrate, oxidisable substances, residue on evaporation, particulate contamination, test for sterility and bacterial endotoxins.

***Uses***: It is used as a solvent for preparing parenteral solutions.

***Storage***: It should be stored in single dose containers of not larger than one liter.

---

### 6.7.8 Filter Aids

Filter aids are special type of filter medium which forms a fine surface deposit that screens out all solids, preventing them from contacting and plugging the supporting filter medium. These are acts by forming a highly porous and non compressible cake that retains solids.

The ideal filter aid produces their effect by mechanically or physically.

***Ideal characteristics of filter aids:***

1. It should be free from impurities.
2. It should be an inert to the liquid material to be filtered.
3. It should have a structure that allows the formation of porous cake.
4. It should be able to remains suspended in the liquid.

Filter aids usually or normally selected to given acceptable filtrate at the highest flow rate.

## Talc

This compound is discussed under **topical agents (protectives)**.

---

## Light Kaolin

This compound is discussed under **topical agents (protectives)**.

---

## Kieshelguhr

Kieselguhr is a pure silicon dioxide and is found as deposits in certain parts of the world. It is otherwise called as diatomaceous earth because it may be formed from diatoms. It is included in the appendix to the pharmacopoeia.

***Preparation*:** The native form of kieselguhr is purified, washed carefully with acids and calcinations to obtain rid of organic matter which is known as purified siliceous earth.

***Physical properties*:** It is neutral in reaction and is a very fine powder, slightly gritty and is capable of absorbing fluid.

It is available in two forms, kieselguhr G and kieselguhr H, Both forms are have a particle size of 10 to 40 μm. Kieselguhr G contains 15% of calcium sulphate hemihydrate. Both forms are present in appendix of Indian pharmacopoeia.

***Uses:***

1. It is extensively used as filtering aid for liquid pharmaceuticals because it does not absorb active ingredients present in the formulations.
2. It is also used in dusting powders up to certain extent.
3. It is used as stationary phases in thin layer chromatography.

---

### Fullers Earth U.S.P.

It is a native hydrated aluminum silicate associated with native calcium carbonate.

***Physical properties:*** It is a fine, white to grey color, odorless, tasteless powder, smooth to touch, insoluble in water and organic solvents, partially soluble in hydrochloric acid.

***Uses:***

1. It is a good adsorbent, due to this property it is used in chromatographic techniques and used as decolorizing agent.
2. It is also used in lotion which are used for eczema, dermatitis and also in powerful insecticidal poisoning.
3. It is used as a filtering aid in industry and it is the one of the ingredient of toilet powders and dusting powders.

## 6.7.9 Preservatives

Preservatives are naturally occurring or synthetic compounds which are added to products such as foods, pharmaceuticals, biological samples, etc. to prevent the decomposition by chemical changes or by microbial growth.

***Types of preservatives*:** Preservatives are classified in to two types.

1. Class I preservatives.
2. Class II preservative.

***Class I preservatives*:** These are naturally occurring substances. For example: Salt, sugar, honey, vinegar, alcohol, hops, castor oil, diatomaceous earth, citrus juice, citric acid and ascorbic acid.

***Class II preservatives*:** These are manufactured by synthetic methods.

| Compound name | Molecular formula |
|---|---|
| Sodium bisulphite | $NaHSO_3$ |
| Sodium meta bisulphite | $Na_2S_2O_5$ |
| Sodium sulphite | $Na_2SO_3.7H_2O$ |
| Sodium propionate | $Na(C_2H_3COO)$ |
| Sodium nitrite | $NaNO_3$ |
| Sodium acetate | $CH_3COONa$ |
| Sodium diacetate | $NaH(C_2H_3O_2)_2$ |
| Potassium nitrate | $KNO_3$ |
| Potassium nitrite | $KNO_2$ |
| Potassium hydrogen sulphide | $KHSO_3$ |
| Carbondioxide | $CO_2$ |
| Sulphur dioxide | $SO_2$ |
| Disodium EDTA | |
| Parabens | |

## 6.7.10 Sclerosing Agents

These are irritants, cause inflammation, coagulation and ultimately fibrosis, when injected into haemorrhoids (piles) or varicose vein mass. Used only for local injection.

*Example:*

1. Phenol (5%) in almond oil (2-5 ml).
2. Polidocanol (3%) (2 ml).

These sclerosing agents, when injected locally to varicose veins and into piles, will cause local inflammation and obliterate these veins.

### Sodium Tetra Decyl Sulphate B.P.

**(Synonym: STS, Sotradecol)**

**Mol. Formula:** $C_{14}H_{29}NaSO_4$ **Mol. Weight:** 316.43

***Preparation*:** It is prepared by treating meristyl alcohol with chlorosulphonic acid which gives the ester of hydrogen sulphate which is neutralized with sodium carbonate.

***Physical properties*:** It occurs as white waxy solid, soluble in water and organic solvents.

***Uses*:**

1. It is commonly used in the treatment of varicose and spider veins of the leg during sclerotherapy. It is used in the concentration of 0.1 to 0.3%.
2. It is also used in anionic surfactants.
3. It is also used as a wetting agent to spread topical antibiotics.

## Hypertonic Saline I.P.

**(Synonym: Sodium chloride hypertonic injection)**

Sodium chloride hypertonic injection is a sterile 1.6% w/v solution of sodium chloride in water for injection. It contains no antimicrobial agents.

It contains not less than 1.52% w/v and not more than 1.68% w/v of sodium chloride.

***Physical properties*:** A clear, colorless solution.

***Test for identification*:** It gives the characteristic reactions of sodium and chloride ions.

***Test for purity*:** It should be tsted for pH, heavy metals, bacterial endotoxins, other tests for parenteral preparations.

***Assay*:** Similar to sodium chloride injection.

***Procedure*:** To an accurately measured volume containing about 0.16 gm of sodium chloride in a glass-stoppered flask add 50 ml of water and 50.0 ml of 0.1M silver nitrate, 5 ml of 2M nitric acid and 2 ml of dibutyl phthalate. Shake well and titrate with 0.1M ammonium thiocyanate using 2 ml of ferric ammonium sulphate solution as indicator, until the colour becomes reddish yellow.

***Storage*:** Similar to sodium chloride injection.

***Use*:** Similar to sodium chloride injection.

## PROBABLE QUESTIONS

1. Define the term antioxidants? Enumerate commonly used antioxidants, their chemistry, properties and specific uses.
2. Write in detail about any two official antioxidants.
3. Explain the method of preparation, properties, assay and uses of hypo phosphorous acid.
4. Write the mechanism of action of antioxidants.
5. Explain about any two sodium compounds which are used as antioxidants.

6. Write briefly about the importance of antioxidants in pharmaceutical substance storage.
7. Explain the assay methods of following compounds.
   (a) Sodium nitrite (b) Sodium thio sulphate
   (c) Sodium bisulphite
8. Define desiccants and explain about silica gel.
9. Define excipients and enumerate the official excipients.
10. Explain about dibasic calcium phosphate and tri basic calcium phosphate.
11. Write about the preparation, properties, test for identification, purity test, assay and uses of magnesium stearate.
12. Enumerate the inorganic excipients used in solid form. Explain their properties and uses.
13. Define suspending agents. List out the official suspending agents.
14. Explain about bentonite.
15. Write the preparation, properties, identification tests, test for purity, assay and uses of the following.
    (a) Colloidal silica (b) Aluminium stearate
16. Write a note on suspending agents.
17. What is meant by colorants explain with examples.
18. Explain in detail about titanium dioxide.
19. Write in detail about two types of ferric oxide and its applications.
20. Define solvent and vehicles with examples?
21. Write about the important method of preparation of purified water?
22. Explain about the following.
    (a) Distillation (b) Ion exchange method or demineralization
    (c) Reverse osmosis
23. Define filter aids.
24. Write in detail about the followings
    (a) Kieselguhr (b) Fullers earth
25. Define preservatives and classify them with examples.
26. List out the important inorganic preservatives used in pharmaceuticals.

## 6.8 MISCELLANEOUS AGENTS

### 6.8.1 Expectorants

**Introduction:** Cough is physiologically useful protective reflex that removes the respiratory irritants and accumulated fluid from the respiratory tract due to infection plural diseases and malignancy. The cough may be protective tenacious cough or non protective cough (day cough). The protective cough is characterized by the presence of excessive sputum due to bronchitis.

Expectorants increase the production of respiratory tract secretions which coats the irritated mucosa. As the secretions become thin and less viscid, they can be easily coughed out. These are also called as 'mucokinetic agents' and are used to treat cough that results from irritation of the respiratory mucosa. They may be act as mentioned below:

Expectorants increases the secretions directly or reflexly according to this, they are classified in to two.

***Direct stimulants*:** When inhaled along with steam, these are increased respiratory tract secretions. Example: Volatile oils such as eucalyptus oil, alcohol and cidar wood oil.

***Reflux stimulants*:** These are gastric irritants and reflexly increase respiratory secretion. These are taken orally.

Ammonium salts like ammonium chloride acts both directly and reflexly to increases respiratory secretion. In large doses of ammonium chloride leads to metabolic acidosis.

#### Potassium Citrate I.P., B.P.

This compound is discussed under **antacids**.

---

#### Potassium Iodide I.P., B.P., U.S.P.

**Mol. Formula:** KI **Mol. Weight:** 166

It contains not less than 99% and not more than 100.5% of potassium iodide, with reference to the dried basis.

***Preparation*:** Potassium iodide is manufactured by the process which is similar to that of potassium bromide and also for sodium iodide.

*Method 1: Industrial preparation:* It is obtained by the action of iodine on moist iron filling to form ferro-ferric iodide, which is then decomposed by potassium carbonate. Ferro ferric oxide is removed by filtration.

$$3Fe + 4I_2 \longrightarrow \underset{\text{Ferro ferric iodide}}{FeI_2.\ 2FeI_3}$$

$$FeI_2.\ 2FeI_3 + 4K_2CO_3 \longrightarrow 8KI + FeO.Fe_2O_3 + 4CO_2$$

The filtrate obtained is evaporated to dryness, potassium iodide gets crystallized out.

*Method 2: From potassium hydroxide:* Potassium iodide is prepared by treating a hot aqueous solution of potassium hydroxide with slight excess of iodine to form potassium iodide and potassium iodate mixture.

$$6KOH + 3I_2 \longrightarrow \underset{\text{Potassium iodide-iodate mixture}}{5KI + KIO_3} + 3H_2O$$

The resulting solution is then treated with excess amount of charcoal powder followed by evaporated to dryness and ignited. The charcoal reduces the iodate to iodide. The product obtained is lixiviated with water. Then it is filtered and crystallized.

$$KIO_3 + 3C \longrightarrow KI + 3CO\uparrow$$

***Physical properties***: It is a colorless, transparent or opaque crystals or white powder, odorless, bitter taste. It is deliquescent in moist air. It is freely soluble in water (1 in 0.7 ml), glycerin, alcohol and acetone. The potassium iodide is added to water for the preparation of its solution, the temperature of the solution is decreased. Iodine is readily soluble in potassium iodide solution due to the formation potassium polyiodide. Potassium iodide is incompatible with metal salts, potassium chlorate, oxidizing agents, mineral acids and alkaloids.

$$KI + I_2 \longrightarrow \underset{\text{Potassium triiodide}}{KI_3} \xrightarrow{I_2} \underset{\text{Potassium polyiodide}}{KI_5}$$

***Test for identification***: The sample solution in carbon dioxide free water gives the characteristic reactions of potassium and iodide ions.

***Test for purity***: It should be tested for color and clarity of the solution, alkalinity, arsenic, heavy metals, iron, barium, cyanide, iodate, sulphates, thiosulphate and loss on drying.

***Test for cyanide***: To the sample solution, add one drop of ferrous sulphate solution and one drop of sodium hydroxide solution, acidified with hydrochloric acid and warm the solution. No blue color is produced.

***Test for thiosulphate***: To the small quantity of sample solution, add one or two drops of starch solution and add 0.005M iodine solution, blue color is produced.

**Assay**

***Principle***: It is assayed by **Andrew's method of titration** (also called iodometry method, redox titration).

In this assay the diluted solution was acidified by treating with hydrochloric acid and titrated with standard potassium iodate solution until the brown colour turns into light brown. At this stage a small amount of chloroform is added to it and the titration continued until the disappearance of colour in chloroform layer and the supernatant layer becomes clear yellow, starch mucilage cannot be used as an indicator due to the use of high concentration of hydrochloric acid, which prevents the hydrolysis of iodine monochloride (ICl). As the oxidation and reduction takes place simultaneously this is called redox titration. In this assay, potassium iodide is oxidized to iodine by potassium iodate in presence of HCl. This liberated iodine is converted to iodine monochloride.

Iodine is more soluble in chloroform than water. After the reaction of free iodine at aqueous layer the iodine may be available at chloroform layer. Hence upon each addition after the aqueous layer becomes colourless, the flask should be shaken well to allow iodine in chloroform layer to react with potassium iodate.

$$2\,KIO_3 + 6\,HCl + KI \longrightarrow 3\,KCl + 3\,ICl + 3\,H_2O$$

***Procedure*:** Weigh accurately about 0.35 gm, dissolve in about 10 ml of water, add 35 ml of hydrochloric acid and 5 ml of chloroform. Titrate with 0.05M potassium iodate until the purple colour of iodine disappears from the chloroform. Add the last portion of the iodate solution drop wise and agitate vigorously and continuously. Allow to stand for 5 minutes. If any colour develops in the chloroform layer continue the titration until the chloroform is decolorized.

***Uses*:**

1. Potassium iodide is mainly used as an anti thyroid, antifungal and expectorant.
2. It is internally used as an iodine source, so it is added to the common salt.
3. It is also finds to used as a saline diuretic.
4. In laboratory, it is used to prepare iodine solutions and reducing agent.
5. It is also used to prepare the reagents containing complex iodides (Potassium mercuric iodide, potassium bismuth iodide etc.).
6. It is the major source of iodine for pre-operative hypothyroidism.
7. Large doses or prolonged uses lead to increased salivation, pain, metallic taste and coryza.
8. It is necessary for the secretion of thyroid hormone.

***Dose*:** As expectorant - 250 to 500 mg.

In preoperative treatment of thyrotoxicosis - 30 to 60 mg

***Storage*:** It should be stored in well closed containers and protected from light and moisture.

---

## Sodium Iodide B.P., U.S.P.

**Mol. Formula:** NaI **Mol. Weight:** 149.9

It contains not less than 99% and not more than 100.5% NaI.

***Preparation*:** It is prepared by treating iodine with slight excess of concentrated sodium hydroxide solution, sodium iodide and sodium iodates are formed. The pale yellow solution formed is evaporated to dryness, and the residue obtained is heated with charcoal to reduce the iodate. It is crystallized above 20 °C.

$$6NaOH + 3I_2 \rightarrow NaIO_3 + 5NaI + 3H_2O$$

$$NaIO_3 + 3C \longrightarrow NaI + 3CO\uparrow$$

***Physical properties***: It occurs as colorless, odourless crystals or white crystalline powder, deliquescent in nature and forms brown tint. It is very soluble in water, freely soluble in alcohol and glycerin.

***Test for identification***: The sample solution gives the characteristic reactions of sodium and iodide ions.

***Test for purity***: It should be tested for alkali, barium, arsenic, cyanide, lead, iodate, sulphate and loss on drying.

**Assay**

***Principle***: Similar to that of potassium iodide solution.

***Procedure***: Dissolve 1.300 gm in water and dilute to 100.0 ml with the same solvent. To 20.0 ml of the solution add 40 ml of hydrochloric acid and titrate with 0.05M potassium iodate until the colour changes from red to yellow. Add 5 ml of chloroform and continue the titration, shaking vigorously, until the chloroform layer is decolorized.

*Uses*:

1. It is mainly used as source of iodine, mostly for hyperthyroidism.
2. It also used as a solvent of iodine in iodine tincture and iodine solution.

***Dose***: 300 mg to 2gm daily by oral route.

1 gm by intravenous infusion.

---

## Ammonium Chloride

This compound is discussed under **acidifiers and alkalinising agents**.

---

## Ammonium Acetate U.S.P.

**Mol. Formula:** $CH_3COONH_4$ **Mol. Weight:** 77

***Preparation***: It is prepared by mixing ammonia solution with acetic acid (neutralization reaction).

$$NH_3 + CH_3COOH \rightarrow CH_3COONH_4$$

***Physical properties***: It occurs as colorless crystals or crystalline masses, deliquescent in nature. It has the odor of acetic acid. It is very soluble in water and alcohol.

***Test for identification***: The sample solution gives the characteristic reactions of ammonium and acetate ions.

***Test for purity***: It should be tested for arsenic, heavy metals, sulphated ash and loss on drying.

***Uses*:**

1. The dilute solution of sample is used as diuretic and mild expectorant.
2. It also shows mild diaphoretic action.

***Storage*:** It should be stored in a well closed container and protected from moisture.

## Ammonium Carbonate

This compound is discussed under **medicinal gases.**

## 6.8.2 Sedatives

***Introduction*:** Sedatives are central nervous system depressants that reduce excitement, tension, and produce relaxation. Hypnotics are drugs that depress the CNS and produce sleep. Same drug can act as sedative and hypnotic. At lower dose, the drug may act as sedative and at a higher dose act as hypnotic.

Sedative and hypnotic drugs are frequently used in preanaesthetic medication and as an adjunctive therapy in psychiatry. Sedatives and hypnotics are also used as the following:

- Muscle relaxants
- General anaesthetics
- Antianxiety agents
- Anticonvulsants
- Adjuvant to anaesthesia
- Co-drugs in the treatment of hypertension

### Potassium Bromide I.P.

**Mol. Formula:** KBr **Mol. Weight:** 119

It contains not less than 98% and not more than 100.5% of KBr which is calculated on dried basis.

***Preparation*:**

*Method 1*: KBr is obtained by adding bromine solution into a concentrated potassium hydroxide solution to yield potassium bromide – potassium bromate complex.

$$6KOH + 3Br_2 \longrightarrow \underbrace{KBrO_3 + 5KBr}_{\text{Potassium bromide-bromate complex}} + 3H_2O$$

The pale yellow solution obtained is evaporated to dryness. The residue obtained is heated with charcoal for reducing potassium bromate to potassium bromide, which is then extracted with water. Filter the solution, evaporate to dryness and collect the crystals.

$$KBrO_3 + 3C \longrightarrow KBr + 3\,CO\uparrow$$

*Method 2*: Potassium bromide is also prepared by treating moist iron foils with bromine.

$$3Fe + 4Br_2 \longrightarrow \underset{\text{Ferroso ferric bromide}}{Fe_3Br_8}$$

The ferroso ferric bromide obtained is boiled with potassium carbonate solution and filtered. The filtrate is evaporated to dryness. The residue obtained is extracted with water and then recrystallized.

$$Fe_3Br_8 + 4K_2CO_3 + 4H_2O \longrightarrow 8KBr + Fe_3(OH)_8 + 4CO_2$$

***Physical properties***: It is a colorless, transparent or opaque crystals or white powder, odorless and has saline, bitter taste. It is deliquescent in moist air. It is freely soluble in water (1 in 0.7 ml), glycerin, alcohol and acetone. It melts at 768 $^0$C, but slowly volatilizes at high temperature with partial decomposition.

***Chemical properties***: *Reaction with silver or mercury or cuprous or lead salts:* Potassium bromide reacts with silver nitrate gives silver bromide.

$$AgNO_3 + KBr \longrightarrow AgBr\downarrow + KNO_3$$

In the presence of acid media, it liberates bromine from bromate.

$$BrO_3^- + 5Br^- + 6H^+ \longrightarrow 3\,Br_2 + 3\,H_2O$$

***Test for identification***: The aqueous solution of sample gives the characteristic reaction of potassium and bromide.

***Test for purity***: It should be tested for arsenic, barium, iron, lead, sodium, bromate, sulphate, alkali and loss on drying.

***Test for bromate***: To the sample solution, add dilute sulphuric acid, no yellow color is produced.

**Assay**

***Principle***: It is assayed by **precipitation method of (Back) titration** by (**Modified Volhard's method**).

In this assay the substance is dissolved in water and acidified with nitric acid and to this a Known Excess Standard (KES) silver nitrate added and silver bromide is precipitated to this nitrobenzene added and the Excess Unreacted (EUR) silver nitrate is back titrated against 0.1N ammonium thiocyanate. Ferric ammonium sulphate (Ferric alum) is used as an indicator. End point is the appearance of brick red colour.

During this assay, potassium bromide reacts with silver nitrate and forms silver bromide. After completion of this reaction, the Excess Unreacted silver nitrate is determined by titrating against ammonium thiocyanate. After the completion of this reaction, further addition of ammonium thiocyanate reacts with the indicator ferric ammonium sulphate and yield brick red colour ferric thiocyanate, which is the end point. Nitrobenzene used in this assay prevents interaction of silver bromide with ferric thiocyanate. As the test substance is converted to a precipitate during this assay this is called precipitation method. The chemical reactions of this assay are shown below.

$$AgNO_3 + KBr \longrightarrow AgBr\downarrow + KNO_3$$

$$AgNO_3 + NH_4SCN \longrightarrow AgSCN\downarrow + NH_4NO_3$$

$$6\,NH_4SCN + Fe(SO_4)_3(NH_4)_2SO_4 \longrightarrow \underset{\text{Brick Red colour}}{2\,Fe(SCN)_3} + 4\,(NH_4)_2SO_4$$

***Procedure***: Dissolve 2.0 gm in water and dilute to 100.0 ml with the same solvent. To 10.0 ml of the solution add 50 ml of water, 5 ml of dilute nitric acid, 25.0 ml of 0.1M silver nitrate and 2 ml of nitrobenzene. Shake. Titrate with 0.1M ammonium thiocyanate, using 2 ml of ferric ammonium sulphate solution as indicator and shaking vigorously towards the endpoint.

***Uses***:

1. It is mainly used as a sedative. The bromide ion is responsible for the central depression effect.
2. It is also used for the treatment of mental excitement. Large doses are producing definite action upon the heart.
3. It is used for the treatment of nervousness, insomnia and seizures of epilepsy.

***Side effects***: Potassium bromide is a toxic substance, slow accumulation of bromide in the body causes excessive depression of central nervous system.

### 6.8.3 Antidotes

**Introduction:** Antidotes may be defined as those substances which react specifically with an ingested poison or toxic substance or an overdose of a potent drug. A 'Poison' is a substance that causes disturbances to organism, usually by chemical reaction or by other action at molecular state, when a sufficient quantity is absorbed. Antidotes act by antagonizing the drug or by neutralizing the poison or by converting toxic drug into a non-toxic metabolite.

***Types of antidotes***: According to their mechanism of action antidotes are classified into three ways.

1. Physiological antidotes
2. Chemical antidotes
3. Mechanical antidotes

***Physiological antidotes***: These agents act by counteracting or neutralizing the effect of poisonous substances or by counteracting the effect of poison. For example, sodium nitrite.

***Chemical antidote*:** These are acts by changing the chemical nature of the poison. Example: Sodium thio sulphate.

***Mechanical antidote*:** These agents act by preventing the absorption of poison in to the body. Example: Activated charcoal, magnesium sulphate and cupric sulphate.

Poisoning into the body occurs due to intentional (suicide), accidental, homicidal or occupational reasons. It includes inhalation of air pollutants (carbon monoxide, ozone, $SO_2$ etc.) or industrial solvents (chloroform, methanol, gasoline, benzene etc.) or insecticides and pesticides or herbicides or environmental hazards (cyanide fumes from burning plastics and asbestos) or heavy metal poisons (lead arsenic, mercury salts etc.).

Inorganic drugs which are used for the treatment of poisoning are sodium nitrite, sodium thiosulphate, EDTA etc. The inorganic chelating agents are also used for the treatment of heavy metal poisoning. For example EDTA, calcium disodium edetate is used as an antidote for lead poisoning.

***Cyanide poisoning*:** Cyanide poisoning occurs by the combination of cyanide ion ($CN^-$) to the ferric ion of cytochrome oxidase which inhibits electron transfer and cellular respiration or oxidation reduction reaction. Antidotes used for the treatment of cyanide poisoning are sodium nitrite and sodium thiosulphate.

***Mechanism of action of sodium nitrite*:** Administration of sodium nitrite by intravenous route causes the oxidation of the ferrous ion of haemoglobin to the ferric ion of methaemoglobin which then combines with serum cyanide that does not entered in to the cell.

Following the sodium nitrite, sodium thiosulphate is given by slow I.V. infusion. The thiosulphate ion reacts with cyanide to gives non toxic thiocyanate ion which is excreted through urine. This is catalyzed by the enzyme rhodanese. This reaction is reversed by thiocyanate oxidase enzyme so the toxic symptoms are reversed during initial antidotal therapy.

$$Na_2S_2O_3 + CN^- \underset{SCN^- \text{ Oxidase}}{\overset{\text{Rhodanese}}{\rightleftharpoons}} \underset{\text{Thiocyanate}}{SCN^-} + Na_2SO_3$$

Dicobalt edetate is a more specific antidote for cyanide poisoning. It directly reacts with cyanide ions to gives a non stable, non toxic cobalt cyanoedetate complex which is excreted through kidney.

***Caution*:** Both of the above drugs (sodium nitrite and dicobalt edetate) are toxic. So their usage is recommended only when cyanide poisoning is confirmed.

## Sodium Nitrite U.S.P.

This compound is discussed under **antioxidants**.

### Sodium Thiosulphate

This compound is discussed under **antioxidants**.

---

### Sodium Thiosulphate Injection

This compound is discussed under **antioxidants**.

---

### Charcoal

This compound is discussed under **adsorbents**.

---

## 6.8.4 Respiratory Stimulants

***Introduction***: These drugs stimulate respiration and can recover patient from coma or fainting. So, they can be used in conditions like

1. Apnoea in premature infant
2. Failure to ventilate spontaneously after general anaesthesia

Organic drugs like Doxapram acts as respiratory stimulants by promoting excitation of central neurons.

### Ammonium Carbonate U.S.P.

This compound is discussed under **medicinal gases**.

---

### Aromatic Spirit of Ammonia U.S.P.

This compound is discussed under **acidifiers and alkalinising agents**.

---

### Dilute Ammonia Solution I.P., B.P.

This compound is discussed under **acidifiers and alkalinising agents**.

---

## 6.8.5 Emetics

**Introduction:** These are inorganic drugs which induces vomiting. Vomiting is a forceful expulsion of gastric contents through mouth due to mass antiperistalsis. It can be valuable and life saving physiological response to remove ingested toxic substances. But it is an unwanted one for chemotherapy. Vomiting mainly occurs due to the stimulation of vomiting center which is present in the lateral medulla efferent from this center, when stimulated leads to stimulation of phrenic nerve supply to the diaphragm and of somatic nerve supply to the muscles of abdomen to induce emesis.

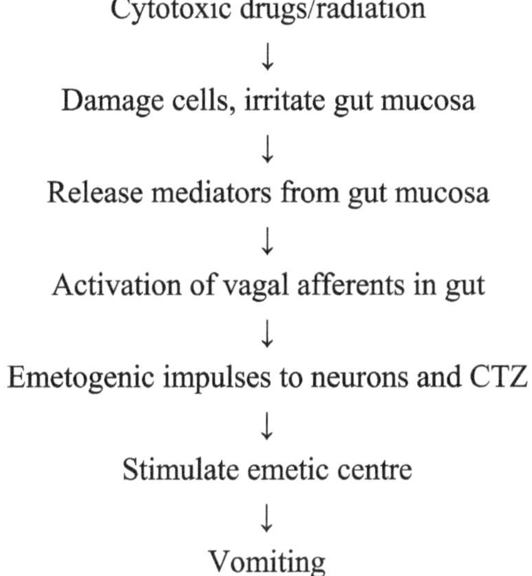


Drugs like apomorphine and Ipecacuanha acts as emetics when given orally or i.v. route by acting on chemoreceptor trigger zone (CTZ). Mostly 'emetics' are used in conditions like drug overdoses, poisoning (heavy metal poisoning, pesticide poisoning and etc.).

## Potassium Antimony Tartarate B.P., U.S.P.
## or
## Antimony Potassium Tartarate
**(Synonym:Tartar emetic)**

**Mol.Formula:** $C_4H_4KO_7Sb.2H_2O$ **Mol. Weight:** 360.96

Chemically it is available in unimolecular or bimolecular formula.

***Structural Formula*:** The approximate composition of this compound is $C_4H_4KO_7$ $Sb.1/2H_2O$.

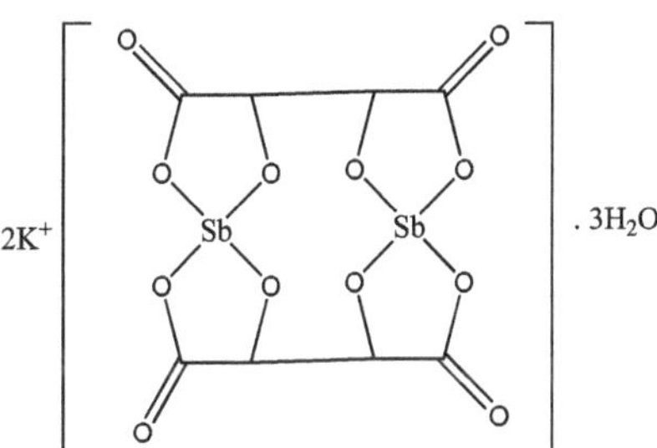


It contains not less than 99% and not more than 103% of potassium antimony tartarate.

***Preparation*:** Antimony potassium tartarate is prepared by mixing 5 parts of antimonous oxide with 6 parts of finely powdered potassium acid tartarate in to a paste with water and kept aside for one day. Then 40 parts of water is added and the mixture is boiled for 15 min, with continuous stirring. The hot liquid is filtered and the filtrate is allowed to crystallize. The crystals are collected on the filter paper and dried at a room temperature. A further crop may be obtained by concentrating the mother liquor.

$$2KHC_4H_4O_6 + Sb_2O_3 \longrightarrow 2K(SbO)C_4H_4O_6 + H_2O$$

***Physical properties*:** It forms colorless crystals, odorless with sweetish taste. It is soluble in 13 parts of water. The advantage of this salt over the other inorganic antimony salt is that this slightly acidic and on dilution it does not deposit as insoluble basic compound or being boiled with water on exposure to air, it effloresces.

***Test for identification*:**

1. The small amount of sample is heated, it chars, emits the odour similar to that of burning sugar and leaves a black residue. When the residue is introduced in to a non luminous flame, the flame is tinted violet.
2. The sample solution acidified with hydrochloric acid and hydrogen sulfide produces an orange red precipitate which is soluble in ammonium sulfide and sodium hydroxide solution.
3. The aqueous solution of the sample gives the characteristic reactions of potassium, antimony and tartarate ions.

***Test for purity*:** It should be tested for acidity or alkalinity, arsenic, lead and loss on drying.

**Assay**

***Principle*:** It is assayed by **iodimetry method of titration** (also called **redox titration**).

In this assay the substance is dissolved in water and treated with sodium bicarbonate or sodium borate and titrated with N/10 iodine solution using starch mucilage as an indicator. End point is the appearance of blue colour. During this titration iodine oxidizes the antimony potassium tartarate (antimonious to antimonic state). The sodium bicarbonate or sodium borate is used to neutralize the acid (hydroiodic acid) formed in the reaction which enables the reaction to complete. As the oxidation and reduction takes place simultaneously this is called Redox titration. The chemical reactions of this assay are shown below.

$$2\,C_4H_4O_7SbK + 3\,H_2O + 2\,I_2 \longrightarrow 2\,KHC_4H_4O_6 + Sb_2O_5 + 4\,HI$$

***Procedure*:** Dissolve about 500 mg of antimony potassium tartarate, accurately weighed, in 50 ml of water, add 5 gm of potassium sodium tartarate, 2 gm of sodium borate, and 3 ml of starch, and immediately titrate with 0.1N iodine until the appearance of blue color.

***Uses*:**

1. It is mainly used as an emetic due to its irritant action on the gastric mucosa.
2. It is also used to treat schistosomiasis and administered by I.V. injection.

***Storage*:** It should be stored in well closed container and protected from light.

---

## Sodium Antimony Tartarate B.P.

**Mol. Formula:** $C_4H_4O_7SbNa$ **Mol. Weight:** 308.8

***Preparation*:** It is prepared by mixing 5 parts of antimonous oxide with 6 parts of finely powdered sodium acid tartarate to make a paste with water, kept aside for one day. Then add 40 parts of water and the resulting mixture is boiled for 15 minutes with continuous stirring. The hot liquid is filtered and the crystals are collected.

$$2NaHC_4H_4O_6 + Sb_2O_3 \longrightarrow 2Na(SbO)C_4H_4O_6 + H_2O$$

***Physical properties*:** It occurs as colorless crystals, freely soluble in water.

***Test for identification*:** The sample solution gives the characteristic reactions of sodium and antimony. After removal of antimony it gives the reactions of tartarate.

***Test for purity*:** It should be tested for acidity or alkalinity, heavy metals, arsenic, lead and loss on drying.

**Assay**

It is assayed by **iodimetry method of titration** (also called **redox titration**).

In this assay the substance is dissolved in water and sodium bicarbonate or sodium borate is added and it is titrated against N/10 iodine using starch mucilage as an indicator. End point is the appearance of blue colour. During this titration antimony is converted to antimony pentoxide and iodine is reduced to hydroiodic acid. The hydroiodic acid can cause the reaction reversible, hence sodium bicarbonate or sodium borate is added to neutralize the formed hydroiodic acid and enable the reaction to complete. As the oxidation and reduction takes place simultaneously this is called Redox titration. The chemical reactions of this assay are shown below.

$$2\ C_4H_4O_7SbNa + 2\ I_2 + 3H_2O \longrightarrow 2\ NaHC_4H_6O_6 + Sb_2O_5 + 4\ HI$$

***Procedure*:** Dissolve about 500 mg of antimony sodium tartarate, accurately weighed, in 50 ml of water, add 5 gm of potassium sodium tartarate, 2 gm of sodium borate, and 3 ml of starch, and immediately titrate with 0.1N iodine until the appearance of blue color.

***Uses*:**

1. It is used as an emetic and reflex expectorant.
2. It is also used as an antischistosomal drug in the treatment of schistosomiasis, filariasis.

***Dose*:** 600 mg to 2 gm/day by intravenous injection.

***Storage***: It should be stored in well closed container.

## Sodium Antimony Tartarate Injection

It contains not less than 95% and not more than 105% of sodium antimony tartarate.

***Preparation***: Antimony sodium tartarate is dissolved in water for injection, filtered and immediately sterilised by filtration or autoclave.

***Test for identification***: The residue obtained after drying the solution gives the characteristic reactions of sodium and antimony. After removal of antimony it gives the reactions of tartarate.

***Test for purity***: It should be tested for acidity or alkalinity, heavy metals, arsenic, lead and loss on drying and it also complies with the test for parenterals.

**Assay**

It is similar to that of antimony sodium tartarate by using the volume of the solution equivalent to 0.5 gm.

***Uses***: It is used as an antischistosomal drug in the treatment of schistosomiasis, filariasis.

***Dose***: 1.5 gm by intravenous injection.

***Storage***: It should be stored in well closed container.

## Zinc Sulphate

This compound is discussed under **astringents**.

## Copper Sulphate I.P.

**(Synonym: Cupric sulphate)**

**Mol. Formula:** $CuSO_4 . 5H_2O$. **Mol. Weight:** 249.7

It contains not less than 98% and not more than 101% of $CuSO_4 . 5H_2O$.

***Preparation:***

1. It is prepared by heating copper with concentrated sulphuric acid in the presence of air. In the absence of air, the sulphuric acid has little action or no action.

$$2Cu + 2H_2SO_4 \longrightarrow 2CuSO_4 + 2H_2$$

   The solution is filtered, evaporated to crystallization when copper sulphate crystals are separated.

2. *Large scale preparation*: In large scale method, copper sulphate is prepared by heating scrap copper with dilute sulphuric acid and simultaneously passing a current of air throughout the liquid.

$$2Cu + 2H_2SO_4 + O_2 \longrightarrow 2CuSO_4 + 2H_2O$$

3. *From sulphide ore:* It is manufactured by roasting copper containing sulphide ore in presence of air or by heating copper in furnace with sulphur. The mixture of copper sulphate and copper oxide formed is treated with dilute sulphuric acid. Then the solution is filtered, concentrated and allowed to crystallize when crystals are separated out.

   Commercial copper sulphate usually contains iron and zinc as impurities.

***Physical properties:*** It occurs in deep blue, triclinic crystals of penta hydrate or as blue crystalline granules or powder. It is soluble in water, very soluble in boiling water, insoluble in alcohol. It is incompatible with alkaloids, phosphates, β-naphthol and sulfathiazole.

***Chemical properties:*** It has been stable to heat at 60 °C, while on heating at 100 °C, loses two molecules of water, at 140 °C loses another molecule of water, and at 200 °C a white anhydrous salt is formed.

$$CuSO_4 . 5H_2O \xrightarrow[100\,^{\circ}C,\ -2H_2O]{\Delta} CuSO_4 . 3H_2O \xrightarrow[140\,^{\circ}C,\ -H_2O]{\Delta} CuSO_4 . 2H_2O \xrightarrow[200\,^{\circ}C,\ -2H_2O]{\Delta} CuSO_4$$

When heated at high temperature, it decomposes into sulphur dioxide, oxygen and black cupric oxide.

$$2CuSO_4 \xrightarrow[\Delta]{<200\,^{\circ}C} 2CuO + 2SO_2 + O_2$$

***Test for identification:*** The aqueous solution gives the characteristic reactions of copper and sulphate ions.

***Test for purity:*** It should be tested for acidity, clarity of the solution, arsenic, iron, lead and zinc. The aqueous solution is acidic to litmus.

**Assay**

***Principle:*** It is assayed by **iodometry method of titration** (also called **redox titration**).

In this assay the substance is treated with sulphuric acid and potassium iodide whereby cupric iodide is formed. As the cupric iodide is unstable it is decomposed to cuprous iodide (CuI) and free iodine is liberated. The liberated iodine is determined by titrating with N/10 sodium thiosulphate using starch mucilage as an indicator. As the decomposition reaction of cupric iodide to cuprous iodide is reversible, potassium thiocyanate is added towards the end of titration to make the reaction to complete. End point is the disappearance of blue colour. During this titration iodine is reduced to sodium iodide and sodium thiosulphate is oxidized to sodium tetrathionate. As the oxidation and reduction takes place simultaneously this is called Redox titration. The chemical reactions of this assay are shown below.

$$CuSO_4 + 2KI \longrightarrow \underset{\text{Cupric iodide}}{CuI_2} + K_2SO_4$$

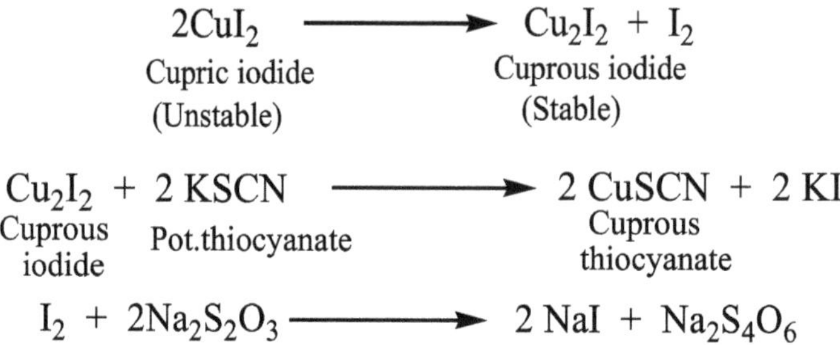


$$I_2 + 2Na_2S_2O_3 \longrightarrow 2\,NaI + Na_2S_4O_6$$

***Procedure:*** Dissolve 0.200 gm in 50 ml of water. Add 2 ml of sulphuric acid and 3 gm of potassium iodide. Titrate with 0.1M sodium thiosulphate, adding 1 ml of starch solution towards the end of the titration.

***Uses:***

1. It is used as an emetic, but it can be dangerous due to large and corrosive doses.
2. It considered as a chemical antidote for phosphorous poisoning.
3. It is used externally as an astringent and also as a fungicide. (1.5% solution)
4. It is one of the ingredients of Benedict's and Fehling's reagent.

***Dose:*** As emetic 300 mg /30 ml water.

***Storage:*** It should be stored in well closed container, and protected from air, heat and moisture.

## 6.8.6 Internal Parasiticides

***Introduction:*** These are the products that are used to control the parasites which attack the organism (human body) internally. Leishmaniasis is caused by a protozoan parasite genus of leishmania which is transmitted to humans through the sand fly bites. These can be given orally or parentally.

***Mechanism of action internal parasiticides:*** It acts by conversion to the trivalent antimony which induces a rapid efflux of glutathione and trypanothione from the protozoal cell and also inhibits trypanothione reductase enzyme which leads to decrease in trypanothione and glutathione level. It also decreases the thiol reduction potential which is important for cellular function of the parasite. Sodium stilbo gluconate is a first choice drug for the treatment of visceral leishmaniasis. Due to the irritant nature, it is administered both IM (or) IV route.

***Common side effect:*** It produces pancreatitis, increase the transamination levels of liver.

### Sodium Antimony Gluconate I.P.

**(Synonym: Sodium Stilbo Gluconate)**

**Mol. Formula:** $C_6H_8O_7SbNa$ **Mol. Weight:** 328

***Structure:***

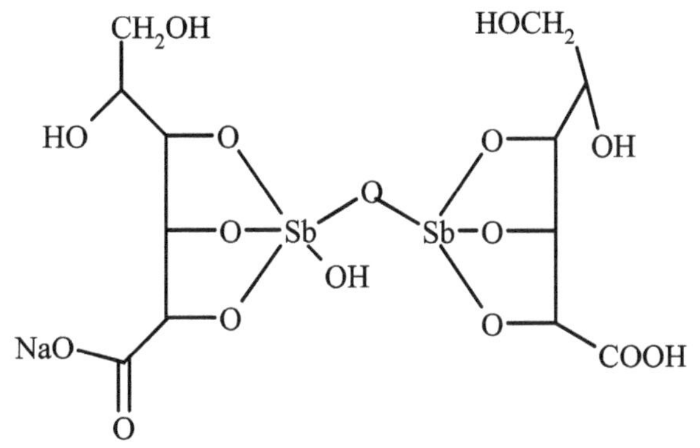

Chemically it is called as the disodium salt of M-oxy-bis(glucanato(3)O[2], O[3], O[4]) hydroxy antimony.

It contains not less than 30.0% and not more than 34.0% of pentavalent antimony calculated with reference to dried and methanol free basis.

***Preparation:*** It is prepared by mixing sodium hydroxide to a mixture of antimony trichloride and gluconic acid solution.

This represents one atom of antimony per mole of gluconic acid and slightly less than 2 atoms of sodium in each mole of the compound.

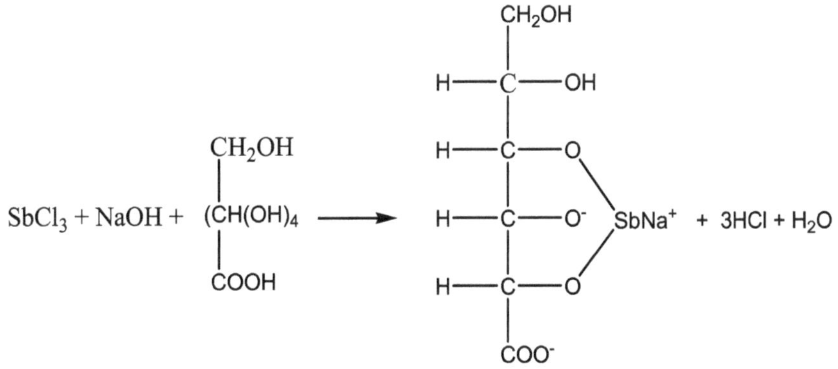

$$SbCl_3 + NaOH + CH_2OH\text{–}(CH(OH))_4\text{–}COOH \longrightarrow CH_2OH\text{–}CH(OH)\text{–}(CH\text{–}O)_3\,SbNa^+\text{–}COO^- + 3HCl + H_2O$$

***Physical properties:*** It occurs as white or colorless, amorphous powder and odorless. It is soluble in water but insoluble in alcohol and solvent ether. Its aqueous solution is cloudy on long standing. The pH of the aqueous solution is 5 to 5.2. The pH of the 2% solution is 9-10, at this pH it is unstable, so the pH should be adjusted to 6-7 by using gluconic acid. The solution should be immediately prepared whenever needed and stored in well closed containers.

***Test for identification:***

1. An aqueous solution of the sample is dextrorotatory.

2. To the aqueous solution of sample, pass hydrogen sulphide gas for 5-10 min. An orange colour precipitate is formed.
3. The required quantity of sample is heated, it chars without melting, produce burnt sugar odour and leaves the residue, that residue gives the characteristic reactions of antimony and sodium ions.

***Test for purity:*** It should be tested for pH, stability of solution, trivalent antimony, chlorides, methanol, undue toxicity and loss on drying.

***Test for methanol:*** It should not be more than 2% w/w, determined by gas chromatography.

***Test for trivalent antimony:*** It is tested by dissolving small amount of sample in required quantity of water, acidified with dilute hydrochloric acid and titrate with 0.00833M potassium bromide using methyl orange as an indicator. The volume of potassium bromide consumed should not more than 1.3 ml.

**Assay**

***Principle:*** It is assayed by **iodimetry method of titration** (also called **redox titration**) for total antimony.

In this assay the substance is first converted into antimony trioxide solution and titrated with N/10 iodine solution using starch mucilage as an indicator. End point is the appearance of blue colour. During this titration iodine is reduced to sodium iodide and antimony is oxidized to antimony pentoxide. As the oxidation and reduction takes place simultaneously this is called Redox titration. The chemical reactions of this assay are shown below.

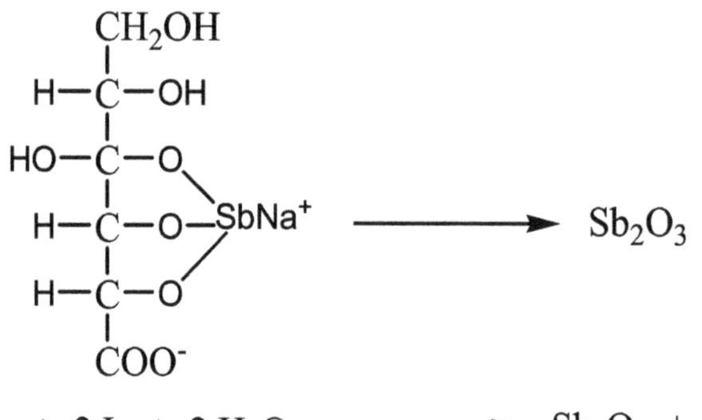

```
        CH2OH
          |
     H—C—OH
          |
    HO—C—O
          |     \
     H—C—O—SbNa+   ——————►   Sb2O3
          |     /
     H—C—O
          |
        COO-
```

$$Sb_2O_3 + 2\,I_2 + 2\,H_2O \longrightarrow Sb_2O_5 + 4\,HI$$

***Uses:***

(i) It is used as an antiprotozoal agent.

(ii) It is also used as systemic leishmaniacidal.

***Advantage:*** It is less toxic than antimony potassium tartarate and antimony sodium tartarate.

***Dose:*** 600 mg – 2 gm daily for 10 to 30 days given by intramuscular or intravenous injection.

***Official formulation:*** Sodium stilbo gluconate injection I.P.

## Sodium Antimony Gluconate Injection I.P.

**(Synonym: Sodium Stilbo gluconate injection)**

It is a sterile solution of sodium stilbogluconate in water for injection. It does not containing any preservatives.

It contains not less than 9.5% w/v and not more than 10.5% w/v of pentavalent antimony.

***Properties:*** It is a clear, colourless or faintly straw colored solution.

***Test for identification, Test for purity, assay:*** Similar to that of sodium antimony gluconate.

***Uses:*** It is used as antiprotozoal agent.

---

## Antimony Potassium Tartarate

This compound is discussed under the topic **emetics**.

---

## Antimony Sodium Tartarate B.P.

This compound is discussed under the topic **emetics**.

---

## Antimony Sodium Tartarate Injection

This compound is discussed under the topic **emetics**.

---

### 6.8.7 Antineoplastic Agents

***Introduction:*** These are the drugs which are used to treat cancer or neoplasm. The term 'cancer' or 'neoplasm' refers to a disease of cells that shows uncontrolled proliferation, differentiation, invasiveness and the ability to metastasis (spread to distal parts of the body).

Apart from the methods like surgical resection and radio therapy which are used to treat cancers, these antineoplastic/anticancer drugs are used as a part of chemotherapy and immunotherapy. The antineoplastic agents acts on the cancerous cells by different mechanisms like cisplatin, interferes with the cell cycle, DNA destruction, etc. The better and proper understanding of cell cycle is essential one for rational use of anticancer drugs Fig. 6.7. It includes 5 phases. They are $G_0$, $G_1$, S, $G_2$, and M phase.

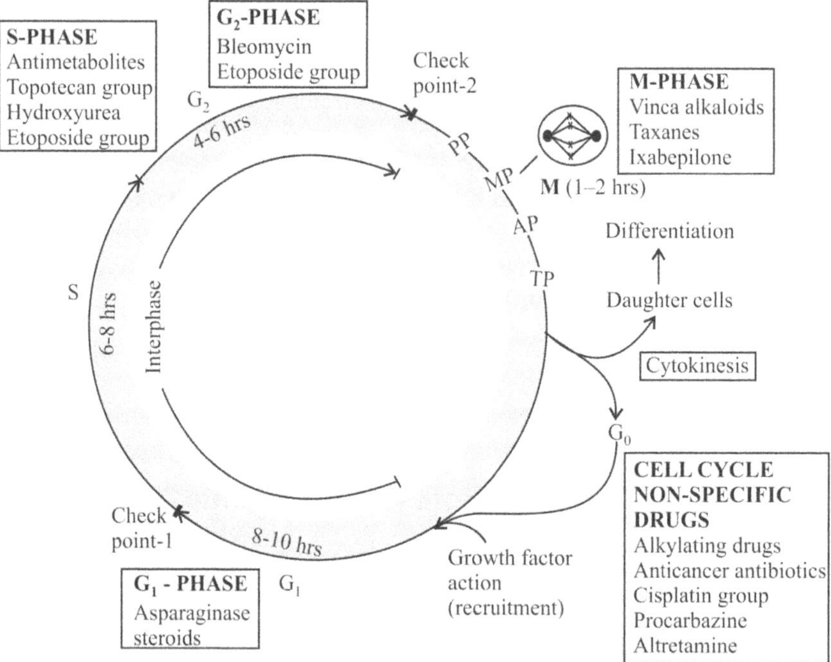


**Fig. 6.7** Different phases of cell cycle

$G_0$ - skeletal muscle, neuron and cardiac muscle

$G_1$ - pre synthetic phase. In which cells are involved in metabolism and production of substances for cell division.

***S phase:*** (synthesis phase)

In this phase, synthesis and replication of DNA occurs.

***$G_2$ (post synthetic phase):*** The cell prepares itself for mitotic division into daughter cells.

***M phases:*** Mitosis of cells are takes place at this stage.

***Mechanism of action of cisplatin:*** It acts in $G_0$ phase, cisplatin binds to DNA at nucleophiles sites of guanine leads to alteration in DNA structure and inhibit DNA synthesis. It is cell cycle non specific agent cross linking of platinum in between adjacent guanine on the same DNA strand leads to primary.

***Common side effect:*** The common side effects of platinum compound are nausea, vomiting, hearing loss and nephrotoxicity.

## Cisplatin I.P., B.P., U.S.P.

**(Synonym: CDDP, Peyrone's salt or Peyrone's chloride)**

**Mol. Formula:** $H_6N_2Cl_2Pt$ **Mol. Weight:** 300

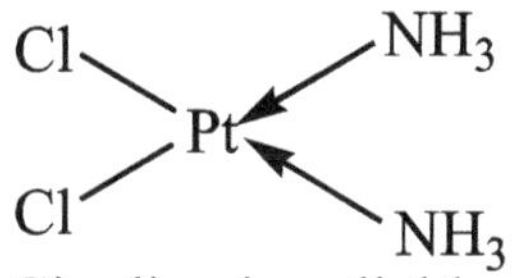

Cl, Cl — Pt ← $NH_3$, $NH_3$

Cis-diamino-dichloro platinum(II)

It contains not less than 97.06% and not more than 102% of cisplatin. The platinum metal has the ability to form co-ordination complex with functional group attached to it and forms a planar configurations. Stereo chemically cisplatin exists in two forms i.e., *cis* and *trans* form.

For example:

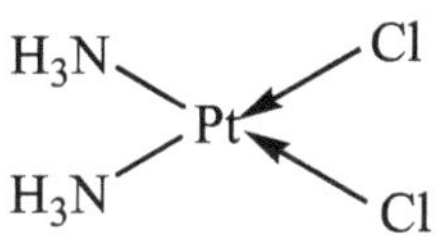

$H_3N$, $H_3N$ — Pt ← Cl, Cl     $H_3N$, Cl — Pt ← Cl, $NH_3$

Cis platin 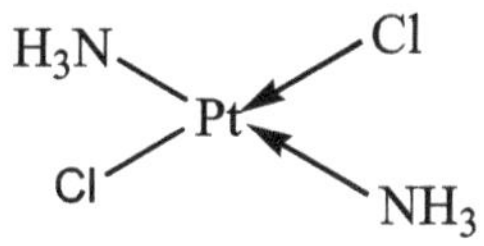     Trans platin

***Preparation:*** It is prepared by the reduction of chloroplatinic acid or the potassium chloroplatinate with hydrazine when tetra chloroplatinic acid or its salt is obtained, which is treated with ammonia – ammonium chloride mixture, the *cis* isomer is precipitated out. The precipitate obtained is filtered, washed and dried.

$$\underset{\text{Chloroplatinic acid}}{2\,H_2PtCl_6} + NH_2NH_2 \longrightarrow \underset{\text{Tetrachloroplatinic acid}}{2\,H_2PtCl_4} + N_2 + 4\,HCl$$

$$H_2PtCl_4 + 2NH_4Cl \longrightarrow \underset{\text{Cis-platin}}{Cl_2Pt(NH_3)_2} + 4\,HCl$$

$$\underset{\text{Potassium chloro platinate}}{2K_2PtCl_6} + NH_2NH_2 \longrightarrow \underset{\text{Potassium tetra chloro platinate}}{2K_2PtCl_4} + N_2 + 4\,HCl$$

$$K_2PtCl_4 + 2NH_4Cl \longrightarrow Cl_2Pt(NH_3)_2 + 2\,HCl + 2KCl$$

***Physical properties:*** It occurs as a yellow powder or orange yellow crystals, slightly soluble in water, sparingly soluble in dimethyl formamide (DMF), and insoluble in alcohol.

***Test for identification:***

1. The isomer cisplatin is identified by IR spectrophotometry.

2. The residue obtained after evaporating the solution with sodium hydroxide, is dissolved in a mixture of nitric acid and hydrochloric acid and evaporate to dryness, the color of the residue is orange. Dissolve the residue in small amount of water and add one or two drops of ammonium chloride solution, a yellow crystalline precipitate are formed.

***Test for purity:*** It should be tested for pH, related substances and silver.

***Test for related substances:*** This test is done by using chromatogram.

***Test for silver:*** It is determined by **atomic absorption spectrophotometry**.

**Assay**

It is assayed by **HPLC**.

***Uses:*** Cisplatin is mainly used for the treatment of testicular and ovarian tumors (anticancer agent).

***Dose:*** 15-20 $mg/m^2$ of body surface daily for 5 days administered by IV injection.

***Toxic effects:*** Platinum compounds are toxic in nature. The toxic symptoms are mainly associated with kidneys, bone marrow, ears and nervous system. So it should be used under medical care.

***Other official formulation:*** Cisplatin injection.

***Caution:*** Cisplatin is potentially cytotoxic. Care should be taken in handling the powder and preparing solutions.

## 6.8.8 Anti Depressants

**Introduction:** Antidepressants enhance alertness and may result in an increased output of behaviour. These agents are used to relieve the symptoms of moderate and severe depression. Lithium carbonate is the first line drug for the treatment of bipolar disorders.

Depression is characterized by feelings of intense sadness or worry, agitation, self-depression, physical changes, such as insomnia, anorexia, loss of enthusiasm, and mental slowing. In general at any given time, about 5%–6% of the population is depressed and estimated 10% of the people may become depressed during their lives. Therapeutically they are used in the following conditions

- Severe anxiety and panic attacks
- Obsessive compulsive disorders
- Moderate to severe depressive illness.

### Lithium Carbonate I.P., B.P., U.S.P.

**Mol. Formula:** $Li_2CO_3$. **Mol. Weight:** 73.9

It contains not less than 98.5% and not more than 100.5% of $Li_2CO_3$.

***Preparation:***

*From lithium sulphate or salts:* It is manufactured by adding ammonium carbonate to lithium sulphate solution.

$$Li_2SO_4 + (NH_4)_2CO_3 \longrightarrow Li_2CO_3 + (NH_4)_2SO_4$$

***Physical properties:*** It is a white or colorless, crystalline powder, odorless, but slight saline taste. It is sparingly soluble in water, soluble in dilute hydrochloric acid.

***Test for identification:***

1. The sample solution gives the characteristic reactions of carbonates.
2. A small quantity of sample is moistened with dilute hydrochloric acid and introduced on a platinum wire; it produces red color to a non-luminous flame.
3. Dissolve small quantity of sample in required amount of hydrochloric acid and boil the solution. To this add small amount of sodium hydroxide solution and add 5 ml of disodium hydrogen phosphate solution, and once again boil the solution. A white precipitate is obtained.

***Test for purity:*** It should be tested for clarity of the solution, arsenic, calcium and magnesium, heavy metals, iron, potassium, sodium, chlorides and sulphates, loss on drying.

**Assay**

***Principle:*** It is assayed by **acidimetry-alkalimetry method (Back) of titration** (also called **neutralization method**).

In this assay the substance is dissolved and a Known Excess Standard (KES) of dilute hydrochloric added and the Excess Unreacted (EUR) acid is determined by titrating with sodium hydroxide, using methyl orange as an indicator. End point is the change of colour from orange to yellow. As the acid and alkali are involved in this assay, it is called as acidimetry-alkalimetry method of titration and the neutralization takes place in this assay during titration hence this assay is also called as Neutralization method.

$$Li_2CO_3 + 2\,HCl \longrightarrow 2\,LiCl + H_2O + CO_2$$

$$HCl + NaOH \longrightarrow NaCl + H_2O$$

***Procedure:*** Weigh accurately about 0.5 gm, dissolve in 25 ml of 1M hydrochloric acid and titrate with 1M sodium hydroxide using methyl orange solution as indicator.

***Uses:***

1. Lithium carbonate is mainly used as antidepressant.
2. It is used for the treatment and prevention of manic depressive disorders. The pharmacological action of lithium is slow, so it is given along with anti psychotic drugs for immediate response in acute manic attacks.

***Toxicity profile:***

1. Lithium toxicity leads to decrease in sodium concentration, so diuretics not given along with lithium therapy.
2. Each gm of lithium carbonate contains 27 mm of lithium. The optimum therapeutic effects are produced with the plasma count ratio of 0.6 to 1.2 mm/L. The plasma concentration if exceeded from 1.5 mm/L is considered as toxic level. So the therapeutic level shows close relations with toxic levels. Hence plasma concentration level is monitored closely during therapy as well as in manic depression condition. Lithium is completely absorbed from liquid preparations but not in tablet form.
3. Sodium bicarbonate (antacid) increases the urinary excretion of lithium, so it acts as an antidote for lithium toxicity.

***Dose:*** 250 mg – 2 gm daily in divided doses.

***Storage:*** It should be stored in well closed container and protected from moisture.

***Official formulations:*** Lithium carbonate Tablets I.P.

---

## 6.8.9 Antirheumatic Agents

***Introduction:*** Rheumatoid arthritis (RA) is a chronic, progressive, autoimmune, inflammatory disease, mainly affecting the joints and periarticular tissues. It is caused by antigen – antibody reactions and release of inflammatory mediators like leukotrienes, prostaglandins. So, the drugs used to treat RA acts in such a way to reduce pain and inflammation (NSAIDS), immuno suppressants like suppressing cell-mediated immunity (Example: Gold Salts).

***Mechanism of action of sodium aurothiomalate:*** It reduces the cell mediated immune reactions by decreases lysosomal enzyme activity. It also reduces the histamine release from the mast cells and suppresses the phagocytic activity of polymorphonuclear leukocytes and inhibits the release of IL – 1TNF.

***Common side effects:*** The unwanted side effects of gold compounds are hepatitis neutropenia, thrombocytopenia etc.

### Sodium Aurothiomalate I.P., B.P., U.S.P.

**Mol. Formula:** $C_4H_4AuNaO_4S$ **Mol. Wt:** 368.09

It is a mixture of mono sodium and disodium salt of aurothiomalic acid.

It contains not less than 44.5% and not more than 46% of gold and not less than 10.8% and not more than 11.8% of sodium calculated with reference to the substance which has been dried in vacuum over $P_2O_5$ for one day.

***Preparation:*** It is obtained by treating sodium thiomalate with aurous iodide. To the above mixture, add sodium chloride, the sodium aurothiomalate is precipitated out. The precipitate is filtered out and dried.

$$\begin{array}{l} CH(SH)COONa \\ | \\ CH_2COONa \end{array} + \underset{\text{Aurous iodide}}{AuI} \xrightarrow[-HI]{} \begin{array}{l} CH(SAu)COONa \\ | \\ CH_2COONa \end{array}$$

Sodium thiomalate — Aurous iodide — Sodium aurothiomalate

***Physical properties:*** It occurs as a fine, pale yellow hygroscopic powder. It is soluble in water and insoluble in organic solvents.

***Test for identification:***

1. The aqueous solution of the sample gives the characteristic reactions of sodium.
2. To the dilute solution of sample, add hydrogen peroxide solution and 1ml of sodium hydroxide solution. Heat the solution to boil for 30 sec. A precipitate is produced that appears in brownish black by reflected light and bluish - green by transmitted light.
3. The residue obtained after ignition is dissolved in hydrochloric acid, diluted to 10 ml and allow stand. The supernatant liquid gives the characteristic reactions of sulphates.

***Test for purity:*** It should be tested for pH, related substances, glycerol and loss on drying, maleic acid, fumaric acid and thiomallic acid.

**Assay**

It is assayed by **gravimetric method**.

***For Au:*** The sample is mixed with sulphuric acid and boiled to get clear solution. After cooling 1 ml nitric acid added drop by drop, boiled, cooled and diluted with water. The residue of gold washed, dried well and ignited at 600 °C for 3 hours and weighed.

***For Sodium:*** The filtrate and washings obtained above for Au are evaporated to dryness, moistened with sulphuric acid, ignited at 600 °C for 3 hr and weighed.

***Uses:***

1. The calcium salt of the substance is used for the treatment of *Lupus erythematosus.*
2. Sodium aurothiomalate finds use in rheumatoid arthritis due to its anti-inflammatory effect. It is specifically used for certain type of arthritis by intramuscular injection.

***Contraindications:*** It is contraindicated in many conditions like kidney disorders, anemia, diabetes and liver diseases. So gold compounds have to be used with great caution.

***Official formulation:*** Sodium aurothiomalate injection I.P.

---

## 6.8.10 Antithyroid Agents

***Introduction:*** These are used in the treatment of hyperthyroidism characterized by increased basal metabolic rate (BMR), heat intolerance, tachycardia, cardiac arrhythmia, menstrual irregularities, muscle weakness, etc. These drugs act by inhibiting the synthesis of thyroid hormones ($T_3$ and $T_4$) by inhibiting iodination of $T_1$, inhibiting thyroid peroxidase, etc., and also radioactive iodine compounds are widely employed in this disorder as they effectively emit $\gamma$ and $\beta$ – particles which destroys the hyperactive thyroid gland. Antithyroids are used in grave's disease, thyrotoxicosis, goiter and thyroid storm.

## Potassium Perchlorate B.P., U.S.P.

**Mol. Formula:** $KClO_4$ **Mol. Weight:** 138.55

It contains not less than 99% and not more than 102% of $KClO_4$.

***Preparation:*** It is prepared by electrolysis of a concentrated solution of potassium chlorate. The chlorate ions are discharged at the anode, and react with water to give chloric acid.

$$ClO_3^- + e \longrightarrow ClO_3$$

$$ClO_3 + KOH \longrightarrow KClO_3 + OH^-$$

The concentration of chloric acid is more than 40%, decomposes in to perchloric acid, chlorine, oxygen and water.

$$3HClO_3 \longrightarrow HClO_4 + Cl_2 + 2O_2 + H_2O$$

The overall reaction is summarized as follows,

$$KClO_3 + H_2O \longrightarrow KClO_4 + H_2$$

***Physical properties:*** It occurs as a white crystalline powder, soluble in water. When heated it evolves oxygen.

***Test for identification:*** When heated, it liberates oxygen with the formation of potassium chloride.

$$KClO_4 \longrightarrow 2O_2 + KCl$$

***Test for purity:*** It should be tested for arsenic, lead, chloride, chlorate and sulphate.

**Assay**

It is assayed by **redox method**.

***Uses:***

1. It is used as an anti thyroid agent where other drugs are not tolerated by patients.
2. It hastens the elimination of radioactive iodide, accumulated in the thyroid gland, which is administered for the treatment or diagnosis of thyroid gland disorders.
3. It also acts as a powerful oxidant.

***Official formulations:*** Potassium per chlorate tablets B.P.

## 6.8.11 Surgical Aids

***Introduction:*** These are referred to a wide range of materials used for dressing of wounds or injured or diseased tissues (surgical dressings); some are used to hold wound edges closely during healing (sutures and ligatures). All these materials are collectively called “Surgical aids”. These are not intended for therapeutic use. As the surgical aids come in direct contact with body parts like skin, they should be prepared, processed and stored carefully without any contamination or deterioration.

## Plaster of Paris (Gypsum) I.P., B.P.

**(Synonym: Dried calcium sulphate, Exsiccated calcium sulphate, Calcium sulphate hemihydrate)**

**Mol. Formula:** $CaSO_4.½ H_2O$ **Mol. Weight:** 145.1

Naturally Calcium sulphate occurs in two molecules of water as monoclinic prisms gypsum and selenite and in granular masses known as alabastar. It is also available in calcium sulphate mineral called as anhydrite.

***Preparation:*** It is prepared by heating powdered gypsum at about 150 °C in a controlled manner (previously powdered) such that it is substantially converted into the hemihydrates about ¾ of the water for crystallization. It may contain accelerators or decelerators.

$$CaSO_4.2H_2O \xrightarrow[\Delta]{150\ ^oC} CaSO_4.1/2\ H_2O + 3/2\ H_2O$$

If the temperature becomes 200 °C, it gives a product which lacks set property and it is unfit for used as a plaster of paris.

***Physical properties:*** It is white or almost white or greyish white powder, odorless, tasteless, hygroscopic, and soluble in water, solubility decreases markedly with increase in temperature, insoluble in alcohol.

When it mixed with water, it forms as mass that "sets quickly". It slowly absorbs moisture from air, changes to granular and loses its setting property.

***Test for identification:*** The sample yields the characteristic reactions of calcium and sulphates.

***Test for purity:*** It should be tested for pH, acid insoluble matter, setting properties and loss on ignition.

***Test for pH:*** The pH of the solution is 6.5 to 9.

***Test for acid insoluble matter:*** It should not be more than that of 5 mg (1%).

***Test for setting properties:*** Required amount of sample is mixed with calculated amount of water at 15 to 20 °C in a cylindrical mould about 2.4 cm diameters. It sets within 4 minutes not more than 6 minutes. After standing for 3 hours, it possesses sufficient hardness to withstand pressure of the finger at all edges and maintain the sharpness of outline and do not crumble under pressure.

***Uses:***

1. It is mainly used to make plaster of paris bandages (surgical aid).
2. In dentistry, it is used for taking impression and in surgery for making casts.
3. It is also used as diluents for the preparation of compressed tablets.

***Storage:*** It should be stored in cool dry place and protected from moisture and heat.

### 6.8.12 Diagnostic Agents

***Introduction:*** These are the chemical substances used to reveal, pinpoint and define the localization of a pathological process. The principal diagnostic agents are X-ray contrast preparations, radioactive isotopes and dyes. X-ray preparations are introduced directly into the organ to be examined (stomach, uterus, heart) or intravenously in examining liver, bile ducts and kidneys. The use of radioactive substances (isotopes) for diagnosis is based on the principle of recording the rays (mainly gamma rays) emitted by them when they are introduced into the body. The diagnostic dyes are given intravenously into organ to be examined.

#### Barium Sulphate I.P., B.P., U.S.P.

**Mol. Formula:** $BaSO_4$ **Mol. Weight:** 233.4

It contains not less than 97.5% of $BaSO_4$

***Occurrence:*** In nature it occurs as barytes $BaSO_4$ or heavy spar and withrite, $BaCO_3$

***Preparation:*** Purification of the natural substances is difficult process, for so the pharmaceutical and other purposes it is prepared by the following method.

1. *From barium chloride:* Medicinally used barium sulphate is prepared by treating barium chloride with any soluble sulphate (sodium sulphate).

$$BaCl_2 + Na_2SO_4 \longrightarrow BaSO_4\downarrow + 2\,NaCl$$

The precipitate is collected, washed and dried in a steam oven.

2. *From barium sulphide:* Barium sulphate is also prepared by the reaction between barium sulphide and sulphuric acid.

$$BaS + H_2SO_4 \longrightarrow BaSO_4 + H_2S$$

Barium sulphate is one of the byproduct of the manufacturing of hydrogen peroxide from barium peroxide, but it is not a pure, so it cannot be used for pharmaceutical purposes.

***Physical properties:*** It is a fine, heavy, white powder, free from gritty particles, odorless, tasteless. It is insoluble in water, dilute acids and alkalis, organic solvents, but it is soluble in concentrated sulphuric acid due to the formation of barium bisulphate.

$$BaSO_4 + H_2SO_4 \longrightarrow Ba(HSO_4)_2$$

***Fusion reaction:*** It reacts with carbonates and gives fused products such as carbonate which readily reacts with acids.

$$2\,BaSO_4 + Na_2CO_3 + K_2CO_3 \longrightarrow 2\,KNaSO_4 + 2\,BaCO_3\downarrow$$

$$BaCO_3 + 2\,CH_3COOH \longrightarrow (CH_3COO)_2Ba + CO_2 + H_2O$$

***Test for identification:***

1. Boil small amount of sample with 50% w/v sodium carbonate solution for 5 minutes, add water and filter. The filtrate is acidified with dilute HCl. It gives the characteristic reactions of sulphates.
2. The residue obtained from the above test is washed repeatedly with water maximum 3 times. To the residue add 5 ml of dilute hydrochloric acid filter it, to the filtrate add one drop of dilute sulphuric acid. A white precipitate is formed which is insoluble in dilute sodium hydroxide solution.

***Test for purity:*** It should be tested for acidity or alkalinity, arsenic, heavy metals, phosphates, sulphide, acid soluble substances, soluble barium salts, bulkiness and loss on ignition.

***Test for sulphide:*** Boil the mixture of equal quantity of sample and dilute hydrochloric acid and required quantity of water for 10 min. Lead acetate paper is introduced into the vapors which discharge from the solution. The paper should be more darken.

***Test for soluble barium salt:*** Residue obtained from the acid soluble substances is treated with water and filter it. To the filtrate add one to two drops of dilute sulphuric acid to clear the filtrate and kept aside for half an hour. No turbidity is produced.

***Test for bulkiness:*** Add 5 gm of sample in 50 ml measuring cylinder to this add 90 ml water. Shake well and allow to stand for 15 minutes. It does not settle below 15 ml mark.

***Test for loss on ignition:*** Not more than 2.5% determined on 1 gm at 600 °C.

**Assay**

***Principle:*** It is assayed by **gravimetric method.**

In this assay barium sulphate is first reacted with sodium carbonate and potassium carbonate whereby all the barium is converted in to barium carbonate. To the barium carbonate is then added solution as a buffer and treated with potassium dichromate followed by urea (Urea is added in this assay to avoid the formation of fine diffusible precipitate. The medium must be made alkaline and buffered to complete precipitation of barium chromate). Now all the barium is precipitated as barium chromate. The precipitate of barium chromate is dried and ignited to a constant weight. From the weight of barium chromate the amount of barium sulphate is calculated. As the test substance is converted to a precipitate, which is used for calculating the actual amount of barium sulphate present this is called Gravimetric assay.

$$2\,BaSO_4 + Na_2CO_3 + K_2CO_3 \longrightarrow 2BaCO_3\downarrow + Na_2SO_4 + K_2SO_4$$

$$2\,BaCO_3 + 4\,HCl \longrightarrow 2\,BaCl_2 + 2\,H_2O + 2\,CO_2\uparrow$$

$$2\,BaCl_2 + K_2Cr_2O_7 + 2\,NH_4OH \longrightarrow 2\,KCl + 2\,NH_4Cl + H_2O + 2BaCrO_4\downarrow$$

***Procedure:*** Weigh accurately about 0.6 gm in a platinum crucible, add 5 gm of sodium carbonate and 5 gm of potassium carbonate and mix. Heat to 1000 °C and maintain at this temperature for 15 minutes. Allow to cool and suspend the residue in 150 ml of water. Wash the crucible with 2 ml of acetic acid and add to the suspension. Cool in ice and filter by decantation, transfer as little of the solid matter as possible to the filter. Wash the residue with successive quantities of a 2% w/v solution of sodium carbonate until the washings are free from sulphate and discard the washings. Add 5 ml of dilute hydrochloric acid to the filter and wash through into the vessel containing the bulk of the solid matter with water. Add 5 ml of hydrochloric acid and dilute to 100 ml with water. Add 10 ml of a 40% w/v solution of ammonium acetate, 25 ml of a 10% w/v solution of potassium dichromate and 10 gm of urea. Cover, digest in an oven at 80 °C to 85 °C for 16 hours and filter while still hot through a sintered-glass filter (porosity No. 4), washing the precipitate initially with a 0.5% w/v solution of potassium dichromate and finally with 2 ml of water. Dry to constant weight at 105°C.

***Uses:***

1. Barium sulphate is used as a diagnostic agent (radio opaque contrast medium).
2. It is also used as a radio opaque contrast medium for x-ray determination of gastro intestinal tract (roentgenographic studies).

***Advantages:*** It is insoluble in gastric juice, hence does not produce any systemic toxic effects.

***Side effects:*** The major side effect associated with barium sulphate is constipation. The accidental entry of this compound into peritoneal or other cavities though perforations has produced some severe inflammations. It is given as suspension forms due to toxic effect of barium ions, U.S.P indicates the following caution.

***Caution:*** When barium sulphate is prescribed, the title always should write out in full to avoid confusion with the poisonous barium sulphide or barium sulphite.

***Dose:*** For oral route = 300 gm (60–450 gm)

For rectal route = 400 to 750 gm.

***Storage:*** It should be stored in well closed containers.

## Barium Sulphate Compound Powder

**(Synonym: Barium meal, shadow meal)**

**Ingredients:**

| | | |
|---|---|---|
| Barium sulphate | = | 1000 gm |
| Saccharin sodium | = | 0.25 gm |
| Vanillin | = | 0.10 gm |

***Preparation:*** Barium sulphate meal is prepared by mixing saccharin and vanillin with barium sulphate and gives to the patients immediately. Saccharin is used as sweetening agent and vanillin is used as flavoring agent.

Remaining all aspects are similar to that of barium sulphate.

### 6.8.13 Disinfectants

***Introduction:*** Disinfectants are chemical substances which are used to destroy or inhibit the growth of pathogenic vegetative bacteria on inanimate (non-living) surfaces such as glass ware or surgical instruments. The disinfectants like phenols, alcohol, formaldehyde acts by precipitating (coagulating) bacterial proteins. Even soaps, caustics and lysol can also be used as disinfectants.

#### Sulphur Dioxide U.S.P.

**Mol. Formula:** $SO_2$ **Mol. Weight:** 64.06

It contains not less than 97% by volume of $SO_2$.

***Preparation:***

*Method 1:* It is prepared by treating bisulphites with dilute mineral acids.

For example, sodium bisulphite is treated with sulphuric acid to give sulphur dioxide.

$$NaHSO_3 + H_2SO_4 \rightarrow NaHSO_4 + SO_2 + H_2O$$

*Method 2:* It is also prepared by burning sulphur in air.

$$S + O_2 \rightarrow SO_2$$

***Physical properties:*** It is a nonflammable gas with strong suffocating odour (smell of burning sulphur). It condenses to a liquid at $-10\ ^0$C. Specific gravity 1.5. It is freely soluble in water and forms sulphurous acid.

***Chemical properties:*** Sulphur dioxide is acting as a strong reducing agent.

*Reaction with iodine solution:* Sulphur dioxide is passed through the aqueous solution of iodine to give hydroiodic acid.

$$SO_2 + I_2 + 2H_2O \rightarrow 2HI + H_2SO_4$$

**Assay**

***Procedure:*** Collect 100 ml of $SO_2$ gas over mercury and note the temperature of the sample and the pressure upon it. Slowly introduce 50 ml of 0.1N sodium hydroxide in to the air space over the mercury, and absorbs the sample in the solution. When absorption is complete, transfer the solution to a 250 ml conical flask, add 3 ml of starch, and titrate with 0.1N iodine until the solution is pale blue in colour.

***Uses:***

1. It is used as an antioxidant.

2. Sulphur dioxide lotion in glycerin is used for sore throat and skin infections.
3. Extensively it is used in industries as a bleaching agent, fumigating grains and to prevent fermentation.

## PROBABLE QUESTIONS

1. What is meant by sclerosing agents?
2. Explain the preparation, properties, assay and uses of sodium tetra decyl sulphate or hypertonic saline.
3. Define expectorants with examples.
4. Write the preparation, assay, test for purity and uses of potassium iodide and sodium iodide.
5. Write a note on following.
   (a) Ammonium acetate
   (b) Ammonium chloride
   (c) Ammonium carbonate
   (d) Zinc sulphate
   (e) Copper sulphate
6. Write in brief about the mechanism of action of expectorants.
7. Explain the role of ammonium compounds as respiratory stimulants.
8. Write an account of preparation, properties, assay and various applications of ammonium chloride.
9. Write the method of preparation and assay for aromatic spirit of ammonia.
10. Define sedatives. Explain the preparation, properties and test for purity, assay and uses of potassium bromide.
11. What is meant by antidotes? List out the official antidote compounds.
12. Write a short note on the type of antidotes.
13. Explain the mechanism of action of sodium thiosulphate in cyanide poisoning.
14. Explain the preparation, properties, test for identification, test for purity, assay, and mechanism of action and specific uses of the following.
    (a) Sodium nitrite
    (b) Sodium thiosulphate
    (c) Charcoal
15. Define inhalants? Write official inhalants.
16. Write in detail about respiratory stimulants with any two ammonium compounds.
17. Define emetics with examples.
18. Write the mechanism of action of emetics.

19. Write the preparation, assay and uses of the following.
    (a) Copper sulphate (b) Zinc sulphate
20. Write a note on antimony sodium tartarate.
21. What is meant by anti neoplastic agents?
22. Write the preparation, properties, test for purity, assay and uses of cisplatin.
23. Define the term antidepressant.
24. Explain in detail about lithium carbonate.
25. Define anti rheumatic agents. Write the chemistry and application of sodium aurothiomalate.
26. Define surgical aids.
27. What is mean by diagnostic agents?
28. Write the preparation, properties, assay and uses of barium sulphate.
29. Define disinfectants.
30. Write in detail about sulphur dioxide.
31. Explain the assay of barium sulphate.

CHAPTER 7

# RADIOPHARMACEUTICALS

## 7.1 INTRODUCTION

In day today life the nuclear conversion of one nucleus (transmutation) in to another one is easily takes place. It occurs mainly by the radioactive reaction. For example, fogging of photographic plates is mainly due to some sort of radiations. Radioactive nuclides exist before the formation of solar system. Some types of short lived radioisotopes are present in the rocks. Another type of nuclides is present in the earth produced by the bombardment of cosmic rays with elements present in the earth crust.

This chapter mainly deals with the fundamentals of radioisotopes like its nature, nomenclature, source, detection methods, measurement of radioactivity and the nature of radioactive reactions whether it occurs within the nuclei of atom or between the nuclides and the inner most electrons. This basic information plays a major role in pharmacy, pharmaceutical industries, medicine, agriculture and other areas.

**History:** In 1896, radioactivity was first discovered by Henri Becquerel by using phosphorescent materials. In 1899, Rutherford discovered the fogging of photographic plates. Later the theory of radioactive disintegration was developed by Ruther ford and Soddy in 1903. The systematic development of this radioactive decay was further continued by Marie Curie and Pierre Curie, to isolate an element polonium and separation of an element radium and barium.

The development, preparation, testing, evaluation and clinical uses of these radio nuclides (radiopharmaceuticals) are studied under the special disciplines known as nuclear medicine and nuclear pharmacy.

### 7.1.1 General Theory of Radioactivity

**Atomic structure:** To understand the concept of radioactivity studies, the basic review of selected properties of atoms are important one.

**Atom:** A neutral charged particle which consists of positively charged nucleus (protons and neutrally charged neutrons) and outer orbital with negatively charged electrons.

**Atomic number (Z):** The number of orbital electrons or the number of protons. Both numbers are equal.

**Neutron number (N):** Number of neutrons in the nucleus.

**Mass number (A):** The sum of the number of protons and neutrons.

**Radius:** The radius of an atom is approximately $10^{-10}$ m or 1 A°.

The determination of mass of the atom was first invented by the scientist Thomson using positive ray analysis method. According to that, some of the nuclei possess the same number of protons but a different number of neutrons, later these are called as isotopes.

**Nuclides:** A nuclide is any one of the more than about 2500 known species of atoms characterized by the number of protons and number of neutrons in the nucleus.

**Isotopes:** The nuclides that contains same atomic number (same number of protons) and different mass number (different number of neutrons). These are possessing same chemical properties but differ in mass. For example: $^{1}H$, $^{2}H$ (deuterium).

**Isobars:** The different nuclides with same mass are called as isobars. For example: $^{3}H$, $^{3}He$.

**Isotones:** The different nuclides with same number of neutrons are called as isotones. For example: $^{3}H$, $^{4}He$.

**Examples for Isotopes:** Isotopes of Neon (8 Isotopes).

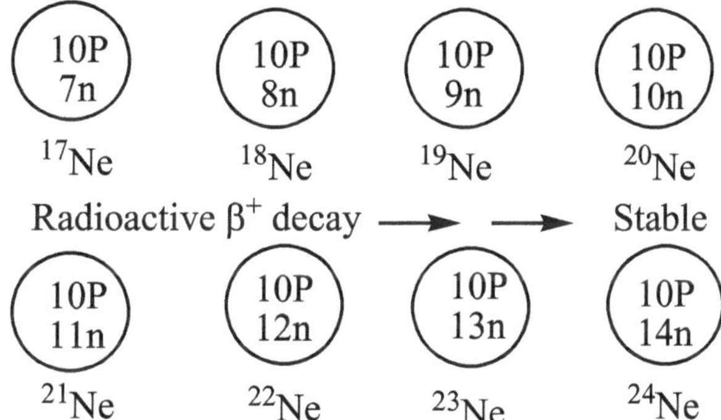


## 7.1.2 Radioactivity and Radiation

Radioactivity is defined as "the phenomenon by which one nuclide is spontaneously transformed into another nuclide with the emission of energy in the form of radiation". Therefore the nuclide which undergoes spontaneous nuclear reaction is called as radioactive. During this spontaneous decay the ratios of protons to neutrons change. After one or more decay process, a stable nucleus is formed.

**Radiations or nuclear reactions:** Several types of radiations may be emitted from radionuclide, each of which is found useful in medicinal field.

The radioactive nuclide frequently emits three types of radiations. They are alpha (α), beta (β), gamma (γ) radiations.

**Alpha particles:** $\left(\alpha,\ {}^{4}_{2}He^{+2}\right)$ These radiations are the heaviest and slowest of all radioactive emissions. Actually the particle is helium nucleus with two protons and two neutrons. It is the more highly charged nuclear species with a charge of +2, and it is having high ionizing power upon interaction with air or other media.

These particles attract electrons to its K-shells and become helium. The range of α - particle in air is about 5 cm and tissue is less than 100 μm.

The emission of alpha particle with radium is shown below.

$$^{226}_{88}Ra \longrightarrow ^{222}_{86}Rn + \alpha \text{ or } ^{4}_{2}He^{+2}$$

**Beta particles:** Beta particles are negatively charged species having the mass of an electron such as approximately $9.1 \times 10^{-28}$ gm. They move faster due to velocity such as 0.9 times the speed of light. Their emissions from the elements do not alter the atomic number. Due to their negative charge produces molecular ionization, when they are passing through the various media. These are having more penetrating power and energy than that of α- particle. These are lighter than α-particle. They move faster due to the interaction with surrounding nuclei leads to acceleration in the β-particle with the energy identical to the EMRS (Electromagnetic radiation source) known as bremsstrahlung or braking radiation. They can penetrate almost 1inch thickness of aluminium or travel from 10 to 15 mm in water.

They are exists in two types since there are two kinds of electrons are present.

1. Negatron ($\beta^-$) = The negative electron.
2. Positron ($\beta^+$) = The positive electron.

The positron is identical with negatron in all aspects except its charge (+1). The positron is also called as anti-particle of electron.

Due to the release of more amount of energy over a short distance, they are locally destructive to tissue, so atoms those emits β particles are used as a therapeutic agents if deposited internally or placed proximity to lesions.

*Example:* For negatron ($\beta^-$) emission with C-14.

$$^{14}_{6}C \longrightarrow ^{14}_{7}N + \beta^-$$

*Example:* For positron ($\beta^+$) emission with Zn-65.

$$^{65}_{30}Zn \longrightarrow ^{65}_{29}Cu + \beta^+$$

**Gamma radiation:** Gamma radiation is different from alpha and beta radiation. Gamma radiation is electromagnetic and α, β-radiations are particulate. These are having the quanta of energy at a velocity of $3.0 \times 10^{12}$ m/sec. They are emitted due to the *nuclear de-excitation* (radioactive nuclei in excited state). The excited nuclei have more energy; they tend to lose excess energy returning to the ground state by emission of gamma radiation.

These are having more penetrating power than that of other types. It can pass easily through more than 25 cm of tissue.

*Example:* For Gamma radiation with $^{60}$Co.

$$^{59}_{27}\text{Co}(n,\gamma) \longrightarrow {}^{60m}_{27}\text{Co} \longrightarrow {}^{60}_{27}\text{Co} + \gamma \longrightarrow {}^{60}_{28}\text{Ni} + \beta^- + 2\gamma$$

The high penetrating power of this radiation increases the chances for secondary ionization.

The gamma emitting radio nuclides are mainly useful for diagnosis. Once they are given internally, they distributed within the body and the photons can penetrate the tissues and can be detected externally by specially designed imaging equipment.

**K-Capture:** A type of radiation similar to gamma rays is present in the emission of X-rays through a process known as K-capture. This radiation is produced by isotopes with an unstable proton/neutron ratio with insufficient energy to emit a positron.

OR

The nucleus captures an electron from the K-shell which combines with a proton to form a neutron; this rearrangement of the orbital electron takes place with the release of energy in the form of X-rays.

Examples of K- capture with mercury.

$$^{197}_{80}\text{Hg} \xrightarrow{\text{K-Capture}} {}^{197}_{79}\text{Au} + \text{X-ray}$$

The energies of all the above radiations emitted by the nuclides can be determined by instrumental techniques. These energies are expressed in terms of million electron volts. (MeV). One electron volt (eV) is defined as the energy acquired by an electron when accelerated through a potential of one volt.

One MeV = 2.3 X $10^7$ kcal/mole

**Nuclear notation:** For writing the symbol of a nuclide, the atomic number is written as a subscript preceding the symbol for the element, and the mass number is written as a superscript.

*Example:* $^{14}_{7}$N

Mass ← A

$X_N$ → Nitrogen nucleus

Atomic number ← Z

**Nuclear equations:** The nuclear reaction is expressed by following way.

$$^{14}_{7}\text{N} + {}^{4}_{2}\text{He} \longrightarrow {}^{1}_{1}\text{H} + {}^{17}_{8}\text{O}$$

In the above reaction, nitrogen with mass number 14 is bombarded with a helium nucleus of mass number 4 to gives oxygen with a mass number 17 and a proton with a mass number 1. The nuclear equations must balance like other chemical reactions. The same equation also represented by short hand notation as follows.

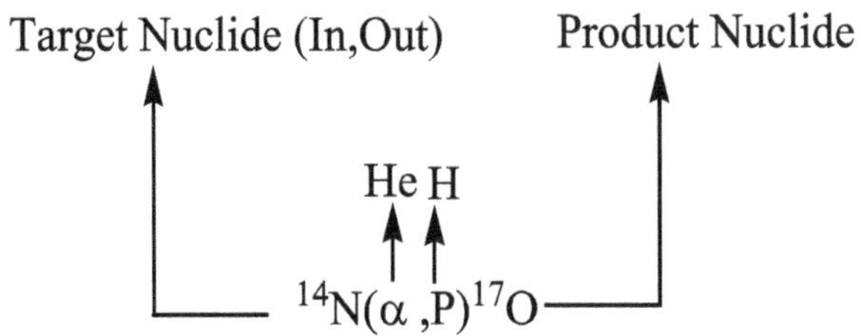


**Kinetic of decay:** Due to spontaneous decay, the concentration of the radioactive sample diminishes with time and the rate of the reaction depending on the concentration of the radioactive atom present (Fig. 7.1).

It is expressed by

$$\frac{-d_N}{d_t} = \lambda N$$

Where, $d_N$ = Change in the number of atoms N

$d_t$ = Change in the time t

$\lambda$ = Proportionality constant (decay constant)

N = number of atoms

The negative sign indicates the decrease in the number of atoms with time.

The radioactive decay depends upon the number of atoms, so it follows first order kinetics.

Integration of the above equation

$$\text{In } N_t/N_o = -\lambda t$$

$N_o$= Number of atoms present at zero time

$N_t$ = Number of atoms present at 't' time

Sometime it is written by exponential form

$$N_t = N_o e^{-\lambda t}$$

It is (Radioactive decay) illustrated graphically

$$-d_N/d_t = \lambda N$$

$$A = \lambda N \ (-d_N/d_t = A = \text{activity})$$

In $A_t/A_o = -\lambda t$ (or) $A_t = A_o e^{-\lambda t}$ (or) $\text{In } A_t = \text{In } A_o - \lambda t$.

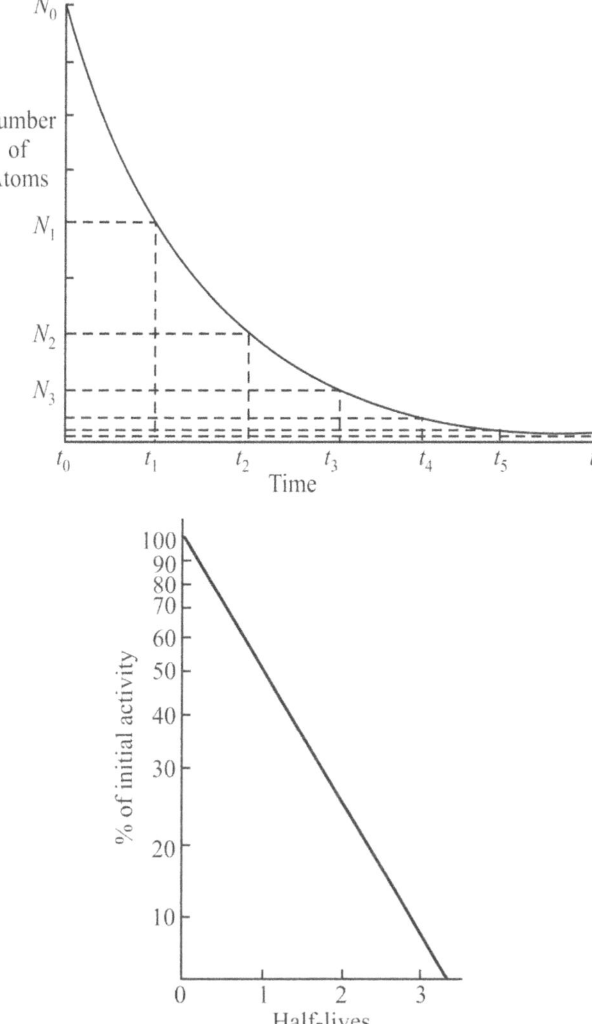


Fig. 7.1 Radioactive decay

**Radioactive decay series**

There are four types of radioactive decay series:

1. 4n series
2. 4n + 1 neptunium series
3. 4n + 2 uranium series
4. 4n + 3 actinium series

***Absolute activity:*** It is expressed as disintegrations per second (d/s) or disintegration per minute (d/m).

***Observed activity:*** It is expressed in counts per second (c/s) or counts per minute (c/m).

***Half-life:*** The half-life of radioactive compound is the time required for one half of a given number of atoms to decay.

$$t_{1/2} = 0.693/\lambda$$

## 7.2 METHODS FOR OBTAINING RADIOACTIVE SUBSTANCES

The radionuclide used in medicine and pharmacy are produced artificially. These are produced by four ways.

1. Nuclear reactor as fission by product.
2. Neutron reaction or activation or transmutation.
3. Use of a particle accelerator such as cyclotron.
4. From radio nuclide generator.

1. **Nuclear reactor as fission by product:** Fission is a radioactive process in which a relatively heavy nucleus is divided in to two nuclei of nearly equal size with the continuous or simultaneous emission of two or three neutrons. The reaction is induced by bombardment of parent nucleus with a neutron.

$$^{235}_{92}U + ^{1}_{0}n \longrightarrow X + Y + 2.5n$$

Where X, Y – Fission products (New nuclei) with z value between 30 and 65.

For each neutron consumed, an average of 2.5 new neutrons are produced that may initiate the fission of other nuclei. This type of reaction is called as chain reaction. Example for fission reaction is shown below

$$^{238}_{92}U + ^{1}_{0}n \longrightarrow ^{131}_{50}Sn + ^{106}_{42}Mo + ^{1}_{0}n + ^{1}_{0}n$$

The $^{131}Sn$ and the $^{106}Mo$ are very radioactive and have very short half-lives. So they immediately undergo series of β decay.

$$^{131}_{50}Sn \longrightarrow ^{131}_{51}Sb \longrightarrow ^{131}_{52}Te \longrightarrow ^{131}_{53}I$$

$$^{106}_{46}Mo \longrightarrow ^{106}_{43}Tc \longrightarrow ^{106}_{44}Ru \longrightarrow ^{106}_{45}Rh$$

Both $^{131}I$ and $^{106}Ru$ are commercially available fission by products.

**Disadvantage:** The separation of desired nuclide produced by this method is too costly and too difficult to produce.

2. **Nuclear reaction or Activation or Transmutation:** Many Radioactive nuclides used in pharmaceuticals are prepared by this method. These are prepared by placing a particular target material in a nuclear reactor where it is bombarded by neutrons.

   *Example:* Preparation of radioactive phosphorous from stable phosphorous by neutron capture.

$$^{31}_{15}P + ^{1}_{0}n \longrightarrow ^{32}_{15}P + \gamma$$

   The main disadvantage of this method is that the radioactive phosphorous is diluted with stable phosphorous.

3. **Use of a particle accelerator such as cyclotron:** The basic principle of this method is, when the particles have been accelerated to a high velocity, they are caused to strike a target containing the atoms to be bombarded. The cyclotron and other similar accelerators are used only with charged particles such as protons, α- particles, electrons or deuterons since the operation of such machine depends upon the electrical/magnetic fields with charge of the particles which are accelerated.

   *Example:* Preparation of sodium 22.

4. **From radio nuclide generators:** For clinical practice the radionuclide are administered internally. So it is advantage to use a nuclide with a short half-life ($t_{½}$) to reduce the radiation source received by the patient. For this type of short half-life ($t_{½}$) radio nuclides are prepared from radionuclide generators, which are working under sequential decay principle.

   Here the short half-life daughter nuclides are prepared from long lived parent nuclide. The daughter nuclide produced is eluted or milked from the generator by using appropriate eluent.

   *Example:* The molybdenum 99/technetium 99m generator (Fig. 7.2) which consists of an alumina ($Al_2O_3$) column on which molybdenum 99 is adsorbed as ammonium molybdate. The technetium 99 formed due to the decay of $^{99}Mo$ is eluted from the column with 0.9% sodium chloride. Upon elution, the $^{99}Tc$ is eluted as sodium pertechneate. Elution is repeated for every 24 hours.

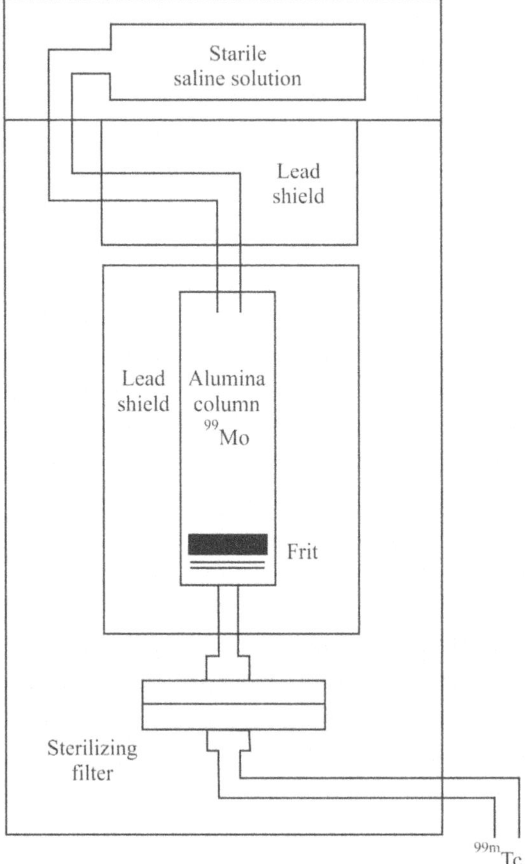


Fig. 7.2 Radio nuclide generator

### 7.2.1 Units of Radioactivity

1. ***Curie:*** The unit of radioactivity is curie which is symbolized as "c". It is defined as the one gram of radioactive substance which undergoes $3.7 \times 10^{10}$ disintegration/second.
2. ***Millicuries:*** $1 \times 10^{-3}$ of curie = $3.7 \times 10^{7}$ disintegration/second ($mc_i$).
3. ***Microcuries:*** $1 \times 10^{-6}$ of curie = $3.7 \times 10^{4}$ disintegration/second ($\mu c_i$).
4. ***RAD (Radioactive Adsorbed Dose):*** It is the unit of adsorbed dose.

$$1 \text{ RAD} = 10^{-2} \text{ J/Kg}$$

## 7.3 MEASUREMENT OF RADIOACTIVITY

The radioactivity of a substance can be measured by two methods.

1. Gas ionization.
2. Scintillation Method (Counting scintillations).

The Gas ionization method includes Geiger Muller counter, Proportional counter, Pulse ionization chamber etc.

The scintillation methods are mainly used for the measurement of gamma radiation.

The method chosen for the measurement of radioactivity depends upon the penetrability of the radiation and the extent of energy dissipation.

### 7.3.1 Gas Ionization

1. **Ionization chambers**

   ***Principle:*** Radiations causes ionization of gas molecules when it passes through gases which lead to the emission of electrons which in turn reveals the changes in electrical current.

   ***Construction:*** These are available in various sizes and shapes. It consists of chambers with two electrodes kept at different electrical potential normally 5 to 10 volts for each centimeter of distance between two electrodes. This chamber is filled with gas. A measuring device attached to the chamber indicate the flow of electric current when the radiation passes to the gas molecules and leads to ionization.

2. **Proportional counters:** These are the modified type of ion chambers.

   ***Principle:*** These are operated by the following principle, when an electrical field strength at the centre electrode in an ionization chamber is increased above the saturation level but decrease in the Geiger region, the size of the pulses from the chamber is increased, but it is proportional to the initial ionization. Amplification of pulse is 1000 times less.

   ***Working:*** A typical example of flow proportional counter is shown below (Fig. 7.3).

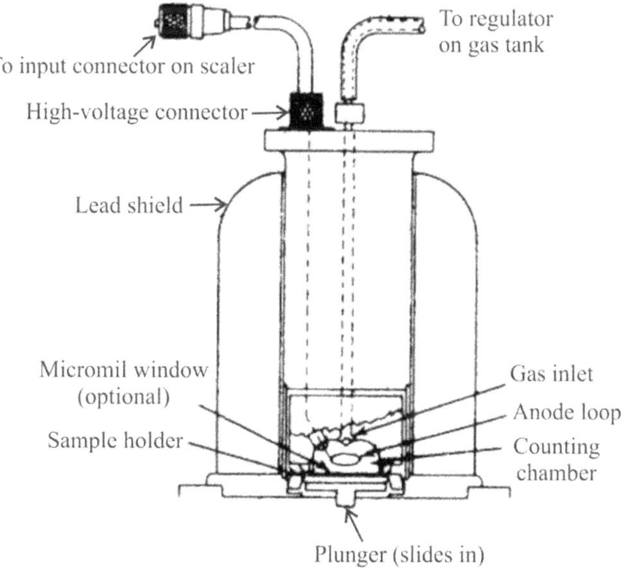


Fig. 7.3 Proportional counter

A small amount of radioactive material to be analyzed is placed inside the active volume of the counter likewise to prevent the losses of sample due to window absorption. Then the steady flow of gas (Argon with 10% Methane) purged to this chamber and steady flow of gas is maintained during counting. It is mainly used to count low energy α and β particles.

3. **Geiger Muller counter:** It is otherwise called as G-M counter or G-M tube in which the ions are produced by the direct ionizing effect of the radiation on the gas molecules in the detector. It is the most popular radiation detector which is used to detect α, β and γ radiation. It is having the efficiency for β particles are near 100% but for γ radiation is only one percent.

***Construction:***

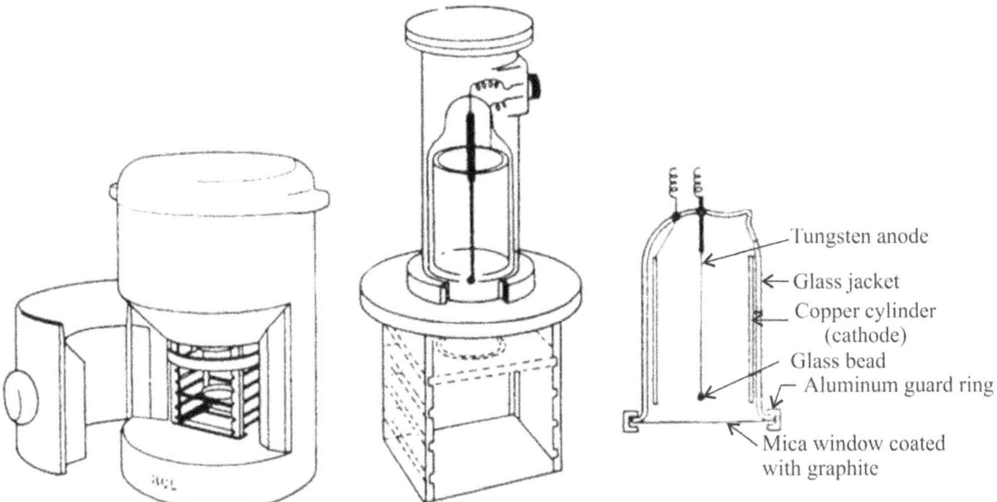


Fig. 7.4 Geiger Muller counter/G-M tube

It consists of central wire anode surrounded by a cylindrical cathode (silver coated glass tube or brass cylinder). The two electrodes are enclosed in gas tight envelope filled with argon gas (80 torr pressure) plus methane or ethanol (20 torr) or chlorine (0.08 torr).

A point of entry of radiation contains a coin made up of mica about 2.5 cm diameter and 2-3 $mg/cm^2$ thick (Fig. 7.4).

***Principle and working:*** When an ionizing radiations or particles enter the active volume of G-M counter, collisions between filling and radiation gas takes place which produces ion pair. These ion pairs are migrated towards the appropriate electrode under the voltage gradient. Due to this potential gradient, the mobility of the electron is quite high and it gets sufficient velocity to produce a new pair of ions upon collision with another atom of argon. This process is repeated several times, each ionizing particle that enters the active volume of counter gives rise to avalanche (sudden large amount) of electrons which traveling towards the central anode and strike the anode, spread the ionization throughout the tube or chamber. These processes produce continuous discharge, each discharge build up to a constant pulse. These pulses are counted by scaling circuits or rate meter without intermediate amplification.

**Paralysis or Dead time of the G-M tube:** After each avalanche, the anode is surrounded by excess number or large number of cations which reduce the potential gradient in the active volume of region and prevent the entry of more ionizing particles. Until the cation has moved a certain distance from the anode no pulses are produced and the G-M tube is insensitive to radiation. This period is known as "dead time" of the G-M counter and is followed by a "recovery time" in which very small pulses are produced. The dead time and the recovery time together make up the paralysis time of the counter during which it does not function.

If the paralysis time is seconds, observed counting rate is N/second and then the corrected counting rate (CCR) is determined by

$$CCR = N/(1\text{-}Nt)$$

Where Nt = No. of counting occurs/seconds.

***Working voltages*:** Normally a potential of 800-2500 V is applied and it depends upon the type of radioactive source.

**Plateau of G-M counter:** The graph is obtained by placing pulse amplitude in y-axis and applied voltage in x-axis (Fig. 7.5).

The design and construction depends upon the purpose for which they required. Different types of G-M counters are available, the most frequently used counter for detecting solid sources is end window type.

In this type, cathode is usually made up of copper which forms the vertical wall of the counter and the end window is made up of mica, aluminium or some alloy of appropriate thickness. The incoming radiation enters the counter through this window and the source is placed beneath it.

A counter used for liquids, contains a metal spiral as cathode. The liquid to be counted is placed in the annual space between the wall of the counter and the outer wall, and the radiation passes through the glass wall of the counter.

**Background radiation:** When measurements are being made, the detector and the source must be shielded from the back ground radiation which is from cosmic and stray radiation like α-radiation from laboratory building materials. This is done by surrounding them with 1½ to 2 inches of "lead caste". For solid counters it is brick shaped, but for liquid counters it is cylindrical shape.

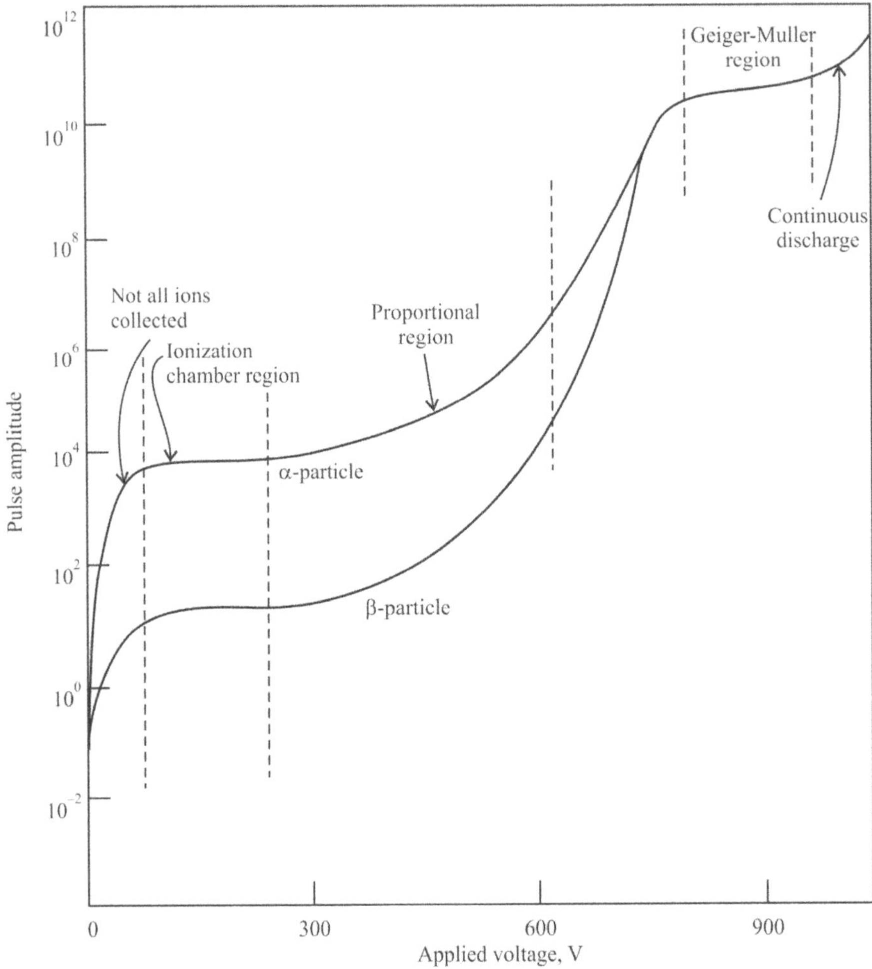


Fig. 7.5 Plateau of G-M counter

## 7.3.2 Scintillation Counters

Scintillators are chemicals which are used to convert radiation energy in to light. When an ionizing particle is absorbed by anyone of several transparent scintillators, the energy acquired by the scintillator is emitted as a pulse of visible light or near UV radiation. This light is observed by photo multiplier tube either by directly or through an internal reflecting optic fiber. The combination of scintillator and photomultiplier tube is called as scintillation counter (Fig. 7.6).

***Construction:*** Scintillation counters consist of

1. A Phosphor
2. A photomultiplier tube (PMT)
3. High voltage supply
4. An amplifier

5. A pulse – height discriminator and
6. A counting system.

The commercial scintillation counters are available in which the phosphor, PMT and amplifier are housed in a light-tight lead shielded container provided with a space for the source. There are large numbers of designs are available, suitable for liquids and other solid forms.

***Phosphor:*** The nature of phosphor used depends upon the types of radiation to be detected.

For α counting, a silver activated zinc sulphide in the form of a thin layer on a clear support is almost used.

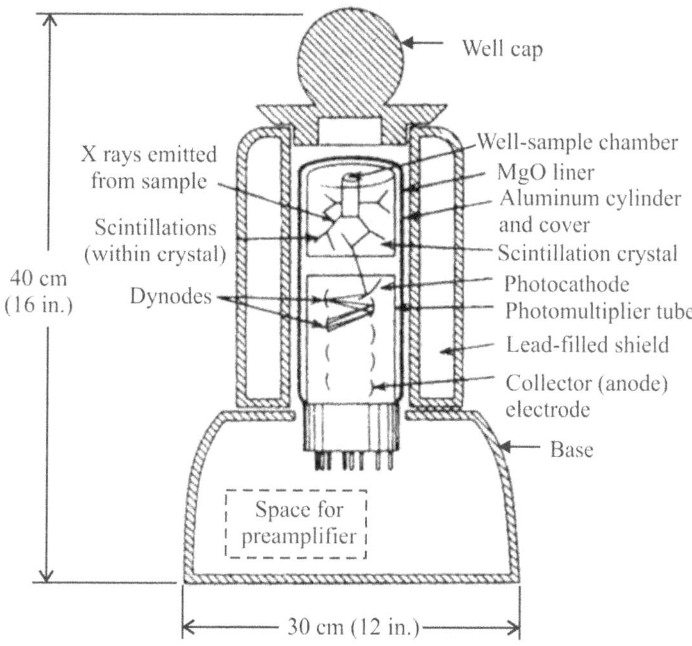


Fig. 7.6 Scintillation counter

For β counting, an organic phosphor like naphthalene or anthracene is used. These are used in the form of large crystals.

For γ counting, thallium activated sodium iodide crystals are more commonly used, sometimes organophosphorous also used.

**Working and principle of scintillation counter**

***Principle:*** The γ photons or charged particles from the radioactive source causes the emission of flashes of light from phosphor (scintillation) which are made to fall on the cathode (light sensitive) of photo multiplier tube. The electrons from the cathode travel to the first dynode which then emit about four electrons for each one it received. Then the electron multiplication effect is takes place between the successive dynodes, so that the number of electrons leave in the last dynode is about $1 \times 10^7$ times.

The electrons are then collected on anode which is connected to the high voltage supply, a sudden decrease in potential occurs which produce a pulse which are passed through an amplifier and then counted by counting equipment.

**Advantages**

1. Scintillation counters do not have a paralysis time, so it can be used in high speed counting.
2. These are more efficient $\gamma$ detectors than G-M counters, so they are specifically used for $\gamma$ - counting and for $\gamma$ energy determinations.

**Disadvantages**

1. Scintillation counters need a well – stabilized high voltage supply.
2. Background counting rates are usually high.

## 7.4 OFFICIAL RADIO ACTIVE PHARMACEUTICALS

The official compounds mentioned below are essential compounds and these are supplied by United Kingdom Atomic Energy Authority (UKAEA). Some compounds which are not official in B.P or U.S.P. also included.

**Labeled Cyanocobalamines**

Cyanocobalamin labeled with cobalt has been used for the diagnosis of pernicious anaemia, determinations of Glomerular Filtration Rate (GFR) and assay of cyanocobalamin by an isotope dilution method.

Here vitamin $B_{12}$ (cyanocobalamin) is labeled with cobalt 57, cobalt 58 or cobalt 60 by biosynthesis using *Streptomyces griseus* on a medium containing appropriate isotope. The labeled vitamin obtained is purified by solvent extraction method and ion-exchange processes and final purification by crystallization.

### Cyanocobalamin ($^{57}Co$)
### (RCC/CT)

It is supplied as freeze dried solid in glass ampoules or in gelatin capsules or as a solution of the vitamin.

***Test for radiochemical purity:*** It should be tested by reverse isotope dilution method.

***Radioactivity assay:*** It is measured by scintillation counter.

***Cyanocobalamin assay:*** By Microbiological assay, using *Lactobacillus Leichmanni.*

***Dose:*** 1 μCi.

***Uses:*** It is used for the diagnosis of pernicious anaemia when the other chemical forms of radioactive cobalt are not absorbed.

## Cyanocobalamin ($^{58}Co$)

In this preparation, cyanocobalamin is labeled with cobalt 58 which is supplied as freeze dried form or in vitamin solution.

***Test for radiochemical purity:*** It should be tested by reverse isotope dilution method.

***Radioactivity assay:*** The activity may be determined by using cobalt 58 standard solution.

***Uses:***

1. For determination of GFR.
2. For absorption and metabolism of cyanocobalamin.

***Dosage:*** For determination of GFR - 2 μCi - given by injection. For absorption and metabolism of cyanocobalamin - 1 μCi given by oral route.

## Cyanocobalamin ($^{60}Co$)

It is a freeze dried cyanocobalamin labeled with cobalt-60. It contains an activity of 0.2 μCi/μg of vitamin.

***Test for radiochemical purity:*** Similar to Cobalt-57.

***Cyanocobalamin assay:*** Similar to Cobalt-57.

***Radioactivity assay:*** The activity may be determined by using cobalt 60 standard solution.

***Dose:***

1. About 1 μCi dose is used for the determination of vitamin $B_{12}$ in culture media, food stuffs, and pharmaceutical products by isotope dilution analysis method.
2. For the investigation of the absorption and metabolism of vitamin $B_{12}$ - 0.5 to 1.0 μCi.
3. All the above compounds contain bacteriostatic agent.

## Ferric Citrate ($^{59}Fe$) Injection (RCG/IFS 2P)

***Introduction:*** Neutron irradiation of iron produces two types of radio isotopes. They are as follows.

1. $^{55}Fe$ with a half-life of 2.7 years.
2. $^{59}Fe$ with a half-life of 45 days.

The isotope $^{59}Fe$ is a β and γ-emitter with energy of 1.1 MeV and 1.29 MeV.

$$^{59}_{26}Fe \xrightarrow{45d} {}^{59}_{27}Co + 1.1MeV\gamma + 1.29MeV\gamma + 0.46MeV\beta^- + 0.271MeV\beta^-$$

The injection is a sterilized isotonic solution of $^{59}Fe$ labeled ferric ion containing 1% of sodium citrate, with pH 6.0 to 8. The specific activity is 3-15 mCi/mg iron.

***Test for radiochemical purity:*** Ferric citrate injection contains ferric ion in sodium citrate solution form. So this test is only of isotopic purity to prove that only $^{59}Fe$ activity is present.

This is done by comparison of γ-spectrum of injection with that of standard $^{59}Fe$ solution. The two spectra must be identical.

***Assay for ferrous ion:*** A sample solution containing 40 μCi iron - 59 must not produce more intense color of thioglycolic acid complex than that of color complex produced by 0.04 mg of ferrous ion. The solution also gives the characteristic reactions of citrate ions.

***Radioactivity assay:*** It is detected by using scintillation counter or standard ion chamber. By this method the activity of injection is compared with the standardized $^{59}Fe$ solution.

***Uses:*** The injection is used for the diagnosis of hematological disorders.

***Dose:*** 5 - 50 μCi.

## Gold ($^{198}$Au) Injection B.P (RCG/GCS 4P 2GGS1P)

It is a sterile, colloidal solution of gold-198, stabilized with gelatin. It contains 12 mg/ml of gold.

***Preparation or Production:*** Gold -198 is produced by the reaction of $^{197}Au$ (n, γ).

$$^{197}Au \xrightarrow[(n,\gamma)]{} 0.960.46Mev\beta^- + 0.412Mev\gamma + {}^{198}_{79}Au$$

The particle size of the injection is ranges between 20 and 30 mμ, for diagnostic use and up to 20 mμ for therapeutic use.

***Properties:*** It is a deep red color, odorless, colloidal solution. The pH of the solution is 4.3 to 7.5. The radiation may cause darkening of the solution and the container over a period of time.

***Radioisotopic purity:*** The absence of isotopes other than $^{198}Au$ and $^{199}Au$ is done by comparing the γ -spectrum with that of a standardized $^{198}Au$ solution or a mixture of $^{199}Au$ and $^{198}Au$ solutions containing the proportion of $^{199}Au$ stated on the label of the injection.

***Radioactivity assay***: The activity of the injection may be determined by comparison of β or γ- ray activity with that of a standardized $^{198}Au$ solution or by using standard ion chamber.

***Uses:***

1. $^{198}$Gold injection is mainly used therapeutically. The solution is administered by intra-cavitary injection into the pleural and peritoneal cavities for aiding the management of pleural effusion (the accumulation of serous fluids in the pleural cavity) and ascites (the accumulation of serous fluid in the peritoneal cavity).
2. It is also used diagnostically to study the blood circulation in the liver.

3. Therapeutically it is used for the treatment of myelogenous leukemia by the irradiation of liver and spleen can be achieved by reducing the production of white cells in these organs.

***Dose:*** For diagnostic dose is 10 to 100 μCi.

For therapeutic dose is 50 to 150 μCi.

## Sodium Chromate ($^{51}Cr$) Solution I.P., B.P.

This is a sterile solution of sodium chromate ($^{51}Cr$) in isotonic saline with a pH of 5-8.

***Physical properties:*** The solution is clear, colorless or faint yellow color solution. It undergoes decay by K-capture and emits γ-radiation also.

***Test for radiochemical purity:*** The activity of chromium ion is not more than 10%.

***Radioactivity assay:*** It should be detected by using scintillation counter.

***Uses:*** It is used to label RBC for the investigation of hematological disorders.

***Dose:*** 20-100 μCi.

***Other formulations:*** Sodium chromate Cr $^{51}$ injection U.S.P.

**Iodine Compounds**

## Sodium Iodide $^{131}I$ Solution I.P., B.P.

$^{131}I$ and $^{125}I$ are two isotopes of iodine used for diagnostic and therapeutic purposes. From above the two isotopes $^{131}I$ is most frequently used.

***Production:*** It may be produced through neutron bombardment of tellurium - 130, giving the $^{131}I$ isotope along with β and γ radiation.

$$^{130}_{52}Te(n,\gamma)\beta \longrightarrow ^{131}_{53}I$$

The $^{131}I$ isotope easily undergoes decay and gives Xenon - 131 along with γ and β emission.

$$^{131}_{53}I \xrightarrow{8.08d} ^{131}_{54}Xe + 0.608\ Mev\beta^- + 0.364\ Mev\gamma$$

The $^{125}I$ undergoes decay gives Tellurium.

$$^{125}_{53}I \xrightarrow[\text{K-Capture}]{60d} ^{125}_{52}Te + 0.027\ MevX \longrightarrow ^{125}_{52}Te + 0.035Mev\gamma$$

Sodium iodide $^{131}I$ solutions are suitable for either oral or I.V. administration.

***Properties:*** It is a clear, colorless solution but for long time storage both the solution and glass may darkens. The pH of the solution is 7.5 to 9.0.

***Test for radio chemical purity:*** It should be tested by chromatography.

***Radioactivity assay:*** The diluted solution of sample (0.1 μCi) is assayed by using scintillation counter.

***Use:*** It is mainly used for the diagnosis and treatment of thyroid disorders. It is given by oral route.

***Dose:***

For detecting thyroid function - 5 to 50 μCi.

For treatment of thyrotoxicosis - 5 to 15 μCi.

For carcinoma of thyroid gland - 60 to 100 μCi.

***Official formulation:*** Sodium iodide $^{131}$I capsule U.S.P., sodium iodide$^{131}$I solution.

## Sodium Iodide ($^{131}$I) Injection B.P.

It is a carrier-free sterilized, isotonic solution of $^{131}$I contains phosphate buffer and sodium thiosulphate. The pH of the solution is 7 to 8.

***Test for radio chemical purity:*** It should be tested by chromatography.

***Radioactivity assay:*** The diluted solution of sample (0.1 μCi) is assayed by using scintillation counter.

***Use:*** It is mainly used for the diagnosis and treatment of thyroid disorders. It is given by oral route.

***Dose:*** For detecting thyroid function - 5 to 50 μCi.

For treatment of thyrotoxicosis - 5 to 15 μCi.

For carcinoma of thyroid gland - 60 to 100 μCi.

***Route:*** It is administered by intravenous route.

## Iodinated $^{125}$I Human Serum Albumin B.P.

It is a sterile, buffered, isotonic solution of human serum albumin, iodinated with $^{131}$I and subsequently free from free iodide. It contains at least 10-20 mg/ml of human serum albumin. The solution is sterilized by filtration.

The iodination is done in mild conditions and introduced not more than 1 gm of iodine per gram of protein molecule. The pH of the solution is 7.5-8.0.

***Test for radio chemical purity:*** It is determined by paper chromatography or paper electrophoresis.

***Protein assay:*** It is determined by Kjeldahl's mehthod.

***Radioactivity assay:*** The diluted solution of sample (0.1 μCi) is assayed by using scintillation counter.

***Uses:***

1. It is mainly used to determine the plasma volume; it is mixed thoroughly and homogenized before 10 to 15 minutes of I.V route of administration.

2. $^{131}I$ human serum albumin is also used to determine the total blood volume along with sodium chromate $^{51}Cr$ and ferrous citrate $^{59}Fe$.
3. It used to study the circulation time and cardiac output.
4. These two isotopes are not found to use in any techniques of thyroid gland investigation.
5. Due to its low energy $\gamma$ radiation property the radiation exposure to the patient is minimized.
6. It is also used to determine the diagnosis of pulmonary blood flow, emphysema, lung and bronchial tumors.

***Dose:*** For blood and plasma volume studies 3 to 20 μCi.

For scanning procedures 200 to 500 μCi.

***Other formulations:*** Iodinated $^{131}I$ serum albumin U.S.P.

## Sodium $^{125}I$ Serum Albumin U.S.P.

This is a solution of albumin labeled with iodine - 125, remaining all are similar to that of $^{131}I$ labeled compound.

***Advantage:*** 1/6 the dose of the injection is enough when compared with $I^{131}$.

***Dose:*** 0.5 to 5 μCi.

## Sodium Iodohippurate $^{131}I$ injections U.S.P.
## Or
## *o*-Iodohippuric acid $^{131}I$ Injection

***Structure of sodium iodohippurate:***

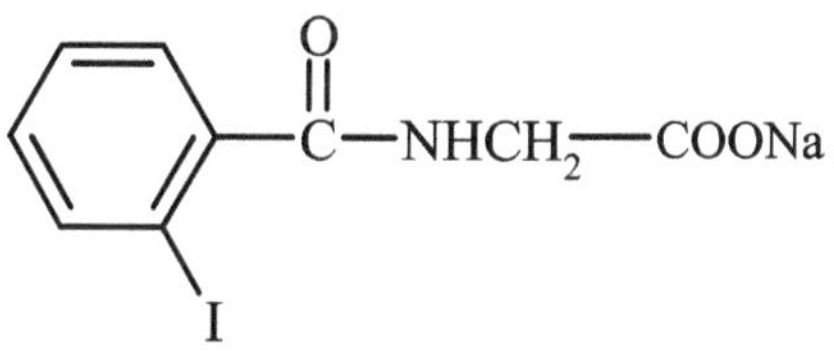

O
||
—C—NHCH$_2$—COONa
I

It is a sterile solution of sodium-*o*-iodohippurate labeled with iodine 131.

***Properties:*** It is a clear, colorless sterile solution. The pH of the solution is 7 to 8.5.

***Test for radio chemical purity:*** It is determined by paper chromatography or paper electrophoresis.

***Radioactivity assay:*** The diluted solution of sample (0.1 μCi) is assayed by using scintillation counter.

***Uses:***

1. It is used for diagnosis of various renal diseases i.e., pyelonephritis (kidney inflammation) and renal hypertension.
2. It is also used to determine renal function by the determination of disappearance rate of the drug from the blood stream.

***Official preparation:*** Hippuran -131, Hipputope.

***Dose:*** 5-30 μCi by I.V route. The dose depends upon the weight of the patient and the type of counting equipment.

## Sodium Rose Bengal $^{131}$I Injection

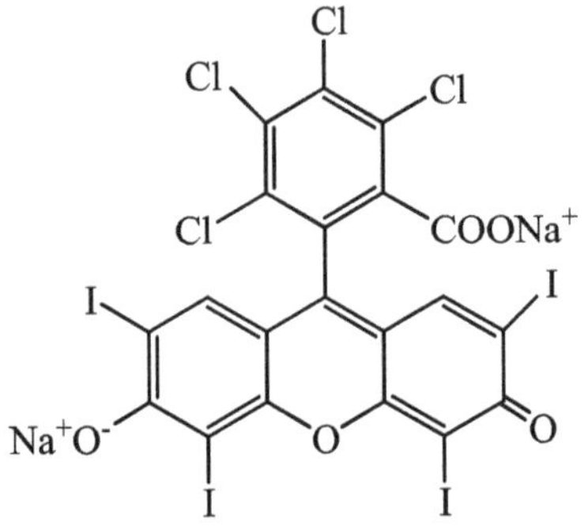

It is a sterile solution of 4,5,6,7-tetrachloro -2',4',5',7' tetraiodo fluorescein disodium salt, which is labeled with $^{131}$I.

This preparation is clear, deep red, sterile solution of sodium rose bengal in which a portion of the molecule is labeled with $^{131}$I. It contains a buffer and pH of solution is between 7 to 8.5.

***Test for radio chemical purity:*** It is determined by paper chromatography or paper electrophoresis.

***Radioactivity assay:*** It is assayed by spectrophotometric method by measuring the absorbance at 550 nm.

***Uses:***

1. Rose bengal is a dye which is used in the colorimetric determination of liver function.
2. Sodium rose bengal labeled with $^{131}$I is used as a radioactive tracer for the diagnosis of liver functions by the disappearance of injected dose from the blood stream and the intestine.
3. The above procedures are used to determine the blood flow, size, location of any abscesses, cysts and tumors present in the liver and also to determine the bile clearance rate.

***Dose:***

1. For Liver Scans: 100 – 200 μCi in adult. For children - 50 μCi.
2. For determination of blood clearance and bile clearance 10 to 25 μCi diluted to 5 ml of normal saline.

## Rose Bengal $^{125}$I Injection

This injection, rose bengal is labeled with $^{125}$I.

Remaining all are similar to sodium $^{125}$I injection.

## Chlormerodrin $^{197}$Hg Injection U.S.P.
## Chlormerodrin $^{203}$Hg Injection U.S.P.

Chemically it is [3-chloromercuri -2-methoxy propyl] urea.

**Mol. Formula:** $C_5H_{11}ClHgN_2O_2$ **Mol. Weight:** 367.2

$$H_2N\text{-}\overset{\overset{\large O}{\|}}{C}\text{-}NH\text{-}CH_2\text{-}\underset{\underset{\large OCH_3}{|}}{CH}\text{-}CH_2\text{-}HgCl$$

***Production:*** Mercury-197 is produced by neutron bombardment of naturally occurring mercury-196.

$$^{196}_{80}Hg_{(n,\gamma)} \longrightarrow {}^{197}_{80}Hg$$

It undergoes radioactive decay and emits gamma radiation by electron capture.

$$^{197}_{80}Hg \xrightarrow[\text{Electron capture}]{2.7d} {}^{197}_{79}Au + 0.077\ Mev\gamma + 0.268\ Mev\gamma$$

***Production of mercury-203:*** It is also produced with target isotope of mercury 202.

$$^{202}_{80}Hg_{(n,\gamma)} \longrightarrow {}^{203}_{80}Hg$$

***Properties:*** Both injections are clear, colorless, sterile solution of chlormerodrin with radioactive mercury.

***Uses:***

1. Both are used as a radioactive tracer for scintillation scans of the kidneys or brain.
2. It is also used for the slow scanning of kidney to locate tumors, cysts or other abnormalities.

***Dose:*** For kidney scanning - 50 to 200 μCi.

For brain scanning - 10 μCi/kg of body weight.

## Sodium Phosphate $^{32}$P Solution U.S.P.

***Production:*** It is prepared by neutron bombardment of sulfur.

$$^{32}_{16}S_{(n,\,p)} \longrightarrow {}^{32}_{15}P$$

Chemically, it is disodium hydrogen phosphate ($Na_2HPO_4$) and sodium dihydrogen phosphate ($NaH_2PO_4$).

***Properties:*** The solution is clear, colorless. The pH of the solution is in between 5 to 6. The solution and the glass container darken upon long time storage.

*Uses:*

1. It is used for the primary diagnosis of intraocular tumors.
2. It is also used for the localization of cerebral tumors.
3. The main therapeutic use of sodium phosphate-32 is the treatment of polycythemia vera (Increase in the number of RBC cells).
4. Sometimes it is used in the treatment of myelocytic leukemia, chronic lymphocytic leukemia.

***Dose:*** For polycythemia vera 2 to 10 μCi.

For diagnostic purpose 125 to 500 μCi.

## Chromic Phosphate - 32

It is a non-official, grayish-green to brown colored colloidal suspension of radioactive chromic phosphate in different types of suspending vehicles.

***Uses:*** It is used in the treatment of pleural effusion and ascites and tumors by intra cavitary injection.

***Dose:*** For pleural effusions - 9 to 12 μCi.

## Technitium$^{99m}$Tc Injection I.P.

It is an artificial element, in which all of its isotopes are radioactive.

***Production:*** It is produced by the decay of molybdenum 99.

$$^{98}_{42}Mo \xrightarrow[(n,\gamma)\ decay]{67\ h} {}^{99m}_{43}Tc + 3\beta^- + 6\gamma$$

The common chemical forms of $^{99m}$Tc are sodium pertechnetate salt and technetium sulfide colloidal preparation and other forms are $^{99m}$Tc labeled serum albumin macro aggregates and $^{99m}$Tc iron ascorbic acid complex.

*Uses:*

1. It is mainly used for the diagnosis of thyroid function studies.
2. Sodium pertechnetate is used for brain scans.

**Other formulations of technetium-99m:** $99^m$ Tc - labeled serum albumin macroaggregates.

$99^m$ Tc - iron ascorbic acid complex.

## Indium - 113m

It is another one artificial element produced by using isotope generators.

***Uses:*** It is used for the renal and brain scanning and also for the determination of plasma volume.

**Miscellaneous Isotopes**

1. **Strontium 85:** $^{85}SrCl_2$

**Fluorine 18:** $^{18}NaF$

Both of the above two compounds are used for the diagnosis of bone metabolism and for bone scanning.

2. ***Calcium* 45, 47:** These are used for the determination of calcium metabolism in diagnosed bone cancer and other bone lesions.
3. ***Selenium* 75:** It is with an amino acid methionine to produce selenomethionine Se - 75. It is used for the synthesis of digestive enzymes. It is also used for the scanning of pancreas and parathyroid gland.
4. ***Ytterbium* 169**

   It is a useful isotope for brain scanning and for the determination of glomerular filtration rate in kidneys.

**Biological Effects of Radiation:** The biological effects of radioactive substances are depends upon various factors includes the related penetration ability of radiation to the tissues, the energy of the radiation, dose rate of radiation and exposed surface area. The destructive effect of radioactivity is directly related to its interaction with tissue molecules to form abnormal amount of free radicals or ions. These chemical species can alter the local pH or initiate free radical chain reactions, results in the formation of peroxides or other toxic compounds. These effect leads to a hostile environment for tissue cells, leads to necrosis and complete destruction of tissue or organ. Water is most abundantly present in the tissues which is the most probable relative species in the path of ionizing radiation leads to the production of different potentially active species which can alter the DNA in cells and leads to the cross linking between certain amino acids in proteins.

$$x\,H_2O \xrightarrow[\text{particles}]{\text{Radio active}} \underset{\substack{\downarrow \\ y\,H_2}}{x\,H\cdot} + \underset{\substack{\downarrow \\ y\,H_2O_2}}{x\,HO\cdot} \longrightarrow \text{Other hazardous species}$$

Any biological effects produced by the radiation must first get entry into tissues which depends upon the penetration power of the radiation. Special and various types of detectors are used to determine the radioactivity of the radiations, which are described previously in this chapter.

***Genetic effects:*** Radiations damage the chromosomes and increase the chances of gene manipulation due to the long term exposure of high intensity X- rays and $\gamma$ rays.

***Somatic effects:*** Cataract, leukemia and severe anemia are produced due to the long term exposure of radiations.

***Skin damages:*** A short term exposure of high intensity radiation leads to erythema. Longer exposure leads to brittleness, dryness and burns if dose is more.

## 7.5 STORAGE AND HANDLING OF RADIOACTIVE MATERIALS

Great care should be taken in handling and storage of radioactive materials for protecting people and personnel who handle it from the emission of harmful radiation.

Radioactive materials must be stored in an area not frequently used by people. Shielding may be done by using thick glass or Perspex containers to protect from the gamma radiations, lead shielding is commonly used. The storage area must be regularly checked for the radioactivity. The working area should not be contaminated with radioactive substances.

Trays with absorbent tissue papers are used for handling radioactive liquids, so that any spillage will get absorbed by paper. Rubber gloves are used when working with liquid radio pharmaceuticals, mouth operated pipettes should not be used. Before making use of glass apparatus, it must be ensured that they must have been inactive. Smoking, eating and drinking should not be done in the premises or labs where the radioactive materials are handled. Disposal of radioactive wastes should be carried out with great care.

Very stringent requirements are prescribed by Department of Atomic Energy (DAE) for the establishment of radioactive isotope facility in hospital pharmacies. These includes

1. Specification of premises and equipments.
2. Working and disposal area maintenance.
3. Personnel training.
4. Storage area.
5. Periodic investigation of leakage or contaminations.

## 7.6 CLINICAL APPLICATIONS OF RADIO PHARMACEUTICALS

Radiopharmaceuticals are used in medicine in four different ways. They are

1. Therapeutic uses
2. Radioactive tracers for diagnosis
3. Sterilization process
4. Radiocarbon dating

Each of these are described below.

1. **Therapeutic uses of radioisotopes:** Radio pharmaceuticals are used for the diseased conditions of extensive cellular metabolic malfunctions. Therapeutic uses of radioactive isotopes depend upon their ability to ionize atoms. The ionization energy is expressed in term of Mev.

   ***$^{60}Co$, $^{58}Co$:*** The cobalt labeled isotopes is majorly used for the treatment of advanced stages of cervic, uterus, bladder and vaginal cancers. It is also used in carcinoma of mouth, tongue and lips.

   ***Gold ($^{198}Au$):*** The $^{198}Au$ solutions are most frequently used in therapeutics. It is mainly used for the management of pleural effusion and ascites. It is also used for the treatment of uterus and urinary bladder carcinoma.

***Sodium Iodide*** $^{131}$***I:*** This isotope is used for the treatment of hyperthyroidism (Thyrotoxicosis), thyroid carcinoma and severe cardiac diseases where the conventional therapy has been failed (congestive cardiac failure and angina pectoris). It is most commonly used to treat any residual thyroid tumor after the surgery (removal of thyroid gland).

***Sodium phosphate*** $^{32}$***P:*** The solution is used for the treatment of various neoplastic diseases and also for the treatment of polycythemia vera, myelocytic leukemia.

2. **Diagnostic uses**

***Sodium chromate*** $^{51}$***Cr:*** It is used diagnostically to determine RBC mass, volume and scanning the spleen.

***Radio chromate serum albumin*** $^{51}$***Cr:*** It is used to localize the position, size etc. of the placenta with less radiation exposure.

***Cyanocobalamin*** $^{57}$***Co (or)*** $^{60}$***Co:*** It is used to diagnose pernicious anemia.

***Ferrous citrate*** $^{59}$***Fe:*** It is used to diagnose iron metabolism and RBC formation.

***Radioactive gold*** $^{198}$***Au colloidal solution:*** It is used to diagnose liver functions.

***Sodium iodide*** $^{131}$***I:*** It is used to study the thyroid gland functions, to determine the size, position and possible tumor location.

**Iodinated** $^{131}$**I serum albumin:** This isotope has the following uses

(a) Determination of plasma volume and also total blood volume along with ferrous citrate $^{59}$Fe and sodium chromate $^{51}$Cr.

(b) Localization of brain neoplasm.

(c) Determination of the cerebrospinal fluid circulation.

(d) Diagnosis of pulmonary blood flow, emphysema and tumors in lungs and bronchioles.

***Sodium Iodohippurate*** $^{131}$***I injection:*** It is used for the diagnosis of renal function.

***Sodium rose Bengal*** $^{131}$***I injection:*** It is used as a colorimetric diagnostic aid in liver function determinations (To determine location, presence of cysts, abscesses and tumors).

***Chlormerodrin*** $^{197}$***Hg:*** It is acts as a radioactive tracer for making scintillation scans of brain or kidneys to find out the presence of cysts, tumors and other abnormalities.

***Sodium phosphate*** $^{32}$***P:*** It is used for the visualization of intraocular and cerebral tumors.

***Technetium*** $^{99m}$***Tc:*** It is used to determine the presence and location of tumors and lesions in brain and liver, spleen and bone marrow (scintillation scans). Tc- labeled human serum albumin is used in lung scans.

***Indium 113m:*** It is used for scanning the brain, renal and for determination of plasma volume.

***Strontium-85 as*** $^{85}SrCl_2$ ***and Fluorine-18 as*** $Na^{18}F$***:*** Both are used to diagnose the bone metabolism and for bone scanning.

***Calcium-45 and calcium-47:*** It is used to study calcium metabolism in diagnosed bone cancer and other bone lesions.

***Ferric chloride solution:*** It is used to determine the iron metabolism.

***Selenium-75 (selenomethionine –$^{75}$Se):*** It is used for the synthesis of digestive enzymes and other proteins as a replacement for methionine. Diagnostically used for the scintillation scanning of pancreas and parathyroid gland.

***Ytterbium-169:*** It is used for the determination of GFR in kidneys.

***Sodium diatrizoate:*** It is used to localize the cerebral angiography (localize and visualization of cerebral blood vessels), urography, pyelography & coronary angiography.

***Sodium iodipamide:*** It is used for visualization of bile duct.

***Iodized oil N.F:*** It is used in visualization of uterus and oviducts.

***Iophendylate U.S.P:*** It is used to diagnose the spinal subarachnoid space.

***Iopanoic acid:*** It is used to diagnose the gall bladder.

***Hydrogen isotopes:*** ($^{2}$H and $^{3}$H) [deuterium and tritium]. These are useful to determine total body water.

***Oxygen*** ($^{17}$O and $^{18}$O): It is used to study the organic synthesis and photo synthesis etc.

***Na-22 and 24:*** These isotopes are used for the estimation of ECF, blood circulation rate, find out the cell permeability, excretion and distribution of water etc.

***Radioactive C-14:*** These isotopes are used to synthesize opium, ergot alkaloids and digitalis glycosides.

***$^{60}$Co (or) cesium-137:*** It is used for sterilizing surgical instruments and sterilizing pharmaceutical products.

***Sterilization uses:*** Thermolabile substances like vitamins, hormones, antibiotics etc. are sterilized by radio isotopes.

## 7.7 RADIO OPAQUE CONTRAST MEDIA

**Introduction:** These are chemical compounds containing high atomic number elements, which will be having the ability to prevent or stop the passage of X-rays. These types of elements are used as diagnostic aids in radiology or roentgenology.

**Roentgenology:** It involves the usage of X-rays which are short wave length electromagnetic radiation, in the imaging or shadowing of various internal organ structures. X-rays are having the capacity to pass through most soft tissues. When a special photographic plate or film is placed on the side of patient opposite to the X-ray source, the plate or film will become darkened which is proportional to the number of X-rays passing through this. Bones and teeth are not allowed for the passage of X-rays due to high concentration of calcium and phosphorous.

The most common radio opaque compounds are barium and iodine but the iodine compounds are covalently bonded organic iodides. These compounds are used to the lesser extent. Example: Sodium iodipamide.

These compounds are mainly used for X-ray examinations of the kidney, blood vessels, heart, brain etc. These are given by I.V injection or retrograde.

The main only one important compound of barium which is useful as radio opaque is barium sulphate due to their lowest atomic number and relatively low toxicity. The opacity to X-rays depends upon their high concentration in the organ.

## Barium Sulphate I.P., B.P., U.S.P.

**Mol. Formula:** $BaSO_4$ **Mol. Weight:** 233.4

It contains not less than 97.5% of $BaSO_4$

***Occurrence:*** In nature it occurs as barytes $BaSO_4$ or heavy spar and withrite $BaCO_3$.

***Preparation:*** Purification of the natural substances are difficult process, so for the pharmaceutical and other purposes it is prepared by the following method.

***From barium chloride:*** Medicinally used barium sulphate is prepared by treating barium chloride with any soluble sulphate (sodium sulphate). The precipitate is collected, washed and dried in a steam oven.

$$BaCl_2 + Na_2SO_4 \longrightarrow BaSO_4\downarrow + 2\,NaCl$$

***From barium sulphide:*** Barium sulphate is also prepared by the reaction between barium sulphide and sulphuric acid.

$$BaS + H_2SO_4 \longrightarrow BaSO_4 + H_2S$$

Barium sulphate is one of the bye products in the manufacturing of hydrogen peroxide from barium peroxide, but it is not a pure one for pharmaceutical purposes.

***Properties:*** It is a fine, heavy, white powder, free from gritty particles, odorless, tasteless. It is insoluble in water, dilute acids and alkalis, organic solvents, but it is soluble in concentrated sulphuric acid due to the formation of barium bisulphate.

$$BaSO_4 + H_2SO_4 \longrightarrow Ba(HSO_4)_2$$

***Fusion reaction:*** It reacts with carbonates and yield fused products such as barium carbonate which readily reacts with acids.

$$2\,BaSO_4 + Na_2CO_3 + K_2CO_3 \longrightarrow 2\,KNaSO_4 + 2\,BaCO_3\downarrow$$

$$BaCO_3 + 2\,CH_3COOH \longrightarrow (CH_3COO)_2Ba + CO_2 + H_2O$$

***Test for identification***

1. Boil small amount of sample with 50% w/v sodium carbonate solution for 5 minutes, add water and filter. The filtrate is acidified with dilute HCl. It gives the characteristic reactions of sulphates.
2. The residue obtained from the above test is washed repeatedly with water maximum 3 times. To the residue add 5 ml of dilute HCl filter it, to the filtrate add one drop of dilute sulphuric acid. A white precipitate is formed which is insoluble in dilute sodium hydroxide solution.

***Test for purity:*** It should be tested for acidity or alkalinity, arsenic, heavy metals, phosphates, sulphide, acid soluble substances, soluble barium salts, bulkiness and loss on ignition.

***Test for sulphide:*** Boil the mixture of equal quantity of sample and dilute hydrochloric acid and required water quantity for 10 minutes. Lead acetate paper is introduced into the vapor which is discharge from the solution. The paper should be more darken.

***Soluble barium salt:*** The residue obtained from the acid soluble substances is treated with water and filter it. To the filtrate add one to two drops of dilute sulphuric acid to clear the filtrate and kept aside for half an hour. No turbidity is produced.

***Bulkiness:*** Add 5 gm of sample in 50 ml measuring cylinder and add 90 ml water. Shake well and allow stand for 15 min. It does not settle below 15 ml mark.

***Loss on ignition:*** Not more than 2.5% determined on 1 gm at 600 °C.

***Uses:*** Barium sulphate is used as a diagnostic agent (radio opaque contrast medium). Also as a radio opaque contrast medium for X-ray determination of gastro intestinal tract (roentgenographic studies). It is insoluble in gastric juice, hence does not produce any systemic toxic effects.

***Side effects:*** The major side effect associated with barium sulphate is constipation. The accidental entry of this compound into peritoneal or other cavities through perforations leads to some severe inflammations. It is given as suspension form due to toxic effect of barium ions. Hence U.S.P indicates the following rule.

***Caution:*** When barium sulphate is prescribed, the title always should write out in full form to avoid confusion with the poisonous barium sulphide or barium sulphite.

***Dose:*** For oral route 300 gm (60 - 450 gm).

For rectal route 400 - 750 gm.

***Storage:*** It should be stored in well closed containers.

**Organoiodine Radioopaque Compounds**

There are many number of iodine compounds which are used in diagnosis by roentgenography. They are as follows.

Meglumine diatrizoate - U.S.P.

Sodium diatrizoate - U.S.P.

Meglumine iodipamide - U.S.P.

Sodium iodipamide - U.S.P.
Iodized oil - N.F.
Iopanoic acid - U.S.P.
Iophendylate - U.S.P.
Calcium ipodate - N.F.
Sodium ipodate - N.F.
} These are cholecystographic agents for oral use.

## PROBABLE QUESTIONS

1. What is meant by radio activity? How was the phenomenon discovered?
2. Explain the general theory of radioactivity.
3. Define the following terms.

   (a) Nuclides (b) Isotopes

   (c) Isobars (d) Isotones
4. Explain the different types of nuclear reactions.
5. Write the emission of α, β- particles with equation.
6. What is meant by Negatron and Positron?
7. What is meant by K-capture and explain it with nuclear reaction?
8. What is the way of writing nuclear equations?
9. Explain the kinetic of radioactive decay with derivation.
10. Define radioactive half life.
11. Write the decay series of radioactivity.
12. Define the following terms

    (a) Observed activity

    (b) Absolute activity
13. Describe the various limits of radio activity.
14. How does the radioactive isotopes are produced. Briefly explain the methods of production.
15. Explain in detail about nuclear fission or neutron reaction.
16. Write a short note on particle accelerator and radionuclide generators.
17. How does the radioactivity of a substance is measured?
18. Write the principle and procedure involved in gas ionization methods.
19. Explain in detail about the working principle, construction, advantages and disadvantages of Geiger Muller counter with neat labeled diagram.
20. What is paralysis (or) dead time of G-M counter?
21. Define corrected counting rate?

22. Explain in detail about scintillation counter & write the advantages and disadvantages.
23. Describe proportional counters.
24. Write in detail about miscellaneous isotopes and their uses.
25. Write in brief about biological effects of radiation.
26. Explain the applications of radio pharmaceuticals.
27. Write in brief about the therapeutic uses of radio pharmaceuticals.
28. Explain the diagnostic uses of radiopharmaceuticals.
29. Define radio opaque contrast media.
30. What is meant by Roentgenology.
31. Write the preparation, properties, assay and uses of barium sulphate.
32. Write a short note on Barium meal.
33. Write a note on organo iodine radio opaque compound.
34. What types of precautions to be taken while handling radioactive materials?
35. Explain about storage of radioactive materials?
36. Write the uses of the following radio-pharmaceuticals
    (a) Chromic phosphate (b) Colloidal gold injection
    (c) Ammonium bromide injection (d) Technetium 99m
    (e) Sodium phosphate (f) Ferric chloride solution
37. Explain the radiopharmaceutical sodium phosphate.
38. Describe sodium iodohippurate 1-131 injection USP.
39. Write in detail about the uses of radioisotopes in research, diagnosis and medicine.
40. Write the radio pharmaceutical ferric citrate.
41. Explain the preparation, radionuclide identification, radiochemical purity, assay, packaging, storage and uses of sodium Iodide 1-131 solution U.S.P.
42. Write the radiopharmaceutical sodium iodide 1-125 solution.
43. Mention the radio-nuclide present in the following commonly used radio pharmaceuticals.
    (a) Sodium chloride injection
    (b) Sodium pertechnetate solution
    (c) Sodium orthophosphate solution
    (d) Cyanocobalamin injection
44. Describe the biological effects of radiation.

CHAPTER 8

# COORDINATION COMPOUNDS

## 8.1 INTRODUCTION

Coordination compounds are the product of a Lewis acid-base reaction, in which neutral molecules or anions (called ligands) bond to a central metal atom or ion by coordinate covalent bonds results in the formation of metal complexes called as coordination compounds. Their structures and properties are important data in pharmacy and medicine. Some of the important definitions in co-ordination chemistry are as follows.

- **Lewis acids**: All electron acceptors are called as Lewis acids.
- **Lewis bases:** All electron donors are called as Lewis bases.
- **Ligands or complexing agents:** These are Lewis bases which contain at least one pair of electrons to donate to a metal atom/ion.
- **Metal atoms/ions:** These are Lewis acids which accept pairs of electrons from Lewis bases.
- **Donor atom:** Within a ligand molecule, the atom that is directly bonded to the metal atom/ion.
- **Complex ion:** The coordination complex carries a net charge is called as a complexing ion.
- **Coordination compounds**: Compounds that contain a coordination complex.

Coordination compounds and complexes are different chemical moieties and their properties and behaviour are different from the metal atom/ion and ligands from which they are formed.

### 8.1.1 History of Coordination Chemistry

Alfred Werner (1866-1919) who has received the Nobel Prize in 1913 is a father of co-ordination chemistry for his invention of theory of transition metal-amine complexes. Inorganic chemistry was not a prominent field until Werner studied the metal-amine complexes such as $[Co(NH_3)_6Cl_3]$.

## 8.1.2 Terms used in Coordination Chemistry

(a) **Coordination entity:** A coordination entity constitutes a central metal atom or ion which is bonded to a fixed number of ions or molecule. Example, $[Co(NH_3)_3Cl_3]$. Here the central cobalt ion is surrounded by three ammonia molecules and three chloride ions. Other examples are $[PtCl_2(NH_3)_2]$.

(b) **Central metal atom/ion (Lewis Acid):** In a coordination moiety, the atom/ion is an electron acceptor to which a fixed number of ions/ neutral groups are bound in a definite geometrical arrangement around it, is called the central atom or ion. For example, the central atom/ion in the coordination moiety of $[Fe(CN)_6]^{3-}$ is $Fe^{3+}$.

(c) **Ligands (Lewis bases):** A ligand is an ion or molecule capable of functioning as an electron donor or the ions/ molecules bound to the central atom/ion in the coordination entity are called ligands. These may be simple ions such as $Cl^-$, small molecules such as $H_2O$ or $NH_3$, larger molecules such as $H_2NCH_2CH_2NH_2$ or N $(CH_2CH_2NH_2)_3$ or even macromolecules, such as proteins.

***Type of Ligands: Unidentate:*** A ligand is bound to a metal ion through a single donor atom ($Cl^-$, $H_2O$ or $NH_3$), then the ligand is called as Unidentate.

***Bidentate:*** When a ligand can bind through two donor atoms, and then the ligand is called as bidentate.

*Example:* $H_2NCH_2CH_2NH_2$, it contains two amino groups which donate a pair of electrons.

Bidentate ligands further classified in to two types according to the number of atoms in the ligands which separates the donor atoms and the size of the chelate ring formed.

1,1-ligands forms four membered chelate ring system.

1,2- ligands forms five membered chelate ring system.

***Polydentate:*** when several donor atoms are present in a single ligand and possessing a closed ring system, then the ligand is called as polydentate.

*Example:* Ethylene diamine tetraacetate ion (EDTA) is an important hexadentate ligand

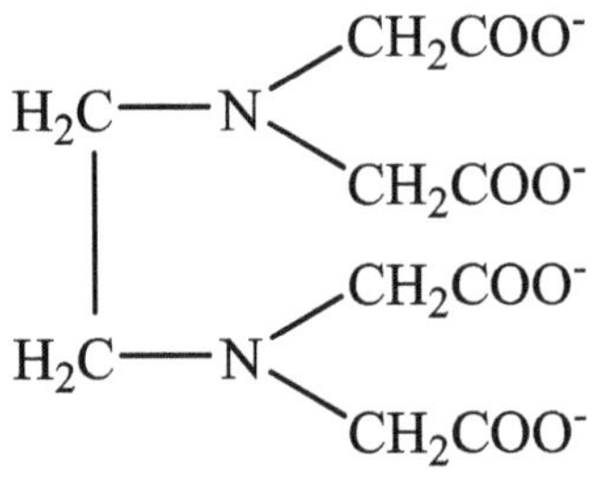

$CH_2COO^-$
$H_2C$—N
$CH_2COO^-$
$CH_2COO^-$
$H_2C$—N
$CH_2COO^-$

***Chelate ligand:*** When a di- or polydentate ligand uses its two or more donor atoms to bind a single metal ion, then the ligand is called as chelate ligand. The number of such ligating groups is called the denticity of the ligand. Such types of complexes are called as Chelate complexes; tend to be more stable than similar complexes containing unidentate ligands.

***Ambidentate ligand:*** Ligand which can ligate through two different atoms.

*Examples:* $NO_2^-$ and $SCN^-$ ions

M ← N(=O)O  M ← O—N=O  M ← SCN  M ← NCS

nitrito-N  nitrito-O  thiocyanato  isothiocyanato

***Macro cyclic proligands*:** Cyclic compounds which contain donor atoms oriented towards a metal ion and which are large enough encircle are called as macro cyclic proligands.

(d) **Coordination number (CN):** The coordination number of a metal ion in a complex is defined as the number of ligand donor atoms to which the metal is directly bonded. For example, $[PtCl_6]^{2-}$ and $[Ni(NH_3)_6]^{2+}$, the coordination number of Pt and Ni are 6 and 4 respectively. It is determined only by the number of sigma bonds formed by the ligand with the central atom/ion. Pi bonds are not counted for this purpose (Table 8.1).

Table 8.1 Some coordination complexes

| Example | Molecular formula | Lewis base/ligand | Lewis acid | Donor atom | Coordination number |
|---|---|---|---|---|---|
| 1. | $[Ag(NH_3)_2]^+$ | $NH_3$ | $Ag^+$ | N | 2 |
| 2. | $[Zn(CN)_4]^{2-}$ | $CN^-$ | $Zn^{2+}$ | C | 4 |
| 3. | $[Ni(CN)_4]^{2-}$ | $CN^-$ | $Ni^{2+}$ | C | 4 |

(e) **Coordination sphere:** The central atom/ion and the ligands bonded to it are enclosed in square bracket and is collectively termed as the coordination sphere

**Counter ions:** The ionisable groups are written outside the bracket, these are called as counter ions. For example, in the complex $K_4[Fe(CN)_6]$, the coordination sphere is $[Fe(CN)_6]^{4-}$ and the counter ion is $K^+$.

(f) **Coordination polyhedron:** The spatial arrangement of the ligand atoms which attached to the central atom/ion explains a coordination polyhedron about the central atom. They are shown in the diagrams.

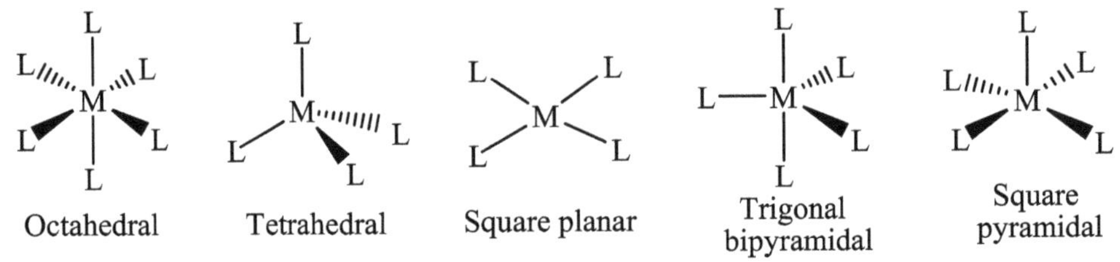

L L L L L L M Octahedral | L L M L L Tetrahedral | L L L L M Square planar | L L L L L M Trigonal bipyramidal | L L L L L M Square pyramidal

(g) **Oxidation number of central atom:** It explains the number of electrons it has lost to form the cation.

The oxidation number of the central atom in a complex is also defined as the charge it would carry if all the ligands are removed along with the electron pairs that are shared with the central atom. It is represented by a Roman numeral in parenthesis followed by the name of the coordination complex. For example, oxidation number of copper in $[Cu(CN)_4]^{3-}$ is +1 and it is written as Cu (I).

(h) **Homoleptic and heteroleptic complexes:** Complexes in which a metal is bound to only one kind of donor groups, e.g., $[Co(NH_3)_6]^{3+}$, are known as homoleptic. Complexes in which a metal is bound to more than one kind of donor groups, e.g., $[Co(NH_3)_4Cl_2]^+$ are known as heteroleptic.

## 8.2 NOMENCLATURE OF COORDINATION COMPOUNDS

Nomenclature is important in coordination chemistry for describing formulas and writing systematic names. The formula and names adopted for coordination entities are based on the recommendations of the International Union of Pure and Applied Chemistry (IUPAC).

### 8.2.1 Rules for the Nomenclature

1. Naming the total complex, the name of the cation given first and the anion name is given second, no matter whether the cation or the anion is the complex species.
2. The name of the ligand or the ligands precedes that of the central atom.
3. A Greek prefix like mono, di, tri, tetra, penta etc. are used to indicates numbers.
4. A Roman numeral or a zero is used in parentheses to indicate the oxidation number of the central metal atom.
5. If the complex is negative ion, the name of the metal ion ends with "ate".
6. If more than one ligand is present in the species, then the ligands are named according to the alphabetical order.
7. If the ligand is negative ion, the name of the ligand is ended with "O" and unmodified the ligand is neutral.

| | | |
|---|---|---|
| $Cl^-$ | chloride | chloro |
| $OH^-$ | hydroxide | hydroxo |
| $O^{2-}$ | oxide | oxo |

| | | |
|---|---|---|
| $CN^-$ | cyanide | cyano |
| $NH_2^-$ | amide | amido |
| $CO_3^{2-}$ | carbonate | carbonato |

8. For neutral ligands, their names are not changed, except the following few:

   $H_2O$, aqua
   $NH_3$, amine

   CO, carbonyl
   NO, nitrosyl

   $NCS^-$, thiocyanate -> thiocyanato-*N*

## 8.3 ISOMERISM IN COORDINATION COMPOUNDS

Isomers are two or more compounds that have the same chemical formula but a different structural arrangement of atoms. They differ in one or more physical or chemical properties. Co ordination compounds exhibit two principal types of isomerism (stereoisomerism and structural isomerism). Each of which can be further subdivided as follows.

**(a) Stereoisomerism**

(i) Geometrical isomerism
(ii) Optical isomerism

**(b) Structural isomerism**

(i) Linkage isomerism
(ii) Coordination isomerism
(iii) Ionisation isomerism
(iv) Solvate isomerism or hydrate isomerism

Stereoisomers have the same chemical formula and chemical bonds but they have different spatial arrangement. A detailed account of these isomers is given below.

**(a) Stereoisomerism**

**(i)** ***Geometrical isomerism or cis–trans isomerism:*** This type of isomerism is possible for square planar and octahedral complexes. In *cis* isomer two identical or similar groups are adjacent to each other whereas *trans* isomer two groups are diametrically opposite to each other. For example,

Cl, Cl, Pt, $NH_3$, $NH_3$ — *cis*

Cl, $H_3N$, Pt, $NH_3$, Cl — *trans*

Geometrical isomers

(ii) ***Optical isomerism:*** Some of the inorganic and organic compounds are having the property to rotate plane polarized light. The compounds which exhibit this property are called optical isomers which are having identical physical and chemical properties.

Optical isomers are mirror images that cannot be superimposed on one another. These are called as enantiomers. According to their rotation of light either left or right, called as levo and dextro respectively.

***For example:*** $[PtCl_2(en)_2]^{12+}$

**(b) Structural isomerism**

(i) ***Linkage isomerism:*** Linkage isomerism is present in ambidentate ligand. These types of ligands are capable of forming more than one coordination bonds. A simple example is compound containing the thiocyanate ligand, $NCS^-$, which may bind through the nitrogen to give M–NCS or through sulphur to give M–SCN. Other examples are

$[Co(NH_3)_5ONO]Cl_2$- nitro isomer-red colour

Pentaminenitritocobalt (III) chloride-O attached

$[Co(NH_3)_5NO_2]Cl_2$-nitroisomer-yellow colour

Pentaminenitrocobalt (III)chloride-N attached

(ii) ***Coordination isomerism:*** This type of isomerism arises from the interchange of ligands between cationic and anionic entities of different metal ions present in a complex. This isomerism occurs where the complex cation and anion contain different metal centres.

| Example: $[Co^{III}(NH_3)_6]$ | $[Co(CN)_6]$ | $[Cr^{III}(NH_3)_6]$ | $[Co^{III}(CN)_6]$ |
|---|---|---|---|
| Hexammine cobalt (III) | Hexacyano cobalt (III) | Hexamine chromium (III) | Hexacyano cobaltate (III) |

(iii) ***Ionisation Isomerism:*** This form of isomerism arises when the coordination compounds having the same molecular formula but forming different ions in solution are called ionisation isomerism.

| Example: $[Co(NH_3)_5Br]SO_4$ | $[Co(NH_3)_5SO_4]Br$ |
|---|---|
| Pentamine bromo cobalt (III) sulphate | Pentamine sulphato cobalt (III) bromide |

(iv) ***Solvate isomerism or Hydrate isomerism:*** This form of isomerism or hydrate isomerism is present in a case where water is involved as a solvent. This is similar to ionisation isomerism. Solvate isomers differ by whether or not a solvent molecule is directly bonded to the metal ion or merely present as free solvent molecules in the crystal lattice.

| Example: $[Cr(H_2O)_6]Cl_3$ (violet) | $[Cr(H_2O)_5Cl]Cl_2.H_2O$ (grey-green). |
|---|---|
| Hexa aqua chromium (III) chloride | Penta aquachloro chromium(III)chloride |

### Bonding in coordination compounds

Nature of bonding in coordination compounds is explained by Werner. But his concept failed to explain about the followings.

1. Only some specific type of compounds is involved in the formation of coordination complexes.
2. Why these bonds are showing directional, optical and magnetic properties.

Many theories are used to explain the nature of bonding in coordination compounds. They are as follows:

Werner's theory

Valence Bond Theory (VBT)

Crystal Field Theory (CFT)

Ligand Field Theory (LFT)

Molecular Orbital Theory (MOT)

### Importance and applications of coordination compounds

Coordination compounds are widely present in the mineral, plant and animal worlds and are known to play many important functions in the area of analytical chemistry, biological systems and medicine.

1. ***Dyes and Pigments:*** Some of the coordination compounds are used as a dyes and pigments in ancient days. For example, madder dye (red in colour) was used by Greeks which is a complex of hydroxy anthraquinone. In analytical chemistry: Coordination compounds are used in many qualitative and quantitative chemical analyses.
2. ***Colour tests:*** The familiar colour reactions given by metal ions with a number of ligands (especially chelating ligands) leads to the formation of coordination entities, form the basis for their detection and estimation by classical and instrumental methods of analysis. ***Examples:*** Formation of red colour complexes of 2,2-bipyridyl and 1,10-phenanthroline as a test for ferrous ion.
3. ***Gravimetric Analysis:*** Here chelating ligands are used to make insoluble complexes. Example: $Ni(DMG)_2$ and $Al(oxine)_3$.
4. ***Determination of hardness of water:*** Hardness of water is estimated by simple titration with disodium EDTA. The $Ca^{2+}$ and $Mg^{2+}$ ions form stable complexes with EDTA. The selective estimation of these ions can be done due to difference in the stability constants of calcium and magnesium complexes.
5. ***Complexometric titrations:*** Coordination complexes are used for the volumetric determination of metal ions in solutions. ***Example*:** $Zn^{2+}$, $Al^{2+}$, $Ca^{2+}$, $Cu^{2+}$ ions etc. EDTA is used as a masking agent for removal of a metal ion which would interfere with the analysis of a second metal present.
6. ***Extraction of metals:*** Some of the metals are leached out from their ores by forming stable complexes. Examples: Ag and Au form a complex with cyanide ion.
7. ***As catalyst:*** Coordination compounds are used as catalysts for many industrial processes. Example: Rhodium complex, $[(Ph_3P)_3RhCl]$, a Wilkinson catalyst, is used for the hydrogenation of alkenes.

8. ***Bio-inorganic chemistry:*** Coordination compounds play an important role in biological process in animals and plants.

   The pigment chlorophyll which is responsible for photosynthesis in plants is a coordination compound of magnesium. Here the modified porphyrin acts as the ligand.

   Haemoglobin, the red pigment of blood which acts as oxygen carrier is a coordination compound of iron.

   Vitamin $B_{12}$, cyanocobalamine, the anti-pernicious anaemia factor, which is a coordination compound of cobalt.

   The other compounds of biological importance with coordinated metal ions are the enzymes like, carboxypeptidase A and carbonic anhydrase catalyst of biological systems.

9. **Therapeutic uses**
   1. Disodium Edetate is used for metal poisoning.
   2. Calcium Disodium Edetate is used for the treatment of lead poisoning.
   3. D-penicillamine and Desferrioxime B is used for copper and iron poisoning by the formation of complexes with the excess ions.
   4. In chemotherapy cisplatin is used as an antitumour drug.

## 8.4 COORDINATION COMPOUNDS USED IN PHARMACY

### Ethylene Diamine Tetra Acetic Acid (EDTA)

**(Synonym: Editic acid)**

**Mol. Formula:** $C_{10}H_{16}N_2O_8$ **Mol. Weight:** 292

***Structure:***

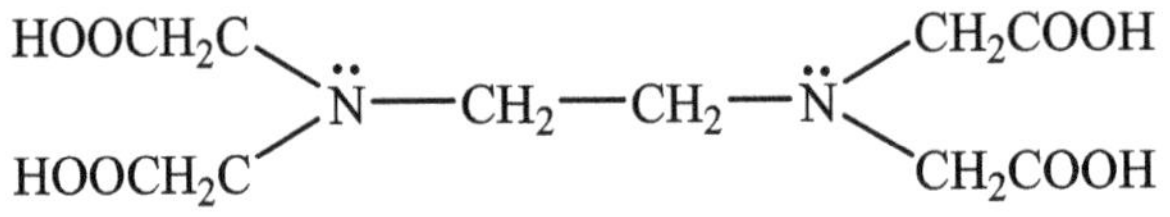

$$(HOOCH_2C)_2\ddot{N}-CH_2-CH_2-\ddot{N}(CH_2COOH)_2$$

***Synthesis:*** It is prepared from ethylene diamine, formaldehyde and sodium cyanide.

$$\underset{\text{Ethylenediamine}}{H_2N\text{-}CH_2\text{-}CH_2\text{-}NH_2} + \underset{\text{Formaldehyde}}{4\,HCHO} + \underset{\text{Sodium cyanide}}{4\,NaCN}$$

$$\downarrow$$

$$4\,NaOH + (CN\text{-}CH_2)_2N\text{-}CH_2CH_2N(CH_2\text{-}CN)_2$$

$$\downarrow \text{HOH}$$

$$\underset{\text{EDTA}}{(COOH\text{-}CH_2)_2N\text{-}CH_2\text{-}CH_2\text{-}N(CH_2\text{-}COOH)_2}$$

***Uses:*** The disodium salt of EDTA is used as a chelating agent.

## Disodium Edetate

**(Synonym: Disodium dihydrogen edetate)**

**Mol. Formula:** $C_{10}H_{14}N_2Na_2O_8.2H_2O$ **Mol. Weight:** 372.2

It is disodium ethylene diamine tetra acetate dihydrate.

It contains not less than 98.5% and not more than 101% of $C_{10}H_{14}N_2Na_2O_8.2H_2O$

***Preparation:*** It is prepared by dissolving EDTA in a hot solution of equivalent quantity of sodium hydroxide. The disodium salt is obtained by crystallization.

$$(HOOCH_2C)_2N{-}CH_2{-}CH_2{-}N(CH_2COOH)_2 + 2\,NaOH \xrightarrow{\text{Hot condition}} (NaOOCH_2C)(HOOCH_2C)N{-}CH_2{-}CH_2{-}N(CH_2COONa)(CH_2COOH)\cdot 2\,H_2O$$

***Physical properties:*** It is a white, crystalline powder, odourless, soluble in water and gives an acidic solution.

***Test for identification:***

1. To the small volume of sample solution, add small amount of lead nitrate solution, shake well and add potassium iodide solution. No yellow color precipitate is formed. Then make the solution to alkaline by using dilute ammonia solution, add ammonium oxalate solution. No precipitate is obtained.
2. It is also identified by Infrared absorption spectrophotometry.
3. The sample solution gives the characteristic reactions of sodium ions.

***Test for purity:*** It should be tested for clarity and color of the solution, heavy metals, iron and other impurities.

***Assay:*** It is assayed by Complexometry method of titration.

***Uses:***

1. It is used as a chelating agent in heavy metal poisoning (lead).
2. It is also used as a pharmaceutical aid.
3. It is primarily used in the treatment of hypercalcaemia.
4. It is also used in treating occlusive vascular disease and cardiac arrhythmias, associated with high levels of calcium in blood.

***Route of administration:*** By Intravenous route.

The official injection containing varying amount of disodium and trisodium salts due to the effects of pH adjustments.

## Disodium Edetate Injection

Disodium Edetate injection is a sterile solution of disodium edetate in water for injection, containing varying amounts of disodium and trisodium salts as a result of pH adjustment.

It contains not less than 90.0% and not more than 110.0% of the stated amount of disodium edetate.

***Test for identification:*** To the sample solution, add required quantity of hydrochloric acid, to adjust the pH to 5 and evaporated to dryness. The residue obtained gives the tests which are described under disodium edetate.

***Test for purity:*** It should be tested for pH, bacterial endotoxin and it should also comply with tests for parenterals.

***Dose:*** By intravenous injection - 50 mg/Kg of body weight upto maximum dose of 3 gm/day.

***Storage:*** It should be stored in single dose containers.

## Calcium Disodium Edetate

**(Synonym: Sodium calcium edetate, Calcium disodium versenate)**

**Mol. Formula:** $C_{10}H_{12}CaN_2Na_2O_8 . x H_2O$ **Mol. Weight:** 374.28

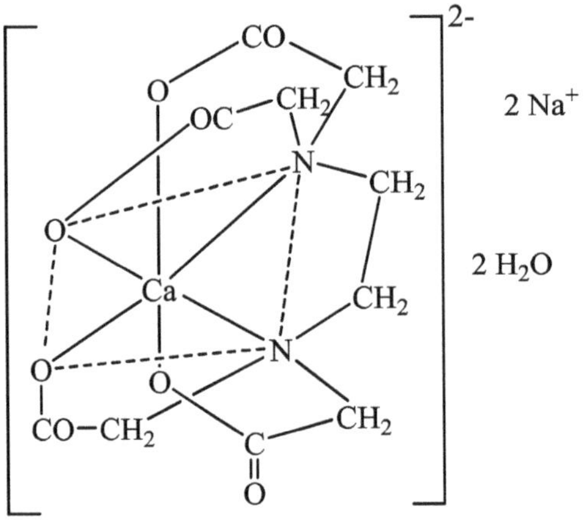

***Preparation:*** It is prepared by boiling disodium edetate solution with powdered calcium carbonate, followed by filtration and concentration. Crystallization is effectively done by the addition of methanol and cooling.

***Properties:*** It is a white, hygroscopic powder, odourless with saline taste, stable in air, very soluble in water, gives weakly acidic solution.

***Mechanism:*** It removes lead from the tissues by forming inactive soluble complex which can be removed from the circulation by the kidneys and excreted in the urine. The I.M route of administration leads to diagnosis of metal poisoning.

***Uses:***

1. It is mainly used in the treatment of lead poisoning (plumbism).

2. It is also used to remove some other heavy metals from the body.
3. It is also used to avoid inducing hypocalcemic states (low serum calcium level).

***Dose:*** By Intravenous infusion

***For Adults:*** 1 gm in 250-500 ml of isotonic solution over a period of one hour, 2 times a day for 5 days.

***For Children:*** 35 mg/kg as 0.2 - 0.4% isotonic solution twice a day.

**By IM route**

***For Adults:*** 75 mg/kg as 20% solution in 0.5% procaine hydro chloride twice a day.

***For Children:*** 35 mg/kg as 20% solution twice a day in divided doses at 8-12 hr interval.

## Penicillamine

**(Synonym: D – Penicillamine)**

**Mol. Formula:** $C_5H_{11}NO_2S$ **Mol. Weight:** 149.2

It is also called as penicillamine -3-mercapto D-valine.

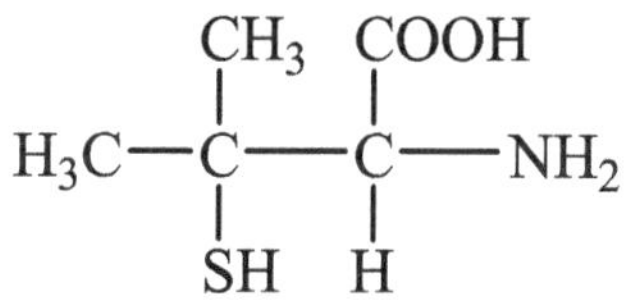

$$\begin{array}{ccccc} & CH_3 & COOH & \\ & | & | & \\ H_3C- & C & -C- & NH_2 \\ & | & | & \\ & SH & H & \end{array}$$

It contains not less than 48.0% and not more than 101.0% of $C_5H_{11}NO_2S$.

***Preparation:*** Penicillamine is obtained by the action of strong acids on penicillins. It was the first degradation product to be obtained as crystalline form.

***Physical properties:*** It is white or almost white crystalline powder.

***Test for identification:***

1. To a small volume of 1% w/v solution of sample, add 2 ml of phosphor tungstic acid solution and heat to boiling. A blue color is produced.
2. To the sample solution, add hydrochloric acid and acetone, warm it, cool in ice and scratch the sides of the test tube with glass rod, to initialise crystallization. Filter it, collect the precipitate, dry it. A 1% solution of the dried material is dextrorotatory.
3. It is also identified by thin layer chromatography.

***Test for purity:*** It should be tested for appearance of solution, pH, specific optical rotation, heavy metals, mercuric salts, penicillamine disulphide, penicillic acid, sulphated ash and loss on drying.

***Assay:*** Non-aqueous titration.

***Uses:***

1. It readily chelates with heavy metals such as mercury or copper and hence it is used for the treatment of heavy metal poisoning.
2. It is also used for the treatment of Wilson's disease and rheumatoid arthritis.

***Dose:***

***For heavy metal poisoning:*** 500 mg - 2 gm daily in divided doses, according to the needs of patients.

***For rheumatoid arthritis:*** 125-250 mg daily before food.

Usual maintance dose 500 - 750 mg daily.

***Storage:*** It should be stored in well closed container and protected from moisture.

## Dimercaprol

**(Synonym: B.A.L. British anti lewisite)**

**Mol. Formula:** $C_3H_8OS_2$ **Mol. Weight:** 124.2

***Structure***

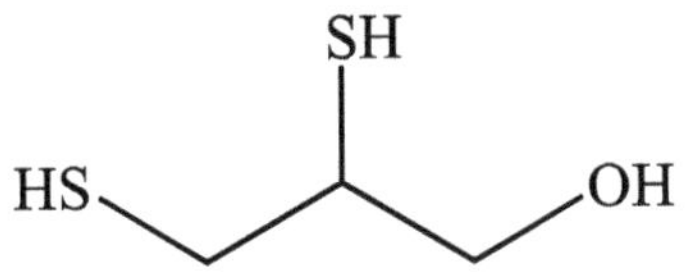

SH

HS OH

Chemically, it is (RS) -2,3- dimercaptopropanol.

***Properties:*** It is a clear, colorless or slightly yellow liquid, strong characteristic odour, and alliaceous.

***Test for identification***

1. To a small quantity of sample in water and add small amount of lead acetate solution, a yellow precipitate is obtained.
2. To a small amount of sample, add 1 ml of 0.05M iodine solution, the color is immediately discharged.
3. To a small amount of sample was added suspension of sodium bismuthate and water in 10% w/w of phosphoric acid solution. Allow to stand for 10 min with concurrent shaking. Collect the supernatant liquid. To the small volume of supernatant liquid, add 5 ml of 0.4% w/v of sodium salt of chromotropic acid in sulphuric acid mix and heat for 15 minutes in a water bath, a violet red color is produced.

***Test for purity:*** It should be tested for appearance of solution, pH, refractive index, specific gravity, iron, halides and stability.

***Uses:*** It is mainly used as an antidote for heavy metal poisoning and metal chelating agent.

***Dose:*** 2-3 mg/kg of body weight every 4 hours in accordance with the needs of the patient.

***Storage:*** It should be stored in well closed containers, in a refrigerator (2-8 °C) and protected from light.

## Calcium Folinate

**(Synonym: Leucovorin calcium)**

**Mol. Formula:** $C_{20}H_{21}CaN_7O_7$ **Mol. Weight:** 511.5

Calcium Folinate is calcium N- (4(2-amino-5-formyl-1,4,5,6,7,8-hexahydro-4-hyrdo-4-oxo-6-pteridinyl methyl amino benzoyl-L-glutamate.

It contains not less than 95% and not more than105% of $C_{20}H_{21}CaN_7O_7$ calculated on dried basis.

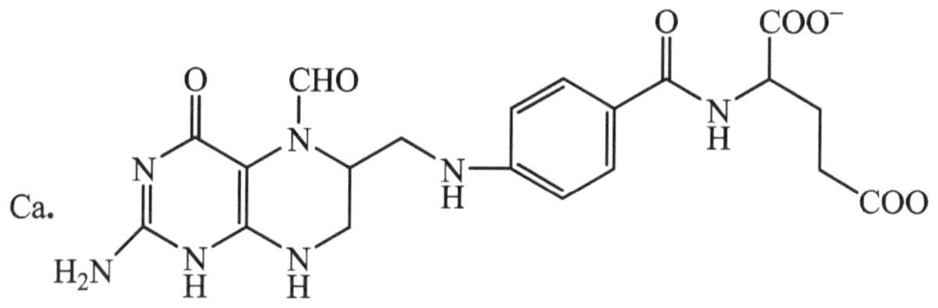

***Properties:*** It occurs as a yellowish white or yellow powder, odourless.

***Test for identification:*** It is identified by infrared absorption spectrophotometry.

***Test for purity:*** It should be tested for heavy metals and water.

***Assay:*** It is assayed by HPLC.

***Uses:*** It is mainly used as an antidote to folate antagonists.

***Dose:*** 120 mg in divided doses within 12-24 hours by IM/IV injection or infusion, followed by 12-15 mg by IM or 15 mg by orally every 6 hours for the next 48 hours.

***Storage:*** It should be preserved in well closed container and protected from light and moisture.

## 1,10-Phenanthroline

**Mol. Formula:** $C_{12}H_8N_2$ **Mol. Weight:** 180

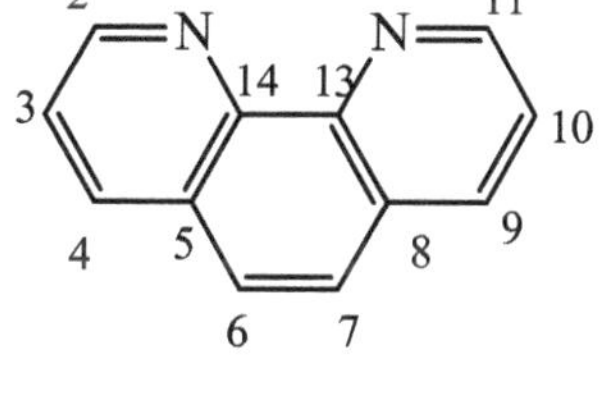

*Uses*

1. It forms complexes with iron, copper, zinc and other metals (cheating agents).
2. It forms complex with ferrous ion called as ferroin, which is mainly used as an indicator for many assay.

## PROBABLE QUESTIONS

1. Define coordination chemistry?
2. Define coordination compounds with any one example.
3. Explain the terms used in coordination chemistry.
4. What are chelates? Write one example.
5. Define the following terms.
   (a) Coordination entity
   (b) Central atom
   (c) Ligands
   (d) Coordination number
6. Describe the different type of ligands with example.
7. Explain the following.
   (a) Coordination polyhedron
   (b) Coordination sphere
   (c) Homoleptic and heteroleptic complexes
8. Explain the isomerism exhibited in coordination compounds.
9. Write the rules for the nomenclature of coordination compounds.
10. Explain ionization and solvate isomerism.
11. Name the theories used to explain the bonding in coordination compounds.
12. Write the therapeutic applications of coordination compounds.
13. Write the applications of coordination compounds in analytical chemistry.
14. Explain the therapeutic uses of coordination compounds.
15. Write any five co-ordination compounds with their molecular formula and therapeutic uses.
16. Explain the method of preparation, properties, assay and therapeutic uses of the following.
    (a) EDTA
    (b) Penicillamine
    (c) Dimercaprol

# SUGGESTED READINGS


1. **Indian Pharmacopoeia** Ministry of health and Family welfare, New Delhi, 2014.
2. **British Pharmacopoeia** Medicines and Healthcare products regulatory agency, London, 2014.
3. **Vogel's Textbook of Quantitative Chemical Analysis** ($6^{th}$ ed.). Pearson Education Limited, Delhi, 2008.
4. **Remington**, **The Science and practice of Pharmacy** ($21^{st}$ ed.). Lippincott Williams and Wilkins, New York, Gennaro, A.R, 2006.
5. **United States Pharmacopoeia** (Asian ed.). United States Pharmacopoeial convention, INC, Twinbrook, Rockville, MD, 2004.
6. Martindale **The Extra Pharmacopoeia** ($30^{th}$ ed.). Reynolds. J.E.F., The Pharmaceutical Press, London, 1993.
7. **British National Formulary No**: 21, British Medical Association and Royal Pharmaceutical Society of Great Britain, London, 1991.
8. Block, Roche, Soine and Wilson. **Inorganic Medicinal and Pharmaceutical Chemistry** ($6^{th}$ ed.). Varghese publishing house, Bombay, 2008.
9. Atherden L.M. **Bentley and Driver's Textbook of Pharmaceutical chemistry** ($8^{th}$ ed.). Oxford medical Publications, New Delhi, 2004.
10. Darrell D. Ebbing. **General chemistry** ($5^{th}$ ed.). A.I.T.B.S. Publishers and Distributors, Delhi, 2002.
11. Patric J Sinko. **Martin Physical pharmacy and pharmaceutical sciences** ($5^{th}$ ed.). Lippincott Williams and Wilkins, Baltimore, MD, 2006.
12. Albert Cotton F, Geoffrey W, Carlos A. Murillo, Manfred B. **Advanced Inorganic Chemistry** ($6^{th}$ ed.). A wiley- interscience publication, John- wiley and sons, Inc, Newyork, 1999.
13. Douglas A. Skoog, Donald M. West, James F. Holler, Stanley R. Crouch. **Fundamentals of Analytical Chemistry** ($8^{th}$ ed.). Engage Learning India Private Limited, Delhi, 2004.
14. Anne Waugh, Allison Grant, Ross and Wilson, **Anatomy and physiology in Health and illness** ($11^{th}$ ed.). Elseivier publications.

15. Cotton F. A, Wilkinson G, Murillo C.A. and Bochmann M. **Advanced Inorganic Chemistry** John Wiley and sons, 2003.

16. Kettle S.F.A, **Co ordination chemistry** The English language book society and Nelson, 1969.

17. Lee J. D. **Concise Inorganic Chemistry** Chapman and Hall, London, 1992.

18. Robin J. Harman. **Hand book of Pharmacy** (Health Care Edition) The Pharmaceutical Press, London 1990.

19. Gary L. Miessler, Donald A. Tarr. **Inorganic Chemistry** (3rd ed.). Pearson Education, Delhi, 2004.

# INDEX

## D

## E

## H



## I

## K



## L

## M

## Q

## R



## S

www.ingramcontent.com/pod-product-compliance
Ingram Content Group UK Ltd.
Pitfield, Milton Keynes, MK11 3LW, UK
UKHW061534190726
13845UKWH00005B/105